BSAVA Manual of Canine and Feline Nephrology and Urology
Second edition

Editors:

Jonathan Elliott
MA VetMB PhD CertSAC DipECVPT MRCVS
Department of Veterinary Basic Sciences,
Royal Veterinary College, University of London,
Royal College Street, London NW1 0TU

and

Gregory F. Grauer
DVM MS DipACVIM (Internal Medicine)
Department of Clinical Sciences,
College of Veterinary Medicine, Kansas State University, 111B Mosier Hall,
Manhattan, KS 66506, USA

Ivan Sosa. Samper.
- Oxford 2009. -

Published by:

British Small Animal Veterinary Association
Woodrow House, 1 Telford Way, Waterwells
Business Park, Quedgeley, Gloucester GL2 2AB

A Company Limited by Guarantee in England.
Registered Company No. 2837793.
Registered as a Charity.

Figure 6.1 was drawn by S.J. Elmhurst BA Hons (www.livingart.org.uk)
and is printed with her permission.

A catalogue record for this book is available from the British Library.

ISBN-10 0905214 93 5
ISBN-13 978 0 905214 93 1

The publishers and contributors cannot take responsibility for information
provided on dosages and methods of application of drugs mentioned in
this publication. Details of this kind must be verified by individual users
from the appropriate literature.

Typeset by: Fusion Design, Wareham, Dorset, UK
Printed by: Replika Press Pvt. Ltd, India

Other titles in the BSAVA Manuals series:

For information on these and all BSAVA publications please visit our website: www.bsava.com

Contents

Contributors

Larry G. Adams DVM PhD DipACVIM
Department of Veterinary Clinical Sciences, Purdue University, West Lafayette, IN 47907, USA

Rick Alleman DVM PhD DipABVP DipACVP
University of Florida, College of Veterinary Medicine, PO Box 100103, Gainsville, FL 32610, USA

Jeanne A. Barsanti DVM MS DipACVIM
Department of Small Animal Medicine and Surgery, College of Veterinary Medicine,
University of Georgia, Athens, GA 30602, USA

Cathy A. Brown VMD PhD DipACVP
Athens Diagnostic Laboratory, College of Veterinary Medicine, University of Georgia, Athens, GA
30602, USA

Scott A. Brown VMD PhD DipACVIM
Department of Small Animal Medicine and Surgery, College of Veterinary Medicine,
University of Georgia, Athens, GA 30602, USA

C.A. Tony Buffington DVM PhD DipACVN
College of Veterinary Medicine, The Ohio State University, 601 Vernon L. Tharp Street, Columbus,
OH 43210, USA

Dennis J. Chew DVM DipACVIM
College of Veterinary Medicine, The Ohio State University, 601 Vernon L. Tharp Street, Columbus,
OH 43210, USA

Ruth Dennis MA VetMB DVR DipECVDI MRCVS
The Animal Health Trust, Centre for Small Animal Studies, Lanwades Park, Kentford, Newmarket,
Suffolk, CB8 7UU

Jonathan Elliott MA VetMB PhD CertSAC DipECVPT MRCVS
Department of Veterinary Basic Sciences, Royal Veterinary College, University of London,
Royal College Street, London NW1 0TU

Julie R. Fischer DVM DipACVIM
Companion Animal Hemodialysis Service, UCVMC, San Diego, CA 92067, USA

Alex German BVSc (Hons) PhD CertSAM DipECVIM-CA MRCVS
Department of Veterinary Clinical Sciences, University of Liverpool Small Animal Hospital,
Crown Street, Liverpool, L7 7EX

Gregory F. Grauer DVM MS DipACVIM
Department of Clinical Sciences, College of Veterinary Medicine, Kansas State University,
111B Mosier Hall, Manhattan, KS 66506, USA

Reidun Heiene DVM PhD MRCVS
Department of Companion Animal Clinical Sciences, Norwegian School of Veterinary Science,
PO Box 8146 Dep 0033, Oslo, Norway

India F. Lane DVM MS DipACVIM
College of Veterinary Medicine, The University of Tennessee, Knoxville, TN 37996, USA

George E. Lees DVM MS DipACVIM
Small Animal Clinical Sciences, College of Veterinary Medicine, 4474 TAMU, Texas A&M University, College Station, TX 77843, USA

Hervé P. Lefebvre DVM PhD DipECVPT
Department of Clinical Sciences, National Veterinary School of Toulouse, Toulouse, France

Jody P. Lulich DVM PhD DipACVIM
Veterinary Clinical Sciences Department, College of Veterinary Medicine, University of Minnesota, 1352 Boyd Avenue, St. Paul, MN 55108, USA

Fraser McConnell BVM&S CertSAM DVR DipECVDI MRCVS
The Animal Health Trust, Centre for Small Animal Studies, Lanwades Park, Kentford, Newmarket, Suffolk, CB8 7UU

Carl A. Osborne DVM PhD DipACVIM
Veterinary Clinical Sciences Department, College of Veterinary Medicine, University of Minnesota, 1352 Boyd Avenue, St. Paul, MN 55108, USA

David F. Senior BVSc DipACVIM ECVIM-CA
Veterinary Clinical Sciences, School of Veterinary Medicine, Louisiana State University, Baton Rouge, LA 70803, USA

Richard A. Squires BVSc, PhD, DVR, DipACVIM, DipECVIM-CA, MRCVS
Institute of Veterinary, Animal and Biomedical Sciences, Massey University, Palmerston North, New Zealand

Rebecca L. Stepien DVM MS DipACVIM
Department of Medical Sciences, University of Wisconsin, School of Veterinary Medicine, 2015 Linden Drive, Madison, WI 53706, USA

Harriet M. Syme BSc BVetMed PhD DipACVIM DipECVIM-CA MRCVS
Royal Veterinary College, Hawkshead Lane, Hatfield, Herts, AL9 7TA

Shelly L. Vaden DVM PhD DipACVIM
College of Veterinary Medicine, North Carolina State University, 4700 Hillsborough Street, Raleigh, NC 27606, USA

Heather Wamsley BS DVM DipACVP
University of Florida, College of Veterinary Medicine, PO Box 100103, Gainsville, FL 32610, USA

A. David J. Watson BVSc PhD FRCVS FAAVPT MACVSc DipECVPT
Sydney, Australia

Foreword

Welcome to this fully updated second edition of the *BSAVA Manual Canine and Feline of Nephrology and Urology*. It brings up to date and enhances the first edition and adds to the continual revision of the enormously popular Manual series. This manual gives a practical and user-friendly overview of conditions routinely and regularly encountered in practice. Diseases of the kidney and bladder are amongst the most common presenting disorders in general practice. This manual reviews them all and offers concise ways of diagnosing and treating them.

In the traditional manner, the text and imagery is clear and concise making it easy for the busy practitioner to dip into but full enough for it to be a source of information to update skills and knowledge.

Led by the two editors, Professors Elliott and Grauer, both giants in the field, this manual has pulled together an impressive array of contributors. It has an international breadth reflecting the ready exchange of ideas and experience from around the world. This manual will be hugely popular and find its way to the library of every veterinary practice, where it will be a regular source of information.

Congratulations to the Editors, Authors and BSAVA Publications team. On behalf of all of the members of BSAVA, many thanks to all those involved in its publication.

Mike K. Jessop BVetMed MRCVS
BSAVA President 2006–2007

Preface

It is 10 years since the publication of the first edition of this manual. It is interesting to reflect on the advances that have occurred over this time and how they have changed clinical practice, and where progress has been slower than predicted a decade ago.

The second edition follows the successful format of the first with sections on presenting problems, diagnostics and therapeutic techniques and management of specific problems. Although the layout will be familiar, the authorship has changed considerably to ensure a completely fresh look has been taken at the subject areas involved. The authorship is truly international and has drawn upon clinical experts from Europe and the United States who are actively publishing original research papers in nephrology and urology. New chapters have been added, particularly in the second section on diagnostic and therapeutic techniques. These include staging chronic kidney disease, measurement of blood pressure, cystoscopy, lithotripsy, dialysis and glomerulonephritis. Whilst some of these techniques are limited to a few highly specialist referral centres, we have taken the view that general practitioners need some knowledge of what can be achieved with these techniques so they can select appropriate cases for referral and communicate effectively with clients and the referral institutions about the cases they refer.

Staging of chronic kidney disease, we feel is a significant development for Nephrology. The IRIS (International Renal Interest Society) System, presented in Chapter 11, has been adopted by the European and American Societies of Veterinary Nephrology and Urology. Linking this staging system to recommended diagnostic efforts and therapy of the chronic kidney disease patient, we feel, will be most useful for practitioners faced with deciding how to investigate and manage individual patients. Chapter 18 does this most effectively and we hope practitioners find this approach helpful.

A major advance in our thinking on kidney disease in general, and feline kidney disease in particular, is the recognition of the importance of proteinuria as a risk factor for progression. The launch of more sensitive patient side and in-clinic quantitative tests for proteinuria over the last two to three years have also brought proteinuria more into focus for practitioners evaluating patients they suspect of having kidney disease.

Chapter 6 (Proteinuria) presents the recent data which support this change in thinking that has resulted in revision of the definition of significant proteinuria and provides a comprehensive discussion of the available diagnostic screening tests. The American College of Veterinary Internal Medicine (ACVIM) Consensus statement on proteinuria issued in 2005 sets out this new thinking and its recommendations have been adopted when monitoring, investigation and therapy is recommended for patients with chronic kidney disease.

When the first edition of this manual was published, measurement of blood pressure was relatively new to small animal veterinary practice with only a small number of practices owning the necessary equipment. Over the last 10 years, clinical specialists have gained much experience in measuring blood pressure in dogs and cats. In Chapter 13 this experience is used to make practical recommendations for the increasing number of practices who have invested in this equipment and who want to use it to make reliable measurements in their patients and interpret their significance. Blood pressure is recognized as an important physiological parameter to assess in the renal patient and is part of the IRIS staging system. The ACVIM Consensus statement on blood pressure is due to be published in 2007 and the views presented in the manual reflect those contained within the consensus statement.

Editing a manual of this size is a hugely enjoyable if time-consuming task as one learns so much in the process. This task has been made as easy as it could be by the efficient editorial team at BSAVA, Marion Jowett, Sabrina Cleevley and Nicola Lloyd, who have supported us so effectively throughout the whole process. We hope the end result will be a useful addition to your practice library.

Jonathan Elliott and Gregory F. Grauer
August 2006

Dysuria and haematuria

A. David J. Watson

Introduction

Dysuria and haematuria often occur together in dogs and cats, but they can also occur separately as signs of disease.

- *Dysuria* is defined as difficult and/or painful urination.
- *Haematuria* denotes the presence of blood in the urine.

Whether occurring separately or together, these signs may be associated with two other abnormalities:

- *Stranguria* (or strangury) indicates slow and painful urination
- *Pollakiuria* is defined as the abnormally frequent passage of urine. When pollakiuria is present, a small volume of urine is passed each time the animal urinates. This pattern must be distinguished from *polyuria*, which refers to an increase in daily urine volume. With polyuria, the animal will also urinate more frequently than usual, but a large volume is passed each time, and the urine is usually dilute (indicated by pale colour and low specific gravity).

Dysuria generally results from disorders of the lower urinary tract (bladder or urethra), the genital tract (prostate or vagina) or both. Haematuria can be more difficult to localize, as bleeding may occur anywhere in the urinary tract, from the kidneys to the urethral meatus, as well as from the prostate, penis or prepuce in the male, and from the uterus, vagina or vulva in the female. When haematuria and dysuria occur together, lower urinary tract disease or a genital lesion is most likely to be present.

Dysuria and its causes

Dysuric animals usually adopt the typical urinating posture, but show obvious effort or difficulty while attempting to pass urine and may appear preoccupied or distressed. If some urine is passed, the flow may be weak, attenuated or intermittent. If little or no urine is passed, either because the bladder is nearly empty or the excretory pathway is obstructed, dysuria may continue for some time, with the animal shifting position repeatedly between attempts.

Veterinary clinicians usually have no difficulty in identifying dysuria, but pet owners do not always recognize dysuria for what it is:

- A dysuric dog or cat that is crouching and straining may be reported as 'constipated'
- An animal with dysuria and pollakiuria may be regarded as 'incontinent' because small amounts of urine are being ejected frequently
- A pet urinating in inappropriate places or at unusual times might be described as 'incontinent' when the problem is really dysuria and pollakiuria
- Ambiguous terminology may create uncertainties – when the owner says their pet is 'going to the toilet', does it relate to urination or to defecation?

Here, as always, care is necessary during the history-taking process to separate the owner's observations from their interpretation, and careful questioning of the owner or direct observation of the pet by the clinician or nurse may be needed to clarify events.

Two distinct processes have the potential to cause dysuria:

- Diseases of the lower urinary or genital tract that result in mucosal irritation or inflammation. Mucosal inflammation can cause pain and urgency to urinate and the bladder wall may spasm, even when the bladder is empty or nearly so. Affected people report painful, burning sensations and presumably dysuric dogs and cats suffer similar symptoms
- Conditions that produce narrowing and obstruction of the urethra or bladder neck. Narrowing is often caused by masses (neoplasms or prostatomegaly) and obstruction by urethral calculi or plugs.

The prevalence of different dysuric disorders differs between dogs and cats:

- In dogs, the two most common causes of dysuria are bacterial infections of the lower urinary tract and urinary calculi
- In cats, the main causes of dysuria are idiopathic cystitis (in males and females) and urethral plugs (males only); both are components of the 'feline urological syndrome' or 'feline lower urinary tract disease' complex.

However, various other conditions cause dysuria in both species (especially in dogs) and care is warranted before excluding them as possible diagnoses. Potential causes of dysuria in dogs and cats are listed in Figure 1.1.

Urinary bladder
Bacterial cystitis
Cystic calculi
Idiopathic cystitis in cats
Neoplasia – transitional cell carcinoma especially (rare in cats)
Bladder rupture
Urinary bladder and urethra
Detrusor – urethral dyssynergia (rare)
Urethra
Calculi
Plugs in cats
Stricture
Bacterial urethritis
Rupture
Neoplasia
Granulomatous urethritis
Prostate (conditions rare in cats)
Benign hyperplasia
Prostatitis
Abscess
Cysts
Transitional cell carcinoma
Other tumours rare
Penis, prepuce, vagina (tumours of external genitalia rarely present as dysuria; bloody discharge or visible mass noted more often)
Transmissible venereal tumour in dogs (mainly in regions with many feral or stray dogs and unregulated breeding)
Squamous cell carcinoma (prepuce)
Mast cell tumour (prepuce)
Leiomyoma, fibroma (vagina)
Vaginitis

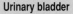 Sites and processes potentially involved in dogs and cats with dysuria.

Haematuria and other causes of reddish urine

Haematuria can arise from blood loss within the renal parenchyma or, more often, from discontinuity of endothelial or epithelial barriers anywhere in the urine collecting system, from the renal pelvis to the external urethral orifice. It can also occur with disorders affecting genital or accessory sex organs.

Gross haematuria

When haematuria is sufficient to be apparent to the naked eye, urine has a brownish to red (occasionally blackish) colour and turbid appearance. This is known as *gross* or *macroscopic haematuria*. Sometimes small blood clots may also be seen. For haematuria to be detected visually, at least 0.5 ml of whole blood must be present per litre of urine, corresponding to about 2500 erythrocytes (RBCs) per microlitre, and >150 RBCs per high-power field (hpf) in urine sediment (Figure 1.2).

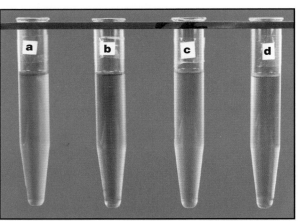

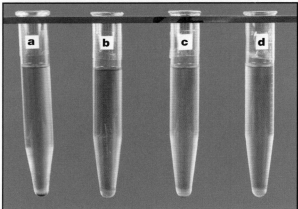

1.2 Urine samples photographed before (upper panel) and after (lower panel) centrifugation. **(a)** Gross haematuria (test strip reaction for blood 'large' in uncentrifuged urine). Note pink colour and turbid appearance before centrifugation; after centrifugation there is red sediment and the supernatant is no longer pink. **(b)** Haemoglobinuria ('large' reaction for blood). Note pink colour and lack of turbidity before centrifugation; the appearance is unchanged after centrifugation, with no visible sediment. **(c)** Occult haematuria ('moderate' reaction for blood). Note lack of pink colour (but slight turbidity when compared with sample d?) before centrifugation; after sedimentation there is sparse red sediment and no turbidity. **(d)** Reference urine ('negative' reaction for blood). Appearance is unchanged by centrifugation. (All tubes contain the same urine, with specific gravity 1.019. Blood was added to give haemoglobin concentrations of 3.10 mg/10 ml of urine in (a) and (b) and 0.52 mg/10 ml in (c). Erythrocytes in (b) were lysed with detergent. Tubes were centrifuged at 3800 *G* for 5 minutes.)

Gross haematuria does not always appear consistently throughout urination. By noting when it *does* occur, i.e. the *pattern* of haematuria, it may be possible to identify potential bleeding sites, as indicated in Figure 1.3. In the author's experience, however, it is not always possible to make firm conclusions on this basis, whether using one's own observations or relying on reports from others. Potential origins and causes of haematuria in dogs and cats are presented in Figure 1.4.

Observation	Possible origin of haemorrhage
Initial haematuria (at beginning of voiding)	Lower urinary tract (bladder neck, urethra, vagina, vulva, penis, prepuce) Extra-urinary (pro-oestrus, metritis, pyometra, prostate, genital neoplasia)
Terminal haematuria (at end of voiding)	Upper urinary tract (bladder, ureters, kidneys; intermittent bleeding allowing RBCs to settle in bladder, to be expelled with final bladder contents)
Total haematuria (throughout voiding)	Upper urinary tract (bladder, ureters, kidneys; bleeding frequent to continuous, or intermittent but mixing occurring because animal is physically active) Diffuse bladder disease Severe prostatic or proximal urethral lesion (blood refluxing into bladder)
Pseudohaematuria (reddish colour throughout urination, no RBCs in urine sediment)	Haematuria absent (suspect haemoglobin, myoglobin, drugs or chemicals; see text)
Bloody fluid dripping from penis or vulva independent of urination	Bleeding distal to urethral sphincter (prostate, urethra, penis, uterus, vagina, vulva)

1.3 Observed patterns of haematuria and possible origins.

Origin	Possible causes	Clinical/historical features
Systemic disorder	Haemostatic defects	Bleeding from other sites, breed or family history suggesting inherited defect, access to anticoagulant rodenticide, strenuous exercise, disseminated intravascular coagulation (DIC) secondary to severe disease
Renal	Blunt trauma, infarction, cysts, renal pelvic haematoma, calculus, telangiectasia (Welsh Corgi), glomerulonephritis, chronic passive congestion, neoplasm, *Dioctophyma renale*, *Dirofilaria immitis* microfilaraemia	Haematuria, gross or microscopic, may occur throughout urination (total haematuria); possibly haemoglobinuria if RBCs lyse in hypotonic urine
Bladder, ureter, urethra	Calculi, bacterial infection, trauma, neoplasm, cyclophosphamide therapy, *Capillaria plica*, feline idiopathic cystitis	Haematuria, gross or microscopic, may occur at beginning or end of urination (sometimes throughout, see Figure 1.3). Dysuria may be concurrent
Genital tract	Prostatic disease, oestrus, subinvolution of placental sites, neoplasia, infection, trauma	Haematuria, gross or microscopic, at beginning of voiding or independent of urination

1.4 Origin, causes and clinical features of haematuria.

Occult haematuria

Haematuria that is present but not visible to the naked eye is known as *occult* or *microscopic haematuria*. Urine from healthy dogs and cats can contain some RBCs without being of concern. Occult haematuria is identified if urine contains >5 RBCs/hpf but is not visibly pink. However, the method of urine collection can affect interpretation; reference values for different techniques are given in Figure 1.5. Interpretation is difficult if catheterization or cystocentesis causes overt trauma.

Sample type	RBCs/hpf
Voided	0–5
Catheterized	0–8
Cystocentesis	0–8

1.5 Suggested reference values for RBCs in urine sediment.

The various conditions that cause gross haematuria can also cause occult haematuria if present in less severe forms. Occult haematuria often accompanies pollakiuria, dysuria and/or stranguria caused by idiopathic cystitis in cats, and bacterial cystitis or urinary calculi in dogs.

Pseudohaematuria

Gross haematuria is not the only process producing red to brownish urine. When this colour change occurs without intact RBCs being found, it is referred to as *pseudohaematuria*. This finding is uncommon in dogs and cats; the most likely cause is haemoglobinuria, but myoglobinuria or chemicals are also potential causes. Important points to note are:

- Turbidity: samples with gross haematuria are turbid, whereas those with pseudohaematuria are not, unless another factor causing turbidity is also present
- Test strip results: the common tests for haematuria react positively to haemoglobin and myoglobin, but negatively if pseudohaematuria is caused by a drug or dye
- After centrifugation: the supernatant remains equally discoloured in pseudohaematuria, whereas with haematuria it becomes less discoloured, or even normal in colour, as RBCs are spun out (see Figure 1.2).

Haemoglobinuria

Haemoglobinuria gives urine a pink to red colour, although this may darken in time with oxidation. Two processes can cause haemoglobinuria:

- *Intravascular lysis of RBCs.* Many processes (e.g. immune-mediated, infectious, toxic, chemical) cause RBCs to lyse within blood vessels. The lysed cells release haemoglobin into plasma, where it forms a complex with haptoglobin. Once the binding capacity of haptoglobin is saturated, free haemoglobin appears in plasma. The plasma becomes visibly pink if the concentrations of free haemoglobin, bound haemoglobin and various derivatives exceed a certain level. Some of the free haemoglobin cleared from plasma by glomerular filtration is taken up by renal tubular cells and metabolized to bilirubin. Haemoglobin appears in urine once this tubular uptake mechanism becomes saturated

- *Lysis of RBCs within the urinary excretory pathway.* When urine is hypotonic (urine specific gravity <1.008), many RBCs may lyse within the excretory pathway. Urine alkalinity (pH >7) also contributes to lysis, both *in vivo* and *in vitro*. In these circumstances, RBCs in urine sediment appear as faint colourless circles ('ghost cells') or become invisible because of lysis.

Intravascular haemolysis should be suspected from the following:

- Haemoglobinuria without RBC ghosts or lysed RBCs in urine sediment
- Haemoglobinaemia (pinkish or red plasma)
- Suggestive changes in RBCs (spherocytes, Heinz bodies, *Babesia* spp., *Mycoplasma haemofelis*)
- Anaemia with bone marrow response (allow 4–5 days for response to appear)
- Exposure to a known haemolytic drug or chemical
- An inherited intrinsic erythrocyte defect known to cause haemolysis in that breed.

Lysis of RBCs within urine should be suspected from the following:

- Haemoglobinuria with RBC ghosts in urine sediment
- Urine is hypotonic and possibly alkaline
- Plasma colour is normal
- Regenerative anaemia is absent.

Myoglobinuria

Myoglobinuria is rarely detected in dogs and cats, but is possible whenever extensive destruction of muscle fibres releases substantial amounts of myoglobin into the plasma. One such condition is 'exertional rhabdomyolysis' (also known as 'tying up' or 'cramping') in unfit racing Greyhounds. Other potential causes are toxic, traumatic, infectious or ischaemic myopathies.

When myoglobinuria is present:

- Active muscle necrosis should be apparent: look for swelling or atrophy of muscles, pain and/or weakness, increased plasma creatine kinase concentration
- Plasma colour is not altered: myoglobin released from myocytes is rapidly eliminated in urine because it does not bind to plasma protein and the renal threshold for myoglobin is low.

Differentiation between myoglobinuria and haemoglobinuria is usually based on plasma colour and the other pointers mentioned previously, but a myoglobin solubility test can be performed as well if required (Figure 1.6).

1. Adjust urine pH to 7.5–8.0 with sodium hydroxide solution.
2. Add 2.8 g of ammonium sulphate per 5 ml of urine and dissolve by mixing – a precipitate will form.
3. Centrifuge the sample: • If supernatant is pigmented, this indicates myoglobin • If supernatant lacks pigment, the colour now being in the precipitate, this indicates haemoglobin • If supernatant and precipitate are both abnormally coloured, both substances are probably present.

1.6 Myoglobin solubility test (Osborne and Stevens, 1999).

Other causes of pseudohaematuria

Other causes of pseudohaematuria are rare. Red, pink, red–brown, red–orange or orange urine testing negatively for haem pigments could indicate the presence of bromsulphthalein or phenolsulphthalein (in alkaline urine), or porphyrins, Congo red, phenazopyridine, phenothiazine, or (in people) various other drugs and chemicals (Bartges, 2005). (Reddish to orange urine can be normal in healthy rabbits.)

Diagnostic approach

As with all clinical problems, a detailed history and thorough physical examination are the cornerstones of diagnosis in patients with dysuria and/or haematuria. Although this discussion will centre on the urinary tract, all body systems and the general health of the patient should be evaluated, to ensure that any contributing factors or systemic consequences are detected. Once basic data have been collected by means of history-taking and physical examination, these findings should be assessed carefully, enabling tentative decisions to be made about the nature of the problem, the diagnostic possibilities, and the diagnostic and/or therapeutic measures required.

History and physical examination

The dysuric patient without haematuria

As outlined above, dysuria usually results from disorders of the lower urinary tract (bladder or urethra), genital tract (prostate or vagina) or both. Some important questions for the owner of a dysuric animal are listed in Figure 1.7.

Is any urine passed? What volume? With what frequency? Is there stranguria? Is the stream interrupted, attenuated or weak? Is there haematuria? Is the urine cloudy or malodorous? Is the animal urinating in inappropriate places? (Also occurs in cats with behavioural problems and dogs with incontinence, polyuria and behavioural problems) Is the animal licking its penis or vulva? How long have the signs been apparent? Have there been any previous episodes? Has there been any previous treatment?

1.7 Important questions to ask about urination in dysuric patients.

Urethral patency: Because urinary obstruction can be life-threatening, urethral patency should be assessed from history and physical examination during the first phase of the investigation. This is especially important if clinical signs suggest uraemia (depression, anorexia, vomiting).

Seeing the animal urinate provides the ideal opportunity to verify urethral patency and confirm the owner's account of events. If urine is passed, a mid-stream sample should be taken for laboratory analysis.

When the bladder is distended and urine is not passed, urethral blockage should be suspected and catheterization attempted:

- If catheterization is easy, this suggests that the cause may be a small urethral plug, easily dislodged, or functional urethral obstruction from detrusor–urethral dyssynergia, wherein sphincter muscle relaxation and detrusor muscle contraction are uncoordinated (see Chapter 3)
- If catheterization is difficult or impossible, cystocentesis could be considered to reduce intravesicular pressure and possibly facilitate catheterization. Another option is hydropulsion (see Chapter 21).

Urine obtained from the bladder should be sent for laboratory evaluation, along with blood for appropriate testing.

Bladder palpation: Palpation of the urinary bladder is very important in dysuric animals, but must be done carefully because a tightly distended bladder can rupture under pressure. It is advisable to palpate the bladder again after emptying, to improve the chances of feeling intraluminal or intramural masses. Findings and interpretation of bladder palpation are summarized in Figure 1.8.

Finding	Interpretation
Small bladder, thickened wall, gentle palpation readily elicits voiding	Bladder inflammation
Large bladder, rather flaccid feel, gentle palpation readily expels urine	Bladder atony
Large bladder, tense wall, urine not easily expressed (be careful!)	Urinary tract obstruction or increased outflow resistance
Irregular, hard masses within lumen, possibly with a grating feeling (easier to appreciate if bladder empty of urine)	Cystic calculi

1.8 Abnormal findings on bladder palpation and their interpretations.

Digital rectal palpation: Ideally, this should be performed in all dysuric animals. Structures that may be thus evaluated include:

- Prostate gland
- Trigone of the bladder
- Pelvic urethra
- Vagina and cervix
- Masses in the caudal abdominal or pelvic region.

Palpation of the prostate and trigone area can often be assisted by pressing upwards and backwards on the caudal abdomen with the other hand at the same time.

Examination of perineum and external genitalia: Inspection and palpation are advisable in both sexes:

- *Males.* Palpate the perineum and urethra. A soft fluctuant perineal swelling could indicate perineal herniation (sometimes causes dysuria) or urine accumulation following urethral obstruction and rupture. Extrude the penis and examine it and inside the prepuce for masses, inflammation, haemorrhage, trauma or discharge. In cats with urethral obstruction, the penis may be partly extruded and red, and a plug may be visible protruding from the urethral meatus
- *Females.* Examine the vulva for swelling, masses, inflammation or discharge and assess for pro-oestrus or oestrus. Consider vaginal digital palpation to identify masses or strictures and abnormalities of the urethral papilla.

The patient with haematuria or pseudohaematuria

It is important to remember that haematuria and pseudo-haematuria can result from systemic disorders as well as from urogenital abnormalities, and to cover both possibilities during history-taking and physical examination. The aspects discussed below should be explored.

Haematuria:

History-taking:

- Consider the possibility of a breed or family haemostatic defect: ask the owner whether bleeding has been noticed from any other sites
- Ask about trauma, exposure to anticoagulant rodenticides and systemic signs suggesting anaemia
- Find out if there is a consistent pattern to urine discoloration that might suggest its origin (see Figure 1.3).

On physical examination:

- Look for haemorrhages at other sites, including abdomen, thorax, subcutis, skin and mucosae (especially mouth, axillae, groin and inside pinnae)
- Examine faeces grossly for blood
- Palpate the kidneys and assess for size, symmetry and discomfort
- Perform digital rectal palpation, assessing structures as suggested for dysuric patients
- Examine external genitalia.

Pseudohaematuria: Urine discoloration here is present throughout urination, as with total haematuria. There are several possibilities to explore:

- Haemoglobinuria: In this breed, is there an inherited erythrocyte defect causing intravascular haemolysis? Has there been exposure to a haemolysin (e.g. drug, chemical, onions). Are there systemic signs suggesting anaemia and/or

jaundice? During physical examination, look for evidence of anaemia and jaundice, and for enlargement of liver, spleen and lymph nodes
- Myoglobinuria: Check history and physical findings for evidence of myopathy
- Other pseudohaematurias: Enquire about exposure to unusual drugs or chemicals.

The dysuric patient with haematuria or haemoglobinuria

Dysuria accompanied by haematuria (gross or microscopic) or haemoglobinuria is most likely to be caused by lesions in the lower urinary tract (bladder or urethra) and/or the genital tract (prostate or vagina). Accordingly, the approach to history and physical examination in these patients should cover all aspects mentioned separately for dysuric patients and for patients with reddish urine.

Making an assessment and planning investigation and treatment

The assessment of individual patients will naturally depend on the findings from history and physical examination. Once a tentative diagnosis or list of diagnostic possibilities is established, this should lead to logical plans for further investigation and treatment.

In patients with urinary tract obstruction and uraemia, establishing urethral patency and instituting appropriate therapy may well take precedence over investigations to establish a definite diagnosis.

In many, but not all, patients with dysuria and/or haematuria, diagnostic aids will be required to confirm the tentative diagnosis or to decide between several diagnostic possibilities. Available options include:

- Urinalysis, either routine or specialized, depending on the case (see Chapter 8)
- Assessment of renal function if renal disease and failure seem likely (see Chapter 9)
- Diagnostic imaging studies, especially to assess involvement of kidneys, urinary bladder and prostate, or to detect urinary tract rupture – for example, ultrasound examination in patients with suspected renal haematuria, urolithiasis or prostatic disease; double-contrast cystography for suspected bladder wall disease; and positive-contrast retrograde urethrography for suspected urethral lesions and/or prostatic disease (see Chapter 10)
- Haematological and blood biochemical tests to evaluate underlying causes of dysuria/haematuria and possible systemic consequences.

Figure 1.9 lists various diagnostic aids that might be used when investigating patients with dysuria/haematuria, together with comments on indications for their use and interpretation of findings. Aspects of treatment for various urinary and prostatic diseases are presented later in this manual.

Test and *indication*	Finding	Interpretation and action
Urine dipstick plus urine specific gravity (SG) (see Chapter 8) *– should be done routinely*	Positive for haem pigment	Could be intact RBCs, haemoglobin or myoglobin – check urine sediment
	Protein positive, urine SG variable	Could be haemorrhage, inflammation, glomerulonephropathy; assess severity of proteinuria using urine SG or protein:creatinine ratio (see Chapter 6)
	Urine alkaline (pH ≥8)	Consider possible infection with urease-producing bacteria (see Chapter 23)
Urine sediment examination (see Chapter 8) *– should be done routinely*	Intact RBCs, exceeding reference values for collection method (see Figure 1.5 and Chapter 8)	Haematuria (but consider possible trauma during sampling)
	No RBCs, but dipstick positive for haem pigment	RBCs haemolysed *in vivo* (check for pink plasma) or haemoglobin/myoglobin (see text and Figure 1.6)
	Leucocytes	Inflammation somewhere in urinary tract (or genital – consider collection method)
	Bacteria	Contamination or infection? Consider collection method
	Casts containing RBCs (or leucocytes)	Bleeding (or inflammation) occurring in kidney(s)
	Epithelial cell clumps with nuclear variability	Neoplasia (commonly transitional cell carcinoma) or dysplastic cells (reaction to severe inflammation)
	Crystalluria	Normal, or might indicate composition of any calculi present
Urine culture ± susceptibility test, sample collected by cystocentesis (see Chapters 8, 22, 23) *– recommended if bacteria and/or leucocytes found in sediment, or signs recurrent*	No growth	Sterile urine, or false-negative result if inappropriate sample or treated animal
	Significant bacteriuria	Indicates bacterial infection somewhere in urinary tract

1.9 Use of ancillary diagnostic aids in patients with dysuria and/or haematuria. (continues) ▶

Test and *indication*	Finding	Interpretation and action
Haematology *– not useful in most cases*	Inflammatory leucogram	Compatible with inflammation, but not usual in lower urinary disorders. Origin renal, prostatic or elsewhere?
	'Stress' leucogram	Suggests severe illness, glucocorticoid therapy or hyperadrenocorticism
Blood biochemical tests *– to assess azotaemia and metabolic effects if uraemia suspected, or detect disorders predisposing to urinary infection or calculus formation*	Increased concentrations of creatinine, urea, phosphate in fasting sample (see Chapter 5)	Azotaemia present – postrenal (urinary obstruction or rupture), renal or prerenal? Check hydration status, urine SG and other findings
	Changes compatible with hyperadrenocorticism, renal failure, diabetes mellitus	May predispose to urinary infection
	Hypercalcaemia or evidence of hepatopathy	May predispose to urolith formation
Prostatic fluid examination (see Chapter 20) *– advisable if any prostatic disease other than uncomplicated benign hyperplasia is suspected*	Leucocytes and bacteria	Prostatitis or prostatic abscess
	Epithelial cell clumps with abnormal appearance	Neoplasia, hyperplasia, squamous metaplasia or reactive change. Fine-needle aspiration biopsy suggested, but may be contraindicated if infection present
Diagnostic imaging (see Chapter 10) *– advisable if: urinary signs recur or persist; uroliths, neoplasia or urinary tract rupture suspected; or to evaluate kidneys, prostate, bladder*	Findings depend on disorder present and techniques used (plain and contrast radiography, ultrasonography)	See Chapter 10

1.9 (continued) Use of ancillary diagnostic aids in patients with dysuria and/or haematuria.

Acknowledgement

In preparing this chapter, I have drawn on the chapters in the previous edition of the Manual by Drs CR Scott-Moncrieff (Dysuria) and AG Torrance (Haematuria).

References and further reading

Bartges JW (2005) Discolored urine. In: *Textbook of Veterinary Internal Medicine, 6th edn*, ed. SJ Ettinger and EC Feldman, pp. 112–114. Elsevier Saunders, St Louis
Grauer GF (2003) Clinical manifestations of urinary disorders. In: *Small Animal Internal Medicine, 3rd edn*, ed. RW Nelson and GC Couto, pp. 568–583. Mosby, St Louis
Osborne CA and Finco DR (1995) *Canine and Feline Nephrology and Urology*. Williams and Wilkins, Baltimore
Osborne CA and Stevens JB (1999) *Urinalysis: a Clinical Guide to Compassionate Patient Care*. Veterinary Learning Systems, Trenton

2

Polyuria and polydipsia

Harriet M. Syme

Introduction

Increased volume of urine production (*polyuria*) and excessive thirst (*polydipsia*) are common presenting problems in small animal veterinary medicine. Water intake is generally easier to quantify than urine output and so is measured more often; polydipsia is defined as an intake of >100 ml/kg/day in the dog. Normal water intake is less in the cat and, as a consequence, the threshold for polydipsia should be lower than this, but no generally accepted cut-off exists. It is important to recognize that the cut-off point serves only as a guide; owners may notice an increase in thirst or urination without this threshold being reached, and the observed increases can have an underlying cause of pathological significance, even if the intake does not exceed 100 ml/kg/day.

A logical approach is required to identify the cause of polyuria/polydipsia (PU/PD) in dogs and cats, without premature recourse to unnecessary, expensive or potentially dangerous diagnostic tests. In many cases, a complete history and physical examination, together with urinalysis and a biochemical profile, will be sufficient for the likely cause of PU/PD to be identified. However, in a few cases, the cause remains enigmatic after these initial diagnostic tests, and, in these cases, a complete understanding of the normal physiological regulation of water balance is required for a logical diagnostic approach to be employed, and the correct diagnosis to be made.

Normal physiology of water balance

The volume of water that is ingested (in both food and water) and produced (as a byproduct of metabolism) each day in the healthy animal is balanced against the water that is lost via insensible means, in sweat and in faeces, and that which is excreted in the urine. Insensible water losses are those that are unnoticed, and occur through evaporative losses from the respiratory tract and the skin. Non-urinary losses of water will increase in some circumstances (e.g. hot environment, exercise, diarrhoea) but are otherwise typically considered to be in the order of 20–25 ml/kg/day. Production of concentrated urine can reduce, but not eliminate, urinary water loss, since some urine has to be produced to enable excretion of toxic waste products (the *minimal urinary void volume*). Provided that water intake and production are sufficient to match these obligatory losses, the homeostatic mechanisms that control the amount of water excreted by the kidneys, if functioning properly, are sufficient to maintain fluid balance within the animal.

Water balance is controlled by the regulation of thirst and urine volume, in response to changes in plasma osmolality (plasma solute concentration) and blood volume. Change in plasma osmolality, detected by osmoreceptors in the hypothalamus, is the more sensitive mechanism. In response to a slight increase in osmolality, antidiuretic hormone (ADH, vasopressin) is secreted from the posterior pituitary gland. ADH has vasoconstrictor actions on vascular smooth muscle, which tend to increase blood pressure, but its most important actions are in the kidney. ADH acts on the cells of the cortical collecting tubules and the collecting ducts, triggering a series of events and ultimately leading to a transient insertion of water-permeable channels (aquaporins) into the tubular membrane of the cells. These channels allow water to move along its osmotic gradient from the lumen of the collecting tubules to the hypertonic renal medulla. Maintenance of this concentration gradient between the collecting ducts and the medulla of the kidney depends upon efficient functioning of the loops of Henlé of the juxtamedullary nephrons and the vasa recta, which together trap solute (sodium chloride and urea) in the medullary interstitium and remove water. The reader is referred to current physiology texts for a more complete discussion of renal concentrating mechanisms.

Stimulation of hypothalamic osmoreceptors, in addition to increasing ADH secretion, also stimulates thirst and so increases water intake. The threshold for stimulation of thirst is higher than that for ADH secretion. However, humans and companion animals habitually drink more than sufficient water to match non-urinary water losses and minimal urinary volume. The concentration of circulating ADH is regulated such that the volume of water excreted by the kidneys matches the amount by which water intake exceeds insensible losses. Thus, a stable extracellular fluid osmolality is maintained.

In summary:

- ADH secretion increases steeply in response to increased plasma osmolality
- The renal response to ADH is to conserve water from the collecting tubules, and hence decrease urine volume

- This is possible only if the kidneys are able to maintain a concentrated medullary interstitium, a function which is dependent on the number of functioning juxtamedullary nephrons
- Increases in plasma osmolality also stimulate thirst.

Pathophysiology

From the above discussion of the normal physiology of the kidney, it is evident that four mechanisms may underlie the clinical presentation of PU/PD, either alone or in combination: lack of ADH secretion; lack of response to ADH; osmotic diuresis; and primary polydipsia (Figure 2.1). Primary polyuria with secondary polydipsia is usually the pathogenic mechanism underlying PU/PD in small animal medicine. If the kidney is unable to conserve water, the animal becomes polyuric and the thirst mechanism is the only means by which water homeostasis can be achieved. Less often, the disease process may cause a primary polydipsia with a secondary polyuria.

Lack of ADH secretion
Central diabetes insipidus (congenital or acquired)

Lack of response to ADH
Primary nephrogenic diabetes insipidus: • Congenital absence of ADH receptors Secondary nephrogenic diabetes insipidus: • Functional inhibition of the effects of ADH at the renal cellular level • Inability of nephrons to generate a concentrated medullary interstitium • Many causes of PU/PD are due, at least in part, to secondary nephrogenic diabetes insipidus, including pyelonephritis, pyometra, hyperadrenocorticism, hypoadrenocorticism, hypercalcaemia, hypokalaemia and hepatic insufficiency

Osmotic diuresis
• Water has to accompany solute particles that the kidneys excrete; when the number of these particles is excessive, polyuria results • Diabetes mellitus and postobstructive diuresis both cause PU/PD via this mechanism • Iatrogenic causes (e.g. mannitol, diuretics or sodium chloride administration) are also common

Primary polydipsia
• Primary 'psychogenic' polydipsia is the classical example of a cause of PU/PD that occurs by this mechanism • May also play a role in PU/PD associated with hepatic encephalopathy, gastrointestinal disease and hyperthyroidism

2.1 Pathogenetic mechanisms of polyuria and polydipsia.

Causes of polyuria/polydipsia

The pathogenesis of, and diagnostic tests for, some of the most important causes of PU/PD are described below. Further causes of PU/PD are listed in Figure 2.2. Many of the conditions that are listed in Figure 2.2 but not described in detail are either very rare or are likely to be associated with other clinical signs in addition to PU/PD, and these will guide the diagnostic approach.

Cats
Common causes
Chronic kidney disease Hyperthyroidism Diabetes mellitus Postobstructive diuresis Iatrogenic (drug, diet or fluid therapy)
Uncommon causes
Liver disease Pyometra Pyelonephritis Hypokalaemia (with renal disease)
Rare causes
Central diabetes insipidus Hypercalcaemia Acromegaly (insulin-resistant diabetes mellitus) Hyperadrenocorticism (insulin-resistant diabetes mellitus) Hypoadrenocorticism Primary hyperaldosteronism
Dogs
Common causes
Chronic kidney disease Pyometra Diabetes mellitus Hyperadrenocorticism Hypercalcaemia Pyelonephritis Iatrogenic (drug, diet or fluid therapy)
Uncommon causes
Liver disease Hypoadrenocorticism Primary polydipsia
Rare causes
Central diabetes insipidus Primary nephrogenic diabetes insipidus Hyperviscosity syndrome Primary glycosuria Fanconi syndrome Acromegaly (insulin-resistant diabetes mellitus) Hypokalaemia Gastrointestinal disease Polycythaemia Phaeochromocytoma Primary hyperaldosteronism Leiomyosarcoma Sudden acquired retinal degeneration syndrome

2.2 Differential diagnoses for polyuria/polydipsia in cats and dogs. Adapted from Hughes (1992) and Elliott (1996).

Diabetes mellitus and other causes of glucosuria

Diabetes mellitus causes PU/PD due to the osmotic diuresis associated with glucosuria. If the plasma concentration of glucose is such that it is filtered at a rate that exceeds the capacity of the proximal tubule to reabsorb it, water will be held in the tubule due to the osmotic forces exerted by the glucose molecules. The renal threshold for glucose is the concentration above which not all will be reabsorbed from the proximal tubules, and glucosuria and polyuria will result. This threshold is 9–12 mmol/l (160–220 mg/dl) for dogs and 11–16 mmol/l (200–280 mg/dl) for cats.

The diagnosis of diabetes mellitus is usually straightforward, at least in dogs. When glucosuria is accompanied by an elevated blood glucose concentration and compatible clinical signs, the diagnosis of diabetes mellitus is supported. Stress-induced hyperglycaemia in the cat may result in blood glucose concentrations that exceed the renal threshold and cause glucosuria. Additional support for the diagnosis of diabetes mellitus in cats can be provided by documenting glucosuria in a urine sample collected in the home environment, or by measuring blood fructosamine or glycosylated haemoglobin concentration as an indication of the prevailing blood glucose concentration over the preceding weeks to months.

Normoglycaemic glucosuria results from defective renal tubular function. The resorptive defect in the proximal tubule may be specific for glucose, or may also result in loss of electrolytes (sodium, potassium, phosphorus, calcium and bicarbonate) and amino acids into the urine, a condition known as Fanconi syndrome. Fanconi syndrome has been reported in numerous breeds but is most frequently encountered in the Basenji. Although the defect is presumed to be inherited in this breed, clinical signs usually do not develop until the dogs are adult. Fanconi syndrome may also develop as a result of an adverse drug reaction, exposure to nephrotoxins, or pyelonephritis; in such cases the syndrome may be transient. Glucosuria may also occur as a sign of generalized proximal renal tubular dysfunction as occurs in acute renal failure, in response to renal toxins, particularly heavy metals, and in end-stage chronic kidney disease.

Kidney disease

Kidney disease is a frequent cause of PU/PD in both the dog and cat. The kidney disease associated with PU/PD is most often chronic in nature, but polyuric forms of acute renal failure do also occur. The PU/PD that occurs with kidney disease results from rapid tubular flow rates, which in turn cause inadequate reabsorption of water from the collecting ducts and inadequate function of the countercurrent mechanism in the loop of Henlé and a loss of medullary hypertonicity. The rapid rates of tubular flow in patients with renal failure are caused by hyperfiltration of the small number of remaining functional nephrons in an attempt to increase the glomerular filtration rate (GFR), and the greatly reduced tubular reabsorption of sodium and chloride that occurs in order to prevent accumulation of these solutes within the body.

In most instances, diagnosis of chronic kidney disease in dogs and cats is quite straightforward. Documentation of azotaemia in an animal with compatible clinical signs, such as PU/PD, supports the diagnosis (see also Chapter 5). However, a specific caveat should be considered before the diagnosis of kidney disease is confirmed in an azotaemic animal, even if an inappropriately dilute urine specific gravity (SG)

(<1.030 in the dog; <1.035 in the cat) is documented concurrently. This is because, if an animal is unable to concentrate its urine for any reason, restricting access to water may result in azotaemia. For example, if a dog that is receiving furosemide and as a result has a urine SG of 1.012, is prevented from obtaining water, its urine SG will remain inappropriately low but, with time, renal perfusion will decrease and the dog will develop azotaemia. Thus it will have both azotaemia and inappropriately dilute urine, a combination of findings that is associated with intrinsic renal disease. In some cases, the only way to ensure that the azotaemia is not prerenal, or does not have a prerenal component, is to evaluate the animal's response to fluid therapy. It is also important to realize that the ability to produce dilute urine depends upon functional tubules to actively transport salt out of the filtrate; a patient that has hyposthenuric urine (SG <1.008; osmolality less than that of plasma) is unlikely to be in renal failure.

Chronic kidney disease may cause PU/PD in the absence of azotaemia. This is because, at least in the dog, fewer nephrons must be lost (approximately 66%) to cause failure of the urine-concentrating mechanism, than must be lost to cause azotaemia (approximately 75%). Documenting that poor renal function is the cause of PU/PD in the absence of azotaemia requires direct measurement of GFR (for details see Chapter 9). In the cat, once sufficient renal function is lost for PU/PD to be noticed, azotaemia is invariably present.

Hyperadrenocorticism

Hyperadrenocorticism, due to excessive endogenous production or exogenous administration of glucocorticoid steroid hormone, is a very common cause of PU/PD in the dog. Many dogs with hyperadrenocorticism will have additional abnormalities in the history or physical examination that point to this diagnosis; however, it is suggested that as many as 30% of dogs with hyperadrenocorticism have PU/PD as their only presenting abnormality (Reusch, 2005). The mechanisms whereby hyperadrenocorticism causes PU/PD are both multifactorial and species-specific; cats do not typically develop PU/PD in response to glucocorticoids (endogenous or exogenous) unless diabetes mellitus develops as a result of insulin resistance. In the main, the PU/PD that occurs in dogs with hyperadrenocorticism is thought to be due to an increase in both the threshold and the slope of ADH release in response to increasing osmolality: a type of partial central diabetes insipidus (Biewenga et al., 1991). In addition, glucocorticoids interfere with the action of ADH on the distal tubule, resulting in a form of nephrogenic diabetes insipidus.

Diagnosis of hyperadrenocorticism is complicated by the fact that no test for the disease has perfect sensitivity or specificity; false-positive and false-negative test results are common. To minimize the likelihood of false-positive test results, testing for this condition should be avoided in patients where the disease is considered unlikely, i.e. in patients for which the pre-test probability of having hyperadreno-corticism is low. Hyperadrenocorticism is uncommon in dogs under 6 years old, so other causes of PU/PD should be considered first in young animals. Hyper-adrenocorticism is unlikely to be the cause of PU/PD in any dog that appears systemically unwell or is inappetant, unless this is due to a secondary compli-cation, such as thromboembolism or an expanding pituitary macroadenoma. Around 90% of dogs with hyperadrenocorticism have elevated alkaline phos-phatase (ALP) activity; thus, if ALP activity is normal, hyperadrenocorticism should be considered less likely, although it cannot be ruled out altogether.

Having determined that hyperadrenocorticism is a possible cause of PU/PD in a dog, further testing is indicated. Numerous screening tests for hyper-adrenocorticism exist, each with inherent advantages and disadvantages. The most frequently employed tests are the adrenocorticotropic hormone (ACTH) stimulation test, low-dose dexamethasone suppres-sion test and urinary cortisol:creatinine ratio (UCCR). The ACTH stimulation test is probably the least sen-sitive of these tests; it is particularly insensitive in patients with adrenal-dependent disease. However, it is quick and easy to perform, and is the only test that will identify patients with iatrogenic hyperadreno-corticism. The sensitivity of the low-dose dexametha-sone suppression test is high in dogs with either pituitary- or adrenal-dependent hyperadrenocorticism. It is also a relatively specific test, provided the dog is not systemically unwell when the test is performed, and is not highly stressed by being hospitalized. The disadvantage of this test is that it takes 8 hours to perform. The UCCR is a sensitive but not very specific test. It is most useful in ruling out hyper-adrenocorticism, rather than confirming the diagno-sis. This test is best performed on a urine sample collected by the owners of the dog at home, prior to any visit to the veterinary clinic. It can be particularly useful in patients that are very stressed by visiting the veterinary clinic and those in which hyperadreno-corticism is considered unlikely, as additional evi-dence for ruling out the diagnosis.

Pyometra

Dogs and cats with pyometra may have PU/PD as a presenting sign. This is because endotoxins produced by the infecting organism, usually *Escherichia coli*, interfere with the actions of ADH on the distal tubule, resulting in a reversible form of nephrogenic diabetes insipidus. Pyometra should be ruled out in any entire female dog or cat presenting for PU/PD, particularly if they are aged. It is most commonly diagnosed 2–12 weeks following oestrus in dogs; in cats the timing relative to oestrus is more variable. Diagnosis is usu-ally made on the detection of an enlarged uterus in a non-pregnant animal by physical examination, radio-graphy or ultrasonography, or by detection of a puru-lent vaginal discharge. Azotaemia, which may be of prerenal or renal origin, is encountered frequently in dogs with pyometra and can result in the PU/PD being wrongly ascribed to renal failure in these patients (Stone *et al.*, 1988).

Pyelonephritis

Pyelonephritis causes PU/PD because interstitial inflammation in the kidney prevents the maintenance of the medullary concentration gradient. The infective agent (particularly if it is *E. coli*) may also interfere with the interaction of ADH with its receptors in the distal nephron, as described above in patients with pyometra. The severity of PU/PD may be very marked, and can occur even if the patient remains non-azotaemic.

The diagnosis of pyelonephritis is not always straightforward. Some patients show concurrent lower urinary tract signs, such as pollakiuria, stranguria, haematuria or urge incontinence, but many do not. Physical examination in patients with pyelonephritis is often unremarkable; classical features of this syn-drome, such as swollen kidneys, fever and lumbar pain, are generally not evident in chronic disease. Similarly, while leucocytosis and neutrophilia with a left shift are suggestive of pyelonephritis in an animal presented for PU/PD, the haemogram is often unre-markable. Abdominal imaging can be helpful in the diagnosis of pyelonephritis (see also Chapter 10); abnormalities that may be observed ultrasonographic-ally include dilation of the renal pelvis and proximal ureter, and a hyperechoic margin to the renal pelvis. Abnormalities that predispose the animal to infection (such as calculi, masses or anatomical abnormalities) may also be observed. Alternatively, dilation of the renal pelvis with blunting or lack of filling of the collect-ing diverticula, dilation of the proximal ureter and decreased renal opacification may also be detected by contrast radiography. Plain radiographs rarely contrib-ute to the diagnosis of pyelonephritis. Unfortunately, in some patients with pyelonephritis, both ultrasonogra-phy and contrast studies may be completely unremark-able (Neuwirth *et al.*, 1993).

Definitive diagnosis of pyelonephritis requires posi-tive cultures of urine collected from the renal pelvis or of aspirates or biopsy specimens of renal tissue. More usually, pyelonephritis is presumptively diagnosed with a positive culture of urine collected by cystocentesis, in a patient that has clinical signs (such as PU/PD) or findings on diagnostic imaging that suggest that infec-tion is not limited to the lower urinary tract. The urine sediment in these animals may or may not be inflam-matory. If the infection is limited to the kidney(s), and especially if the PU/PD is very profound resulting in dilution of any cellular components, the urine sediment examination may be unremarkable. The limitations of the currently available tests for pyelonephritis mean that urine culture is mandatory in the diagnostic work-up of all dogs and cats with PU/PD and that, in many cases, even if culture is negative, a trial with empirical antibiotic therapy is often advisable before discounting pyelonephritis as a possibility. More details on the diagnosis and treatment of urinary tract infections are given in Chapter 23.

Hypercalcaemia

Increases in the concentration of ionized calcium de-crease the ability of the cells of the distal tubule to respond to ADH – a form of nephrogenic diabetes insipidus. In addition, hypercalcaemia can cause damage to the renal tubules, resulting in a reduced capacity for water and electrolyte reabsorption. Thus, complete resolution of hypercalcaemia, if it has been severe or of long standing, may not totally resolve the PU/PD, since the resulting renal dysfunction may be permanent. In patients that are presented with both hypercalcaemia and azotaemia, a conundrum may develop as to which came first, since hypercalcaemia may cause renal failure and *vice versa*. If available, measurement of ionized calcium can be very helpful in these situations, since it is the total calcium concentration that is increased in patients with chronic kidney disease (because calcium forms complexes with retained organic and inorganic anions) and ionized calcium concentrations are usually normal or low.

Identifying hypercalcaemia as the cause of PU/PD is typically just the start of the diagnostic work-up in affected patients. The most common cause of hypercalcaemia in dogs is malignancy, with lymphoma and apocrine gland adenocarcinoma being the most frequently encountered forms (Figure 2.3). If the cause of hypercalcaemia is not evident from the history and a complete physical examination, including a rectal examination, the diagnostic work-up in these patients is likely to include thoracic and abdominal imaging, aspirates of peripheral lymph nodes and possibly examination of bone marrow. Measurement of parathyroid hormone (PTH) and PTH-related peptide concentrations may also be helpful by distinguishing primary from secondary hyperparathyroidism.

Neoplasia
Lymphoma
Apocrine gland adenocarcinoma
Thymoma
Multiple myeloma, plasma cell tumours
Lymphocytic leukaemia
Primary or metastatic bone tumours
Other tumours, primarily carcinomas
Squamous cell carcinoma (cats)
Primary hyperparathyroidism
Toxicity
Rodenticides containing vitamin D
Antipsoriasis creams
Others
Renal failure
Hypoadrenocorticism
Granulomatous disease
Angiostrongylus vasorum
Idiopathic (cats)

2.3 Causes of hypercalcaemia.

Hyperthyroidism

Hyperthyroidism is one of the most common causes of PU/PD in the cat. The mechanisms whereby hyperthyroidism causes PU/PD are not completely understood. Hyperthyroidism induces natriuresis through stimulation of the sympathetic nervous system, which increases blood flow within the vasa recta and so reduces medullary hypertonicity. It is also suggested that an additional cause for PU/PD is primary polydipsia, possibly related to heat intolerance.

Hyperthyroidism is such a common disease that testing for this condition is recommended in all but the youngest cats that are presented for investigation of PU/PD. Most hyperthyroid cats will have palpable goitres. In addition, increases in liver enzyme levels (particularly alanine aminotransferase; ALT) are common abnormalities associated with hyperthyroidism. Documentation of an increased circulating thyroxine (total T4) concentration gives a definitive diagnosis in most instances. Some cats have total T4 values that are at the high end of the laboratory reference range, but are not definitive for the diagnosis of hyperthyroidism. The simple approach to such cases is to repeat the T4 measurement in 2–3 weeks. Other methods for confirming a diagnosis of hyperthyroidism include the T3 suppression test, thyrotropin-releasing hormone (TRH) stimulation test, or measurement of free T4 by equilibrium dialysis. Of these, the measurement of free T4 is the most frequently employed, but care is necessary because of the relatively high rate of false-positive tests that occur when this test is used in isolation; however, the combination of 'high-normal' total T4 (>40 nmol/l) and elevated free T4 concentration appears to be both sensitive and specific for the diagnosis of hyperthyroidism (Peterson *et al.*, 2001).

Hypoadrenocorticism

PU/PD may be a historical finding in dogs and cats with hypoadrenocorticism at the time of diagnosis. The PU/PD is thought to result from a lack of medullary hypertonicity due to hyponatraemia. In most instances, dogs with hypoadrenocorticism will be presented with clinical signs that overshadow the significance of the observed PU/PD. Dogs with hypoadrenocorticism may also be presented due to PU/PD when they are receiving treatment; this is usually due to excessive glucocorticoid effects, either through administration of glucocorticoids directly (e.g. prednisolone), or the glucocorticoid effects of fludrocortisone. If signs of hyperadrenocorticism persist when the dog is receiving fludrocortisone alone, desoxycorticosterone pivilate (DOCP) can be substituted. This drug has no glucocorticoid activity so signs of hyperadrenocorticism should resolve, although this also means it has to be supplemented with a small dose of glucocorticoid, usually in the form of prednisolone. DOCP is not available in the UK and a Special Treatment Authorisation (STA) must be obtained from the Veterinary Medicines Directorate (VMD) to obtain it.

Hepatic dysfunction

The cause of PU/PD in animals with hepatic dysfunction is multifactorial. Low urea concentrations result in decreased medullary hypertonicity. Hepatic encephalopathy may cause primary 'psychogenic' polydipsia. In addition, increased glucocorticoid concentrations, resulting from inefficient hepatic metabolism and increases in ACTH concentrations, contribute to PU/PD.

Hepatic dysfunction sufficient to result in PU/PD will usually result in abnormalities in a routine biochemistry profile. Definitive documentation of hepatic dysfunction requires measurement of fasting ammonia, or pre- and postprandial bile acid concentrations.

Central diabetes insipidus

Central diabetes insipidus (CDI) is a rare cause of PU/PD. It results from a complete or partial lack of ADH release from the posterior lobe of the pituitary (neurohypophysis). Tumours of the pituitary or hypothalamus are common causes of CDI in middle-aged to older dogs. Primary pituitary neoplasms are most common, but meningiomas, craniopharyngiomas and metastatic lesions have also been reported. Severe head injury and intracranial surgery may disrupt the pituitary stalk, resulting in CDI. Sometimes this condition is only temporary, with spontaneous remission occurring due to regeneration of axons emanating from the hypothalamus. Idiopathic forms of CDI also occur in which no lesion is demonstrable in the pituitary or hypothalamus. Idiopathic CDI is most common in young animals.

Diagnosis of CDI requires specialist diagnostic tests, which should not be considered until other causes for PU/PD have been effectively ruled out. Urine SG in dogs with CDI is often very low; those with complete CDI will have hyposthenuric urine (<1.008), although those with partial CDI may have higher urine specific gravities. Other abnormalities in the results of routine urinalysis and serum/plasma biochemistry are normally absent. Plasma osmolality and its main determinant, the plasma sodium concentration, are often at the high end of the laboratory reference range in dogs with CDI, due to a failure to totally replenish renal water loss. Any dog or cat suspected of having CDI should have a complete neurological examination before any other diagnostic testing is performed. If the neurological examination is abnormal then advanced imaging of the hypothalamus and pituitary using magnetic resonance imaging (MRI) is often more appropriate to the diagnostic work-up of the case than further tests of urine-concentrating ability.

The diagnosis of CDI is usually confirmed by performing tests of urine-concentrating ability: either the water deprivation test or response to trial therapy with exogenous ADH analogues. Measurement of ADH secretion in response to hypertonic saline infusion has also been used in the research setting. However, it cannot be overemphasized that these tests are rarely necessary in the work-up of a patient with PU/PD and they are often performed prematurely. Following diagnosis of CDI, advanced imaging of the pituitary should be considered, particularly in middle-aged and older animals; if a mass is identified these patients may benefit from radiation therapy.

If a diagnosis of CDI is confirmed then treatment with desmopressin (DDAVP, 1-deamino, 9-D-arginine vasopressin), a synthetic analogue of ADH, should result in resolution of PU/PD. The aqueous solution (marketed for intranasal use in humans) has been given as an eye drop in dogs and cats with CDI. This approach has generally been replaced by the use of desmopressin tablets; total dose of 0.05–0.1 mg per dog, according to its size, two to three times daily as needed to control clinical signs. If, due to financial reasons, CDI is not treated, adverse consequences other than PU/PD should not occur, provided that free access to water is maintained at all times. Untreated patients with CDI will require special care if they develop a concurrent problem that limits their water intake, even for short periods (e.g. acute gastric upset resulting in vomiting), since severe dehydration can develop very quickly in these animals.

Nephrogenic diabetes insipidus

Primary nephrogenic diabetes insipidus (primary NDI) is an extremely uncommon clinical problem. To date, congenital NDI has been diagnosed in only a small number of dogs. It has never been diagnosed in the cat. Primary NDI occurs when there is a defect in the binding of ADH to its receptor (the V_2 receptor in the cortical and medullary collecting tubules), in the coupling of this receptor via adenylate cyclase to the insertion of water channels (aquaporins) into the luminal membrane, or in the structure of the water channels themselves. Secondary NDI has a multiplicity of causes (see Figure 2.1) and cannot be distinguished from primary NDI by performing tests of urine-concentrating ability. Therefore, testing for NDI should only be considered once all possible causes of secondary NDI have been excluded.

Primary polydipsia

In this condition, excessive water intake occurs with secondary polyuria to maintain stable plasma osmolality (psychogenic or primary polydipsia). This condition is relatively uncommon. It is most frequently encountered in hyperactive young dogs, particularly those that are left unattended for large parts of the day. Environmental modification resolves the PU/PD in some of these dogs. Some cases in human medicine have been associated with lesions in the hypothalamus, and this may also occur in dogs.

Diagnosis of primary polydipsia has traditionally been confirmed by proving that urine can be adequately concentrated during a water deprivation test (WDT). However, dogs with primary polydipsia may have a very variable urine concentration during the course of the day, including some samples with SG >1.025 (or osmolality >1000 mOsm/kg), negating the requirement for a WDT. It is recommended that, before performing a WDT in a patient suspected to have primary polydipsia, the owners are instructed to collect multiple urine samples, including at times when the dog is very active and thus may be less inclined to be polydipsic, such as at the weekends or other times when the dog is not left alone. If randomly collected urine samples, without water restriction, have a SG >1.025, then CDI is effectively ruled out and a diagnosis of primary polydipsia can be made.

Treatment of patients with primary polydipsia consists of restricting water intake to a near normal daily volume (80 ml/kg/day). Gradual restriction is recommended to prevent the development of other undesirable behaviours. Changes in the dog's environment may also be helpful.

Initial diagnostic work-up

History

An accurate and full history is of great importance in the investigation of all medical problems. It is important to be sure that the animal is indeed polyuric and does not simply have a problem of increased frequency of urination or of urinary incontinence, leading to urination in the house at night. Whilst either of these problems may be present concurrently in a dog or cat that is polyuric, they can also be presenting complaints in many disorders of the lower urinary tract (see Chapters 1 and 3). Quantification of the amount of water drunk by the animal may be necessary in some cases to confirm that PU/PD is truly a significant problem. In most cases, close questioning of the owner will confirm the significance of the PU/PD.

Next, it is important to rule out iatrogenic causes of polyuria and polydipsia. The most frequently encountered of these are listed in Figure 2.4.

Fluid therapy
Diuretics
Loop diuretics (e.g. furosemide) Thiazide diuretics (e.g. hydrochlorothiazide) Aldosterone antagonists (e.g. spironolactone) Carbonic anhydrase inhibitors (e.g. acetazolamide) Osmotic diuretics (e.g. mannitol)
Steroid hormones
Oral and injectable glucocorticoid preparations Topical steroids (aural, ophthalmic, cutaneous medications) Fludrocortisone and other drugs given for their mineralocorticoid properties
Anticonvulsants
Phenobarbital Phenytoin
Dietary composition
Dry *versus* moist diets Salt-supplemented diets (e.g. for management of urolithiasis) Protein-restricted diets (e.g. for management of hepatic failure, urolithiasis)
High ambient temperature and humidity

2.4 Iatrogenic causes of polyuria and polydipsia.

Consideration of the patient's signalment (age, sex and breed) will be of help in prioritizing the differential diagnoses in patients with PU/PD (Figure 2.5). In addition, many of the diseases that cause PU/PD are multisystemic and will also cause other clinical signs. It is therefore necessary to take a full clinical history. The problem-oriented approach to the investigation of animals that present with PU/PD allows diseases that can account for more than one problem to be investigated concurrently and ruled in or out first, thus saving time and money in the diagnostic work-up. Examples of such problems or historical findings and their potential diagnostic significance are presented in Figure 2.6.

Patient characteristics	Differential diagnoses
Entire female: In season recently (in dioestrus on presentation)	Pyometra Diabetes mellitus Acromegaly (dogs) Pyelonephritis
Irregular seasons or anoestrus	Hyperadrenocorticism
Immature animal	Juvenile nephropathy Congenital portosystemic shunt Juvenile diabetes mellitus Primary glucosuria Primary nephrogenic diabetes insipidus Congenital central diabetes insipidus
Older animal	Pyometra Hyperthyroidism Chronic kidney disease Intrinsic liver disease, acquired portosystemic shunts Hyperadrenocorticism Hypercalcaemia (apocrine gland adenocarcinoma and other neoplasms) Hypercalcaemia (primary hyperparathyroidism) Acquired central diabetes insipidus (neoplasia) Acromegaly
Breed predisposition [a]	Basenji: Fanconi syndrome Keeshond: primary hyperparathyroidism Norwegian Elkhound: primary renal glucosuria Scottish Terrier: primary renal glucosuria Many breeds: familial nephropathies (see Chapter 7 for details)

2.5 Diagnostic significance of the signalment of animals presenting with polyuria/polydipsia.
[a] Only diseases that are uncommon in the general population are listed; for example, some breeds are predisposed to development of diabetes mellitus, but these are not listed here since this condition is common in the population at large.

Problem or historical finding	Differential diagnoses
Weight loss with polyphagia	Diabetes mellitus Hyperthyroidism
Weight loss with poor appetite	Chronic kidney disease Pyelonephritis Hypercalcaemia Liver disease Hypoadrenocorticism
Polyphagia without weight loss	Hyperadrenocorticism Acromegaly
Weakness, exercise intolerance but bright and alert	Hyperadrenocorticism
Weakness, depression (systemically ill – may be vomiting)	Chronic kidney disease (advanced) Pyometra Diabetes mellitus (ketoacidotic) Hypercalcaemia Hypoadrenocorticism Hypokalaemia Liver disease

2.6 Diagnostic significance of common historical problems in animals presenting with polyuria/polydipsia. Adapted from Elliott (1996). (continues) ▶

Problem or historical finding	Differential diagnoses
Behavioural abnormalities/ central nervous system signs (ataxia, blindness, stupor, seizures)	Hepatic encephalopathy Pituitary neoplasm: • Hyperadrenocorticism (macroadenoma) • Acromegaly • Acquired central diabetes insipidus Sudden acquired retinal degeneration syndrome
No clinical signs other than PU/PD	Pyelonephritis Hyperadrenocorticism Chronic kidney disease (mild) Hypercalcaemia (primary hyperparathyroidism) Primary renal glucosuria Fanconi syndrome Central diabetes insipidus Nephrogenic diabetes insipidus

2.6 (continued) Diagnostic significance of common historical problems in animals presenting with polyuria/polydipsia. Adapted from Elliott (1996).

Physical examination

A thorough physical examination may identify problems which, when combined with history findings, may be highly suggestive of the underlying disease, thus reducing the number of further tests required to confirm the diagnosis. The physical findings of significance and the disease processes of which they are suggestive are presented in Figure 2.7.

Routine diagnostic tests

The history and physical findings may suggest a particular cause for PU/PD, which can be confirmed by selected routine haematology, biochemistry and urinalysis tests. In most instances, at least if the owner of the dog or cat wishes to pursue treatment for the condition underlying PU/PD, full plasma/serum biochemistry and urinalysis is indicated. This approach may increase the confidence in the diagnosis and reveal concurrent problems that affect the prognosis. Similarly, urine culture is almost always advisable, as urinary tract infections are commonly associated with several common causes of PU/PD.

Complete urinalysis

Examination of the urine is an important part of the diagnostic work-up of an animal presenting with PU/PD. As a minimum, this should consist of measurement of urine SG (or osmolality), testing for the presence of abnormal urine constituents (by a dipstick test), and examining the urine sediment microscopically. Urinalysis is described in detail in Chapter 8. Ideally, urine should be obtained by cystocentesis to ensure contamination from the lower urinary tract does not affect the interpretation of the results and certainly should be collected before any therapy (fluid or drug) has been administered. The exception to this rule is in unspayed females that could have pyometra; these animals should only have samples collected by cystocentesis if this can be done under ultrasound guidance, otherwise a voided sample will have to suffice.

Organ/system examined	Abnormality found	Possible disease indicated
Eyes	Cataracts Jaundiced sclera Corneal lipidosis Anterior uveitis Tortuous retinal vessels Papilloedema Hyphaema, retinal haemorrhage, detachment or oedema Blindness (without apparent ocular lesions)	Diabetes mellitus Liver disease Hyperadrenocorticism Lymphoma (hypercalcaemia) Hyperviscosity syndromes Pituitary neoplasm Systemic hypertension (chronic kidney disease, hyperthyroidism, hyperadrenocorticism, phaeochromocytoma) Hypothalamic or pituitary mass, hepatic encephalopathy, sudden acquired retinal degeneration syndrome
Mucous membranes	Pale Congested Jaundiced Sticky/dry	Chronic kidney disease, hypoadrenocorticism Toxaemia (pyometra), polycythaemia Liver disease Dehydration
Mouth	Ulceration, stomatitis Tonsillar hyperplasia Increased interdental spaces	Chronic kidney disease (advanced) Malignant lymphoma Acromegaly
Lymph nodes	Enlargement	Lymphoma
Neck	Thyroid mass	Hyperthyroidism, hyperparathyroidism (parathyroid adenomas are usually not palpable in dogs but may be palpable in cats)
Thorax	Tachypnoea, panting Tachycardia Bradycardia Heart murmur Muffled or displaced heart sounds	Hyperthyroidism, hyperadrenocorticism, mediastinal mass (lymphoma) Hyperthyroidism, toxaemia (pyometra), hypovolaemia Hypoadrenocorticism, hyperkalaemia (secondary to renal failure) Hyperthyroidism, acromegaly, chronic kidney disease (systemic hypertension) Mediastinal mass (lymphoma)

2.7 Physical examination findings and their significance in animals presenting with polyuria/polydipsia. Note that most animals that have primary polyuria and secondary polydipsia will be dehydrated to a certain extent (although this is often subclinical). In those patients that are systemically ill the dehydration may be particularly marked. Adapted from Elliott (1996). (continues)

▶

Organ/system examined	Abnormality found	Possible disease indicated
Skin and hair coat	Thin skin, comedones, non-pruritic alopecia Calcinosis cutis Skin tears (related to minor trauma) Unkempt hair coat Resolution of allergic skin disease	Hyperadrenocorticism Hyperadrenocorticism Hyperadrenocorticism, especially in cats Hyperthyroidism Hyperadrenocorticism
Abdomen	Abdominal enlargement Hepatomegaly Small kidneys Large kidneys Enlarged uterus Lymphadenomegaly	Hyperadrenocorticism, liver disease (ascites), nephrotic syndrome (ascites) Diabetes mellitus, hyperadrenocorticism, liver disease (infiltrative) Chronic kidney disease (interstitial nephritis), congenital hypoplasia Pyelonephritis, polycystic kidney disease, renal lymphoma, feline infectious peritonitis Pyometra (care on palpation) Lymphoma
Nervous system	Neurological deficits	Hypothalamic or pituitary mass, hepatic encephalopathy
External genitalia	Vaginal discharge	Open pyometra
Rectal examination	Anal sac mass Sublumbar lymph node enlargement	Apocrine gland adenocarcinoma Apocrine gland adenocarcinoma (metastasis), lymphoma

2.7 (continued) Physical examination findings and their significance in animals presenting with polyuria/polydipsia. Note that most animals that have primary polyuria and secondary polydipsia will be dehydrated to a certain extent (although this is often subclinical). In those patients that are systemically ill the dehydration may be particularly marked. Adapted from Elliott (1996).

Urine specific gravity: In general, urine with a SG >1.030 in the dog or >1.035 in the cat indicates that a concentrating defect is not likely and the observed polydipsia is replacing non-renal losses. Most patients with significant PU/PD will have urine specific gravities <1.025. In some instances significant PU/PD is only evident in the animal's home environment; in the hospital the patient does not drink as much – due to fear, anxiety or reduced access to water – even though this may result in the development of dehydration (which is often subclinical). If the SG of urine samples collected while the animal is hospitalized does not support PU/PD, it is a good idea to review the history and ensure that pollakiuria or inappropriate urination is not actually the problem. If the history is definitely one of PU/PD, it may be necessary to get the owner to collect urine samples at home. In dogs suspected to have primary polydipsia it is often helpful to collect multiple urine samples, both when the patient is hospitalized and at home, because these dogs will often have intermittently concentrated urine. If this can be confirmed then a WDT becomes unnecessary.

Urine SG can be used to refine the differential diagnosis. SG in the fixed, or isosthenuric, range (1.008–1.012) indicates excretion of urine with the same osmolality as plasma. If urine SG is <1.008 (hyposthenuria), the early part of the distal tubule of the nephron is able to absorb salt from the tubular fluid and thus produce dilute urine; hence, tubular function is still present. The production of hyposthenuric urine effectively excludes chronic kidney disease as the cause. Cases of CDI, primary NDI and primary polydipsia usually present with hyposthenuria. Urine concentrations in patients with secondary nephrogenic diabetes insipidus (e.g. due to hypercalcaemia, pyelonephritis, pyometra, hyperadrenocorticism) are more variable and may be hyposthenuric, isosthenuric or minimally concentrated. Figure 2.8 illustrates the typical SG of urine from dogs and cats presenting with the common causes of PU/PD.

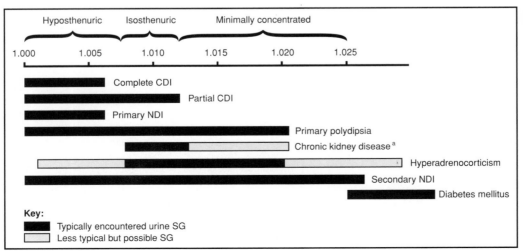

2.8
Urine specific gravities typically found in patients with polyuria/polydipsia due to different causes. [a] Range refers to dogs only. Cats with chronic kidney disease may have a urine specific gravity that is much greater than this; it may exceed 1.035. CDI = Central diabetes insipidus; NDI = Nephrogenic diabetes insipidus.

Osmolality: Measurement of urine osmolality rather than SG produces a more accurate assessment of urine-concentrating ability. Osmolality (usually measured by freezing point depression) is a colligative property and, as such, reflects the number of particles present regardless of their nature or size. SG is determined by the refractive index of a fluid, a property which depends not only on the number of particles present within a solution but also on the nature of those particles. With significant proteinuria, urine SG will be relatively higher than urine osmolality. Measuring urine osmolality and plasma osmolality of samples taken at the same time is particularly useful (see Modified water deprivation test, below).

Glucosuria: Urine SG is often >1.025 (and osmolality is also high) in patients with significant glucosuria. This is because the glucose molecules themselves will increase the SG measurement. Thus it is always essential to check for glucosuria (by performing dipstick analysis) at the same time as measuring SG. The significance of glucosuria in a patient presented for investigation of PU/PD is discussed above.

Proteinuria: This is discussed as a separate problem in Chapter 6. The finding of significant proteinuria in an animal presented for PU/PD may indicate that pyometra, protein-losing nephropathy (glomerulonephritis, amyloidosis and certain familial proteinuric nephropathies), pyelonephritis or hyperadrenocorticism is the cause. However, proteinuria may also be noted due to a lower urinary tract infection. Lower urinary tract infections do not cause PU/PD unless accompanied by pyelonephritis; however, they are relatively common secondary complications of other diseases that cause PU/PD, notably chronic kidney disease, diabetes mellitus and hyperadrenocorticism. Microscopic examination of the urine sediment and urine culture should always be performed to assist in the interpretation of the dipstick proteinuria. If urine culture is negative, proteinuria can be more accurately quantified by determining the protein:creatinine ratio.

Urine sediment examination: This is discussed in detail in Chapter 8. The presence of white blood cell casts is indicative of tubular inflammatory lesions and may be seen in pyelonephritis, although these are not always present. The presence of leucocytes or bacteria usually indicates an infection, although, as discussed above, this does not always signify pyelonephritis as many other causes of PU/PD predispose to the development of urinary tract infection.

Urine culture: This is mandatory in all patients with proteinuria and/or inflammatory urine sediment. Arguably, urine culture should be part of the minimum database of all patients that present with PU/PD, since production of a very large volume of urine dilutes any cellular components, making their recognition difficult. Cell lysis may also occur due to the hypotonicity of the urine. Furthermore, in patients with hyperadrenocorticism the inflammatory response is suppressed making recognition of infection without culture difficult. Diagnosis and management of urinary tract infections is discussed in detail in Chapter 23.

Haematology and biochemistry

Figures 2.9 and 2.10 present abnormalities that may be encountered in a routine haematology and biochemistry screen, respectively, with the significance of the findings in an animal presenting with PU/PD.

Parameter	Change observed	Disease state
Erythrocytes	Polycythaemia	Dehydration/haemoconcentration Hyperadrenocortism Polycythaemia vera
	Anaemia (non-regenerative)	Chronic kidney disease Liver disease Hypoadrenocorticism Lymphoma (marrow infiltration)
	Anaemia (regenerative)	Lymphoma (secondary immune-mediated haemolytic anaemia)
	Microcytosis	Portosystemic shunts
Leucocytes	Stress leucogram (mature neutrophilia, monocytosis, eosinopenia, lymphopenia)	Hyperadrenocorticism
	Absence of a stress leucogram	Hypoadrenocorticism
	Neutrophilia with left shift	Pyometra Pyelonephritis
	Lymphocytosis	Lymphocytic leukaemia Lymphoma (stage V)
	Neutropenia	Lymphoma (marrow infiltration)
Thrombocytes	Thrombocytopenia	Lymphoma (immune-mediated destruction, marrow infiltration)
	Thrombocytosis	Hyperadrenocorticism

2.9 Haematological findings and their significance in animals presenting with polyuria/polydipsia. Adapted from Elliott (1996).

Parameter	Change observed	Disease state
Albumin	Increased	Dehydration (together with globulin)
	Decreased	Liver disease Nephrotic syndrome Hypoadrenocorticism Compensatory (hyperglobulinaemia)
Globulin	Increased	Dehydration (together with albumin) Hyperviscosity syndrome Liver disease
Creatinine and urea	Increased	Chronic kidney disease Dehydration (prerenal azotaemia) Drugs (diuretics, leading to prerenal azotaemia) Hypoadrenocorticism Hypercalcaemic nephropathy
Urea	Decreased	Liver disease Diuresis (PU/PD not associated with renal failure) Low-protein diet
Phosphate	Increased	Chronic kidney disease Vitamin D toxicosis Severe dehydration Hypoadrenocorticism Hyperthroidism
	Decreased	Primary hyperparathyroidism Hypercalcaemia of malignancy (Hypophosphataemia accompanying hypercalcaemia is only found in the absence of evidence of renal dysfunction; i.e. if creatinine and urea are elevated, plasma phosphate may be normal or elevated) Hyperadrenocorticism
Calcium	Increased	See Figure 2.3
	Decreased	Chronic kidney disease Hypoalbuminaemia (causes a lowering of the total plasma calcium concentration, as 50% of the total calcium is bound to albumin. The free ionized calcium is the important fraction physiologically)
Alkaline phosphatase	Increased	Hyperadrenocortcism Diabetes mellitus Liver disease Hyperthyroidism Drugs (glucocorticoids, anticonvulsants)
Alanine aminotransferase	Increased	Hyperthyroidism Diabetes mellitus Hyperadrenocorticism (less marked than elevation of alkaline phosphatase) Liver disease Drugs (glucocorticoids, anticonvulsants)
Total bilirubin	Increased	Cholestatic liver disease
Cholesterol	Increased	Hyperadrenocorticism Diabetes mellitus Nephrotic syndrome Cholestatic liver disease
	Decreased	Liver failure Portosystemic shunt Hypoadrenocorticism
Glucose	Increased	Diabetes mellitus Acromegaly Hyperadrenocorticism Stress (cats) Drugs (glucocorticoids, progestogens)
	Decreased	Hypoadrenocorticism Liver failure Polycythaemia Leukaemia

2.10 Plasma biochemical findings and their significance in animals presenting with polyuria/polydipsia. Adapted from Elliott (1996). (continues) ▶

Parameter	Change observed	Disease state
Sodium and chloride	Increased	Primary nephrogenic diabetes insipidus Central diabetes insipidus (Dehydration; most causes of dehydration have lost both water and electrolytes in roughly equal proportions, thus plasma sodium and chloride concentration do not change (or may even fall). In diabetes insipidus (central or primary nephrogenic) water loss is the primary problem and plasma sodium and chloride ion concentrations may rise)
	Decreased	Hypoadrenocorticism Ketoacidotic diabetes mellitus (Psychogenic polydipsia)
Potassium	Increased	Chronic kidney disease (end-stage) Hypoadrenocorticism Diabetic ketoacidosis Drugs (ACE inhibitors, potassium-sparing diuretics)
	Decreased	Postobstructive diuresis Diabetes mellitus Chronic kidney disease Hyperaldosteronism Drugs (furosemide)

2.10 (continued) Plasma biochemical findings and their significance in animals presenting with polyuria/polydipsia. Adapted from Elliott (1996).

It is important to recognize that many sick and dehydrated animals may present with increased urea, creatinine and, perhaps, phosphate if renal perfusion has been compromised (prerenal azotaemia). This is particularly the case where the polyuric animal becomes anorexic or vomits and so water intake does not meet the excessive urinary losses. Such animals have no defence against dehydration so the development of azotaemia can be particularly rapid. This is discussed above with reference to diagnosing chronic kidney disease in patients that are presented with PU/PD.

Further diagnostic work-up

In most patients with PU/PD a complete history, physical examination, urinalysis and routine haematological and biochemical analysis will reveal the underlying cause, or indicate what further testing is required. However, in a minority of patients, further testing will be required to identify the cause of PU/PD. Figure 2.11 outlines a potential diagnostic approach in these patients. This is not meant to be prescriptive; based on the signalment, history, physical examination and results of the initial diagnostic tests described above,

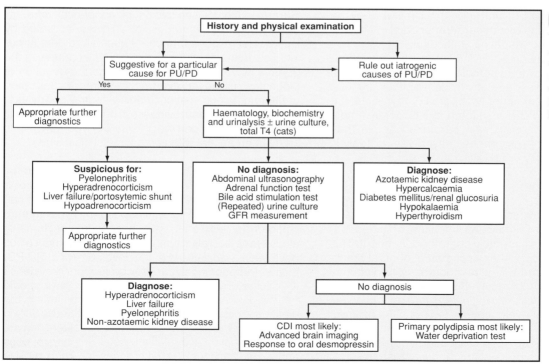

2.11 The diagnostic approach to cases presenting with documented polyuria/polydipsia.

suspicions may be raised and the sequence of further diagnostic tests altered accordingly. This is the practice of good, problem-oriented medicine. However, the tests described below are usually appropriate before considering a test of urine-concentrating ability, which should only be performed once every cause of PU/PD other than CDI, primary NDI and primary polydipsia has been conclusively ruled out.

Diagnostic imaging

Diagnostic imaging may be helpful in supporting or confirming the diagnosis of the underlying cause of PU/PD or in directing further diagnostic testing in a patient in which the results of initial diagnostic tests (history, physical examination, haematology, biochemistry and urinalysis) have proved uninformative.

Radiography

Abdominal radiography can be used to confirm the presence of an enlarged uterus, e.g. in pyometra. Liver size can also be assessed. Hepatomegaly may support the diagnosis of hyperadrenocorticism, diabetes mellitus or infiltrative disease giving rise to liver failure. A small liver may indicate chronic liver disease caused by cirrhotic change, or, if found in a young animal, may indicate the presence of a portosystemic shunt. Renomegaly has also been noted in these animals. In cases where kidney disease is suspected, assessment of kidney size by radiography may assist in patient evaluation, although ultrasonography is replacing this imaging modality as it also allows assessment of the internal renal architecture. Small or large kidneys may be evident in dogs and cats with renal disease; this finding is discussed in detail in Chapter 4. Occasionally abdominal radiography may also allow visualization of adrenal gland masses (particularly if they are calcified), although it is important to remember that the adrenal glands are sometimes mineralized in normal cats. Uroliths may be evident in patients with hyperadrenocorticism, hyperparathyroidism or hepatic insufficiency.

Thoracic radiography is indicated in the investigation of patients with hypercalcaemia, since a cranial mediastinal mass is a relatively common finding, due to the presence of either lymphoma or thymoma. If a suspicion of multiple myeloma exists, for example due to hypercalcaemia and hyperglobulinaemia, then skeletal survey radiographs may reveal osteolytic bone lesions.

Ultrasonography

Ultrasonography is replacing radiography as the primary imaging tool for the abdomen (see Chapter 10). Unfortunately, a significant limitation of ultrasonography is that it is extremely operator-dependent. This means that although many competent general practitioners are able to use ultrasonography to diagnose pyometra, and to identify the bladder to facilitate cystocentesis, evaluating patients for the subtle changes that indicate that pyelonephritis is present or for mild, bilateral adrenomegaly consistent with a diagnosis of pituitary-dependent hyperadrenocorticism, remains, for the most part, the preserve of the specialist.

Pyometra: Ultrasonography is valuable in confirming the presence of pyometra, particularly when results of radiographic studies are inconclusive. Ultrasonography allows determination of uterine size, thickness of the uterine wall, the presence or absence of fluid within the uterine lumen and the presence or absence of fetuses within the fluid. The presence of a convoluted, fluid-filled uterus, without fetuses, in a patient with PU/PD is consistent with a diagnosis of pyometra. However, the ultrasonographic findings in pyometra and cystic endometrial hyperplasia with fluid accumulation (mucometra or hydrometra) are essentially indistinguishable; one must rely on the results of other diagnostic tests to distinguish these conditions. Stump pyometra may be detected as a hypoechoic or mixed-echogenicity mass located caudodorsal to the urinary bladder.

Liver: The liver architecture can also be evaluated using ultrasonography, but estimates of total hepatic size are most easily made from abdominal radiographs. A diffuse increase in hepatic echogenicity may be noted with diabetes mellitus and hyperadrenocorticism, although this cannot be definitively distinguished from diffuse infiltrative disease as occurs in patients with lymphoma. Paradoxically, lymphoma has also been associated with diffuse uniform hypoechogenicity or normal echogenicity of the liver. It also may cause nodular or multinodular hypoechoic parenchymal lesions. None of these appearances of lymphoma is pathognomonic for the disease, and the diagnosis must be confirmed by the collection of samples for cytological or histopathological evaluation. Changes in hepatic architecture may be noted in patients with chronic hepatitis or cirrhosis, but regenerative nodules, when present, are not always visible. Ascites may be present in patients with hepatic failure and this is easily detected and sampled using ultrasonography.

Shunts: Direct visualization of congenital intra- or extrahepatic shunts is possible. This is facilitated by Doppler techniques that can be used to detect turbulent flow in the caudal vena cava and increases in the portal flow velocity, and to determine the direction of blood flow. However, even without direct visualization of the anomalous vessel, imaging a small poorly vascularized liver, without evidence of hepatic parenchymal disease, might support the presence of a portosystemic shunt in an animal with compatible clinical signs.

Adrenal glands: Careful evaluation of the adrenal glands can form a valuable part of the work-up of a patient with PU/PD. The finding of an adrenal mass can be compatible with adrenal-dependent hyperadrenocorticism, or less often, with phaeochromocytoma or aldosterone-secreting tumours. All of these tumour types have been associated with the development of PU/PD. Bilateral adrenomegaly can provide supportive evidence for pituitary hyperadrenocorticism, although it should not be used as the sole method for confirming the diagnosis; normal adrenal glands are reported to vary in thickness from 3–7.5 mm, but these values were derived from examination of a relatively small numbers of dogs and do not account for differences in breed or size

(Barthez *et al.*, 1995). The shape and echogenicity of the adrenal glands in dogs and cats with pituitary-dependent hyperadrenocorticism would be expected to be normal, whereas functional adrenal tumours (of whatever histological type) often have an irregular rounded shape with mixed echogenicity.

Lymph nodes: Abdominal ultrasonography should include careful assessment of lymph node size in all patients, but particularly those with hypercalcaemia. Enlargement of multiple lymph nodes should increase suspicion of lymphoma, which may be confirmed by needle aspirate. Lymphoma of the spleen may produce focal to multifocal hypoechoic lesions or diffuse hypoechoic splenomegaly. The medial iliac lymph nodes, which are relatively straightforward to image lying alongside the trifurcation of the terminal aorta, are frequently enlarged in animals with metastatic apocrine gland adenocarcinoma.

Parathyroid glands: Ultrasonography of the parathyroid glands is becoming a very valuable tool in preoperative assessment of patients with hypercalcaemia due to primary hyperparathyoidism, allowing the affected gland(s) to be identified in many instances. This is of particular value when the parathyroid gland that is enlarged has an intrathyroidal location, which may be difficult to identify intra-operatively.

Kidneys and bladder: Ultrasonography of the kidneys and bladder may be useful in the assessment of a patient with PU/PD. The normal and abnormal appearances of these organs is described in detail in Chapter 10. Careful assessment of renal architecture is of particular value in dogs in which the cause of PU/PD has not been identified following history, physical examination and routine blood tests. Two important differentials in these patients are pyelonephritis and non-azotaemic chronic kidney disease. Abnormal ultrasonographic appearance of the kidneys may support further diagnostics be performed to rule out these conditions.

Advanced imaging techniques
Advanced imaging techniques, such as magnetic resonance imaging (MRI), are indicated in the evaluation of patients with CDI, especially those that are middle-aged or older at presentation. Documentation of a pituitary or hypothalamic mass will have significant prognostic and therapeutic implications.

Thyroid function testing
Hyperthyroidism is such a common problem in middle-aged and older cats that, arguably, measurement of total T4 concentration should form part of the minimum database in all cats. Alternative approaches that can be employed if total T4 concentration is within the laboratory reference range but hyperthyroidism is suspected based on historical or physical examination findings are discussed above. A more detailed discussion of thyroid function tests can be found in the *BSAVA Manual of Canine and Feline Endocrinology*. Hyperthyroidism is very uncommon in dogs but should be considered if a mass is palpable in the neck.

Ruling out pyelonephritis
If a urine culture was not performed as part of the initial work-up this should now be performed in an attempt to rule out pyelonephritis as a potential cause for PU/PD. If it was performed, and was negative, there may be an argument for repeating the culture, particularly if antibiotic therapy was only discontinued shortly before the sample was taken. A single negative urine culture does not rule out pyelonephritis. If diagnostic imaging reveals changes consistent with pyelonephritis but urine culture is negative then further measures are necessary; if the renal pelvis is dilated then ultrasound-guided aspiration of urine from the renal pelvis is possible. Alternatively, empirical antibiotic therapy may be appropriate.

Liver function tests
In most instances there will be indications from diagnostic imaging and/or the results of routine biochemical analysis that a patient may have hepatic dysfunction. It is important in this regard to remember that liver enzyme activities (ALT and ALP) may be normal in patients with significant hepatic dysfunction. This is because these enzymes indicate that significant hepatocellular injury is occurring; this may not be the case in patients with very little functional liver tissue remaining (e.g. in cirrhosis) or in patients with portosystemic shunts. The findings on a routine chemistry that are suggestive of hepatic dysfunction or portosystemic shunts are decreased concentrations of glucose, albumin, urea and/or cholesterol. To rule out liver disease as a cause of PU/PD, measurement of pre- and post-prandial bile acids is recommended.

Adrenal function testing
Hyperadrenocorticism is one of the most frequent causes of PU/PD in dogs. Hyperadrenocorticism is much less common in the cat and would only be expected to cause PU/PD when secondary diabetes mellitus develops. Diagnostic tests for hyperadrenocorticism are discussed above. Further details of these are given in the *BSAVA Manual of Canine and Feline Endocrinology*. The results of diagnostic imaging may also lend support to a diagnosis of hyperadrenocorticism. It is important to recognize that none of the commonly employed endocrine tests for hyperadrenocorticism is 100% sensitive (or specific) and if the history, physical examination, results of routine blood work or diagnostic imaging result in an increased suspicion for hyperadrenocorticism then more than one test may need to be performed if the first does not support the diagnosis. This is especially true of the ACTH stimulation test, which has a relatively low sensitivity.

Hypoadrenocorticism should be ruled out in any patient with hyponatraemia and/or hyperkalaemia by performing an ACTH stimulation test.

Measurement of ionized calcium concentration
In most instances significant hypercalcaemia, sufficient to result in PU/PD, will be reflected in the total calcium concentration. However, it is possible to have increases in ionized calcium, the physiologically active and thus significant fraction, while total calcium

concentration remains within the laboratory reference range. Measurement of ionized calcium concentration can be performed using in-house blood gas analysers, which now are available in many larger veterinary hospitals and particularly in emergency practices. It is also possible for samples to be collected for measurement of ionized calcium concentrations at a remote site, such as a reference laboratory, provided that special attention is paid to sample handling. Blood samples must be handled anaerobically because if exposed to air the carbon dioxide concentration will decrease, increasing the pH and decreasing the concentration of ionized calcium in the sample.

Measurement of glomerular filtration rate

Most animals with a primary kidney disease leading to renal insufficiency will present with elevations of blood urea and creatinine. Such animals are likely to be less intensely polydipsic than is typically the case in animals suffering from diabetes insipidus or primary polydipsia, which may have hyposthenuric urine. It is possible for dogs with renal dysfunction to have dilute urine (typically in the minimally concentrated range, 1.012–1.025) and not be azotaemic. This scenario should be suspected particularly in dogs with significant proteinuria or with ultrasonographic changes to the renal architecture. In these cases there is merit in assessing their GFR (as described in Chapter 9) before performing further diagnostic tests. Withholding water from animals with compensated renal insufficiency may precipitate a worsening of the disease, thus if there is any suspicion of renal disease, measurement of GFR is indicated before performing a WDT. Cats with chronic kidney disease do not develop dilute urine until the disease is relatively advanced, thus it would be expected that if renal disease is the cause of PU/PD, the cat would be azotaemic and so measurement of GFR is unlikely to be necessary.

Provocative tests of urine-concentrating ability

The test of urine-concentrating ability that has been employed traditionally in veterinary medicine is the WDT. Recently, an alternative approach – evaluation of the response to orally administered desmopressin – has been advocated as an alternative. The rationale and protocol for performing these tests is outlined below. It cannot be overemphasized that neither of these tests is indicated until almost all causes of PU/PD have already been ruled out (see Figure 2.11).

Water deprivation test

The principle of the modified WDT is that if an animal is deprived of water such that it loses 5% of its body weight, the increase in plasma osmolality that occurs will stimulate maximal ADH secretion and therefore maximal concentration of urine. Administration of exogenous ADH (or a synthetic analogue) to this dehydrated animal should not result in a further increase in the concentration of the urine as the kidney has already been fully stimulated by endogenous ADH. A protocol for a modified WDT is presented in Figure 2.12.

Prior to the test

- Consider gradual water restriction prior to the test (see text for details).
- Fast for 12 hours prior to the period of water deprivation.
- Start water deprivation early in the day since animals undergoing this test must be evaluated frequently.

Phase I – Water deprivation

1. Empty the bladder and measure urine specific gravity and, preferably, osmolality. Placement of an indwelling urinary catheter is recommended to facilitate complete emptying of the urinary bladder.
2. Take a plasma/serum sample to measure creatinine and sodium concentration and preferably osmolality.
3. Weigh the animal accurately.
4. Collect urine samples for measurement of specific gravity (and if possible osmolality) every 1–2 hours, according to the severity of polyuria. Ensure that the urinary bladder is completely emptied at each collection. Weigh the patient following urine collection. Evaluate sodium and creatinine concentrations periodically (every 2–4 hours).
5. Observe the animal for signs of depression/dehydration.
6. Stop this phase if:
   - The animal loses 5% of its body weight
   - Urine specific gravity increases to >1.030
   - Neurological signs develop
   - Hypernatraemia or azotaemia develop.
7. Check urine specific gravity and plasma/serum creatinine and sodium concentrations (and if possible urine and plasma/serum osmolality) at this time.

Phase II – Response to exogenous ADH

1. Administer aqueous vasopressin (2–5 IU total dose) or aqueous desmopressin (1 μg/kg to a maximum of 20 μg) by intravenous injection. Absorption following subcutaneous injection is inconsistent and not recommended during the water deprivation test.
2. Catheterize and empty the bladder every 30 minutes for 2 hours. It is possible that response to desmopressin injection will require longer than 2 hours, but extreme caution is required before continuing water deprivation beyond this time if continued dehydration is developing.
3. Take urine for osmolality and specific gravity every 30 minutes.
4. Take plasma for measurement of osmolality at same time.
5. Check hydration and CNS status regularly.

Phase III – End of test

1. Introduce small amounts of water every 30 minutes for 2 hours.
2. Monitor for vomiting and CNS depression.
3. Return to water *ad libitum* after 2 hours if patient is well.

2.12 Protocol for the modified water deprivation test.

Animals with primary polydipsia are likely to have a low concentration gradient in their renal medullas (*renal medullary washout*) and because of this will not concentrate their urine very efficiently when deprived of water. It has been suggested that to reduce the problem that this creates in the interpretation of the modified WDT, water should be withheld gradually over 3–5 days (to a minimum of 80–100 ml/kg/day given in 6–8 aliquots throughout the day) before depriving the animal of water completely. Caution is required, however, since restriction of water in this manner is likely to induce dehydration in patients with complete CDI and severe obligatory polyuria. Restriction of water in patients that are extremely polydipsic should only be performed in the hospital environment where careful, frequent, assessment of hydration status is possible.

Interpretation of the WDT is only really straightforward in patients with either primary polydipsia or complete CDI. In these patients, measurement of urine SG throughout the WDT is likely to be adequate for its subsequent interpretation. However, particularly in patients with partial CDI, measurement of serum and urine osmolality at frequent intervals throughout the test will be required. This is because interpretation of test results in these animals requires recognition that the osmolality has reached a plateau (changes of <30 mOsm between consecutive measurements), with further water deprivation resulting in no further increase in osmolality. Unfortunately, when using SG to assess urine concentration, 'false' plateaus are known to occur. Commercial laboratories, university hospitals and local human hospitals may be able to provide measurements of osmolality.

Normal: When deprived of water, normal dogs concentrate their urine to a mean peak osmolality of 2290 mOsm/kg (range 1700–2700 mOsm/kg) (urine SG of 1.062; range of 1.050–1.075) and do not respond to exogenous ADH or desmopressin injected once their urine is maximally concentrated (urine osmolality fluctuates by about 10% once a stable osmolality has been reached in response to water deprivation (Hardy and Osborne, 1979)). In the face of medullary washout, the increase in urine osmolality in response to water deprivation is likely to be of lower magnitude but should still exceed 1100 mOsm/kg and an SG of 1.030. If urine concentration increases to an SG between 1.020 and 1.030, the response is equivocal.

Similar figures for the cat are not available but one would normally expect the cat to concentrate its urine even more efficiently than the dog in the face of water deprivation and a urine SG >1.035 on water deprivation (or in a dehydrated cat) would be expected if the renal concentrating capacity is adequate.

Primary polydipsia: Animals with primary polydipsia can concentrate their urine to an osmolality greater than that of plasma (up to a urine SG of 1.030). These animals have a normal response to dehydration in terms of secretion of ADH, thus injection of vasopressin or desmopressin, once they have lost 5% of their body weight, leads to little (typically <10%) change in the urine osmolality.

Central diabetes insipidus: Animals with complete CDI, when deprived of water, will not increase their urine osmolalities above that of plasma (290–310 mOsm/kg), even when they have lost 5% of their body weight. When vasopressin is administered, urine osmolality should increase by between 50 and 800% of the pre-injection value. If the deficiency of ADH secretion is only partial, an increase in urine osmolality above that of plasma may be possible and a further 10–50% increase in urine osmolality may follow

vasopressin administration. Use of urine SG alone makes the result of this test less clear cut. If urine SG remains at or below 1.012 after water deprivation and increases to >1.025 after desmopressin administration, a diagnosis of severe CDI can be made. Increases in urine SG to 1.012–1.020 on water deprivation and further increases to >1.025 following administration of desmopressin would indicate partial CDI.

Nephrogenic diabetes insipidus: Animals with primary NDI are unable to increase urine osmolality above that of plasma even when they have lost 5% of their body weight due to water deprivation (urine SG stays <1.012). Furthermore, following injection of vasopressin or desmopressin, no further rise in urine osmolality or SG occurs. Primary NDI appears to be a very rare congenital abnormality in dogs and so far has not been recorded in the cat. If a result of the modified WDT is obtained which suggests the diagnosis of nephrogenic diabetes in an adult animal, one should consider that the animal has acquired (secondary) NDI and review the routine diagnostic work-up to identify an underlying cause (e.g. hypercalcaemia, hypokalaemia, pyometra, pyelonephritis). To further confuse matters, animals with secondary NDI may often have results of the WDT that are equivocal, with a slight rise in osmolality and SG in response to dehydration and no response or a further slight increase when vasopressin or desmopressin is administered. In some instances results of a WDT in animals with secondary NDI will be difficult to distinguish from those of partial CDI. This is an additional reason why it is essential to rule out all possible causes of secondary NDI before proceeding with a WDT. Reasons for not carrying out a WDT are listed in Figure 2.13.

- Biochemical evidence of azotaemia (absolute contraindication).
- Animal is already dehydrated (although evaluating response to vasopressin/desmopressin administration can be considered, provided no adverse clinical signs are evident).
- Basline plasma osmolality >310–315 mOsm.
- Failure to rule out all possible causes of secondary NDI first. Animals with pyelonephritis, chronic kidney disease, hypoadrenocorticism or hypercalcaemia could decompensate when dehydration is induced during a water deprivation test.
- Inadequate trained staff or facilities to perform labour-intensive, time-consuming test.
- Common things are common. Conditions that can be diagnosed by a water deprivation test (CDI, primary NDI and primary polydipsia) are all rare.

2.13 Reasons for not performing a water deprivation test.

Response to oral desmopressin

The response of animals to treatment with oral desmopressin (0.05–0.2 mg/dog q8h) for 5–7 days has been advocated as an alternative to the WDT. The owner of the dog monitors the patient for any resolution of PU/PD over this period. Evaluation of urine SG from samples collected before and after treatment should also be performed to confirm and quantify the magnitude of any clinical response. Essentially, this is a test for CDI; an animal with CDI will respond to the exogenous ADH (desmopressin) and concentrate its urine SG to >1.025 as a result. Dogs with hyperadrenocorticism may also concentrate their urine during this test, since one mechanism for polyuria in dogs with this condition is inadequate release of ADH in response to osmotic stimuli; thus, when desmopressin is administered the urine will become more concentrated. Animals with primary polydipsia or (primary or secondary) NDI will not respond to desmopressin treatment. Thus, as with the WDT, it is essential that this test only be performed once all possible causes of secondary NDI have been ruled out.

A theoretical complication of this test is that an animal with primary polydipsia could develop water intoxication due to a decrease in urine output following desmopressin administration in the face of continued polydipsia. This complication has, however, not yet been reported. A comparison of the WDT and oral response to desmopressin is given in Figure 2.14.

Water deprivation test
Advantages:
Differentiation of primary polydipsia and primary NDI
Restriction of water intake can be safely implemented following the diagnosis of primary polydipsia with this test
Disadvantages:
Labour-intensive
Hospitalization required
Potentially dangerous
Relatively expensive
Response to oral desmopressin
Advantages:
Easy out-patient procedure
Relatively cheap
Simplifies diagnosis of CDI
Disadvantages:
Potential of water intoxication
Unable to differentiate NDI and primary polydipsia

2.14 Comparison of water deprivation test and response to oral desmopressin.

Case examples

Case 1

Signalment
8-year-old, female entire English Springer Spaniel.

History
Polyuria and polydipsia with nocturia of 3–4 weeks duration. Slight lethargy and inappetence. Last in season 5 weeks prior to presentation and there was a possible misalliance with a GSD. No vulval discharge has been noticed by the owner. Mammary mass removed last year; no histopathological examination.

Physical examination
Bright and excitable, quite obese. Pea-sized mass felt in right caudal mammary gland. Vaginal examination revealed scant amount of creamy white discharge.

Haematology
Unremarkable.

Serum biochemistry
- Mild hypercalcaemia (2.86 mmol/l; reference range 2.1–2.7 mmol/l).
- Hyperalbuminaemia (39.9 g/l; reference range 28–39 g/l).
- Hypercholesterolaemia (9.4 mmol/l; reference range 3.3–8.9 mmol/l).
- Increase in alkaline phosphatase activity (309 IU/l; reference range 19–285 IU/l).

Urinalysis
Urine SG 1.015, pH 8.0; inactive sediment.

Diagnostic imaging
Thoracic radiographs and abdominal ultrasonography unremarkable.

Outcome
The finding of an increase in total calcium could have resulted in a futile search for a paraneoplastic cause. However, the associated increase in albumin concentration suggested that the ionized calcium concentration would be normal, which it was, thus ruling out hypercalcaemia as a cause. The history of PU/PD in an intact bitch should always lead to a suspicion of pyometra. In this instance, abdominal imaging did not substantiate this. Development of diabetes mellitus was ruled out by the observation of normoglycaemia and the absence of glycosuria, but was an important differential diagnosis given that the bitch had developed clinical signs a few weeks after her 'heat'.

There is always a great temptation to perform adrenal function tests in animals presenting for PU/PD. However, it should be remembered that all of the available tests are subject to both false-positive and false-negative results. For this reason these tests are never indicated unless compatible clinical signs are present. This bitch was obese and had PU/PD; signs consistent with hyperadrenocorticism, but she also had a decreased appetite, which is incompatible with the diagnosis (except in cases with an expanding pituitary macroadenoma). The mild increase in alkaline phosphatase activity could be consistent with hyperadrenocorticism but is a relatively non-specific finding.

Pyelonephritis was considered as the cause of this bitch's clinical signs. Although there was nothing on abdominal ultrasound examination to support this diagnosis, abnormalities are not always noted. The urine sediment examination was unremarkable in this case but, again, a localized infection does not always result in an inflammatory urine sediment. The raised urine pH could be incidental (old sample, postprandial collection) but could support the presence of infection. A urine culture yielded a pure growth of *Escherichia coli* >10^6 cfu/ml, sensitive only to enrofloxacin and trimethoprim/sulphonamide.

The dog was treated with enrofloxacin 2.5 mg/kg orally q12h for 6 weeks. The PU/PD resolved within the first week of treatment. Subsequent urine cultures 1 week into treatment and 1 week after discontinuing antibiotic therapy were both negative. She returned to the hospital for ovariohysterectomy and removal of the mammary masses, which were benign.

Case 2

Signalment
7-month-old, male entire English Springer Spaniel.

History
3-week history of acute-onset PU/PD. Reported to have always been somewhat quiet for a puppy. Increase in respiratory rate and effort, which preceded the onset of PU/PD and was not the owner's main concern.

Physical examination
Harsh lung sounds, most notable on inspiration, in all lung fields. Respiration rate 16 breaths/min.

Haematology
Not performed due to financial constraints.

Serum biochemistry
Mild hypercalcaemia (2.73 mmol/l; reference range 2.1–2.7 mmol/l). The accompanying comment from the clinical pathologist was that this degree of hypercalcaemia is not unusual in a dog of this age.

Urinalysis
SG 1.010; otherwise unremarkable.

Thoracic radiography
Patchy alveolar lung pattern in the periphery of the lung fields and a perihilar bronchointerstitial pattern.

Outcome
Angiostrongylus infestation was considered as a possible cause of both PU/PD (due to hypercalcaemia) and the respiratory pathology. This diagnosis was confirmed by measuring ionized calcium (1.66 mmol/l; reference range 1.13–1.33 mmol/l) and performing a faecal Baermann test, which yielded >2000 larvae per gram of faeces. Treatment was initiated with fenbendazole (50 mg/kg q24h for 14 days) and prednisolone (0.5 mg/kg q12h for 5 days, then rapidly tapered). The prednisolone was given to reduce the severity of the hypercalcaemia and in an attempt to prevent an exacerbation of the dog's respiratory signs as the lungworm were killed. He responded very well to this treatment and when rechecked after 2 weeks his PU/PD had resolved, ionized calcium concentrations were normal, and no lungworm larvae were found in the faeces.

References and further reading

Barthez PY, Nyland TG and Feldman EC (1995) Ultrasonographic evaluation of the adrenal glands in dogs. *Journal of the American Veterinary Medical Association* **207**, 1180–1183

Biewenga WJ, Rijnberk A and Mol JA (1991) Osmoregulation of systemic vasopressin release during long-term glucocorticoid excess: a study in dogs with hyperadrenocorticism. *Acta Endocrinologica* **124**, 583–588

Elliott J (1996) Polyuria/polydipsia. In: *Manual of Canine and Feline Nephrology and Urology*, ed. J Bainbridge and J Elliott, pp. 28–41. BSAVA Publications, Cheltenham

Ettinger SJ and Feldman EC (2005) *Textbook of Veterinary Internal Medicine, 6th edn.* Elsevier Saunders, St. Louis

Feldman EC and Nelson RW (2004) *Canine and Feline Endocrinology and Reproduction, 3rd edn.* Elsevier Saunders, St. Louis

Guyton AC and Hall JE (2006) *Textbook of Medical Physiology, 11th edn.* Elsevier Saunders, St. Louis

Hardy RM and Osborne CA (1979) Water deprivation test in the dog: maximal normal values. *Journal of the American Veterinary Medical Association* **174**, 479–483

Hughes D (1992) Polyuria and polydipsia. *Compendium on Continuing Education for the Practicing Veterinarian* **14**, 1161–1175

Mooney CT and Peterson ME (2004) *BSAVA Manual of Endocrinology, 3rd edn.* BSAVA Publications, Gloucester

Neuwirth L, Mahaffey M, Crowell W *et al.* (1993) Comparison of excretory urography and ultrasonography for detection of experimentally induced pyelonephritis in dogs. *American Journal of Veterinary Research* **54**, 660–669

Peterson ME, Melian C and Nichols R (2001) Measurement of serum concentrations of free thyroxine, total thyroxine, and total triiodothyronine in cats with hyperthyroidism and cats with nonthyroidal disease. *Journal of the American Veterinary Medical Association* **218**, 529–536

Reusch CE (2005) Hyperadrenocorticism. In: *Textbook of Veterinary Internal Medicine, 6th edn*, ed. SJ Ettinger and EC Feldman, pp. 1592–1611. Elsevier Saunders, St. Louis

Stone EA, Littman MP, Robertson JL and Bovee KC (1988) Renal dysfunction in dogs with pyometra. *Journal of the American Veterinary Medical Association* **193**, 457–464

3

Incontinence and urine retention

Julie R. Fischer and India F. Lane

Introduction

Normal micturition consists of a *urine storage phase*, when the bladder slowly fills and relaxes while the urethra remains closed, and a *urine voiding phase*, when the bladder contracts and urine is expelled through a relaxed urethra. Appropriate urine storage and voiding depend on the intricate and coordinated interaction of the nervous system, urinary bladder and urethra. Disorders of urine storage usually manifest clinically as *urinary incontinence*, while disorders of urine voiding usually manifest as *urine retention*. Successful treatment of micturition disorders depends foremost on accurate localization and description of the problem, as well as an understanding of the basic associated neurophysiology.

Lower urinary tract anatomy

The key anatomical components of the lower urinary tract include:

- The *detrusor muscle*, the smooth muscle which forms the body and neck of the bladder
- The *internal urethral sphincter* (IUS), comprised of the smooth muscle of the urethrovesicular junction
- The *external urethral sphincter* (EUS), which includes striated muscle encircling portions of the urethra distal to the IUS (position of the EUS varies somewhat by sex and species)

- The *ureterovesicular junction*, normally located proximal to the IUS, at the junction of the bladder body and neck.

The urethral closure mechanism, consisting of the bladder neck and the smooth and striated urethral musculature, is often collectively referred to as the 'outflow tract' or 'outlet' (Figure 3.1).

Neurophysiology of micturition

The urine storage phase of micturition occurs chiefly under sympathetic (adrenergic) nervous control (Figure 3.2). The hypogastric nerve (arising from spinal segments L1–4 in the dog, L2–5 in the cat) stimulates detrusor beta adrenoceptors, inducing smooth muscular relaxation and permitting filling under low pressure. In contrast, sympathetic stimulation of the alpha-1 adrenoceptors of the bladder neck and urethral smooth muscle (the IUS) induces smooth muscle contraction, closing the outlet and maintaining continence. Sympathetic input also modulates and minimizes parasympathetic-mediated contraction of the detrusor muscle. Voluntary input to the striated urethral musculature (the EUS) is supplied via the pudendal nerve (arising from spinal segments S1–3) (Figure 3.3). During the storage phase, this input stimulates nicotinic cholinergic receptors in the EUS, causing contracture and additional closure of the outlet when needed (e.g. during coughing or sneezing reflex closure occurs; voluntarily to over-ride the urge to void when inappropriate).

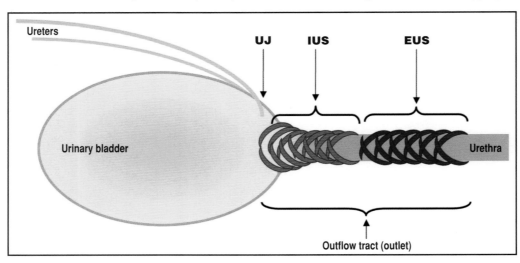

3.1

Basic anatomy of the lower urinary tract. EUS = External urethral sphincter; IUS = Internal urethral sphincter (smooth muscle); UJ = Ureterovesicular junction.

Ureters

UJ   IUS   EUS

Urinary bladder   Urethra

Outflow tract (outlet)

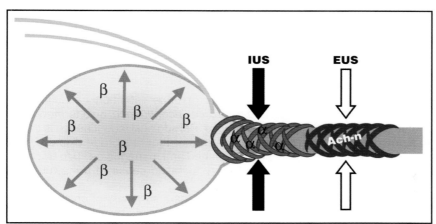

3.2 The urine storage phase of micturition. Sympathetic input to the beta adrenoceptors in the bladder stimulates detrusor relaxation; sympathetic input to the alpha adrenoceptors in the IUS stimulates smooth muscle contraction. Voluntary input to the nicotinic cholinergic receptors (Ach-n) in the EUS stimulates striated muscle contraction. During the storage phase, outlet resistance must exceed intravesicular pressure to maintain continence.

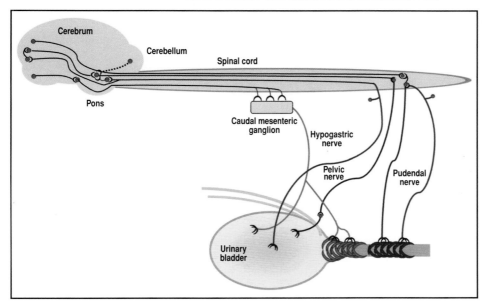

3.3 Schematic representation of central nervous system input to the lower urinary tract. Sympathetic input is supplied to the bladder and proximal urethra via the hypogastric nerve (grey); parasympathetic input is supplied via the afferent pelvic nerve (dark red) and sensation of stretch is relayed to higher centres via the afferent pelvic nerve (dark red). The afferent (dark red) and efferent (blue) branches of the pudendal nerve relay somatic input to and from the external urethral sphincter. Voiding is coordinated in the pontine micturition centre, with input from cerebrocortical centres.

As bladder filling progresses, information from stretch receptors in the detrusor muscle is passed to higher centres via the pelvic (filling sensation, need to void) and hypogastric (pain, overdistension) nerves. The urine voiding phase of micturition occurs chiefly under parasympathetic (cholinergic) control. The pelvic nerve (arising from spinal segments S1–3) stimulates muscarinic cholinergic receptors in the detrusor muscle, stimulating contraction and raising the intravesicular pressure. Simultaneously, sympathetic input to the outlet is inhibited at the level of the micturition centre in the pons, allowing IUS and EUS relaxation. When intravesicular pressure exceeds outlet closure pressure, voiding occurs (Figure 3.4). After complete voiding, the system is 'reset' for the filling stage to begin again.

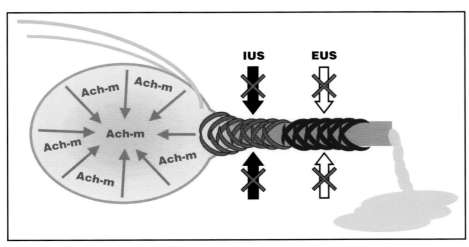

3.4 The urine voiding phase of micturition. Parasympathetic stimulation of muscarinic cholinergic receptors (Ach-m) causes contraction of the detrusor muscle. Parasympathetic inhibition of sympathetic input to the IUS and voluntary inhibition of EUS contraction cause passive relaxation of the outflow tract and cause intravesicular pressure to exceed outlet pressure, permitting urine voiding.

Incontinence

Urinary incontinence is defined as the involuntary leakage of urine through the urethra. Incontinence is most common in bitches, but is also clinically recognized in male dogs and in cats. Most often incontinence is due to failure of the storage phase of micturition, meaning that the urethral closure mechanism is defective, bladder filling is restricted, or an anatomical abnormality bypasses normal structures. In some patients, multiple mechanisms contribute to urinary incontinence.

Causes

Causes of urinary incontinence (Figures 3.5 and 3.6) are traditionally divided into neurogenic and non-neurogenic disorders:

- *Neurogenic* causes usually involve the sacral spinal cord, and cause lower motor neuron signs
- *Non-neurogenic* causes are associated with anatomical or functional disorders of the urinary tract.

Many causes of urine retention can ultimately result in *paradoxical incontinence*, also termed *overflow incontinence*. Paradoxical incontinence is truly a voiding disorder rather than a storage disorder, and must be approached and managed as such by determination of the underlying cause of urine retention (see later).

Figure 3.7 provides a summary of characteristics and useful diagnostics associated with common causes of incontinence.

Neurogenic
Sacral fracture
Pelvic nerve or pelvic plexus trauma
Lumbosacral disease:
Intervertebral disc disease
Lumbosacral stenosis
Neoplasia
Sacral malformation (Manx cats)
Feline leukaemia virus-associated
Generalized peripheral lower motor neuron disease
Dysautonomia

Non-neurogenic
Urethral sphincter mechanism incompetence
Urethral hypoplasia
Lower urinary tract inflammation:
Bacterial cystitis
Sterile cystitis
Urolithiasis
Detrusor instability
Ectopic ureter
Partial outflow obstruction:
Uroliths
Neoplasia
Polyps
Patent urachus
Vestibulovaginal stenosis/septum
Primary detrusor atony with overflow

3.5 Causes of urinary incontinence in small animals.

Adult bitches
Urethral sphincter mechanism incompetence
Detrusor instability (bladder storage dysfunction)
Vaginal pooling
Lower urinary tract inflammation
Neurogenic disorders

Adult male dogs
Prostatic disease
Urethral sphincter mechanism incompetence
Detrusor instability
Neurogenic disorders

Juvenile dogs
Ectopic ureter
Urethral or bladder hypoplasia
Congenital urethral sphincter mechanism incompetence
Vaginal anomalies
Intersex disorder
Patent urachus

Cats
Feline leukaemia virus-associated
Urethral sphincter mechanism incompetence
Overflow
Neurogenic disorders

3.6 Common causes of urinary incontinence by signalment.

Disorder	Characteristics	Diagnostic methods
Acquired urethral sphincter mechanism incompetence (reproductive hormone-responsive or 'spay' incontinence)	Medium to large-breed adult dogs, usually female Prior ovariohysterectomy Intermittent urine leakage Resting urinary incontinence Otherwise normal	Response to treatment Urethral pressure profile
Urinary bladder storage dysfunction (detrusor instability, urge incontinence, overactive bladder)	Intermittent urine leakage Pollakiuria May appear behavioural or voluntary May be associated with excitement or activity	Response to treatment Cystometrography Cystourethrography
Ectopic ureter	Affected since birth Often continuous urine leakage	Contrast radiography/computed tomography Urethrocystoscopy Vaginourethrography Surgical exploration

3.7 Characteristics of common disorders causing urinary incontinence. (continues) ▶

Disorder	Characteristics	Diagnostic methods
Congenital urethral incompetence or hypoplasia	Severe or continuous urine leakage Juvenile animal Wide or short urethra in some cases Ectopic ureter not demonstrated	Cystourethrography Urethral pressure profile
Vaginal abnormality or urine pooling	Urine leakage at rest or when rising Urine leakage following voiding Recurrent or persistent vaginitis Vestibulovaginal stenosis/septum on digital examination	Vaginal examination and vaginoscopy Vaginourethrography
Prostatic disease (male dogs)	Intact or neutered Other signs of prostatic disease or concurrent dysuria Hindlimb weakness/stiff, stilted gait	Abdominal radiography Ultrasonography Contrast urethrography Prostatic brushing, aspirate or biopsy
FeLV-associated urinary incontinence	Intermittent urine leakage Anisocoria	FeLV test

3.7 (continued) Characteristics of common disorders causing urinary incontinence.

Neurogenic causes

In dogs with neurogenic incontinence, it is rarely the sole neurological abnormality on physical examination. For these dogs, treatment of the incontinence and prognosis for resolution or clinical control depend primarily on diagnosis and management of the underlying cause (e.g. surgical management of intervertebral disc herniation, fixation of sacral fracture).

Non-neurogenic causes

Urethral sphincter mechanism incompetence: USMI is the most common non-neurogenic cause of incontinence in dogs. This type of urethral dysfunction occurs most often in neutered, medium to large-breed adults, but can also be seen congenitally. Several structural and physiological factors may play a role in the development and degree of USMI in a given patient (Lane and Fischer, 2003):

- Ageing and/or relative oestrogen lack may affect the collagenous support structures of the urogenital region, decreasing intrinsic tone
- Abnormal positioning or morphology of the bladder or urethra can contribute to functional failure
- Urethral alpha-adrenergic receptors can decrease in availability and/or responsiveness

- Obesity and/or vaginal structural abnormalities can be contributory
- Breed predispositions suggest underlying genetic factors
- Other hormonal alterations or interactions may play a role in this multifactorial disorder.

In an otherwise healthy, neurologically normal dog with concentrated urine and without lower urinary tract inflammation, a diagnosis of USMI can be confirmed by positive response to pharmacotherapy aimed at increasing outlet resistance. Both castrated and sexually intact male dogs can acquire USMI, though this is uncommon. Incontinence due to acquired USMI is usually intermittent and is most frequent in recumbency, particularly during sleep. Sympathomimetic agents (e.g. phenylpropanolamine, ephedrine), which target alpha adrenoceptors (commonly termed alpha-agonists), and oestrogen compounds (e.g. diethylstilbestrol, estriol, conjugated oestrogens) are the drugs most often used to control USMI. The significant majority (75–90%) of mature bitches with USMI will respond very well to one or a combination of these therapies (Forrester, 2005). Since these agents are synergistic, combining their use may produce good clinical effect in a patient that does not respond to either agent alone. Clinical characteristics of sympathomimetic agents and reproductive hormones are compared in Figure 3.8.

Parameter	Sympathomimetic agents	Oestrogens
Effectiveness	75–90% excellent results	40–65% excellent results
Indications	Males or females, dogs or cats Poor response to oestrogen	Bitches Combination with alpha-agonists Recurrent UTI or vaginitis?
Administration frequency	q8–24h	q2–14d
Residual effects	Short	Possibly prolonged
Adverse effects	Hyperactivity, hypertension, anxiety, tachycardia, anorexia, weight loss	Behavioural change, bone marrow toxicity (rare), oestrus, exacerbation of immune-mediated disease?

3.8 Comparison of sympathomimetic agents and reproductive hormones in the management of urinary incontinence.

Contraindications for sympathomimetic therapy include hypertension, some cardiac diseases and anxiety disorders. Oestrogens are generally contraindicated for male dogs and intact bitches, and for cats; sympathomimetic agents are the drugs of choice for these patients. Oestrogens are also contraindicated in pregnant bitches. Male dogs may be treated with injectable testosterone, either alone or in combination with an sympathomimetic. Testosterone therapy is contraindicated in dogs that have been castrated for behavioural issues or for testosterone-mediated diseases (e.g. non-neoplastic prostatic disease, perineal hernia). Response rate in males is lower than that of females; medical control of USMI in male dogs is effective in <50% of dogs treated.

Therapy with depot formulations of gonadotropin-releasing hormone (GnRH) analogues has shown promise in management of USMI refractory to sympathomimetics and oestrogen compounds. The GnRH analogues cause down-regulation of the production and secretion of follicle-stimulating hormone and luteinizing hormone, and may contribute to restoration of continence by several mechanisms. In a recent study (Reichler *et al.*, 2003), therapy with depot GnRH analogues or depot GnRH analogues plus phenylpropanolamine restored continence within 5–10 days to 12 of 13 dogs with either USMI refractory to sympathomimetics and oestrogen compounds, or an inability to take sympathomimetics.

Endoscopic submucosal injection of biocompatible substances (initially Teflon paste, now collagen or extracellular matrix) into the proximal canine urethra is a promising emerging therapy for USMI. These bulking agents protrude into the urethral lumen and improve outflow resistance. Recent reviews of this technique (Barch *et al.*, 2005; Wood *et al.*, 2005) show good long-term results in dogs that were refractory to, or had intolerable side effects from, conventional medical therapies.

Several surgical procedures have been used for management of refractory USMI, including colposuspension, cystourethropexy and creation of a seromuscular urethral sling. These procedures have relatively high success rates (approximately 50–55% continent and 25–35% clinically improved) immediately following surgery, but continence rate drops significantly over time, and postoperative complications include urine retention severe enough to require reoperation. The reader is referred to the Further reading list for further information regarding surgical management of USMI.

Detrusor instability: Detrusor instability (*urge incontinence*) represents a failure of the bladder to remain relaxed during the urine storage phase. Instability and incontinence associated with involuntary, uninhibited detrusor contraction is now termed *overactive bladder* in human patients. This disorder is less common than USMI and is characterized by intermittent incontinence that may be associated with activity or excitement. This type of incontinence may be difficult to discriminate from pollakiuria, or even inappropriate urination, since dogs will often posture to urinate when stimulated by detrusor contraction. Detrusor instability is rare in small animals, but can occur alone or in combination with USMI in male or female dogs. Bladder storage dysfunction is treated with antimuscarinic (anticholinergic) agents (e.g. imipramine, oxybutynin, dicyclomine) that help to increase bladder capacity and decrease spasticity (Lane, 2000; Lane and Fischer, 2003).

Ectopic ureter: Ureteral termination that bypasses the bladder trigone is termed *ectopic*. Incontinence occurs when the ureter tunnels to a point distal to, or empties distal to, the trigone, allowing urine to flow into the proximal urethra or the vagina instead of the bladder. Dogs with ectopic ureters usually demonstrate continuous urine leakage that has occurred since birth, and often have failed to respond to medications prescribed for either USMI or urinary tract infection (UTI). Surgical correction of the ectopic ureter(s), either by nephrectomy and ureterectomy (if unilateral and the associated kidney is severely hydronephrotic) or by ureteral reimplantation into the bladder (if bilateral or the associated kidney is salvageable), is required for clinical improvement of the incontinence (see *BSAVA Manual of Canine and Feline Abdominal Surgery*).

Ureteral ectopia may be unilateral or bilateral, and other anatomical or functional abnormalities are commonly observed concurrently (e.g. reduced bladder capacity, USMI). Thorough evaluation of the urinary tract, including urodynamic assessment prior to surgery when available, is recommended to refine the prognosis and predict the need for additional medical management (Cannizzo *et al.*, 2003; Samii *et al.*, 2004). A significant percentage of animals with surgically corrected ectopic ureters will require postoperative pharmacological treatment to maintain continence. Ectopic ureters occur most often in bitches, but are also diagnosed occasionally in male dogs and in cats.

Prostatic disease: Incontinence in male dogs is frequently associated with prostatic disease. Incontinent males should be closely screened for bacterial prostatitis, prostatic neoplasia and other prostatic disease, via rectal palpation, urine/prostatic fluid analysis and ultrasonography (see Chapter 20).

Cats
Urinary incontinence is a rare clinical problem in cats. Causes include congenital anatomical anomalies, neurological injury or malformation, viral disease and urethral incompetence. Juvenile cats should be screened for ectopic ureters and vaginoureteral abnormalities. Adults should be tested for feline leukaemia virus (FeLV), once lower urinary tract inflammation and polyuria are excluded. Sympathomimetic agents are occasionally effective in adult cats with non-neurogenic urethral incompetence. Both urinary and faecal incontinence can occur in the Manx breed due to congenital malformation of the sacrum.

Diagnostic approach

History and physical examination

History-taking and physical examination (including observed voiding) provide the basis for diagnosis of the cause of incontinence in many small animal patients; signalment alone will narrow down the differential list (see Figure 3.6). The physical examination for incontinence should include a rectal examination and careful bladder palpation before and after voiding. Problem-specific historical questions and physical examination guidelines are listed in Figure 3.9.

History (incontinence)

When does leakage occur?
- Nocturnally/when resting or recumbent?
- Continuously?
- With excitation?
- Upon rising?

How old was the patient when the problem began?
- Was it related to neutering surgery?

Is the leakage worsening, constant or improving?
Is the pet able to void normally?
Is the pet conscious of the dribbling?
Is the problem worse with a full bladder?
Is urine volume increased in general?
Are lower urinary tract signs present (pollakiuria, stranguria, haematuria)?
Are there any systemic signs of illness?
What is the estimated daily water consumption?
Is there any history of prior urinary tract problems?
Has there been any recent abdominal, pelvic or urogenital surgery or trauma?

History (urine retention)

How old was the patient when the problem began?
- Was it related to neutering surgery?

Have there been any previous medical problems?
What is the estimated daily water consumption?
Is there any history of prior urogenital disorders (e.g. urinary tract infections, urolithiasis, urethral obstructions)?
Are there any systemic signs of illness?
Has there been any previous back surgery or trauma?
Has there been any recent abdominal, pelvic or urogenital surgery or trauma?
How frequent are voiding attempts?
Is any urine passed during voiding attempts?

Physical examination

Is the bladder large or small?
Is it firm or soft?
Are the urethra and prostate/vagina normal on palpation?
Is perineal/preputial urine staining/scald present?
Is the neurological examination normal?
- Mentation and cranial nerves
- Conscious proprioception, spinal reflexes, tail and anal tone, perineal reflexes, bulbourethral/vulvar reflex
- Pupillary light reflexes

Is the bladder expressible?

Observed voiding

Can the patient initiate and maintain a normal urine stream?
What is the residual urine volume following voiding attempts?

3.9 Problem-specific historical questions and physical examination guidelines for patients with urinary incontinence or urine retention.

Laboratory tests

The minimum database for incontinent animals should include urinalysis, with urine culture if indicated by the presence of pyuria, bacteriuria or lack of concentration. Polyuria may precipitate or exacerbate incontinence by overwhelming bladder capacity; poorly concentrated urine (specific gravity (SG) <1.025 in dogs, <1.035 in cats) should be confirmed and investigated, if persistent. If the animal exhibits any signs of systemic illness, a complete blood count and serum biochemistry evaluation should also be performed.

Diagnostic imaging

Most dogs presented for incontinence do not require imaging as part of the diagnostic approach. Imaging is, however, recommended for:

- Incontinent juvenile dogs or cats (<1 year of age)
- Incontinent male dogs
- Dogs or cats whose incontinence closely follows a surgical procedure
- Dogs or cats with continuous urine leakage
- Dogs or cats with urine leakage from an anatomically abnormal site
- Dogs or cats with concomitant recurrent UTI, recurrent vaginitis, haematuria, crystalluria or azotaemia
- Dogs or cats for whom surgical correction of incontinence is considered.

The choice of imaging modality depends on the signalment and clinical signs (see Chapter 10). Survey radiography will detect radiopaque uroliths and gross malformations of the urinary bladder, vertebrae or pelvis. Excretory urography (including radiography (Figure 3.10) and computed tomography), vaginourethrography (Figure 3.11) and/or urethrocystoscopy are helpful in identifying anatomical abnormalities of the ureters and urethra, such as ectopic ureter. Ultrasonography of the prostate is recommended for any incontinent male dog; ultrasonography can also help rule out a trigonal mass interfering with normal outlet closure. Digital vaginal examination, vaginoscopy (Figure 3.12) and/or a

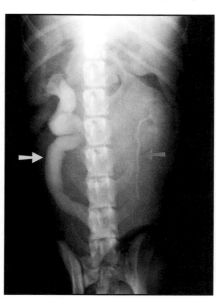

3.10

Excretory urogram. The yellow arrow indicates the massively dilated right ectopic ureter, while the red arrow indicates the relatively normal left ureter of this incontinent young dog. (Courtesy of UC Davis Veterinary Medical Teaching Hospital.)

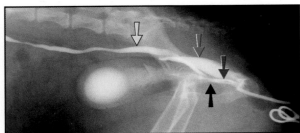

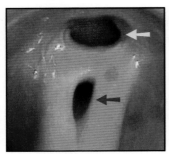

3.11 Retrograde vaginourethrocystogram. A Foley catheter was inflated just inside the vaginal opening, and contrast material injected to fill the vaginal vault. The contrast medium enters the urethral orifice and then the ectopic ureteral orifice, delineating well both the abnormally caudal entry site of the ureter and its pathologically dilated state. An additional finding of this study is the caudal placement and 'gourd-like' shape of this classic pelvic bladder. This young bitch had multiple anatomical abnormalities that contributed to her incontinence. The yellow arrow indicates the dilated ectopic ureter. The red arrow indicates the vagina. The blue arrrow indicates the urethra. The black arrow indicates the ectopic ureteral interface with the urethra. (Courtesy of UC Davis Veterinary Medical Teaching Hospital.)

3.12 Vaginoscopy. The yellow arrow indicates the ectopic ureteral opening in this continuously incontinent juvenile bitch. The blue arrow indicates the normal urethral orifice within the vestibule. (Courtesy of UC Davis Veterinary Medical Teaching Hospital.)

contrast vaginogram will help to evaluate the presence, position and severity of vestibulovaginal stenosis, or the presence of vaginal urine pooling. The reader is referred to the Further reading list for further discussion of the advantages and disadvantages of imaging methods in lower urinary tract disorders.

Specialized urodynamic studies
Urodynamic studies may be indicated and can be helpful in some patients.

Urethral pressure profilometry: UPP measures pressure along the length of the outflow tract and urethra (Figure 3.13). In some complicated incontinence or urine retention cases, UPP may be useful for:

- Evaluation of suspected USMI refractory to traditional medical therapies
- Evaluation of urethral function in patients with anatomical abnormalities (e.g. ectopic ureter)
- Perioperative evaluation of surgical treatment of USMI (e.g. urethral bulking, colposuspension)
- Confirmation/localization of urethral spasm.

Cystometrography: CMG measures the pressure within the bladder as it is filled with fluid or gas (Figure 3.14). Bladder capacity and compliance may be estimated from calculations of infused volume and the pressure slope during filling. Bladder overactivity is diagnosed if early or repeated detrusor contractions are observed in response to filling. Underactivity (or atony) of the bladder is more difficult to assess, as many dogs will inhibit bladder contractions during the study. An atonic bladder, however, would be expected to have an expanded capacity and fill to large volumes

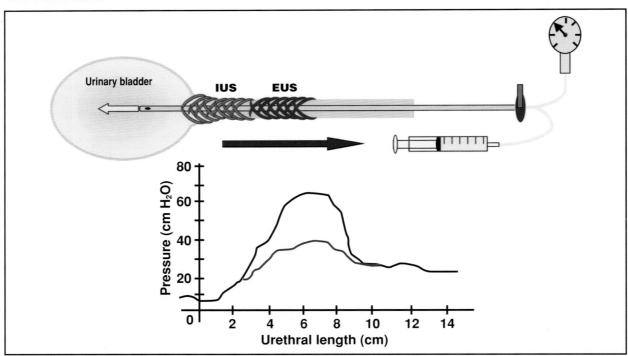

3.13 Schematic urethral pressure profiles. It is preferable for the patient to be conscious. A flexible urethral catheter with a side hole is inserted through the urethra into the bladder and is connected to a pressure transducer via a saline column. Saline is infused into the catheter via a syringe pump as the catheter is withdrawn from the urethra at a constant rate. The transducer continuously measures the pressure exerted on the saline column along the urethral length during withdrawal. The black trace represents a normal profile. The blue trace represents the profile of a dog with USMI.

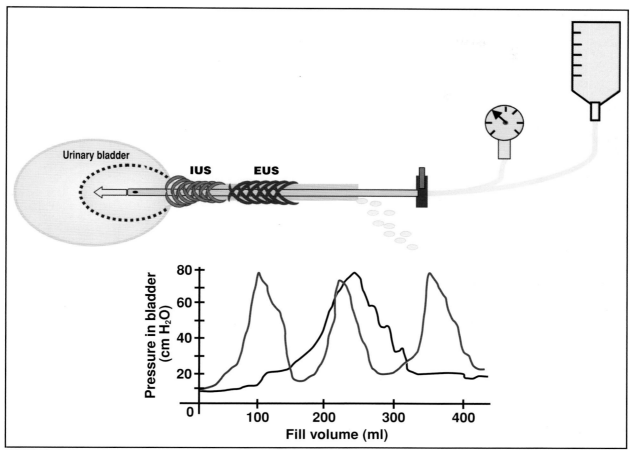

3.14 Schematic cystometrograms. A flexible urethral catheter is inserted into the bladder of a sedated patient and connected as before to a pressure transducer. As the bladder is slowly filled with saline, the transducer measures the intravesicular pressure and the point of spontaneous detrusor contraction with consequent bladder emptying. The black trace represents normal bladder filling under relatively low pressure until detrusor contraction is stimulated (at about 200 ml fill volume here). The blue trace represents filling of an abnormally reactive or non-compliant bladder. Pressures rise quickly and precipitously, and detrusor contraction is repeatedly stimulated at only 50–75 ml fill volume.

at low pressure. In complicated incontinence or urine retention cases, CMG may be useful for:

- Evaluation of suspected USMI refractory to traditional medical therapies
- Diagnosis of suspected bladder overactivity
- Evaluation of bladder contractile function in neurogenic disorders
- Evaluation of incomplete voiding and bladder contractile function in suspected detrusor atony.

Relapsing or refractory incontinence

In many incontinent animals, particularly those with uncomplicated early USMI, incontinence is easily controlled with pharmacological treatment (Figure 3.15). Other dogs respond initially and later relapse, whereas a small percentage fail to achieve satisfactory remission of clinical signs. Suggested reasons, as well as additional diagnostic and therapeutic options, for relapsing or refractory incontinence are presented in Figure 3.16.

Agent	Classification	Recommended dosage	Possible adverse effects	Contraindications	Comments
Diethylstilbestrol[a] (DES); stilbestrol[a]	Reproductive hormone	Bitch: 0.1–1.0 mg/dog orally q24h for 5–7 days, then weekly or as needed	Oestrus, behavioural change, myelosuppression, pyometra in intact female	Males Cats Pregnancy	
Stilbestrol[a] (alternative regimen)	Reproductive hormone	Bitch: 0.04–0.06 mg/dog orally q24h for 7 days, reduced weekly to 0.01–0.02 mg/dog/day	Oestrus, behavioural change, myelosuppression, pyometra in intact female	Males Cats Pregnancy	

3.15 Formulary of agents useful in the management of urinary incontinence. Note that oestrogens (marked [a]) are not recommended in male dogs nor in cats. [b] Doses for the GnRH analogues are from Reichler *et al.* (2003) and were extrapolated from the human doses designed to maintain continence for 6 (deslorelin), 3 (leuprolide) or 2 (busrelin) months. Duration of effect of the depot preparations varied in that report from 1.5 months to 5 years; most of the dogs were treated with deslorelin. (continues) ▶

Agent	Classification	Recommended dosage	Possible adverse effects	Contraindications	Comments
Premarin[a]	Conjugated oestrogen	Bitch: 0.02 mg/kg orally q24h for 5–7 days, then q2–4d or as needed	Oestrus, behavioural change, myelosuppression, pyometra in intact female	Males Cats Pregnancy	
Estriol[a]	Reproductive hormone	Bitch: 0.5–1.0 mg/dog orally q24h for 5–7 days, then q2–3d as needed	Oestrus, behavioural change, myelosuppression, pyometra in intact female	Males Cats Pregnancy	
Estriol[a] (alternative regimen)	Reproductive hormone	Bitch: 2.0 mg/dog orally q24h for 7 days, then reduce daily dose by 0.5 mg each week to establish minimal effective daily dose; then try q48h administration	Oestrus, behavioural change, myelosuppression, pyometra in intact female	Males Cats Pregnancy	
Testosterone cypionate	Reproductive hormone	Dogs: 2.2 mg/kg i.m. every 4–8 weeks	Behavioural change, perianal adenoma, perineal hernias, prostatic disorders, aggression	Cardiac, renal or hepatic disease	
Testosterone propionate	Reproductive hormone	Dogs: 2.2 mg/kg i.m. q2–3d	Behavioural change, perianal adenoma, perineal hernias, prostatic disorders, aggression	Cardiac, renal or hepatic disease	
Phenylpropanolamine (PPA)	Sympathomimetic	Dogs: 1.5 mg/kg orally q8–12h, or 12.5–75 mg orally q8–12h	Anxiety, aggression, anorexia, hypertension, tachycardia	Some cardiac disease Hypertension ± anxiety disorders	
Ephedrine	Sympathomimetic	Dogs: 1.2 mg/kg orally q8h	Anxiety, aggression, anorexia, hypertension, tachycardia	Some cardiac disease Hypertension ± anxiety disorders	
Pseudoephedrine	Sympathomimetic	Dogs: 0.2–0.4 mg/kg (practically, 15–60 mg total dose per dog) orally q8–12h	Anxiety, aggression, anorexia, hypertension, tachycardia	Some cardiac disease Hypertension ± anxiety disorders	
Imipramine	Antimuscarinic, neuronal uptake blocker	Dogs: 5–15 mg orally q12h	Sedation, dry mouth, urinary retention, gastrointestinal upset	Seizure disorders Use of other anticholinergic or CNS depressants Glaucoma Gastrointestinal obstruction Renal or hepatic disease Cardiac arrhythmias	
Oxybutynin	Antimuscarinic	Cats and small dogs: 0.5–1.25 mg total dose Larger dogs: 2.5–3.75 mg total dose	Sedation, dry mouth, urinary retention, gastrointestinal upset	Glaucoma Gastrointestinal obstruction Renal or hepatic disease Cardiac arrhythmias Hypertension	
Dicyclomine	Antimuscarinic	Dogs: 5–10 mg/dog orally q8h	Sedation, dry mouth, urinary retention, gastrointestinal upset	Glaucoma Gastrointestinal obstruction Renal or hepatic disease Cardiac arrhythmias Hypertension	
Depot leuprolide[b]	GnRH analogue	Dogs: 11.25 mg/dog			May be re-dosed as needed May be used in combination with sympathomimetics
Depot deslorelin[b]	GnRH analogue	Dogs: 5–10 mg/dog			May be re-dosed as needed May be used in combination with sympathomimetics
Depot buserelin[b]	GnRH analogue	Dogs: 6.3 mg/dog			May be re-dosed as needed May be used in combination with sympathomimetics

3.15 (continued) Formulary of agents useful in the management of urinary incontinence. Note that oestrogens (marked [a]) are not recommended in male dogs nor in cats. [b] Doses for the GnRH analogues are from Reichler *et al.* (2003) and were extrapolated from the human doses designed to maintain continence for 6 (deslorelin), 3 (leuprolide) or 2 (busrelin) months. Duration of effect of the depot preparations varied in that report from 1.5 months to 5 years; most of the dogs were treated with deslorelin.

Cause or complicating factor	Possible solution(s)
Inadequate dosage or frequency of medication	Increase dosage within recommended range Increase frequency of sympathomimetic (up to q8h) or oestrogen (up to q48h) as tolerated
Inappropriate medication	Consider change from oestrogen to sympathomimetic administration Consider addition of oestrogen to sympathomimetic administration
Poor owner compliance	Consider switch to long-acting sympathomimetic or to oestrogens to improve compliance
Underlying urinary tract infection	Monitor for infection and treat appropriately
Underlying polyuria	Evaluate for common, treatable polyuric disorders (e.g. hyperadrenocorticism, diabetes mellitus)
Mixed disorder of micturition	Consider addition of or trial treatment with anticholinergic agent
Underlying anatomical abnormality	Investigate anatomy with contrast radiography Consider surgical management of ectopic ureter, pelvic bladder or vaginal/vulvar abnormality
Underlying neurological lesion	Investigate for subtle lumbosacral disorder with neurological examination and imaging studies
Behavioural component or senility	Consider treatments for behavioural disorders or cognitive dysfunction
Refractory urethral incompetence	Consider combinations of medications or surgical treatment to enhance medical management Consider trial of GnRH analogue or duloxetine Consider urethral bulking agents

3.16 Potential causes and possible solutions for refractory or relapsing urinary incontinence.

Urine retention

Urine retention usually represents a failure of the urine voiding phase of micturition (*voiding dysfunction*). For normal and complete voiding to occur, intravesicular pressure must rise quickly and exceed outlet pressure until the bladder is empty. In contrast to patients presented for incontinence, the clinical signs associated with voiding disorders usually include stranguria or dysuria; the patient with urine retention may make frequent attempts to void with little or no success. Stringent efforts should be made to determine the aetiology of urine retention, since early correction of the underlying cause greatly improves prognosis for recovery of normal voiding function. Management strategies may include temporary urinary catheterization to facilitate bladder emptying and surgical procedures to correct or bypass obstruction. Pharmacological manipulation of detrusor function and/or outlet resistance is often used along with other procedures, or as sole therapy for functional disorders (Lane and Fischer, 2003; Labato, 2005).

Causes

Urine retention is caused by failure of detrusor contraction or by inappropriately high outlet resistance during voiding, or both (Figure 3.17). Detrusor atony may be primary or may be secondary to chronically increased outlet resistance. Increased outlet resistance may be neurogenic in origin or due to obstruction (either anatomical or functional). As with incontinence, causes of urine retention can be divided into neurogenic and non-neurogenic categories.

Disorder	Characteristics	Diagnostics
Neurogenic causes		
Lesions of sacral spinal cord (lower motor neuron)	Distended, flaccid urinary bladder Bladder easily expressed Depressed genitoanal reflexes Lumbosacral pain Possible overflow incontinence	Neurological examination Myelography, epidurography or CT/MRI
Lesions of suprasacral spinal cord (upper motor neuron)	Distended, firm urinary bladder Bladder not easily expressed Incomplete voiding possible Gait and proprioceptive deficits	Neurological examination Myelography, epidurography or CT/MRI
Detrusor–urethral dyssynergia	Distended, firm urinary bladder Bladder not easily expressed Incomplete voiding possible; stream may be initiated but cannot be maintained Patient is otherwise normal	Observation, measurement of residual urine volume Urethral pressure profilometry ± cystometrography Response to alpha-antagonists
Primary detrusor atony	Distended bladder Weak or absent urine stream Caused by dysautonomia, damage to hypogastric nerve	Observation, measurement of residual urine volume Response to treatment Cystometrography

3.17 Characteristics of common disorders causing urine retention. (continues) ▶

Disorder	Characteristics	Diagnostics
Non-neurogenic causes		
Anatomical urethral obstruction	Difficult urethral catheterization Dysuria and stranguria ± haematuria Caused by uroliths, neoplasia, blood clots, urethral plugs (cats)	Urethral catheterization Radiography/contrast cystourethrography Ultrasonography
Functional urinary obstruction	Distended bladder, difficult to express Easy urethral catheterization Voiding may be initiated, then interrupted Usually male dogs and cats Idiopathic or caused by urethral irritation or previous obstruction Rarely and transiently occurs following abdominal, pelvic or pelvic limb surgery	Exclusion of anatomical or neurogenic causes Response to treatment with alpha-antagonists Urethral pressure profile
Primary detrusor atony	Distended bladder Weak or absent urine stream Caused by overdistension from any cause of obstruction, muscle weakness, drugs	Observation, measurement of residual urine volume Response to treatment Cystometrography
Medications (e.g. opioids, anticholinergics/antispasmodics, tricyclic antidepressants, calcium channel blockers)	Easy urethral catheterization Variable presentation otherwise	Medication history Exclusion of anatomical or functional obstruction Response to withdrawal of medication

3.17 (continued) Characteristics of common disorders causing urine retention.

Neurogenic causes

Lower motor neuron disorders: Disruption of sacral spinal cord segments, or of the pelvic nerve or pelvic plexus, results in detrusor atony and sphincter areflexia. Clinically, patients with lower motor neuron (LMN) disorders usually exhibit loss of perineal reflexes, and have distended bladders that are easily expressed. Overflow incontinence may be seen when the bladder is full. Causes of LMN disorders include cauda equina syndrome, sacroiliac luxation, intervertebral disc disease, sacrococcygeal separation or fracture ('tail-pull' injury) and neoplasia.

Treatment for complete neurogenic detrusor atony and sphincter areflexia is generally unsuccessful unless the underlying cause is correctable. Parasympathomimetic agents, such as bethanechol, may be administered to help increase strength of detrusor contraction if partial function is present, but are ineffective if pelvic nerve function is absent. Patients can be managed at home with scrupulous bladder and nursing care, including manual bladder expression 3–4 times daily and cleaning to prevent urine scald. Patients should be monitored routinely for UTI and treated when infection is documented.

Upper motor neuron disorders: Upper motor neuron (UMN) lesions result from disruption of the spinal cord between the sacral segments and the pontine micturition centre, and cause reflex detrusor contraction with concurrent uninhibited sphincter spasticity. Patients with UMN disorders often have overt paresis or paralysis of the hindlimbs and usually cannot urinate voluntarily. On physical examination, the bladder is large, turgid and usually very difficult or impossible to express early in the course of disease. Aggressive attempts to express the bladder manually should be avoided at this point, due to the risk of bladder rupture. Intermittent aseptic urinary catheterization several times daily is preferred to reduce risk of bladder trauma and ensure complete emptying.

After days to weeks, local spinal reflexes may resume and allow for some voiding activity. Involuntary bladder emptying is typically initiated when threshold capacity is reached. This phenomenon is termed an *automatic* or *reflex bladder*. When automatic bladder activity occurs, management with manual expression may be possible, since stimulation of detrusor contraction now should result in sphincter relaxation and partial to complete emptying. Urethral smooth muscle relaxants, such as alpha-antagonists (e.g. phenoxybenzamine, prazosin) and skeletal muscle relaxants (e.g. baclofen, diazepam, dantrolene), may facilitate complete bladder emptying by relaxing the internal and external urethral sphincters, respectively. As with LMN disorders, patients should be monitored routinely for UTI and treated when infection is documented.

Detrusor–urethral dyssynergia: A dyssynergic state results when initiation of detrusor contraction stimulates simultaneous contraction of the urethral musculature (either the internal or external sphincter), resulting in the bladder contracting against markedly increased outlet pressure. The condition may be caused by a partial lesion of the reticulospinal tract, a lesion cranial to the caudal mesenteric ganglion or idiopathic (non-neurogenic) causes. This is most often a disorder of male dogs and may be exacerbated by excitation and sympathetic nervous system stimulation. Dogs can often initiate a urine stream that is quickly attenuated. Severe cases may present with any degree of detrusor atony; such cases should be initially managed with indwelling catheterization to permit restoration of bladder function.

Documentation of dyssynergia in clinical practice is difficult, since it requires simultaneous assessment of detrusor and sphincter muscle activity during voiding. Practically, however, the diagnosis can be made after careful physical examination, observation and exclusion of obstructive causes. Results of UPP studies may include markedly increased outlet pressure.

Management of detrusor–urethral dyssynergia involves decreasing internal and/or external urethral sphincter resistance (see UMN disorders). Parasympathomimetic agents are not chronically indicated; therapy should focus on decreasing outlet resistance and decreasing sympathetic stimulus. In difficult cases, periodic or daily aseptic home catheterization may be required in addition to medication to ensure bladder emptying. Residual urine volume should be quantified periodically to assess success of therapy. Patients should be monitored routinely for UTI, and treated when infection is documented.

Dysautonomia: Dysautonomia is a rare and often generalized dysfunction of the autonomic nervous system. It is chiefly reported in cats in Great Britain and dogs in the midwestern United States, but has been recognized in dogs and cats worldwide. Overflow incontinence due to bladder atony and sphincter areflexia may be the chief presenting clinical sign, but other signs of autonomic dysfunction (e.g. dilated nonresponsive pupils; xerostomia; nictitans prolapse; absent anal sphincter tone) are frequently apparent on clinical examination. Diagnosis is strongly suggested by physical examination and may be further supported with specific clinical testing. Management is generally unrewarding if the gastrointestinal tract is affected (e.g. ileus, megaoesophagus), but may be possible with parasympathomimetic agents and bladder expression or catheterization if signs are largely confined to the urinary tract.

Non-neurogenic causes

Anatomical outflow obstruction: Any intraluminal or extraluminal partial or complete obstruction of the outflow tract can cause voiding dysfunction. The most common causes of anatomical obstruction include urolithiasis, trigonal, prostatic or urethral neoplasia, severe urethritis or stricture and mucoid or crystalline urethral plugs (in cats). Treatment and prognosis depend on the underlying cause.

Functional outflow obstruction: This is usually the result of increased sympathetic stimulation of urethral musculature and may sometimes have a neurogenic component. The increased sympathetic input increases sphincter tone and inappropriately raises outlet pressure, restricting or precluding urine flow during voiding attempts. Functional obstruction due to urethral spasm is a common occurrence in cats following relief of anatomical urethral obstruction.

Management of functional obstruction includes treatment or prevention of bladder atony from overdistension, with indwelling catheterization if necessary, while decreasing internal and/or external urethral sphincter resistance (see UMN disorders). Anxiolytic therapy may be helpful to decrease stress and consequently sympathetic input to the lower urinary tract. Prognosis is variable, but may be good for situations involving acute urethral irritation (e.g. cats with urethral spasm following obstruction).

Detrusor atony from overdistension: Any cause of persistent outlet obstruction can lead to detrusor atony from bladder overdistension. Excessive stretch separates the tight junctions in the detrusor muscle, resulting in weak, uncoordinated or absent contraction. Animals with detrusor atony from overdistension may be presented for stranguria, anuria or overflow (paradoxical) incontinence, and have large, flaccid bladders on physical examination. The bladder remains distended after partial or weak voiding attempts. Perineal reflexes are intact but the detrusor contraction is diminished or absent.

For such patients, maintenance of an indwelling urinary catheter for 3–14 days may be required to re-establish tight junctions and permit detrusor function to return. Although parasympathomimetic agents may help restore detrusor contractions, it is essential that they not be given without establishing a low-resistance outflow conduit, either with indwelling catheterization, removal of an anatomical obstruction or with pharmacological agents that relax the urethral outlet (in the case of functional obstruction). Urethral relaxants alone are usually not sufficient to ensure outflow patency in the initial stages of recovery from detrusor atony. Prognosis is dependent on cause and reversibility of obstruction, but is good for recovery of detrusor function in relatively acute cases. Chronic detrusor atony from any cause carries a guarded prognosis for return to full function.

Diagnostic approach to urine retention

History and physical examination
As for most micturition disorders, history-taking and physical examination provide the basis for diagnosis. Problem-specific historical questions related to urine retention are listed in Figure 3.9. Most animals with urine retention will have a distended bladder that is readily palpable on physical examination, and some will have evidence of overflow incontinence. Critical assessment of neurological status, particularly of the hindlimb reflexes and reflexes testing the sacral arc (e.g. perineal, bulbospongiosus/vulvar), is specifically indicated.

The diagnostic approach to urine retention is designed to:

* Rule out neurological and obstructive disorders
* Assess the status of the urinary bladder contractile force and urethral outlet resistance
* Investigate possible underlying aetiologies for the primary disorder.

Observation of voiding behaviour is an important part of the initial assessment. Particular attention should be given to the patient's ability to initiate and maintain a urine stream. Patients with anatomical obstruction typically strain and produce little to no urine. Functionally obstructed animals may initiate a stream that is quickly attenuated. Animals with bladder atony may slowly initiate a weak stream that sometimes increases with manual abdominal compression. Some animals with more chronic atony will not attempt to void at all. The bladder should normally be nearly empty following voiding attempts, even in male dogs. If there is palpable distension following voiding, manual expression should be gently attempted. Inability to express a distended bladder manually indicates a likely anatomical or functional outlet obstruction.

Catheterization

Catheterization of the urinary bladder following voiding allows assessment of anatomical outlet obstruction and residual urine volume. In healthy animals, resistance to the urethral catheter is encountered at the urethral flexure in male cats and the distal os penis and pelvic brim of male dogs. Urethral catheters also may easily pass by small uroliths and some soft tissue lesions; ability to catheterize the urethra does not fully rule out anatomical obstruction. Normal residual urine volume in dogs is 0.2–0.4 ml/kg, or <10 ml in total. Serial measurement of residual urine volume also can be used to assess response to therapy.

Diagnostic imaging

Additional imaging procedures are usually required to identify positively or rule out anatomical obstruction. Plain radiography will demonstrate most mineralized obstructions (Figure 3.18), and thoracic radiographs are indicated if neoplasia is suspected or confirmed. Ultrasonography is an excellent modality for demonstration of trigonal and proximal urethral lesions (Figure 3.19). Contrast urethrocystography will delineate the location and extent of many obstructive lesions (Figure 3.20), and in some cases urethrocystoscopy will be useful for visualization and/or biopsy of obstructing structures.

Urethroscopy has proved valuable for detection of urethral lesions that do not appear on conventional imaging studies; however, the procedure could disrupt neoplastic cells and seed them elsewhere along the

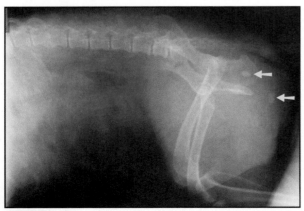

3.18 Right lateral radiograph. Yellow arrows indicate urethroliths clearly visible in this castrated male Schnauzer presented for anuria.

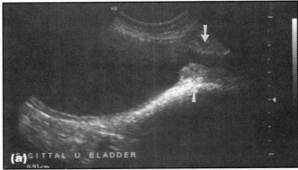

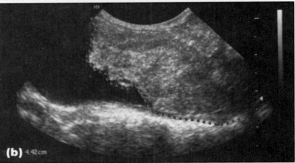

3.19 Ultrasound still images. **(a)** A small, partially obstructive trigonal mass (yellow arrows) in a spayed female Beagle. **(b)** A very large, fully obstructive trigonal mass in a spayed female Toy Poodle. The extent of the mass into the bladder lumen is outlined by the broken blue line.

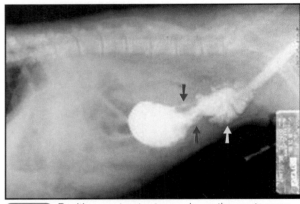

3.20 Positive-contrast retrograde urethrocystogram in a male dog. Reflux of contrast material into a diseased prostate gland (yellow arrow) is apparent, as are filling defects at the trigone (blue arrows) that were later determined to be transitional cell carcinoma.

urinary tract. Advanced imaging of the spinal cord (e.g. myelography/epidurography, computed tomography, magnetic resonance imaging) may be necessary to confirm or localize subtle neurological lesions.

Advanced urodynamic evaluation

Advanced urodynamic evaluation may be useful in some cases to document bladder and urethral function (see Specialized urodynamic studies, above).

Treatment

A formulary of pharmacological agents commonly used for the management of urine retention is presented in Figure 3.21.

Agent	Mechanism	Recommended dosage	Possible adverse effects	Contraindications	Comments
Urethral relaxants					
Acepromazine maleate	Skeletal muscle relaxation via neuroleptic effect; smooth muscle relaxation via alpha-antagonism	Up to 0.1 mg/kg i.v. q12–24h (doses as low as 0.02 mg/kg i.v. may be effective) 1.1–2.2 mg/kg orally q12–24h	Hypotension, sedation, exacerbation of seizure disorder, disinhibition	Hypovolaemia Cardiac disease Seizure disorder	
Baclofen	Skeletal muscle relaxation	Dogs: 1–2 mg/kg orally q8h Cats: not recommended	Weakness, gastrointestinal upset, pruritus		
Dantrolene	Skeletal muscle relaxation via direct effects	Dogs: 1–5 mg/kg orally q8–12h Cats: 0.5–2.0 mg/kg orally q8h 1.0 mg/kg i.v.	Weakness, sedation, gastrointestinal upset, hepatotoxicity	Cardiac disease	
Diazepam	Skeletal muscle relaxation via central effects (benzodiazepine)	Dogs: 2–10 mg/dog orally q8h Cats: 1–2.5 mg/cat orally q8h or as needed	Sedation, paradoxical excitation, idiopathic hepatic necrosis (with oral use in cats only), polyphagia	Pregnancy Hepatic disease	
Phenoxybenzamine	Smooth muscle relaxation via non-specific alpha-antagonism	Dogs: 0.25 mg/kg orally q8–12h or 2.5–20 mg/dog orally q 8–12h Cats: 1.25–7.5 mg/cat orally q8–12h	Hypotension, tachycardia, gastrointestinal upset	Cardiac disease Hypovolaemia Glaucoma Renal failure Diabetes mellitus (type II)	
Prazosin	Smooth muscle relaxation via alpha-1 antagonism	Dogs: 1 mg/15 kg orally q8–12h Cats: 0.25–0.5 mg/cat orally q12–24h	Hypotension, mild sedation, ptyalism	Cardiac disease Renal failure	
Terazosin	Smooth muscle relaxation via alpha-1 antagonism	Dogs: 0.5–5.0 mg/dog q12–24h Cats: not determined	Hypotension, mild sedation, ptyalism	Cardiac disease Renal failure	
Anxiolytic agents					
Acepromazine maleate	See above	See above	See above	See above	
Alprazolam	Centrally acting anxiolytic benzodiazepine	Cats: 0.125–0.25 mg/cat orally q12h	As for diazepam, except idiopathic hepatic necrosis has not been documented		May be a good alternative to diazepam if oral therapy is needed
Amitriptyline	Tricyclic antidepressant, anxiolytic, alpha-antagonist, antihistamine, analgesic, anticholinergic	Cats: 1–2 mg/kg/day orally or 2.5–10 mg/cat/day orally	Sedation, neutropenia, thrombocytopenia, urine retention, weight gain	Do not use if bladder atony is suspected	Use cautiously and discontinue if worsening of urine retention is suspected
Diazepam	See above	See above	See above	See above	
Detrusor muscle contractile agents					
Bethanechol	Parasympathomimetic	Dogs: 5–25 mg orally q8h Cats: 1.25–5 mg orally q8h	Ptyalism, vomiting, diarrhoea	Outlet obstruction or high outlet resistance Gastrointestinal obstruction	Atropine is antidotal
Cisapride [a]	Prokinetic, may enhance acetylcholine release	Dogs: 0.5 mg/kg orally q8h Cats: 1.25–5 mg/cat orally q8–12h	Diarrhoea, possible abdominal pain	Gastrointestinal obstruction	Reduce dose with hepatic insufficiency

3.21 Formulary of agents useful in the management of urine retention. [a] Not available in the UK.

References and further reading

Arnold S and Weber U (2000) Urethral sphincter mechanism incompetence. In: *Current Veterinary Therapy XIII*, ed. JD Bonagura, pp. 896–899. WB Saunders, Philadelphia

Barch A, Reichler IM, Hubler M *et al*. (2005) Evaluation of long-term effects of endoscopic injection of collagen into the urethral submucosa for treatment of urethral sphincter incompetence in female dogs: 40 cases (1993–2000). *Journal of the American Veterinary Medical Association* **226**, 73–76

Barsanti JA, Coates JR, Bartges JW *et al*. (1996) Detrusor–urethral dyssynergia. In: *Veterinary Clinics of North America: Small Animal Practice* **26**, 327–338

Cannizzo KL, McLoughlin MA, Mattoon JS *et al*. (2003) Evaluation of transurethral cystoscopy and excretory urography for diagnosis of ectopic ureters in female dogs: 25 cases (1992–2000). *Journal of the American Veterinary Medical Association* **223**, 475–481

Fischer JR, Lane IF and Cribb AE (2003) Urethral pressure profile and hemodynamic effects of phenoxybenzamine and prazosin in non-sedated male beagle dogs. *Canadian Journal of Veterinary Research* **67**, 30–38

Forrester SD (2005) Urinary incontinence. In: *Textbook of Veterinary Internal Medicine, 6th edn*, ed. SJ Ettinger and E Feldman, pp. 109–111. Elsevier Saunders, St. Louis

Hoelzler MG and Lidbetter DA (2004) Surgical management of urinary incontinence. *Veterinary Clinics of North America: Small Animal Practice* **34**, 1057–1073

Labato MA (2005) Micturition disorders. In: *Textbook of Veterinary Internal Medicine, 6th edn*, ed. SJ Ettinger and E Feldman, pp. 105–109. Elsevier Saunders, St. Louis

Lane IF (2000) Use of anticholinergic agents in lower urinary tract disease. In: *Current Veterinary Therapy XIII,* ed. JD Bonagura, pp. 899–902. WB Saunders, Philadelphia

Lane IF and Fischer JR (2003) Symposium: A diagnostic approach to micturition disorders, treating urinary incontinence, and medical treatment of voiding dysfunction in dogs and cats. *Veterinary Medicine,* **January,** 49–74

Rawlings C, Barsanti JA, Mahaffer MB and Bement S (2001) Evaluation of colposuspension for treatment of incontinence in spayed female dogs. *Journal of the American Veterinary Medical Association* **219**, 770–775

Reichler IM, Hubler M, Jöchle W *et al.* (2003) The effect of GnRH analogs on urinary incontinence after ablation of the ovaries in dogs. *Theriogenology* **60**, 1207–1216

Samii VF, McLoughlin MA, Mattoon JS *et al.* (2004) Digital fluoroscopic excretory urography, digital fluoroscopic urethrography, helical computed tomography, and cystoscopy in 24 dogs with suspected ureteral ectopia. *Journal of Veterinary Internal Medicine* **18**, 271–281

Scott L, Leddy M, Bernay F and Dovot JL (2002) Evaluation of phenylpropanolamine in the treatment of urethral sphincter mechanism incompetence in the bitch. *Journal of Small Animal Practice* **43**, 493–496

Silverman S and Long CD (2000) The diagnosis of urinary incontinence and abnormal urination in dogs and cats. In: *Veterinary Clinics of North America: Small Animal Practice* **30**, 427–448

Williams JM and Niles JD (2005) *BSAVA Manual of Canine and Feline Abdominal Surgery.* BSAVA Publications, Gloucester

Wood JD, Simmons-Byrd A, Spievack AR and Badylak SF (2005) Use of a particulate extracellular matrix bioscaffold for treatment of acquired urinary incontinence in dogs. *Journal of the American Veterinary Medical Association* **226**, 1095–1097

4

Abnormal renal palpation

Alex German

Introduction

When renal disease is suspected, abdominal palpation is critical to the initial physical examination. Abdominal palpation will reveal changes in renal morphology that accompany various pathological processes, but it is important to recognize that no direct information on renal function can be derived (see Chapter 9 for details on assessment of renal function).

The normal kidneys are bean-shaped organs that lie in a retroperitoneal position ventral to the sublumbar musculature. The right kidney lies cranial to the left. Anatomical relations of the right kidney are:

* Cranioventrally it is deeply recessed in the liver (renal notch)
* Medially and cranially are the right adrenal gland and vena cava
* Laterally are the last rib and abdominal wall.

Increased size
Reduced size
Altered number
Altered shape
Altered consistency
Altered position
Pain

4.1 Summary of abnormal findings on renal palpation.

The left kidney is positioned more caudally than the right. Anatomical relations of the left kidney are:

* Cranially is the spleen
* Medially are the left adrenal gland and aorta
* Laterally is the abdominal wall and ventrally the descending colon.

In dogs, the normal left kidney can be palpated in most animals, whilst the right kidney is only palpable in thin subjects. Relative to body weight, feline kidneys are larger than those of the dog; the normal left kidney and caudoventral surface of the right kidney are readily palpable in most animals. Kidneys are also more mobile in cats; both kidneys (but the left in particular) can be easily displaced from their normal positions on palpation.

When normal kidney morphology is altered it usually implies a pathological process, but some changes can be physiological. The main palpable abnormalities include enlargement (renomegaly), decreased size and abnormal shape, whilst changes can be unilateral or bilateral (Figure 4.1). Other abnormalities include altered number of kidneys (usually decreased, e.g. renal agenesis), abnormal position (e.g. renal ectopia), altered renal consistency and the presence of pain. Since a number of consequences can arise as a result of morphological abnormalities of the kidney (Figure 4.2), prognosis is variable.

Disorder	Azotaemia?	Unilateral (U) or bilateral (B)	Prognosis

Physiological:
  Acromegaly
  Nephrectomy
  Portovascular anomalies
	Y/N	
		B
		U
		B
			Variable

Acute pyelonephritis	Y/N	U or B	Guarded. Can resolve with appropriate treatment
Perinephric pseudocysts	N	B>U	Good
Primary renal neoplasia	N	U unless cystadenocarcinoma	Guarded
Renal lymphoma	Y/N	B usually	Guarded short term Poor long term
Feline infectious peritonitis (FIP)	Y/N	B	Poor
Metastatic neoplasia	N	U/B	Poor

4.2 Effects of selected diseases on kidney morphology. All of these diseases/disorders lead to renomegaly with the exception of chronic kidney disease and selected congenital diseases, which give rise to small kidneys. (continues) ▶

Disorder	Renal failure?	Unilateral (U) or bilateral (B)	Prognosis
Polycystic kidney disease	Y/N	B	Guarded to poor if multiple cysts and azotaemia develop
Hydronephrosis	Y/N	U/B	Guarded if unilateral Very poor if bilateral, unless obstruction can be relieved
Congenital	See Chapter 7	U/B	See Chapter 7
Subcapsular haematoma	N	U	Good
Chronic kidney disease	Y	B	Guarded
Urolithiasis	N unless bilateral	U>B	Good unless bilateral
Trauma	N unless bilateral	U>B	Variable
Acute nephrosis	Y/N	B	Guarded. Can resolve with appropriate treatment

4.2 (continued) Effects of selected diseases on kidney morphology. All of these diseases/disorders lead to renomegaly with the exception of chronic kidney disease and selected congenital diseases, which give rise to small kidneys.

Increased size

Renomegaly may be physiological or pathological. Unilateral nephrectomy, congenital unilateral renal agenesis and other conditions which result in loss of function in one kidney induce compensatory physiological hypertrophy of the remaining kidney. Unilateral renomegaly is always a pathological finding if the remaining kidney is present and functional. Bilateral renomegaly usually implies renal pathology, although compensatory renal hypertrophy can be seen in animals with portovascular anomalies (PVA). Technically, renomegaly secondary to acromegaly is a physiological response to excess growth hormone and insulin-like growth factor-1 (IGF-1) production.

Several diseases which cause renomegaly occur more frequently in cats than in dogs (detailed in Figure 4.2). These include renal lymphoma, feline infectious peritonitis (FIP), idiopathic polycystic kidney disease (PKD) and perinephric pseudocysts. Renal lymphoma occurs occasionally in dogs, PKD is uncommon but is hereditary in certain breeds (West Highland White Terriers, English Bull Terriers), whilst a canine equivalent of FIP has not been reported. Other causes of renomegaly, such as hydronephrosis, acute pyelonephritis, some of the diseases leading to acute uraemia (e.g. nephrotoxicosis, renal ischaemia, obstructive uropathy), PVA, renal neoplasia, subcapsular haematomas and acromegaly, are less species-specific. In the dog, bilateral renomegaly is often accompanied by acute rather than chronic kidney failure, whereas in the cat, some of the diseases causing bilateral renomegaly can lead to chronic kidney failure (see Chapter 5 for further discussion).

Reduced size

Reduced renal size can occur in both dogs and cats, and usually suggests a chronic rather than acute cause. In contrast to renomegaly, small kidneys are usually abnormal whether unilateral or bilateral. Chronic kidney disease (see Chapter 18) is the most common cause, but other differential diagnoses are possible, including congenital diseases (dysplasia, familial nephropathies) and renal atrophy (e.g. as a long-term consequence of ureteral obstruction). The latter are usually unilateral rather than bilateral.

Altered number

Congenital diseases, although rare, are the most common reason for alterations in kidney number (Figure 4.3). Decreased number is seen with renal agenesis and fused (horseshoe) kidneys; increased renal number can be seen with renal duplication. Although many breeds can be affected, agenesis and duplication have been reported as familial diseases in Beagles and English Bull Terriers, respectively. Agenesis can be unilateral or bilateral, and is usually accompanied by ureteral aplasia. Not surprisingly, bilateral agenesis is invariably fatal and is a potential cause of fading puppy syndrome. The main acquired cause of decreased kidney number is prior nephrectomy. Renal duplication is the only, rare, abnormality that causes an increased number of kidneys, and this is usually an incidental finding.

Decreased number

Congenital:
- Renal agenesis
- Fused (horseshoe) kidneys

Acquired:
- Nephrectomy

Increased number

Congenital:
- Renal duplication

4.3 Causes of altered kidney number.

Altered shape

Many of the diseases which alter the shape of the kidney (Figure 4.4) also lead to changes in size. Examples include renal dysplasia, congenital renal fusion (horseshoe kidney), perinephric pseudocysts, renal neoplasia, subcapsular haematomas and PKD.

Altered consistency

Palpable changes in consistency include kidneys that have a fluctuant feel, and those that are firmer than normal (Figure 4.5). The former is most often noted with perinephric pseudocysts, subcapsular haematomas, cystic tumours and hydronephrosis; the latter

Congenital
Renal fusion – horseshoe kidney
Renal dysplasia
Perinephric pseudocysts
Neoplasia
Primary renal neoplasia
Renal lymphoma
Metastatic neoplasia
Polycystic kidney disease
Chronic kidney disease (small and deformed)
Hydronephrosis
Congenital
Acquired

4.4 Causes of altered renal shape.

Fluctuant kidneys
Perinephric pseudocyst
Subcapsular haematoma
Cystic tumour
Hydronephrosis
Firm kidneys
Neoplasia
Chronic kidney disease

4.5 Causes of altered renal consistency.

is often detected with neoplasia (usually large, abnormally shaped, and/or asymmetrical) and chronic kidney disease (usually small, may be abnormally shaped).

Altered position

Causes of altered kidney position are listed in Figure 4.6. Renal ectopia is a congenital condition, which arises as a result of failure of normal embryonic ascent of the kidney. The condition is usually incidental, and the kidney can be identified either as a caudal abdominal, sublumbar or pelvic mass. Altered position can also accompany renomegaly (the enlarged kidney becomes displaced ventrally)

Renal ectopia
Enlarged kidney
Displaced kidney
Enlargement of adjacent organ:
Adrenal gland tumour
Splenomegaly
Hepatomegaly
Alimentary tract disease
Sublumbar disease
Obesity

4.6 Causes of altered kidney position.

and conditions which result in enlargement of an adjacent structure, e.g. hepatomegaly and adrenal gland tumours. In obese subjects, kidneys are displaced ventrally and often embedded within large amounts of fat. However, this finding is rarely documented on abdominal palpation.

Pain

Renal pain is most often seen with pyelonephritis, acute nephrosis, renal abscesses, neoplasia and in the early stage of hydronephrosis (Figure 4.7).

Pyelonephritis
Urolithiasis:
Renal calculi
Ureteric calculi causing obstruction
Acute nephrosis
Hydronephrosis
Stretching of renal capsule:
Renal trauma (e.g. subcapsular haematoma)
Amyloidosis?
Trauma
Referred pain:
Spinal disease
Other abdominal disease
Abscesses
Neoplasia

4.7 Causes of kidney pain.

Diagnostic approach to abnormal renal morphology

As with diagnosis of a disease in any body system, a problem-oriented approach is recommended, taking into account information compiled from a minimum database of signalment, history, physical examination and a range of further diagnostic tests. Some diseases involve other body systems in addition to the renal system (e.g. lymphoma, FIP, PVA, metastatic neoplasia and acromegaly), whilst others are organ-specific, e.g. PKD, hydronephrosis, perinephric pseudocysts, acute pyelonephritis and acute uraemia. From the minimum database, a problem list and set of differential diagnoses can be constructed. With subsequent diagnostic evaluations, the problem list is refined and the differential diagnoses are narrowed.

Signalment

Breed, gender and age predispositions are evident in some of the diseases that cause morphological renal abnormalities, allowing the clinician to prioritize the preliminary list of differential diagnoses. Examples of diseases where breed predispositions exist include PKD (Persian cats, Figure 4.8; Cairn Terriers, West Highland White Terriers and English Bull Terriers), basement membrane disorders (Dobermanns, English Cocker Spaniels and Samoyeds) and amyloidosis (Beagles, English Foxhounds, Shar Peis and Abyssinian cats) (see Chapter 7). Diseases with a gender

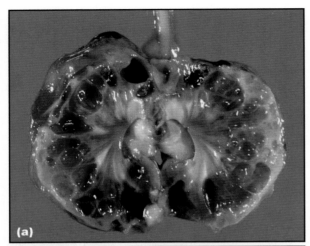

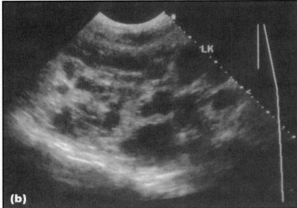

4.8 Example of PKD in a Persian cat. **(a)** The renal cortex is distorted with multiple fluid-filled cysts. **(b)** These cysts can readily be detected by ultrasonographic examination. (Courtesy of the Feline Advisory Bureau.)

Historical and physical findings	Possible diagnostic implications
Signs of renal failure: buccal ulceration, uraemic breath, dehydration, poor concentrating ability and oliguria/polyuria (acute or decompensated chronic). Pallor and emaciation (additional findings which suggest a chronic problem)	Acute nephrosis: ischaemic, toxic, infectious Bilateral pyelonephritis Bilateral hydronephrosis Chronic kidney disease
Lymphadenopathy	Lymphoma
Anterior uveitis and/or chorioretinitis	FIP
Neurological/encephalopathic signs	Renal encephalopathy Portovascular anomaly FIP Lymphoma (Acromegaly – pituitary neoplasm)
Haematuria without dysuria	Renal neoplasia Pyelonephritis Nephrolithiasis Acute nephrosis? Trauma Telangiectasia
Dysuria and haematuria	Hydronephrosis: urinary calculi, renal or ureteral trauma Pyelonephritis with lower urinary tract infection Portovascular anomaly with ammonium biurate urolithiasis
Urinary calculi	Hydronephrosis (renal calculi) Portovascular anomaly with ammonium biurate urolithiasis
Urinary incontinence with urine scalding	Congenital anatomical defect causing incontinence and hydronephrosis/pyelonephritis
Microhepatica	Portovascular anomaly
Hepatomegaly	Acute tubular nephrosis (leptospirosis) Acromegaly and secondary diabetes mellitus Amyloidosis in Siamese cats
Enlargement of the skull, mandible *(prognathia inferior)* and tongue in an adult animal	Acromegaly
Enlargement/malformation of the mandibles in a young animal	Osteodystrophy associated with chronic kidney disease
Signs of systemic sepsis: fever, depression, tachycardia, vomiting, petechiation	Acute tubular nephrosis Leptospirosis Acute pyelonephritis Sepsis
Skin nodules	Renal cystadenocarcinoma In German Shepherd Dogs associated with dermatofibrosis

4.9 Significance of physical findings when associated with morphological abnormalities.

predisposition include acromegaly (male cats, and neutered bitches) and the basement membrane disorder in male Samoyeds (X-linked recessive), whilst diseases with an age predisposition include congenital PVA (young animals) and most neoplastic diseases (older individuals). In contrast, German Shepherd Dogs have an inherited predisposition for nodular dermatofibrosis combined with renal cystadenocarcinomas (Lingaas *et al.*, 2003).

History

A full medical history should be obtained in all cases. Signs of disease in other body systems may be evident and, in some cases, concurrent acute or chronic azotaemia may be present (Figure 4.9). Further, there are some historical findings which, when present, may suggest the specific underlying cause. Cases of unilateral hydronephrosis and perinephric pseudocysts have simple histories of progressive abdominal enlargement, often with no systemic signs. In contrast, the history of acute pyelonephritis may be poorly defined, although pyrexia, anorexia, lethargy, dehydration and weight loss may be present. In severe cases there may be sublumbar pain and signs of systemic sepsis.

Physical examination

Physical examination provides the opportunity to evaluate the renal system indirectly (e.g. with abdominal palpation), and to assess the rest of the systemic health of the animal. Systematic abdominal palpation provides information on most aspects of renal morphology (size, shape and position), as well as providing evidence of other organ involvement. The following questions should be addressed:

- Are two kidneys palpable, and in their normal position? If not, is there evidence to suggest an alteration in kidney number or position?
- Are there alterations in renal size, e.g. either renomegaly or decreased size?
- Are the renal contours smooth or irregular?
- Are the abnormalities documented unilateral or bilateral?
- Are other abdominal masses present?
- Is there renal or sublumbar pain?
- Are there any other abnormalities present?

Other physical examination findings which may be relevant to the diagnosis are presented in Figure 4.9.

Further diagnostic tests

In some circumstances altered renal morphology is physiological and an incidental finding (e.g. renomegaly associated with PVA, acromegaly and physiological hypertrophy of the remaining kidney after nephrectomy). However, in most cases it indicates a significant pathological process, which requires further diagnostic evaluation (see also Chapters 5 and 9). The initial approach is to collect baseline clinicopathological data:

- *Haematology*. Complete blood count and blood smear evaluation are recommended
- *Serum biochemical analysis*. A complete profile including electrolytes is recommended
- *Urinalysis*. This should include gross examination, dipstick, sediment examination and measurement of specific gravity by refractometer
- *Virology*. Serological tests for feline leukaemia virus (FeLV) antigen and anti-feline immunodeficiency virus (FIV) antibody should be performed in all cats, whilst coronavirus serology should also be considered.

In some cases, the above database is sufficient to obtain a definitive diagnosis. However, on occasion additional procedures may be warranted, including bacterial culture of urine, diagnostic imaging, tests of renal function, cytological examination and histopathological assessment of biopsy material.

Bacterial culture of urine

Cystocentesis is the preferred method of urine collection if bacterial culture is required, and it is recommended that a laboratory is chosen which provides information on minimum inhibitory concentration (MIC) to assist in antibiotic selection if appropriate (see Chapter 9). The presence of intracellular bacteria confirms that an active infection exists. The presence of white blood cell casts is strongly suggestive of pyelonephritis (see Chapter 8).

Diagnostic imaging

In cases of renomegaly, some form of diagnostic imaging is always recommended in order to characterize better the reason for renal enlargement (see also Chapter 10). In contrast, for cases presenting with small kidneys, it is debatable as to whether diagnostic imaging will yield further information.

Survey radiographs of the abdomen and thorax are recommended, and both lateral and ventrodorsal views should be taken if ultrasonography is not available. The ventrodorsal view can be used to measure renal size, although this is greatly facilitated by the use of contrast radiography (see below). The clinician should be aware that the kidneys are magnified on the resulting image. A complete ultrasonographic evaluation of the abdomen is indicated, paying particular attention to the kidneys. Renal size can be evaluated by plain radiographs taken in dorsal recumbency, even though some degree of magnification occurs. Size is better evaluated by ultrasonography, which avoids this problem of magnification, and ranges for normal renal size have been reported (Figure 4.10). Parameters have been devised for assessing renal size from contrast radiographs and ultrasonographic images:

- Excretory urogram in the ventrodorsal view:
  - Dog: normal kidney length = 2.5–3.5 x L2 (length of second lumbar vertebra)
  - Cat: normal kidney length = 2.4–3.0 x L2
- Maximal sagittal dimension on ultrasonographic images:
  - Cat = 38–44 mm
  - In the dog, kidney length is directly proportional to body weight (Figure 4.10).

Weight range (kg)	Number of kidneys evaluated	Renal length (cm)		
		Range	Mean	Standard deviation
0–4	2	3.2–3.3	3.2	0.09
5–9	16	3.2–5.2	4.4	0.5
10–14	10	4.8–6.4	5.6	0.6
15–19	20	5.0–6.7	6.0	0.4
20–24	20	5.2–8.0	6.5	0.72
25–29	44	5.3–7.8	6.9	0.58
30–34	32	6.1–8.7	7.2	0.6
35–39	24	6.6–9.3	7.6	0.72
40–44	12	6.3–8.4	7.6	0.54
45–49	8	7.6–9.1	8.5	0.46
50–59	6	7.5–10.6	9.1	1.27
60–69	4	8.3–9.8	9.0	0.63
90–99	2	8.6–10.1	9.4	1.06

4.10 Relationship between kidney length and body weight in dogs.

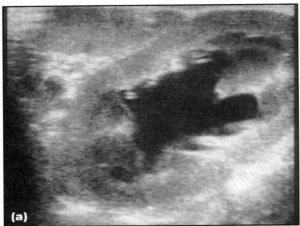

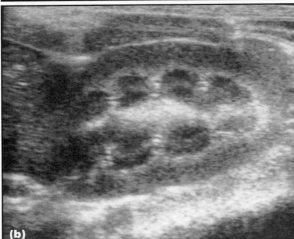

Renal ultrasonography can also provide excellent detail on internal architecture, and many lesions, such as cysts, mass lesions, subcapsular fluid accumulation and renal pelvis dilation, can be readily identified (Figures 4.11 and 4.12). Changes in echogenicity are also associated with certain diseases. Increased echogenicity is seen in acute nephrosis and FIP, while lymphoma can increase or decrease echogenicity. Focal lesions are, thus, readily recognized. Ultrasonography can also facilitate fine needle aspiration cytology and percutaneous collection of biopsy material (see Chapters 10 and 12).

Advanced imaging techniques include excretory urography (Figures 4.13 and 4.14), antegrade pyelography, renal scintigraphy, computed tomography (CT), magnetic resonance imaging (MRI) and advanced ultrasonographic techniques. With the advent of

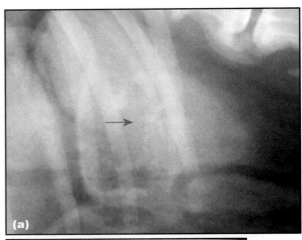

4.11 Ultrasonography demonstrating hydronephrosis. Ultrasonogram of a 3-year-old female (recently neutered) Chihuahua, presenting shortly after routine ovariohysterectomy. **(a)** Longitudinal image of the left kidney shows the hyperechoic fat of the renal pelvis markedly separated by anechoic fluid, consistent with severe hydronephrosis. The outline of the kidney is expanded, the normal architecture of the renal medulla is compressed, but the cortex is relatively normal. **(b)** Longitudinal view of the right kidney in the same dog showing normal renal architecture. (Courtesy of Anna Newitt, University of Liverpool.)

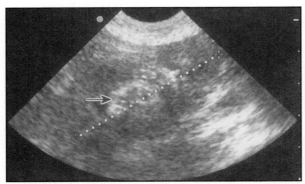

4.12 Ultrasonography demonstrating nephrolithiasis. Ultrasonogram of the left kidney of a 7-year-old male Dalmatian, presenting with apparent sublumbar pain. Hyperechoic shadowing regions are present in the renal pelvis (arrowed), consistent with nephrolithiasis (probably urate given the breed). (Courtesy of Anna Newitt and Alistair Freeman, University of Liverpool.)

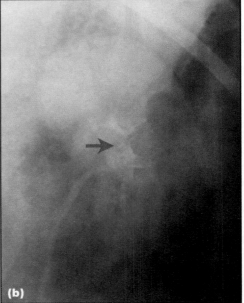

4.13 Excretory urography demonstrating nephrolithiasis in a 7-year-old male Dalmatian, presenting with apparent sublumbar pain (same dog as in Figure 4.12). **(a)** Nephroliths (probably urate) are evident on the plain right lateral abdominal radiograph (arrowed). **(b)** Filling defects can be seen during subsequent excretory urography (arrowed). (Courtesy of Anna Newitt and Alistair Freeman, University of Liverpool.)

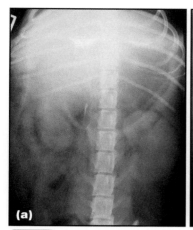
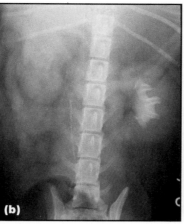
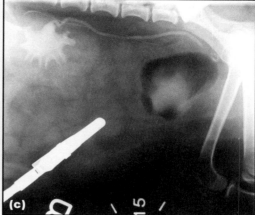

4.14 Excretory urography demonstrating hydronephrosis. Excretory urography in a 3-year-old female (recently neutered) Chihuahua, presenting shortly after routine ovariohysterectomy (same dog as in Figure 4.11). There is evidence of: **(a)** left-sided renomegaly, **(b)** dilation of the left renal pelvis and **(c)** left ureter dilation. The findings are suggestive of hydronephrosis secondary to iatrogenic ureteric ligation. (Courtesy of Anna Newitt, University of Liverpool.)

abdominal ultrasonography, the indications for intravenous urography have declined. However, if ultrasonography is not available, this is the only alternative method to provide information on the size, shape, position and internal architecture of the kidney. Antegrade pyelography can be used to localize the site of ureteral obstructions.

Although CT and MRI undoubtedly provide superior three-dimensional information to other techniques, they are still not widely available. However, advanced ultrasonographic techniques may be of more use, not least because abdominal ultrasonography has become commonplace in most small animal practices. In human medicine, intrarenal blood flow impedance, expressed as the *renal resistive index* (RRI) and obtained by duplex Doppler ultrasonography, has been used to aid in diagnosis and prognosis of renal failure (Rivers *et al.*, 1997). Increased RRI is seen in a variety of diseases, including acute tubular necrosis (ATN) and glomerulopathy, and the RRI can return to normal upon successful treatment. Furthermore, after the administration of either mannitol or furosemide, RRI remains unchanged in non-obstructed kidneys but is increased in obstructed kidneys (Choi *et al.*, 2003). Further details of these advanced imaging techniques can be found in Chapter 10.

Tests of renal function
The initial database provides some information on renal function, e.g. serum creatinine and urine specific gravity. However, given the insensitivity of these methods, other techniques may be necessary in some cases. Examples of function tests include measurement of water intake, water deprivation test and assessment of glomerular filtration rate (GFR), all of which are covered in detail in Chapter 9.

Renal cytology
Fine needle aspiration can be performed blind, if the kidney can be palpated and readily immobilized for the procedure. However, samples should ideally be taken under ultrasound guidance if at all possible;

this enables appropriate sites to be chosen, renal vasculature to be avoided and specific lesions to be targeted. Cytology is potentially useful for assessing mass lesions, although, with neoplastic lesions such as lymphoma, cells often do not readily exfoliate, and samples usually have marked blood contamination.

Renal biopsy
Renal biopsy should only be considered when the information obtained is likely to alter the approach to management of a particular case (see Chapter 12). Biopsy is more commonly indicated for assessment of renomegaly and changes in renal architecture, than for small kidneys, since the latter are almost invariably associated with end-stage disease. Diseases such as lymphoma, other types of neoplasia, ATN, FIP and familial nephropathy can all be diagnosed by renal biopsy (Figures 4.15 and 4.16).

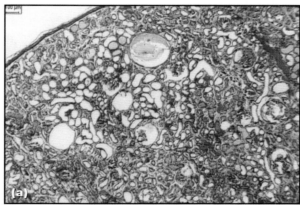

4.15 Histopathological pictures of renal parenchyma from an 11-month-old Cocker Spaniel bitch with familial nephropathy. Bowman's spaces are dilated and empty; some contain components of vascular glomerular tufts and proteinaceous material, whilst scattered tubules contain proteinaceous material. There is multifocal calcification of Bowman's capsules, tubular basement membrane and glomerular basement membranes. **(a)** H&E stain (original magnification X100). (continues) ▶

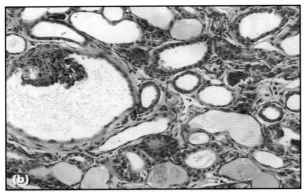

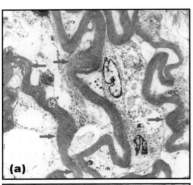

4.15 (continued) Histopathological pictures of renal parenchyma from an 11-month-old Cocker Spaniel bitch with familial nephropathy. Bowman's spaces are dilated and empty; some contain components of vascular glomerular tufts and proteinaceous material, whilst scattered tubules contain proteinaceous material. There is multifocal calcification of Bowman's capsules, tubular basement membrane and glomerular basement membranes. **(b)** H&E stain (original magnification X400).

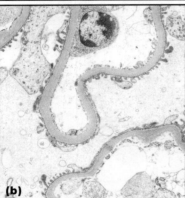

4.16

Transmission electron micrographs of glomeruli, from **(a)** an 11-month-old Cocker Spaniel bitch with familial nephropathy and **(b)** a normal dog. In the affected dog, there is evidence of basement membrane thickening (red arrows) and splitting (green arrows). (Original magnification X5400.)

Conditions causing abnormal renal morphology

Acute uraemia

Acute uraemia is defined as sudden, often catastrophic, failure of the kidney to meet the excretory, metabolic and endocrine demands of the body. The condition can arise secondary to disruptions to a number of renal functions, including haemodynamic, filtration, tubular and outflow tract disruptions. The causes, consequences and clinical signs of acute uraemia are discussed in Chapters 5 and 17 and the management of this syndrome is discussed in Chapter 17. Affected kidneys are either normal or enlarged regardless of the cause of the acute uraemia unless a pre-existing chronic kidney disease is evident. They often have a turgid feel to them and may be painful on palpation.

The mechanisms which underlie the renomegaly depend upon the underlying cause. In obstructive uropathy, the enlargement is due to dilation of the renal pelvis and development of hydronephrosis (see below). In contrast, in cases of acute nephrosis (nephrotoxicosis, renal ischaemia, etc.) the enlargement is the result of the parenchymal damage associated with the insult, which leads to a pathogenetic process involving three stages (initiation, maintenance and recovery; see Chapters 5 and 17).

Amyloidosis

Amyloidosis involves the extracellular deposition of fibrils formed by polymerization of proteins with a β-pleated sheet tertiary structure. Although several different types of protein have been recognized in human amyloidosis, fewer types are noted or reported in companion animals. The protein usually involved is amyloid A, which is produced from the polymerization of the *N*-terminal portion of serum amyloid A. Serum amyloid A is an acute phase protein predominantly synthesized in the liver. Therefore, amyloidosis is usually a sequel to a variety of chronic inflammatory disorders. Amyloid can be deposited in a number of organs, but the kidney is most often involved. Renal amyloidosis is more common in dogs than in cats and older animals are most often affected. The disease affects females more commonly than males. An increased incidence is reported in some breeds (e.g. Shar Pei, Beagle, English Foxhound, Walker Hound), and the disease is thought to be familial in most of these cases. Although amyloidosis is uncommon in cats, certain breeds are reportedly predisposed, e.g. Abyssinian and Siamese.

In most breeds of dog, the glomerulus is the most common site of renal amyloid deposition, and hence the most common abnormality is proteinuria. However, in Shar Peis and Abyssinian cats, amyloid is predominantly deposited in the renal medulla and proteinuria is less commonly observed. Diagnosis requires renal biopsy and histopathological examination, where the amyloid can be readily identified if special staining procedures are employed, e.g. Congo red or Sirius red. Specific treatment options are limited because the β-pleated sheet conformation is naturally resistant to breakdown. Suggested therapies have included colchicine (some success in Shar Peis) and dimethylsulfoxide. However, in most cases response is poor, especially after chronic kidney disease has developed. The prognosis is generally poor.

Chronic kidney disease

Chronic kidney disease is the most common disorder involving the kidneys of dogs and cats, and is defined as the presence of functional or structural abnormalities of one or both kidneys (see Chapters 5 and 18). It is characterized by irreversible loss of functional nephrons, and leads ultimately to decreased renal function. In order to define that a particular patient has chronic kidney disease, either renal damage or reduced renal function (e.g. decreased GFR) must have been present for at least 3 months. Chronic kidney disease can be the result of a number of initiating causes, and in many patients the factor(s) responsible is not clear. Whatever the inciting insult and irrespective of where in the nephron it develops, the whole nephron eventually becomes involved, leading to destruction of the complete structure and replacement with non-functional connective tissue. Initially, any potential decrease in renal size resulting from such nephron loss is counteracted by compensatory hypertrophy of remaining (functional) nephrons. However, as nephron loss progresses, the overall kidney mass eventually declines and end-stage kidneys result. Therefore, in most cases of chronic kidney disease, the kidneys are small and this is a helpful finding in differentiating chronic from acute kidney disease. Nevertheless, some chronic kidney disease patients have kidneys that are of normal size or even enlarged (see above for examples).

Definitive diagnosis of chronic kidney disease theoretically involves renal biopsy, although this is seldom performed or indicated in most cases. Treatment is supportive and/or renoprotective (see Chapter 18), and prognosis depends upon duration, aetiology and rate of progression of the disease.

Congenital renal disease and familial nephropathies

The details of congenital and familial renal disorders are given in Chapter 7. Most of such disorders develop at a young age (e.g. less than 5 years), but some can arise in older individuals. Most of such diseases ultimately lead to chronic renal insufficiency, although the severity and rate of progression is variable. Therapeutic options are limited to conservative therapy only, and the prognosis is usually guarded to poor.

The key features of these conditions with regard to renal palpation are as follows:

- Amyloidosis – variable
- Tubular dysfunction – none?
- Basement membrane disorder – decreased size
- Glomerular disorders – decreased size
- Polycystic kidney disease – increased size ± altered shape
- Renal dysplasia – decreased size
- Unilateral renal agenesis – decreased number
- Cystadenocarcinoma – altered size and shape (occasionally normal)
- Telangiectasia – none or altered size and shape
- Agenesis – decreased number
- Fusion (horseshoe kidney) – decreased number ± altered shape and position.

Hydronephrosis

Obstruction of urine flow causes a progressive dilation of the renal pelvis (see Figures 4.11 and 4.14). In bilateral ureteric or urethral obstruction, the patient will die from acute postrenal renal failure before significant atrophy of renal parenchyma occurs; in cases of unilateral ureteric obstruction, compensation by the unobstructed kidney will allow the development of gross hydronephrosis. The renal pelvis progressively dilates

causing pressure atrophy of the renal parenchyma and eventually the kidney becomes a distended, fibrous, fluid-filled sac. In the early stages, the distension of the renal capsule will induce signs of renal pain, but in many cases the first indication of hydronephrosis is progressive abdominal enlargement due to a large, unilateral, abdominal mass. Obstructive lesions may be congenital or acquired. Congenital obstructions include ureteral atresia, stenosis, torsion and ureterocele. These abnormalities may be seen in association with ectopic ureters. Acquired causes of obstruction include neoplasms, blood clots, uroliths, trauma, inflammatory masses and inadvertent ureteral ligation.

Because bilateral hydronephrosis presents with acute renal failure, rapid diagnosis and urgent therapy are required if renal function is to be re-established. For unilateral cases, diagnosis is usually made by imaging, with ultrasonography providing the best information. Treatment depends upon the cause and duration of the condition. Unfortunately, most unilateral cases are not diagnosed until the condition is long-standing, and the only recourse is surgical resection of the affected kidney.

Infectious disorders

Feline infectious peritonitis
Renomegaly can be seen in the non-effusive form of FIP. Affected kidneys have multiple granulomas on the renal surface extending into the cortex and cytological aspirates have mixed lymphocytes, plasma cells, neutrophils and macrophages. Pathological change is usually also present in the liver, mesenteric lymph nodes, central nervous system and eyes. FIP should be suspected in patients presenting with enlarged irregular kidneys, ocular lesions and central nervous system signs.

Leptospirosis
Leptospirosis is a systemic infection which causes renal enlargement and acute uraemia in dogs. Several different forms are recognized, depending upon the infecting serovar, and can be peracute, subacute or chronic. Most animals affected by the peracute form die from the complications of systemic sepsis and disseminated intravascular coagulation, while subacute cases may develop renal enlargement, acute uraemia, hepatitis and jaundice.

Pyelonephritis
Pyelonephritis is interstitial inflammation of the kidney associated with bacterial infection. In acute cases, one or both kidneys may be enlarged. Chronic pyelonephritis causes structural damage, fibrosis and scarring and is associated with reduced renal size. Most cases in the dog are caused by ascending urinary tract infection, but the importance of ascending infection has not been fully established in the cat. Other possible mechanisms of infection include haematogenous spread or septic embolization in animals with bacteraemia or septicaemia, e.g. in cases of bacterial endocarditis, discospondylitis and pyometra. Pyelonephritis can also occur secondary to immunosuppression, e.g. hyperadrenocorticism.

Signs of acute pyelonephritis may be quite vague but include mild renomegaly, renal pain, fever, anorexia, dehydration, weight loss, polyuria, polydipsia and vomiting. Diagnosis is usually made from a combination of tests, including diagnostic imaging (especially ultrasonography) and laboratory findings (haematology, serum biochemistry and urinalysis) (Figure 4.17). Ultrasonographic findings in acute pyelonephritis are variable (see Chapter 10). There may be:

- Dilation of the renal pelvis
- A hyperechoic mucosal line within the renal pelvis
- Focal hypoechoic areas in the medulla
- Focal hyper- or hypoechoic cortical lesions.

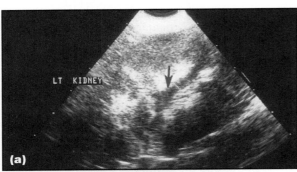

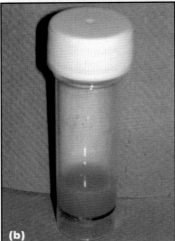

4.17

Pyelonephritis in a 9-year-old neutered Weimaraner bitch. **(a)** Ultrasonogram of the left kidney, demonstrating dilation of the renal pelvis (arrowed), and poor corticomedullary definition. (Courtesy of Annette Kerins, University of Liverpool.) **(b)** Specimen of urine demonstrating gross turbidity.

Ultrasonography may also facilitate the collection of cytological specimens, by fine needle aspiration, from the renal parenchyma or from a dilated renal pelvis.

Neutrophilic leucocytosis may be noted on haematological examination, whereas serum biochemical analysis may reveal azotaemia if renal insufficiency has developed. Urinalysis may demonstrate haematuria, pyuria, evidence of sub-optimal concentrating ability (specific gravity usually within the hypersthenuric range, but not markedly concentrated, e.g. 1.015–1.025; often in the face of azotaemia) and a positive urine culture (see Chapter 8). The source of urinary tract infection may be difficult to localize, but the presence of white blood cell casts confirms the presence of inflammation in the upper urinary tract. Unfortunately, the absence of white cell casts does not rule out pyelonephritis. A definitive diagnosis can be made by renal biopsy, although this technique carries the risk of iatrogenic

spread of infection within the abdomen. Further, taking a biopsy of the cortex might miss the diagnosis since this region can be unaffected in pyelonephritis.

Perinephric pseudocysts

A small number of cats have been described with large fluid accumulations in fibrous pseudocysts surrounding one or both kidneys. The cysts are termed pseudocysts because they are not lined by epithelium and develop between the renal parenchyma and the renal capsule. The kidneys, which are enclosed within the cyst, are usually of normal size and fully functional. The pathogenesis is not understood, but trauma with subcapsular urine leakage has been suggested. Older intact male cats are most often affected and there are few clinical signs except progressive abdominal enlargement. The cyst fluid is a transudate and, after surgical resection and drainage of the cyst, there was no recurrence in cats followed up for 2 years.

Portovascular anomalies

Renomegaly is a relatively common finding in dogs and cats with congenital PVA. The increase in renal size is thought to be related to increased renal workload, to increased delivery of trophic factors to the kidneys and to increased renal blood flow. There is some evidence that exposure of renal cells to high ammonia concentrations causes hypertrophy; increased renal gluconeogenesis can also develop secondary to systemic hypoglycaemia and this can also cause hypertrophy. Renal enlargement can additionally occur secondary to increased GFR, which can be seen in animals with PVA. PVA are usually diagnosed with a combination of laboratory analyses (including dynamic bile acids) and diagnostic imaging (ultrasonography and portovenography).

Renal neoplasia

Tumours are important causes of unilateral renomegaly in the dog (Figure 4.18). Lymphoma is the most common renal neoplasm in the cat and is usually, but not invariably, bilateral (Figure 4.19). Other metastatic neoplasms, such as haemangiosarcoma, may also

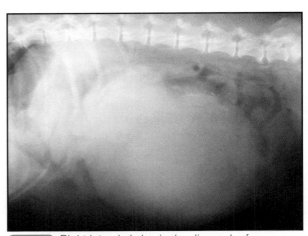

4.18 Right lateral abdominal radiograph of an anaplastic sarcoma causing dramatic unilateral renomegaly, altered shape and altered position in a 7-year-old Bassett Hound bitch. (Courtesy of Anna Newitt and Laura Blackwood, University of Liverpool.)

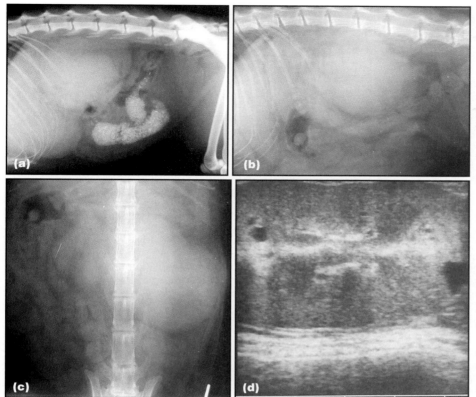

4.19 Renal lymphoma. **(a)** Right lateral abdominal radiograph of a domestic shorthair cat with bilateral renomegaly caused by lymphoma. Small intestinal impaction (from ingestion of cat litter) was the result of concurrent pica. (Photograph: Dr Penney Barber.) **(b)** Right lateral and **(c)** ventrodorsal abdominal radiographs of a 14-year-old domestic shorthair cat with unilateral renomegaly caused by lymphoma. (Courtesy of Anna Newitt and Rachel Steen, University of Liverpool.) **(d)** Ultrasonogram of the left kidney of an 11-year-old neutered male Persian cat with bilateral renal lymphoma. There is renomegaly (left kidney 5.6 cm) and poor corticomedullary definition. Two cysts are also present within the renal cortex, probably secondary to concurrent PKD. (Courtesy of Anna Newitt and Dan Batchelor, University of Liverpool.)

induce bilateral renomegaly. Primary renal malignancies, such as renal cell carcinoma and transitional cell carcinoma, are relatively rare in both species and vary in their behaviour. Some tumours are highly invasive locally and cause erosion of the renal artery and vein while others are quite static. Some metastasize early, whereas others are curable by excision. The presence of an irregular mass involving part or all of one kidney should always prompt careful evaluation for local and distant metastasis.

Renal lymphoma is relatively common in cats, and usually affects both kidneys, which may have an irregular outline (Figure 4.19). As a result, signs of renal insufficiency are common. Renal lymphoma may be accompanied by involvement of other abdominal organs and lymph nodes (peripheral, abdominal and mediastinal). In cats presenting with renal lymphoma, subsequent progression to central nervous system lymphoma is common, whilst cases with nasopharyngeal lymphoma may subsequently progress to renal lymphoma. The initial response to chemotherapy may be good but the long-term prognosis is guarded.

Hereditary multifocal renal cystadenocarcinoma and nodular dermatofibrosis (RCND) is an inherited disorder in German Shepherd Dogs, and is transmitted in an autosomal dominant fashion. As the name suggests, affected dogs can develop renal cystadenocarcinomas accompanied by cutaneous and subcutaneous nodules. Affected entire bitches can also develop uterine leiomyosarcomas. The disease has similarities with RCND in people, and a disease-associated mutation in exon 7 of the Birt-Hogg-Dube protein has recently been described (Lingaas *et al.*,

2003). The condition is usually seen in middle-aged to older animals, and clinical signs include polydipsia, weight loss and anorexia.

Prognosis of diseases causing abnormal renal morphology

The overall prognosis for patients with morphological renal abnormalities is variable, and depends upon the specific cause (see Figure 4.2). Some abnormalities are incidental findings (e.g. renal duplication, ectopic kidney) and have no major consequences for the patient. In others the prognosis is favourable, as long as appropriate therapy is provided; examples include unilateral hydronephrosis, perinephric pseudocysts and localized renal neoplasms, which are all amenable to surgical correction. In contrast, many (if not most) diseases have a guarded prognosis, although the rate of progression can be variable. Given such a spectrum of possible outcomes, it is important for the clinician to obtain a definitive diagnosis, so that correct advice can be given to the owner, and correct therapy can be provided.

In summary, abdominal palpation is a key step in the initial examination of any patient with suspected renal disease. Changes in renal morphology can be recognized, which may provide information on the underlying pathological processes of a particular disease condition. Such alterations most commonly imply a pathological process, and the most common abnormalities include renomegaly, decreased size and abnormal shape. In most cases, if a morphological abnormality is identified, further investigations are warranted in order to determine the exact cause and, ultimately, the prognosis.

Case examples

Case 1

Signalment
6-year-old neutered male domestic shorthair cat.

History
24–36-hour history which started with altered behaviour, ataxia, hysterical vocalization and tremors. Polydipsia, vomiting and collapse developed in the last 24 hours.

Physical examination
Marked bilateral renomegaly, with smooth contours.

Haematology
No abnormality detected.

Serum biochemistry

* Marked azotaemia (urea 164 mmol/l; reference range = 3.5–6.0 mmol/l; creatinine 3290 µmol/l; reference <140 µmol/l).
* Hypocalcaemia (2.03 mmol/l; reference range = 2.10–2.60 mmol/l).
* Hyperphosphataemia (6.70 mmol/l; reference range = 1.10–2.30 mmol/l).
* Mild hyperkalaemia (5.65 mmol/l; reference range = 3.80–5.30 mmol/l).

Urinalysis
Specific gravity 1.015, suggesting inappropriate renal concentrating ability in the face of such marked azotaemia. Sediment analysis revealed calcium oxalate crystals.

Acid–base status
High anion-gap metabolic acidosis.

Abdominal radiography
Bilateral renomegaly (Figure 4.20a).

Abdominal ultrasonography
Again bilateral renomegaly with some loss of corticomedullary definition (Figure 4.20b).

Outcome
At this stage the most likely differential diagnosis was ethylene glycol intoxication causing acute nephrosis (e.g. compatible history, presence of hypocalcaemia, presence of high anion-gap metabolic acidosis and findings on abdominal ultrasonography). Given that clinical signs had been evident for >8 hours, specific therapy for ethylene glycol was not indicated; instead, symptomatic therapy (e.g. intravenous fluids, antibacterials, gastric protectants, etc.) was administered. There was little change 24 hours after admission, and the owner elected to have the cat euthanased, and submitted for postmortem examination. The owners subsequently located a potential source of ethylene glycol exposure.

Postmortem examination
This revealed a mild to moderate periglomerular mixed inflammatory cell infiltrate; there was mild vacuolation of tubular epithelial cells, and multiple pale yellow crystals were evident within the tubular lumen (Figure 4.20c). Such findings confirmed acute nephrosis, secondary to ethylene glycol intoxication.

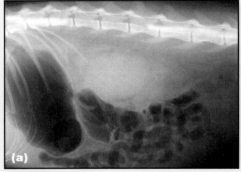 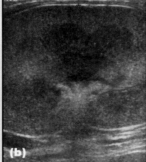 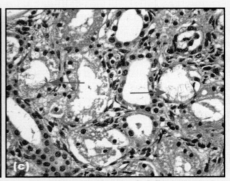

4.20 Images from a 6-year-old neutered male domestic shorthair cat with ethylene glycol toxicosis. **(a)** Right lateral abdominal radiograph demonstrating bilateral renomegaly. **(b)** Ultrasonogram of the left kidney, demonstrating renomegaly with some loss of corticomedullary definition. **(c)** Photomicrograph demonstrating mild vacuolation of renal tubular epithelial cells, and elongated pale yellow crystals within the tubular lumen (blue arrows). (H&E stain; original magnification X400.) ((a) and (b) courtesy of Anna Newitt, (c) courtesy of Gail Leeming, University of Liverpool.)

Case 2

Signalment
9-year-old neutered female Weimaraner.

History
Marked polydipsia and polyuria, nocturia and anorexia.

Physical examination
Discomfort on palpation of the craniodorsal abdomen.

Haematology
No abnormality detected.

Serum biochemistry
Mild azotaemia (urea 6.8 mmol/l; reference range = 3.5–6.0 mmol/l; creatinine 124 µmol/l; reference range = 20–110 µmol/l).

Urinalysis
Urine was collected by cystocentesis and was turbid on gross examination (see Figure 4.17b). Biochemical assessment demonstrated:

* pH 9.0
* Blood (+++)
* Protein 0.3 g/l
* An active sediment containing massive numbers of leucocytes (neutrophils) and bacterial rods and cocci (see Figure 4.17b). Intracellular bacteria were present in some of the leucocytes.

Case 2 continues ▶

Case 2 continued

Bacterial culture demonstrated a heavy, pure growth of haemolytic *Escherichia coli*, resistant to ampicillin and clindamycin, but sensitive to other antibiotics, including fluoroquinolones.

Abdominal ultrasonography

Renal pelvis dilation was evident in both kidneys, and both had poor corticomedullary definition.

Outcome

A presumptive diagnosis of pyelonephritis was made. The dog was treated with a 4-week course of enrofloxacin. Clinical signs rapidly resolved, and follow-up urine culture was negative both 7 days after the commencement of treatment, and 7 days after discontinuation.

References and further reading

Barr FJ, Holt PE and Gibbs C (1990) Ultrasonographic measurement of normal renal parameters. *Journal of Small Animal Practice* **31**, 180–184

Choi H, Won S, Chung W *et al.* (2003) Effect of intravenous mannitol upon the resistive index in complete unilateral renal obstruction in dogs. *Journal of Veterinary Internal Medicine* **17**, 158–162

Cowgill LD and Francey T (2005) Acute uremia. In: *Textbook of Veterinary Internal Medicine, 6th edn,* ed. SJ Ettinger and EC Feldman, pp. 1731–1751. WB Saunders, St. Louis

Ettinger SJ and Feldman EC (2005) *Textbook of Veterinary Internal Medicine, 6th edn.* WB Saunders, St. Louis

Hood JC, Savige J, Hendtlass A *et al.* (1995) Bull Terrier hereditary nephritis: a model for autosomal dominant Alport syndrome. *Kidney International* **47**, 758–765

Lees GE, Helman RG, Kashtan CE *et al.* (1998) A model of autosomal recessive Alport syndrome in English Cocker Spaniel dogs. *Kidney International* **54**, 706–719

Lingaas F, Comstock KE, Kirkness EF *et al.* (2003) A mutation in the canine BHD gene is associated with hereditary multifocal renal cystadenocarcinoma and nodular dermatofibrosis in the German Shepherd Dog. *Human Molecular Genetics* **12**, 3043–3053

Rivers BJ, Walter PA, Polzin DJ and King VL (1997) Duplex Doppler estimation of intrarenal Pourcelot resistive index in dogs and cats with renal disease. *Journal of Veterinary Internal Medicine* **11**, 250–260

Watson ADJ, Lefebvre HP, Concordet D *et al.* (2002) Plasma exogenous creatinine clearance test in dogs: comparison with other methods and proposed limited sampling strategy. *Journal of Veterinary Internal Medicine* **16**, 22–33

Young AE, Biller DS, Herrgesell EJ, Roberts HR and Lyons LA (2005) Feline polycystic kidney disease is linked to the PKD1 region. *Mammalian Genome* **16**, 59–65

Zheng K, Thorner PS, Marrano P, Baumal R and McInnes RR (1994) Canine X chromosome-linked hereditary nephritis: a genetic model for human X-linked hereditary nephritis resulting from a single base mutation in the gene encoding the alpha 5 chain of collagen type IV. *Proceedings of the National Academy of Sciences USA* **91**, 3989–3993

5

Uraemia

Richard A. Squires

Introduction

Uraemia may be defined as the constellation of adverse clinical effects that develops as a consequence of severe renal excretory failure (Figure 5.1). Uraemia should be distinguished from azotaemia. Azotaemia is defined as an increase in the concentration of non-protein nitrogenous waste products in blood. Creatinine and urea are examples of non-protein nitrogenous substances that are commonly measured in blood samples to assess renal excretory function. Azotaemia may arise as a consequence of:

- Inadequate renal blood perfusion (prerenal azotaemia)
- Intrinsic renal failure (renal azotaemia)
- Postrenal obstruction or rupture of the urinary tract (postrenal azotaemia).

Renal disease
Damage or functional impairment of the kidneys. Can vary in severity from very mild, to severe enough to cause uraemia
Renal insufficiency (stage I and early stage II kidney disease)
Renal functional impairment not severe enough to cause azotaemia, but sufficient to cause loss of renal reserve. These patients have a reduced ability to compensate for dehydration. Their urine-concentrating ability may be diminished
Azotaemia
An abnormal increase in the concentration of non-protein nitrogenous wastes (such as creatinine and urea nitrogen) in blood
Renal failure (late stage II to stage IV kidney disease)
Renal functional impairment sufficient to cause azotaemia. Urine-concentrating ability is usually impaired
Uraemia (usually stage III and stage IV kidney disease)
The constellation of adverse clinical signs caused by advanced renal failure, or (occasionally) other causes of severe azotaemia
Glomerular filtration rate (GFR)
The total volume of fluid filtered by all of the glomeruli in both kidneys per unit time. The GFR is directly proportional to the number of functioning nephrons and, therefore, the remaining functional renal mass

5.1 Definitions of terms used in nephrology and urology. See Chapter 11 for further details on the IRIS staging system for renal disease.

Mildly azotaemic patients do not have sufficient renal impairment to show signs of uraemia. For example, it is very unusual for uncomplicated prerenal azotaemia to be sufficiently severe to cause uraemia. However, all uraemic patients are azotaemic. The severity of uraemia depends not only upon the degree of renal impairment, but also upon the rate of deterioration. Rapid deterioration to a given degree of renal impairment will cause more severe clinical signs than gradual progression. Although azotaemia is a useful indicator of the presence of renal failure, it is important to remember that it is only a part of the complex metabolic and endocrine derangements that lead to uraemia.

Advanced chronic renal failure is the most common cause of uraemia. However, other conditions, such as acute renal failure, lower urinary tract obstruction and rupture of the urinary tract, occasionally cause it. Regardless of its cause, a profound reduction in renal excretory function leads inevitably to a characteristic clinical syndrome with disturbed function in many organ systems. Uraemia is not caused solely by the accumulation of metabolic waste products. Impairment of other important metabolic and endocrine renal functions contributes substantially to the observed clinical signs. Figure 5.2 lists clinical features associated with uraemia in dogs and cats.

There are many causes of uraemia. Having established that it is present, the clinician must try to identify a

Fluid, electrolyte and serum biochemical disturbances
Polyuria/polydipsia
Dehydration
Azotaemia
Hyperphosphataemia
Metabolic acidosis (acute >> chronic)
Elevated carbamylated haemoglobin (chronic > acute)
Hyperkalaemia or hypokalaemia
Hypercalcaemia or hypocalcaemia
Gastrointestinal disturbances
Anorexia
Vomiting (dogs >> cats)
Halitosis
Oral ulceration/stomatitis (Figure 5.3)
Gastritis, gastric ulceration, gastrointestinal bleeding

5.2 Clinical features associated with uraemia. (continues) ▶

Haematological disturbances

Normocytic, normochromic, non-regenerative anaemia

Platelet dysfunction/haemostatic disorder

Lymphopenia

Neutrophilia (with hypersegmentation)

Endocrine–metabolic disturbances

Negative nitrogen balance, with tissue protein catabolism and weight loss

Secondary hyperparathyroidism with enlarged parathyroid glands

Osteodystrophy

Peripheral insulin resistance and glucose intolerance

Hypertriglyceridaemia

Low triiodothyronine (T3)

Normal or slightly increased plasma cortisol and adrenocorticotropic hormone (ACTH) levels

Cardiovascular and pulmonary disturbances

Systemic arterial hypertension

Uraemic pneumonitis

Neuromuscular disturbances

Weakness

Lethargy

Depression

Hypokalaemic polymyopathy (cats)

Uraemic encephalopathy (poorly characterized)

Peripheral polyneuropathy (poorly characterized)

5.2 (continued) Clinical features associated with uraemia.

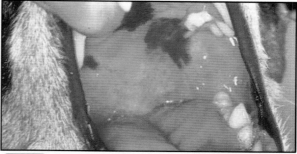

5.3 Dog with stomatitis secondary to acute and severe uraemia. (Courtesy of M Herrtage, University of Cambridge.)

specific underlying cause, in order to choose appropriate therapy and increase the accuracy of prognosis. The first requirement is to determine whether a particular patient's uraemia is due to intrinsic renal failure or some other cause, such as postrenal obstruction or rupture of the urinary tract. Most uraemic patients have intrinsic renal failure. If intrinsic failure is present, the second step is to determine whether it is acute or chronic, as this influences treatment and prognosis. Historical and physical examination findings, along with the results of various other diagnostic tests, are helpful in making the distinction. Once the cause of uraemia has been categorized as acute renal failure (ARF), chronic renal failure (CRF) or postrenal disease, the range of differential diagnoses is substantially narrowed and a specific diagnosis is much more easily approached. Figure 5.4 shows some frequently encountered pathways that lead to uraemia. Figure 5.5 lists a selection of differential diagnoses for uraemia categorized using the popular 'DAMNIT' scheme.

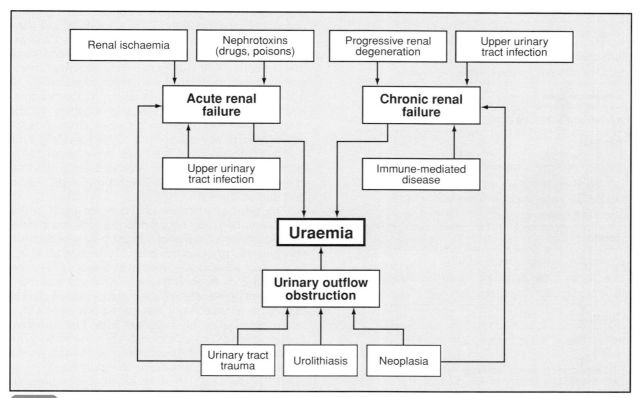

5.4 Principal pathways leading to the development of uraemia.

Degenerative
Advanced chronic interstitial nephritis → chronic renal failure
Renal infarcts → chronic renal failure
Congestive heart failure → chronic renal failure

Developmental
Familial renal dysplasia → chronic renal failure

Allergic
Anaphylactic shock → acute renal failure

Metabolic
Hypoadrenocorticism → hypovolaemic shock → acute renal failure
Hypercalcaemia → chronic renal failure
Metabolic disease → urolith formation → urinary outflow obstruction

Neoplastic
Bilateral renal lymphoma or carcinomas → chronic renal failure
Urethral or bladder neck transitional cell carcinoma → urinary outflow obstruction

Iatrogenic
Excessive vitamin D supplementation → hypervitaminosis D → hypercalcaemia → renal failure
Deep anaesthesia → arterial hypotension → renal ischaemia → acute renal failure
Relative or absolute overdose of nephrotoxic drugs (e.g. doxorubicin (in cats), aminoglycosides, cisplatin, amphotericin B, non-steroidal anti-inflammatory drugs) → renal failure
Surgical error: ligation of ureters during ovariohysterectomy → postrenal urinary obstruction

Idiopathic
Renal amyloidosis → chronic renal failure
Some forms of glomerulonephritis → chronic renal failure

Immune-mediated
Immune complex-mediated glomerulonephritis → chronic renal failure

Infectious
Pyelonephritis → chronic renal failure
Lyme (borreliosis) nephropathy → acute and chronic renal failure
Leptospirosis → acute and subacute renal failure
Septic shock → acute renal failure

Toxic
Ethylene glycol ingestion → acute renal failure
Easter lily, day lily, tiger lily ingestion → acute renal failure (cats)
Raisin/grape ingestion → acute renal failure (dogs)

Traumatic
Ruptured bladder, avulsed or ruptured ureters or urethra → urine retention
Fractured kidneys or haemorrhagic shock → acute renal failure

5.5 Examples of possible causes of uraemia categorized according to the 'DAMNIT' scheme.

Normal physiology and pathophysiology

The primary role of the kidneys is to maintain fluid and electrolyte homeostasis and to excrete nitrogenous wastes and excess acid (Michell, 2004). This is achieved in the normal animal by a process that involves ultrafiltration of large volumes of plasma, followed by selective reabsorption of more than 99% of the filtered fluid. The relatively small volume of residual filtrate that is not reabsorbed contains high concentrations of waste substances and is excreted as urine. The process of filtration and selective reabsorption is carried out by more than 400,000 functional units (termed nephrons) in each canine kidney and 190,000 in each feline kidney. Each nephron consists of a well vascularized glomerulus and a convoluted tubule. The glomerulus is the primary filtering unit of the nephron and the convoluted tubule is responsible for selective reabsorption of the glomerular ultrafiltrate. A variable amount of filtered water and solutes can be reabsorbed by the renal tubules, depending upon the needs of the body. If there are a sufficient number of functional tubules, urine can be substantially concentrated or diluted compared with plasma.

The overall *glomerular filtration rate* (GFR) of the kidneys is a useful measure of renal excretory capacity (see Chapter 9). If inadequate filtration occurs, nitrogenous wastes will accumulate in the body. As renal disease progresses towards renal failure, the number of functional nephrons and, therefore, the GFR decline. A normal animal has substantially more nephrons than are necessary for good health. Indeed, the number of functional nephrons and the GFR must fall below one third of normal before urine-concentrating ability is noticeably impaired. If the GFR declines to less than about 25% of normal, azotaemia develops. Uraemic patients frequently have a GFR that is less than 10% of that of a normal animal. Figure 5.6 shows how progression of renal damage usually leads sequentially to a loss of urine-concentrating ability, azotaemia and, eventually, to uraemia (see also Chapter 11 for details on staging of kidney disease). Dogs in renal failure are typically isosthenuric (urine specific gravity 1.008–1.012) whereas most cats retain some ability to concentrate urine and have urine specific gravities in the range 1.015–1.030 (DiBartola *et al.* 1987; Elliott and Barber, 1998).

The term uraemia, which connotes urine in the blood, was originally adopted to describe the clinical consequences of advanced renal failure because it was believed that accumulation of urea and other byproducts of protein metabolism was responsible for the observed clinical abnormalities. Although excretory failure is of prime importance in producing the clinical syndrome of uraemia, it has become apparent that other factors play an important role. For example, accumulation of 'uraemic toxins' may occur, not only as a result of excretory failure, but also as a consequence of the physiological responses to renal failure. Parathyroid hormone (PTH) is an example of a uraemic toxin that accumulates as part of a compensatory response to renal phosphorus retention (Barber and

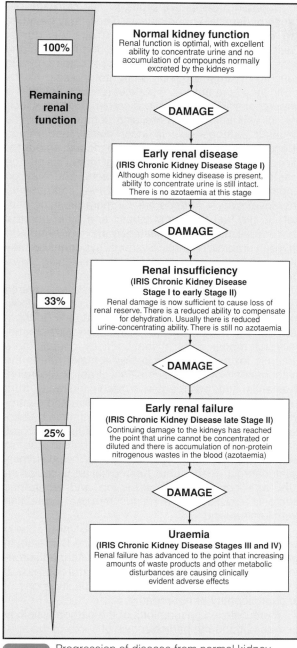

<table>
<tr><td>100%</td></tr>
</table>

Normal kidney function
Renal function is optimal, with excellent ability to concentrate urine and no accumulation of compounds normally excreted by the kidneys

DAMAGE

Early renal disease
(IRIS Chronic Kidney Disease Stage I)
Although some kidney disease is present, ability to concentrate urine is still intact. There is no azotaemia at this stage

DAMAGE

Renal insufficiency
(IRIS Chronic Kidney Disease Stage I to early Stage II)
Renal damage is now sufficient to cause loss of renal reserve. There is a reduced ability to compensate for dehydration. Usually there is reduced urine-concentrating ability. There is still no azotaemia

33%

DAMAGE

Early renal failure
(IRIS Chronic Kidney Disease late Stage II)
Continuing damage to the kidneys has reached the point that urine cannot be concentrated or diluted and there is accumulation of non-protein nitrogenous wastes in the blood (azotaemia)

25%

DAMAGE

Uraemia
(IRIS Chronic Kidney Disease Stages III and IV)
Renal failure has advanced to the point that increasing amounts of waste products and other metabolic disturbances are causing clinically evident adverse effects

Remaining renal function

5.6 Progression of disease from normal kidney function to advanced uraemia. See Chapter 11 for further discussion of the IRIS staging system.

Elliott, 1998). Compounds that accumulate in uraemia and are thought to contribute to the clinical syndrome are itemized in Figure 5.7. Although experiments intended to investigate the pathophysiological effects of isolated uraemic toxins are instructive, it is important to realize that uraemic toxins act together in a complex fashion to produce the broad repertoire of abnormalities that constitutes the uraemic syndrome.

Synthesis of the hormone calcitriol (active vitamin D_3; 1,25 dihydroxycolecalciferol) is normally completed by the renal proximal tubules. Failing kidneys synthesize an insufficient amount of calcitriol; in part because hyperphosphataemia inhibits its formation and in part because renal failure is associated with a loss of

Accumulating substance	Proposed adverse effects
Urea	Weakness, anorexia, vomiting, glucose intolerance, haemostatic disorder
Guanidino compounds: Guanidine (Di)methylguanidine Creatinine Creatine Guanidinoacetic acid Guanidinosuccinic acid	Weight loss, platelet dysfunction Guanidinosuccinic acid is thought to interfere with platelet factor III release
Aliphatic amines: Dimethylamine Trimethylamine	Uraemic breath odour, encephalopathy
Polyamines Spermine Spermidine	Spermine reduces erythropoiesis
'Middle molecules'	Uncertain, speculative role, many adverse effects have been hypothesized. 'Middle molecules' are poorly defined middle-sized molecular substances, with molecular weights in the range 500–2000 Daltons. They are larger than most of the other substances mentioned in this table. Their role in uraemia is uncertain. It has been hypothesized that middle-sized molecules are important uraemic toxins because peritoneal dialysis has been reported to be more efficacious than haemodialysis in the treatment of uraemia in some patients. Peritoneal dialysis is more effective than haemodialysis for the removal of middle-sized molecules, whereas haemodialysis is more effective for the removal of small molecules
Peptides and polypeptide hormones: Parathyroid hormone	Osteodystrophy, nephrotoxicity, impaired erythropoiesis, cardiotoxicity
Insulin	Hyperinsulinism may lead eventually to islet cell exhaustion and diabetes mellitus
Glucagon	Insulin resistance/glucose intolerance
Growth hormone	Insulin resistance/glucose intolerance
Gastrin	Hypergastrinaemia contributes to gastritis
Myoinositol	Neuropathy
Ribonuclease	Impaired erythropoiesis, decreased cellular proliferation
Cyclic adenosine monophosphate (cAMP)	Abnormal platelet function
Derivatives of the aromatic amino acids: Tryptophan Tyrosine Phenylalanine	Anorexia

5.7 Substances that accumulate in uraemia and are thought to contribute to the clinical syndrome.

proximal tubule cells. Calcitriol deficiency leads to impaired gastrointestinal calcium absorption, a tendency towards hypocalcaemia and compensatory renal secondary hyperparathyroidism. (See Nagode *et al.*, 1996; Polzin *et al.*, 2005; and Chapter 18 for further discussion of the pathological effects of PTH accumulation and the potential benefits of calcitriol therapy in renal failure.)

Erythropoietin synthesis is another endocrine function normally carried out by the kidneys. Failing kidneys sometimes synthesize and secrete an insufficient amount of this hormone. Since erythropoietin is essential for normal erythropoiesis, this relative or absolute deficiency leads eventually to anaemia, which is typically normocytic, normochromic and non-regenerative (King *et al.* 1992). Supplementation with exogenous human recombinant erythropoietin can help to correct the anaemia of chronic renal failure in dogs and cats (Polzin *et al.*, 2005) but use of this human protein, which differs somewhat from that found in dogs and cats, may lead to the development of erythropoietin-neutralizing antibodies and consequent refractory anaemia. Other less important causes of anaemia in uraemic patients include shortened red blood cell lifespan, inhibitors of erythropoiesis in uraemic plasma and gastrointestinal blood loss.

Failure of the kidneys to catabolize several polypeptide hormones can lead to hormone excess in uraemic patients, with consequent endocrine and metabolic derangements. Several peptides, polypeptides and small protein hormones are normally filtered by the glomerulus, reabsorbed by proximal tubule cells, and there degraded to their constituent amino acids. Gastrin, insulin, glucagon and growth hormone are examples of peptide hormones that accumulate because of failure of renal catabolism. Hypergastrinaemia may predispose to uraemic gastritis. Accumulation of glucagon and growth hormone contributes to the insulin resistance and postprandial hyperglycaemia seen in some uraemic patients.

Abnormal kidneys are known to play a primary role in the initiation and maintenance of systemic arterial hypertension in some mammalian species, but a detailed understanding of their role in pathogenesis remains elusive. Several studies suggest that systemic hypertension is a common complication of chronic renal disease in cats and, perhaps to a lesser extent, in dogs. Striking ocular manifestations of systemic hypertension (such as retinal detachment and choroidal and retinal haemorrhages) are sometimes observed during routine physical examination of hypertensive, uraemic cats and dogs. Indeed, hypertensive cats in chronic renal failure very often have ocular lesions that can be detected either during routine physical examination or fundoscopically (Syme *et al.*, 2002). Recent work suggests that systemic hypertension may worsen the prognosis for animals with chronic renal failure. Systemic hypertension is undoubtedly an important complication of renal disease in some dogs and cats, although its prevalence in uraemic animals remains uncertain because, in part, of differing opinions about suitable cut-off values (Michell *et al.*, 1997; Jacob *et al.*, 2003; see also Chapter 13).

Uraemic patients are prone to haemorrhage because of defective haemostasis. There may be bruising of the skin and bleeding from the gums. Gastrointestinal haemorrhage (causing melaena and occasionally haematemesis) is also common, with concurrent uraemic gastropathy contributing to the blood loss (see below). A platelet function defect is a feature of this haemostatic disorder. Platelet–blood vessel wall interactions are also compromised. The detailed pathogenesis is incompletely understood (Boccardo *et al.*, 2004). Typically, a modest amount of blood is lost from the gastrointestinal tract. This may be insufficient to cause obvious melaena and may go undetected. However, over time, it may contribute to the development of anaemia. Of more pressing concern is the fact that renal biopsy and other surgical procedures may be complicated by excessive haemorrhage in uraemic patients. Systemic hypertension may also contribute to the potential for life-threatening haemorrhage after biopsy in some patients.

Uraemia causes important gastrointestinal adverse effects. Vomiting is a frequent finding in uraemic dogs, but is less commonly seen in affected cats. Inappetence is seen in both species. Stimulation of the chemoreceptor trigger zone in the brain by one or more uraemic toxins is thought to play a major role in the pathogenesis of uraemic vomiting. Uraemic ulcerative stomatitis and gastroenteritis result indirectly from an increased urea concentration in saliva and gastrointestinal fluid. Urea is degraded to ammonia by bacterial urease and then ammonia causes mucosal damage. Other factors thought to contribute to uraemic ulcerative lesions in the alimentary tract include hypergastrinaemia, inadequate haemostasis, vascular injury with consequent obstruction and ischaemic necrosis, and defective gastric mucosal protection from luminal acid.

Uraemic encephalopathy and polyneuropathy are well recognized features of advanced uraemia in humans, seen in a minority of patients. Although uraemic dogs and cats are frequently weak and depressed, they do not typically manifest more specific signs of encephalopathy or neuropathy.

More detailed descriptions of the pathophysiology of uraemia and the pathogenesis of some of the specific disease syndromes that can cause uraemia (acute renal failure, chronic renal failure) have been previously published in the veterinary literature (Cowgill and Francey, 2005; Polzin *et al.*, 2005).

Diagnostic approach

Signalment
Although male and female cats and dogs of all ages and breeds may develop uraemia, consideration of the signalment of a uraemic patient (age, breed, sex and neutering status) can be instructive when attempting to determine the underlying cause(s) of the problem. For example, certain canine and feline breeds are prone to inherited familial nephropathies, which can cause proteinuria, uraemia or both (Figure 5.8) (DiBartola, 2005). In many familial nephropathies, the

Breed	Nature of the nephropathy
Abyssinian cat	Renal medullary amyloidosis. Usually presented at 1–5 years of age for signs of renal failure. Probably autosomal dominant inheritance with incomplete penetrance
Basenji	Fanconi syndrome (renal tubular defect). Usually presented at 1–5 years of age for PU/PD. May be seen with glucosuria and aminoaciduria before azotaemia develops. May develop acute renal failure or pyelonephritis
Beagle	Unilateral renal agenesis. Predisposes to the development of uraemia, if function of the solitary kidney is sufficiently compromised **also** Renal amyloidosis leading to progressive renal failure in some older Beagles (5–11 years)
Bull Terrier	Autosomal dominant hereditary nephritis (a homologue of human autosomal dominant Alport syndrome). Causes proteinuria and renal failure in dogs of variable age (11 months to 8 years)
Cairn Terrier	Congenital polycystic renal and hepatic disease. Usually presented at about 6 weeks of age for abdominal distension due to hepatomegaly and renomegaly, rather than for uraemia. Probably autosomal recessive
Cocker Spaniel	Tubular basement membrane collagen defect (Alport syndrome homologue). Usually presented at 6 months to 2 years of age for signs of uraemia
Dobermann	Basement membrane disorder. Usually presented at 1–2 years of age for signs of uraemia. May also manifest signs of nephrotic syndrome
Lhasa Apso and Shih Tzu	Progressive nephropathy. Usually presented at <6 years of age for signs of early renal failure or uraemia. Rate of progression of disease is very variable
Norwegian Elkhound	Glomerulopathy with interstitial fibrosis. Usually presented at 8 months to 5 years of age for signs of uraemia. May be glucosuric, despite normal blood glucose concentration
Persian cat	Autosomal dominant polycystic kidney disease (PKD). This has been reported to affect approximately 38% of Persian cats worldwide. Causes renal failure at 3–10 years of age. Can be diagnosed ultrasonographically in young cats
Samoyed	Progressive nephropathy. More common and more severe in males than females. Males are usually presented for signs of uraemia at less than 1 year of age; females for mild renal failure at about 5 years
Shar Pei	Renal amyloidosis. Usually are presented for signs of renal failure or uraemia at 1–6 years. Renal medulla and sometimes glomeruli are infiltrated
Soft-Coated Wheaten Terrier	Disorder of renal maturation with thin cortices and cortical cysts. Usually are presented at 5–30 months for signs of renal failure. Other SCWTs may be presented for signs of PLN and nephrotic syndrome, without uraemia
Standard Poodle	Cystic glomerular atrophy with immature glomeruli and tubular dilation/atrophy. Presented at 3 months to 2 years of age for signs of renal failure

5.8 Some breeds affected by familial nephropathies. This is not intended to be a comprehensive list (see Chapter 7 for further details). PLN = Protein-losing nephropathy; PU/PD = Polyuria/polydipsia; SCWT = Soft-Coated Wheaten Terrier.

kidneys are thought to be relatively normal at birth, with progressive deterioration in structure and function over the first months to years of life. Thus, patients with familial nephropathy tend to be relatively young when renal failure and uraemia ensue, although some familial diseases do not manifest until quite late in life. In contrast, patients with uraemia caused by various degenerative and neoplastic renal disorders tend to be middle-aged or older.

Severe upper urinary tract infection can cause or worsen uraemia. Bitches are more susceptible to bacterial urinary tract infections (UTI) than are male dogs. Cats with chronic renal failure are much more susceptible to UTI than cats with normal renal function. Less commonly, bacterial prostatitis can lead to pyelonephritis and, eventually, to uraemia in sexually intact male dogs.

History

A carefully elicited history may help not only to provide information that indicates the presence of uraemia, but to identify its underlying cause. A complete history will also help the clinician to identify any other health problems unrelated to renal function that might have a bearing on the overall prognosis for the patient.

The owner should be asked questions concerning the duration of the illness. A history of prolonged illness in a uraemic patient is more compatible with chronic renal failure than with acute failure, postrenal obstruction or rupture of the urinary tract. The owner of a dog or cat with chronic renal failure may report that the animal has had increased thirst and drinking (polydipsia) for some time, passes large volumes of pale-coloured urine (polyuria), and has begun to need to urinate in the middle of the night (nocturia). Later on, weight loss, inappetence, lethargy, halitosis and vomiting may be noticed. Often these problems progressively worsen over the weeks prior to presentation. The vomiting, in particular, may increase in frequency from once every few days to several times daily in uraemic dogs. Uraemic cats are less prone to vomit. Vomiting, when it occurs, is usually on an empty stomach. In some cases, the owner may not notice anything abnormal until the patient has advanced chronic renal failure. Such patients are usually presented for an apparently acute onset of anorexia, lethargy and vomiting; signs identical to those seen in acute uraemia (Cowgill and Francey, 2005). Further diagnostic evaluation will usually help to distinguish acute from chronic uraemia in such patients (discussed later in this chapter).

When patients are presented with acute signs, the owner should be carefully questioned about potential access to nephrotoxic substances. Ethylene glycol (in automotive antifreeze fluid) is a well known example of a highly nephrotoxic substance that has a sweet taste. Both dogs and cats will occasionally drink it, if allowed the opportunity. Malicious poisoning of dogs and cats with antifreeze fluid has occasionally been suspected or observed. Intoxication with this substance may cause vomiting and neurological signs (similar to drunkenness) 1–3 days before acute oliguric renal failure develops. Bear in mind that an owner may be completely unaware that an animal has had access to antifreeze fluid.

Several interesting new nephrotoxins have been identified recently (Stokes and Forrester, 2004). For example, ingestion of various lilies (day lily, tiger lily, Easter lily) has been shown to lead to acute renal failure in cats (Hadley *et al.*, 2003). Intriguingly, ingestion of large quantities of raisins and grapes has occasionally been associated with the development of acute renal failure in dogs (Gwaltney-Brant *et al.*, 2001).

Certain medications can cause acute renal failure and uraemia, especially if used inappropriately. The owner should be asked whether any medications have been used in the days and weeks preceding presentation with signs of uraemia. Drug data-sheets can be very useful when assessing the nephrotoxic potential of unfamiliar drugs, although manufacturers of some of the newer non-steroidal anti-inflammatory drugs (NSAIDs) may underplay the nephrotoxic potential of their products. Well known potentially nephrotoxic drugs include:

- Aminoglycoside antibiotics (e.g. gentamicin, amikacin)
- NSAIDs (both COX-1 and COX-2 inhibitors)
- Intravenous radiographic contrast agents
- Certain antineoplastic chemotherapeutic agents (e.g. cisplatin in dogs, doxorubicin in cats).

High-dose glucocorticoids and certain other immunosuppressant and antineoplastic drugs may predispose to upper urinary tract infection and consequent renal failure. See Cowgill and Francey (2005) for a more comprehensive list of potentially nephrotoxic medications.

General anaesthesia may be associated with a period of systemic arterial hypotension and impaired renal perfusion. This can lead to acute renal failure. A history of recent anaesthesia, or of any other potential cause of renal hypoperfusion (such as a recent traumatic event or a period of severe dehydration) should prompt the clinician to consider a diagnosis of acute renal failure in a patient showing signs of uraemia.

Evidence of lower urinary tract inflammation or obstruction may be apparent from the history. Straining to pass urine (stranguria), dramatically increased frequency of urination (pollakiuria) and apparent discomfort upon urination (dysuria) are signs of lower urinary tract disease. Uraemia in patients showing these clinical signs may be a consequence of urinary obstruction, or extension of disease from the lower to the upper urinary tract. Haematuria is less common in uraemic patients and less helpful in localizing the cause of uraemia, since it may be caused by disorders at all levels of the urinary tract. Some animals will bleed only at the very end of their urine stream, or drip blood from the vulva or penis at times other than urination; these signs reflect lower urinary tract or genital tract disease.

Some owners of animals with suspected uraemia may report that the animal shows signs of back pain. This can be caused by renal, perirenal or ureteral inflammation or obstruction.

Uraemic patients are frequently anaemic, and the owner may notice weakness or (less commonly) tachycardia and mucous membrane pallor. In patients with substantial gastrointestinal ulceration and haemorrhage, there may be a history of blood in the vomitus (haematemesis) or black, digested blood in the faeces (melaena). Diarrhoea is observed relatively infrequently. Patients with advanced protein-losing nephropathy and renal failure may be uraemic and may have peripheral subcutaneous oedema, ascites or pleural effusion (see also Chapter 6). The owner may notice swelling of the distal limbs, abdominal enlargement or dyspnoea. However, many dogs and cats with all of the other consequences of heavy proteinuria fail to develop oedema or body cavity effusions.

Systemic arterial hypertension can complicate uraemia and may cause a patient to develop intraocular haemorrhage. The owner may notice blood inside the eye or acute blindness.

Physical examination

A complete physical examination is essential in all patients suspected to be uraemic. Patients with chronic uraemia typically have a poor hair coat and evidence of loss of muscle mass. These signs are much less likely to be present in patients with acute uraemia, unless their acute uraemia is superimposed upon chronic illness. Uraemic patients usually have a normal or slightly low rectal temperature. Fever should prompt the clinician to consider pyelonephritis, urosepsis, neoplasia and other related or unrelated inflammatory disorders as differential diagnoses.

Uraemic patients are frequently dehydrated at the time of presentation, because of vomiting, anorexia, decreased water intake and continuing obligatory urinary losses in the face of an inability to concentrate urine maximally. Poor skin turgor, sunken eyes and pale, tacky mucous membranes are found in severely dehydrated animals. Pale mucous membranes may also be present in uraemic patients because of anaemia. Evaluation of the packed cell volume (PCV) and total plasma protein (TPP) will help to determine the relative contributions of anaemia and dehydration to any observed pallor (see below).

In addition to dryness and pallor, the oral mucous membranes may show areas of vascular injection and uraemic ulcers. The ulcers are most often found on those parts of the buccal mucosa that overlie the premolar and molar teeth. In dogs, there may also be necrosis and ulceration of the lateral margins and tip of the tongue. Some clinicians are able to smell a distinctive, acrid, metallic breath odour in uraemic patients.

Young, growing puppies with chronic uraemia (for example, caused by a familial nephropathy) may show evidence of fibrous osteodystrophy in their maxilla and mandibles. On palpation, the poorly mineralized bones are usually dramatically thickened compared with normal. Despite their increased thickness, the bones are abnormally flexible. The mandibles can be sprung together (so called 'rubber jaw') and the maxilla can be twisted sideways. These changes are not usually found in animals that become uraemic as adults.

Abdominal palpation may reveal kidneys of an abnormal size or shape. One or both of the kidneys may be found to be abnormally large on palpation. Possible explanations include:

- Renal neoplasia (lymphoma is usually bilateral, renal carcinoma is more likely to be unilateral)
- Hydronephrosis
- Perirenal cysts or haemorrhage
- Polycystic kidneys
- Renal haematoma
- Unilateral compensatory hypertrophy (if the other kidney is absent or hypofunctional)
- Acute renal inflammation (often associated with acute renal failure).

If the kidneys are abnormally small, chronic kidney disease should be suspected. Chronic interstitial nephritis, renal infarcts and consequent fibrosis are associated with a gradual reduction in renal size. Kidneys may be lumpy or irregular in shape because of neoplastic masses, cysts, haematomas, abscesses and infarcts. One or both of the kidneys may be painful. Pyelonephritis, acute hydronephrosis, large renal calculi or ureteral obstruction may cause pain on palpation of the kidneys or dorsal abdomen. Lower urinary tract inflammatory disorders often cause sufficient irritation that the patient will tense its abdomen and pass urine during palpation of the bladder. After emptying, the bladder feels extremely tight and small.

The bladder may feel abnormal in size, shape or consistency. Acute, complete urethral obstruction obviously leads rapidly to bladder distension. Postrenal azotaemia and uraemia follow within 24–72 hours. In this situation, the bladder is almost perfectly round and is very firm on palpation. Patients with a ruptured bladder usually (but not invariably) have an impalpable or empty bladder. Dehydrated, uraemic patients often have a large, normal-shaped bladder on palpation. This is because the bladder is full of dilute urine much of the time in these polydipsic, polyuric patients. Patients dehydrated for other reasons are less likely to have a big, full bladder. If there is any question about urethral patency, urethral catheterization should be carried out as an adjunct to the physical examination.

A rectal examination should be part of the physical examination of every animal with polydipsia, polyuria or suspected uraemia. The anal sacs should be palpated for the presence of a mass. Anal sac adenocarcinomas are not usually visible on direct, external inspection of the anus, but are readily appreciated on rectal palpation. These tumours usually cause paraneoplastic hypercalcaemia that can, in turn, cause polydipsia, polyuria, renal failure and uraemia. The pelvic floor should be examined for the presence of a urethral, prostatic or bladder neck mass. The sublumbar area should be palpated for the presence of lymphadenopathy. Calculi in the urinary bladder may be detected during caudal abdominal palpation. In medium to large dogs, carrying out bladder and rectal palpation simultaneously may increase the probability of detecting bladder calculi by palpation.

Fundoscopic examination will allow detection of hypertensive retinal lesions, if they are present. Dilation and tortuosity of retinal blood vessels, retinal haemorrhages, retinal detachments and hyphaema are features of severe systemic arterial hypertension. If such lesions are found, arterial blood pressure should be measured and other causes of the retinal lesions should be considered and ruled out. Ideally, arterial blood pressure should be measured as an adjunct to the physical examination in every patient with suspected renal disease (see Chapter 13).

Diagnostic tests

The history and physical examination may provide presumptive evidence that uraemia is present. Further diagnostic tests are required to confirm the presence of uraemia, determine its severity and discover its underlying cause. In patients suspected to be uraemic, it is particularly important to obtain samples of blood and urine *prior to* the initiation of any fluid therapy. Samples obtained later will not accurately reflect the urine-concentrating ability of the animal, nor the degree of azotaemia. Figure 5.9 shows a list of initial tests recommended for patients suspected to be uraemic, followed by some additional tests that may be indicated for particular patients. Figure 5.10 is a flow chart that offers a diagnostic approach to suspected uraemia.

Initial tests
History
Physical examination (including retinal and rectal examinations)
Urinalysis
Serum chemistry profile
Routine haemogram
Abdominal imaging (ultrasonography, radiography)
Arterial blood pressure measurement
Additional tests that may be indicated, depending upon the results of the initial tests
Urine bacterial or fungal culture
Screen for infectious agents: • FeLV ⎫   • FCoV ⎬ cats   • FIV ⎭   • *Leptospira* spp. (dogs)
Urine protein:creatinine ratio
Ultrasonography of the parathyroid glands
Chest radiographs
Excretory urography
Fractional excretions
Serum PTH and ionized calcium
Renal biopsy

5.8 Diagnostic tests indicated for canine and feline patients strongly suspected to be uraemic
FCoV = Feline coronavirus; FeLV = Feline leukaemia virus; FIV = Feline immunodeficiency virus; PTH = Parathyroid hormone.

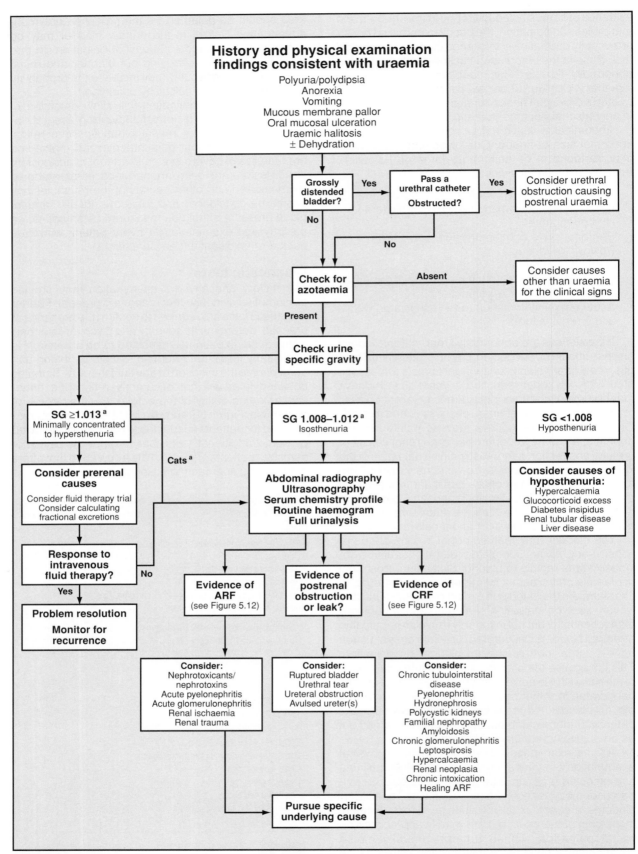

5.9 Initial diagnostic approach to suspected uraemia. [a] Many uraemic cats have urine specific gravity in the range 1.015–1.025 and a few are higher still. Therefore, a urine SG ≥1.013 in a cat should not impede the clinician from investigating for primary, intrinsic renal causes of uraemia. ARF = Acute renal failure; CRF = Chronic renal failure; SG = Specific gravity; UTI = Urinary tract infection.

Initial assessment

Shortly after a patient with suspected severe uraemia is presented, a urine sample should be collected (preferably by cystocentesis) and blood should be drawn for a routine haemogram and serum chemistry profile. If a microhaematocrit centrifuge or other suitable equipment is available in the practice, PCV/TPP should immediately be measured, to help assess hydration status and check for anaemia. Dipsticks are available for rapid measurement of blood urea and are still used in some practices. Although these are relatively inaccurate, they can be useful in an emergency setting to confirm or refute the presence of azotaemia within seconds. Samples from uraemic animals usually produce a very intense colour reaction compared with those from normal animals. The dipstick result can later be confirmed by serum chemistry profile.

Thus, within a few minutes of patient presentation, the clinician may have strong preliminary evidence that uraemia is present, and may have some hypotheses about its cause. In all cases, azotaemia should be present. The physical examination and PCV/TPP can help in the detection of anaemia and dehydration. The history and physical examination findings are likely to help distinguish patients with postrenal azotaemia from the others. The history, physical examination and urine specific gravity may help to rule in or rule out chronic renal failure. Most uraemic patients have chronic renal failure and will be severely azotaemic at presentation. Dogs in chronic renal failure are very likely to be isosthenuric whereas cats will be unable to concentrate their urine maximally, but may have a urine specific gravity of up to 1.025, and occasionally higher. Those with acute failure may be polyuric, oliguric or anuric; their urine specific gravity is uninformative. However, if they are acutely uraemic, such patients are likely to be feeling very ill indeed, so the history and physical examination can be diagnostically useful.

Urinalysis

Most uraemic patients are to some extent dehydrated. A dehydrated patient with normal renal function should be making concentrated urine. The finding of dilute, *isosthenuric* urine (urine with specific gravity 1.008–1.012, similar to that of plasma) in a dehydrated patient with historical and physical examination findings consistent with uraemia is strongly suggestive of renal failure. A urine sample should be collected early in the evaluation of patients suspected to be uraemic. For the purpose of measuring specific gravity, a free catch, catheter or cystocentesis sample is satisfactory. If the bladder is palpable, cystocentesis is a rapid,

clean means of obtaining urine from the bladder (see Chapter 8 for details). In patients with ascites, cystocentesis should be avoided or done under ultrasound guidance. The risk of significant haemorrhage from cystocentesis is small, even in patients with advanced uraemia.

A refractometer should be used for the measurement of urine specific gravity. Although dipsticks are available for urine specific gravity measurement, they are less reliable than refractometry. Patients with signs of uraemia and isosthenuric urine should undergo further diagnostic evaluation of renal function (see below). A dehydrated patient with highly concentrated urine is probably not in renal failure, so causes of prerenal azotaemia should first be considered. Trial fluid therapy should resolve or substantially improve the azotaemia if there is a significant prerenal component.

There are a few exceptions to the rule that isosthenuric urine in the face of dehydration indicates renal failure. Water-deprived patients with normal GFR, but deficient urine-concentrating ability, would have to be considered. Intrinsic renal tubular disease, diabetes insipidus, pyometra, hypercalcaemia, glucocorticoid excess, potent diuretic therapy and hypoadrenocorticism can all cause selective loss of tubular concentrating ability, despite normal glomerular filtration. The screening tests described in the following sections help to rule out these disorders. Sometimes the urine is *hyposthenuric* (specific gravity <1.008) in patients with these disorders. Hyposthenuria is evidence of active dilution of the glomerular filtrate by the renal tubules, and is not typical of renal failure or uraemia.

Apart from the essential specific gravity measurement, a full urinalysis is recommended for patients suspected to be uraemic (see Chapter 8 for details). Urine dipstick and sediment examination may reveal a cause of uraemia. Urine bacterial culture and, less commonly, fungal culture should be carried out if bacteriuria (bacteria in the urine), funguria (fungal elements in the urine) or unexplained pyuria (excessive numbers of white blood cells in the urine) is discovered on examination of the sediment of a cystocentesis or catheter-derived urine sample. Urine bacterial culture is indicated in patients with a completely normal urine sediment, especially if the urine is dilute, if urinary tract infection is suspected for other reasons. Patients with acute renal failure and uraemia are more likely to be glucosuric than patients with chronic failure (Gerber *et al.*, 2004), although glucosuria is by no means a consistent feature of acute failure. Figure 5.11 lists some urinalysis findings and their possible significance in patients suspected to be uraemic.

Finding	Significance
Hypersthenuric (concentrated) urine, SG >1.030	The patient probably does not have renal failure. If azotaemia is present, it is probably prerenal. If signs suggestive of uraemia are present, it is possible, but very unlikely, that the patient is uraemic because of severe prerenal azotaemia or peracute renal failure. First consider other causes for the signs that suggest uraemia
Minimally concentrated urine, 1.030≥ SG >1.012	The patient may have renal failure, particularly if it is a cat. If azotaemia is present, consider prerenal causes; also consider causes of reduced concentrating ability and other causes for the signs that suggest uraemia

5.11 Urinalysis findings and their significance in patients suspected from the history and physical examination to be uraemic. SG = Specific gravity; UPC = Urine protein:creatinine ratio; UTI = Urinary tract infection. (continues) ▶

Finding	Significance
Isosthenuric urine, 1.012≥ SG ≥1.008	If the patient is azotaemic, has signs of uraemia and does not have another identifiable cause for failure to concentrate urine, it is almost certainly in renal failure. The next step is to determine the cause
Hyposthenuric urine, SG <1.008	The renal tubules are actively diluting the glomerular filtrate, making renal failure less likely. Consider other causes of hyposthenuric urine, especially if the SG is well below 1.008. These include hypercalcaemia, hyperadrenocorticism, central diabetes insipidus and severe liver disease
Heavy proteinuria on the dipstick	Check the rest of the dipstick and the urine sediment. The patient may have a protein-losing nephropathy that has progressed to renal failure and uraemia. A UPC is indicated to confirm and build upon the dipstick result (see Chapter 6)
Glucosuria	In animals with normal blood glucose and signs of uraemia, glucosuria may indicate proximal renal tubular dysfunction. It is seen in some dogs with familial renal tubular disorders. Otherwise, it is more likely to be seen in patients with acute than chronic uraemia
Bacteria and white blood cells on urine sediment examination (cystocentesis or catheter-derived urine sample)	In a patient with signs of uraemia, bacterial UTI may be the cause of renal failure (pyelonephritis) or may be a secondary complication. Urine culture and sensitivity is indicated. Antibiotic therapy (with a broad-spectrum drug) should be started, pending the results
Cylindruria (excessive numbers of casts on urine sediment examination)	Casts are cylindrical moulds of the renal tubular lumina, made of proteins and cells. Toxic, infectious, ischaemic and traumatic renal lesions can lead to cast formation. In general, casts suggest an active, acute cause of uraemia. Hyaline casts usually indicate heavy albuminuria (see Chapter 8)

5.11 (continued) Urinalysis findings and their significance in patients suspected from the history and physical examination to be uraemic. SG = Specific gravity; UPC = Urine protein:creatinine ratio; UTI = Urinary tract infection.

Serum chemistry profile

When the serum chemistry profile results become available, the most important parameters to evaluate are:

- Creatinine
- Urea
- Phosphorus
- Potassium
- Calcium.

Urea and creatinine: Serum urea and creatinine concentrations are commonly measured in clinical situations to determine renal function. Both creatinine and urea are excreted by glomerular filtration, thus the concentration of each in blood, plasma or serum tends to vary inversely with the GFR. Urea is produced in the liver from ammonia and its serum concentration tends to increase in various catabolic disease states, after high-protein meals and after gastrointestinal haemorrhage. Serum urea concentration is decreased in liver failure, after prolonged fasting and after feeding a low-protein diet. These changes are unassociated with changes in renal function, and tend to diminish the accuracy of serum urea concentration as a predictor of GFR. Another problem is that urea is reabsorbed by the renal tubules, particularly in dehydrated patients. This means that evaluation of serum urea alone may lead to a tendency to underestimate the GFR, and to overestimate the degree of renal functional impairment in dehydrated patients.

The serum concentration of creatinine is less affected by dietary and other non-renal factors. Creatinine is produced at a constant daily rate from muscle. It is freely filtered by the glomeruli and excreted in urine. Since a constant amount is produced and excreted daily, the serum creatinine concentration (SC) more accurately reflects GFR than does serum urea. However, in advanced renal failure, a small amount of renal tubular secretion of creatinine occurs in male dogs; and in both dogs and cats, some creatinine may be catabolized in the large intestine. Cachectic animals produce less creatinine daily because of their reduced muscle mass. Under these circumstances of advanced renal failure, SC may slightly underestimate the degree of renal failure.

The magnitude of serum creatinine and urea elevation should not be relied upon to distinguish the various causes of uraemia; however, a few points are worthy of note. Uncomplicated prerenal azotaemia tends not to become quite so severe as the renal and postrenal forms. SC rarely exceeds 600 µmol/l (6.78 mg/dl) in this form of azotaemia. Of course, animals with severe prerenal azotaemia frequently go on to develop acute intrinsic renal failure unless they are appropriately treated; if this happens SC can become much higher. Complete postrenal obstruction can lead to a staggeringly high SC – the highest value the author recalls was 2640 µmol/l (29.8 mg/dl) in a male cat with urethral obstruction. Patients with chronic renal failure are usually first presented for veterinary attention with uraemic signs when their SC is in the range 260–700 µmol/l (2.9–7.9 mg/dl) (stage III–IV renal disease). The severity of clinical signs does not correlate well with the SC within this range. Animals with acute renal failure generally appear more ill at a given SC than animals with chronic failure and the same degree of azotaemia.

Phosphorus: Hyperphosphataemia can be a feature of all forms of azotaemia. Its association with metabolic bone disease (renal osteodystrophy) is a feature of chronic kidney disease and should be treated appropriately (see Chapter 18).

Potassium: Hyperkalaemia is a feature of advanced postrenal azotaemia, and oliguric or anuric acute renal failure. It is also seen in end-stage chronic renal failure. If severe, this electrolyte disturbance is life-threatening and requires prompt attention (see Chapter 17).

Hypokalaemia is present in some patients with chronic renal failure, particularly cats. It causes weakness, inappetence and occasionally polymyopathy (Dow *et al.*, 1987). Hypokalaemia should be treated using parenteral or enteral potassium supplementation.

Calcium: The total serum calcium may be high, low or normal in uraemic patients. Total calcium does not always accurately reflect the physiologically active ionized calcium fraction in this patient group. Complexed forms of calcium increase in the plasma of uraemic patients, so that the ionized calcium fraction may be low or normal in the face of a slightly elevated total calcium concentration. Usually the serum total calcium concentration is sufficiently close to normal that it does not justify further investigation. A serum total calcium concentration over 3.3 mmol/l (13.2 mg/dl) in a uraemic patient warrants further investigation, in case hypercalcaemia is the cause rather than a consequence of renal failure.

Haemogram

Haematological findings may help to guide the clinician towards one or other of the possible causes of uraemia. Chronic renal failure is frequently associated with a moderately severe, normocytic, normochromic, non-regenerative anaemia. Acute renal failure and postrenal causes of azotaemia are less frequently associated with anaemia, although anaemia may develop as a consequence of acute uraemic gastrointestinal bleeding. The anaemia of chronic renal failure is primarily due to a failure of red blood cell production, rather than accelerated destruction or loss. Given the relatively long lifespan of a red blood cell, anaemia of renal failure may take weeks to months to develop.

Although the PCV of a patient with chronic uraemia may be normal at the time of initial presentation, it frequently declines into the low range after correction of dehydration. Assessment of the TPP at the same time as the PCV will allow early recognition of anaemia in dehydrated patients, assuming they do not have concurrent hypoproteinaemia. The lymphopenia and mild neutrophilia seen in some uraemic patients are not useful in discriminating different causes of uraemia. Moderate to severe neutrophilia, particularly if toxic changes are evident in the neutrophils, may indicate an upper urinary tract infection or urosepsis.

Imaging studies

Abdominal radiography or ultrasonography is indicated in the investigation of all patients suspected to be uraemic. Kidney size is the first parameter to assess. Small kidneys are typical of advanced chronic renal failure whereas normal-sized or slightly large kidneys are typically found in patients with acute failure. Small kidneys may be normal in shape, or

may be irregular in outline as a consequence of cysts, infarcts and areas of fibrosis. If one or both of the kidneys is abnormally large, acute renal inflammation, renal haematoma, renal neoplasia, hydronephrosis and various forms of renal and perirenal cysts should be considered as diagnoses. Abdominal ultrasonography is extremely useful for distinguishing the various causes of abnormally sized and shaped kidneys since it permits evaluation of the internal architecture of the kidneys. Certain causes of uraemia (for example ethylene glycol intoxication) produce very characteristic ultrasonographic changes (see Chapter 10).

Abdominal images should be scrutinized for the presence of urinary calculi. Cystic calculi are not usually associated with uraemia in dogs and cats, but bilateral ureteral calculi occasionally cause hydroureter, urinary outflow obstruction and postrenal azotaemia. In one recent study, 76% of cats diagnosed with *unilateral* ureteral calculi were azotaemic at presentation (Kyles *et al.*, 2005a,b). Prerenal azotaemia or pre-existing, bilateral renal disease were considered possible causes. The contralateral kidney was found to be small in 56% of those cats that were checked, and dilation of the contralateral renal pelvis or ureter was observed in 37%, strengthening an argument that pre-existing damage was present in the contralateral kidney. Although serum creatinine concentration decreased in most of the cats that were treated, it remained high in approximately half of treated cats 6–12 months later. Taken together, these findings indicate that postobstructive or primary parenchymal disease is often present in the contralateral kidneys of cats presented for unilateral ureterolithiasis. These observations are important because calcium oxalate ureterolithiasis has been diagnosed with increasing frequency in recent years.

Renal calculi may be associated with pyelonephritis. Radiolucent urinary calculi can be imaged ultrasonographically or by positive- or double-contrast excretory urography.

Ultrasonography can be used to assess the size of the parathyroid glands, if a suitable high-resolution transducer is available. Dogs with chronic renal failure have been found to have larger glands than dogs of a similar body weight that were clinically normal, or in acute renal failure (Reusch *et al.*, 2000).

Abdominal imaging is also useful for the detection of leakage from the urinary tract. If the bladder or cranial urethra is ruptured, there may be evidence of intrapelvic soft tissue swelling, caudal peritonitis and (later) gross ascites. A ruptured or avulsed ureter may, in addition, cause retroperitoneal swelling. Positive-contrast radiographic studies and ultrasonography can help to localize the source of leakage.

Chest radiographs are indicated if cardiorespiratory signs are present or if renal neoplasia is suspected. Systemic arterial hypertension may cause cardiac enlargement. Advanced uraemia is occasionally associated with diffuse pulmonary calcification and a form of pneumonitis characterized by patchy alveolar and diffuse interstitial pulmonary infiltrates.

Fractional excretions and 'test' fluid therapy

Whenever uraemia is suspected, it is essential to try to categorize it as prerenal, renal or postrenal in origin. Combinations of these are also encountered in some patients. In most cases categorization is relatively straightforward but clinicians will occasionally encounter a uraemic patient with non-renal illness(es), or unknown or unconsidered drug exposure, which presents a greater diagnostic challenge than usual. In particular, drugs and non-renal illnesses that cause isosthenuria in the face of dehydration may mislead the unwary clinician into diagnosing intrinsic renal failure when the problem is, in fact, prerenal.

Calculation of the fractional excretion (FE) of various substances in urine (e.g. sodium) has long been suggested as a way to distinguish acute intrinsic renal failure from severe prerenal azotaemia (see Chapter 9). The formula for this calculation is as follows:

$$FE_x = \frac{[U]x \times [P]\text{creatinine}}{[P]x \times [U]\text{creatinine}}$$

Classically, prerenal azotaemia is associated with avid retention of sodium and low FE. However, it is important to emphasize that some non-renal illnesses and drugs can cause prerenal azotaemia combined with excessive natriuresis (renal sodium loss). Renal sodium wasting (i.e. a high FE of sodium, FE_{Na}) is one of the diagnostic criteria commonly listed as useful for identifying acute intrinsic renal failure and distinguishing it from prerenal azotaemia. To complicate matters further, there are several forms of acute intrinsic renal failure that are associated with a low or normal, rather than a high, FE_{Na}. Here are a few examples from human medicine, not all of which have been confirmed in dogs and cats:

- Radiographic contrast agent-induced nephropathy
- Acute glomerulonephritis
- Sepsis-induced acute tubular necrosis
- Obstructive uropathy.

Clinicians should therefore be careful not to accept uncritically FE_{Na} test results and should not narrow down on a diagnosis of acute intrinsic renal failure without thoroughly excluding the possibility of polyuric prerenal disease or drug exposure.

Fortunately, prerenal azotaemia can be distinguished from acute intrinsic renal failure in many patients simply by providing generous intravenous fluid therapy and monitoring to see whether the azotaemia promptly and completely resolves. If it does so in 24–48 hours, the problem was most likely prerenal. If it is considered inappropriate or unsafe to use 'test' fluid therapy in a particular patient (for example, one with unstable congestive heart failure) then other approaches can be taken. The urine:serum creatinine ratio should be >20 in animals with prerenal azotaemia and <10 in animals with acute intrinsic renal failure. In human medicine, the fractional excretion of urea (FE_{Urea}) has recently been found to be superior to FE_{Na} for distinguishing patients with prerenal azotaemia that are receiving loop diuretics from those with acute intrinsic renal failure caused by renal tubular necrosis (Carvounis *et al.*, 2002).

Renal biopsy

Renal biopsy allows the collection of tissue for histopathological and (less commonly) microbiological assessment. It is the most reliable way to obtain a specific diagnosis and prognosis. Like many diagnostic tests, renal biopsy should be reserved for situations in which it is considered likely that the results will alter the approach to patient management. In uraemic dogs and cats, renal biopsy is best reserved for the following situations:

- Renal neoplasia is suspected
- Acute renal failure has been diagnosed but the cause remains obscure
- Severe acute renal failure has been diagnosed and the owner needs a more accurate prognosis to help decide about further management
- History, physical examination and other diagnostic tests have failed to elucidate whether the patient has acute renal failure, chronic renal failure or acute failure superimposed on chronic renal disease
- A familial nephropathy is suspected and there are considerations beyond the needs of the individual animal
- The patient is heavily proteinuric as well as uraemic and the owner is seriously considering specific, biopsy-tailored therapy for the protein-losing nephropathy, despite the fact that renal failure is already well advanced.

Occasionally, in challenging diagnostic situations, renal biopsy may be needed to help distinguish acute from chronic renal failure, or to establish whether chronic renal disease underlies acute failure. If the patient is known to be in acute failure, biopsy results can sometimes be useful to identify a specific diagnosis and help prognosticate. Histological examination of the renal tubular basement membranes can help with prognostication. Infrequently, sequential biopsies may be used to monitor patient progress and response to therapy; however, this is rarely appropriate in uraemic animals.

Renal biopsy is usually carried out by the percutaneous route under ultrasound guidance (see Chapter 12). Since the procedure carries a certain risk of haemorrhage and other complications, it is best carried out by an experienced individual and should only be done after the informed consent of the owner has been obtained. Biopsy specimens can be submitted for histopathological examination and (if appropriate) for bacterial or fungal culture.

Unfortunately, renal biopsy results often have little positive impact on patient management because uraemic dogs and cats often have quite advanced, irreversible renal disease at the time of first presentation. Renal biopsy is discussed in detail in Chapter 12.

Screening for infectious diseases

In cats, feline leukaemia virus (FeLV), feline immunodeficiency virus (FIV) and feline coronavirus (FCoV; causes feline infectious peritonitis, FIP) can all cause renal disease and, eventually, uraemia. FeLV may cause immunodeficiency, predisposing to pyelonephritis, or may induce renal lymphoma. However, most cats with renal lymphoma show no clinical evidence of infection with FeLV. Human immunodeficiency virus (HIV) infection is associated with a distinctive protein-losing nephropathy with rapid progression to uraemia (Schwartz and Klotman, 1998). There is gathering evidence that FIV may produce a similar disease in cats (Poli *et al.*, 1995a,b). FCoV can cause a non-effusive form of disease, characterized by granulomatous inflammation in several organs. The kidneys are frequently involved. Serological testing for these infectious agents may be helpful in the diagnosis of some uraemic cats. However, renal biopsy will be required to confirm the diagnosis in most cases.

Several 'exotic' serovars of *Leptospira interrogans* and *L. kirschneri* have been implicated as causes of acute and subacute renal failure in dogs (Ward *et al.*, 2004a,b). Affected patients may have no icterus or other evidence of hepatic involvement. In one report, glucosuria was detected in more than half of the affected dogs, suggesting proximal renal tubular damage. Diagnosis is usually based upon serological evidence, often with the support of renal biopsy findings. Leptospirosis should be considered in the differential diagnosis of all canine patients with acute and subacute renal failure, regardless of vaccination status. Appropriate precautions should be taken by veterinary staff and owners handling urine from these animals.

In some parts of the world, *Borrelia burgdorferi* has been reported to cause a rapidly progressive nephropathy characterized by heavy proteinuria, worsening azotaemia and, eventually, uraemia (Dambach *et al.*, 1997).

Prognosis

The prognosis for uraemic patients is heavily dependent upon the underlying cause. The diagnostic process described above should enable the clinician to categorize the uraemia as prerenal, renal or postrenal.

Prerenal uraemia (which is rare) responds well to intravenous fluid therapy and carries a good prognosis for complete recovery. This is true so long as acute intrinsic renal failure has not supervened as a consequence of renal ischaemia.

Postrenal uraemia carries a good prognosis, as long as the urinary outflow obstruction can be relieved, and the patient can be successfully managed through the uraemic crisis. Hyperkalaemia and acidosis can be life-threatening in this situation, and must be managed appropriately (see Chapter 17). Like prerenal causes of uraemia, postrenal disorders can lead to acute intrinsic renal failure. If this happens, the prognosis is worsened substantially.

Intrinsic renal causes of uraemia should be divided into acute renal failure and chronic renal failure. Figure 5.12 shows clinical features that help in distinguishing one from the other. Acute renal failure carries a better prognosis than chronic renal failure for recovery of renal function, since there is a chance that tubular regeneration will occur in the days and weeks following the crisis. However, patients with acute renal failure are often extremely ill at the time of presentation and can be challenging to manage through the crisis. The prognosis for acute renal failure patients depends upon the severity and the nature of the acute renal damage. Response to therapy is the most reliable prognostic indicator. In oliguric or anuric patients, failure to produce urine after appropriate fluid therapy and rehydration is a strong negative prognostic indicator. Renal biopsy can help to determine the probability of recovery from acute renal failure. If the renal tubular basement membranes are destroyed, there is little chance of renal tubular regeneration. Unfortunately, this sort of determination may require electron microscopy. Overall, the prognosis for patients with acute renal failure is guarded to poor.

Acute	Chronic
There is often a history of perfect health until very recently. There may be a history of recent anaesthesia, or exposure to a toxin or nephrotoxic drug	A history of weeks to months of polyuria/polydipsia can often be elicited. Low-grade vomiting (several times a week) may also have been occurring for some time
The patient is usually in good body condition, but feels extremely ill relative to the degree of azotaemia	Chronic history of weight loss and relatively mild clinical signs for the degree of azotaemia
Kidneys are usually normal-sized or large. They may be swollen and/or painful	The kidneys are usually (but not invariably) small and non-painful
Anaemia is not usually present, unless acute gastrointestinal haemorrhage occurs	Non-regenerative anaemia is often a feature
Hyperkalaemia and metabolic acidosis are often present.	Hyperkalaemia is absent until terminal acute exacerbation occurs. Metabolic acidosis is mild or absent
Urine sediment is often very 'active' with casts, cells, debris etc., coming from the kidneys	Usually the urine sediment is inactive although hyaline casts may be seen in dogs where chronic failure is complicated by heavy proteinuria
These patients are often anuric or oliguric, but aminoglycoside overdose and other intoxications can cause *polyuric* acute renal failure. Urine specific gravity is NOT helpful in distinguishing acute from chronic failure	These patients are usually polyuric until the very terminal stages. Urine specific gravity is NOT helpful in distinguishing chronic from acute failure
Acute renal failure may be reversible, if the patient can be supported through the crisis	Chronic renal failure is irreversible, although correction of any prerenal component may reduce the degree of azotaemia and other management steps can substantially improve quality of life

5.12 Clinical features that help in distinguishing acute from chronic renal failure.

Chronic renal failure is associated with irreversible, usually progressive, renal damage, so the prognosis for improvement of renal function is poor. Despite this, medical management of chronic renal failure can substantially reduce the severity of uraemia and improve length and quality of life. There is often a substantial prerenal component to the azotaemia in newly presented chronic renal failure patients, so rehydration may help to reduce the severity of the uraemic signs. Identification and treatment of any complicating factors (such as urinary tract infection and systemic arterial hypertension) are important and will improve the long-term prognosis. Once these complicating factors are dealt with, the prognosis for good quality life depends on the extent or *stage* of chronic renal disease. Staging of chronic renal disease is covered in Chapter 11 and elsewhere (Polzin *et al.*, 2005). Medical management of chronic renal failure is discussed in Chapter 18 and elsewhere (Krawiec, 1996; Cowgill, 2003; Fischer *et al.*, 2004; Lane, 2005; Langston and Ludwig, 2005; Polzin *et al.*, 2005). Renal transplantation, an emerging management option for intrinsic renal failure, is described elsewhere (Langston and Ludwig, 2005).

Editors' note

With the exception of Chapters 5 and 9, the term chronic renal failure has been discarded in favour of the term chronic kidney disease. Where the severity of the chronic kidney disease needs quantification, this has been provided using the IRIS system (see Chapter 11). This Chapter uses renal failure (both acute and chronic) to indicate the presence of uraemia. In both Figures 5.1 and 5.6 we have indicated how these terms relate to the IRIS classification of chronic kidney disease.

References and further reading

Barber PJ and Elliott J (1998) Feline chronic renal failure: calcium homeostasis in 80 cases diagnosed between 1992 and 1995. *Journal of Small Animal Practice* **39**, 108–116

Boccardo P, Remuzzi G and Galbusera M (2004) Platelet dysfunction in renal failure. *Seminars in Thrombosis and Hemostasis* **30**, 579–589

Carvounis CP, Nisar S and Guro-Razuman S (2002) Significance of the fractional excretion of urea in the differential diagnosis of acute renal failure. *Kidney International* **62**, 2223–2229

Cowgill LD (2003) Advanced therapeutic approaches for the management of uraemia - 'the met and unmet needs'. *Journal of Feline Medicine and Surgery* **5**, 57–67

Cowgill LD and Francey T (2005) Acute uremia. In: *Textbook of Veterinary Internal Medicine, 6th edn,* ed. SJ Ettinger and EC Feldman, pp. 1731–1751. Elsevier Saunders, St. Louis

Dambach DM, Smith CA, Lewis RM and Van Winkle TJ (1997) Morphologic, immunohistochemical, and ultrastructural characterization of a distinctive renal lesion in dogs putatively associated with *Borrelia burgdorferi* infection: 49 cases (1987–1992). *Veterinary Pathology* **34**, 85–96

DiBartola SP (2005) Familial renal disease in dogs and cats. In: *Textbook of Veterinary Internal Medicine, 6th edn,* ed. SJ Ettinger and EC Feldman, pp. 1819–1824. Elsevier Saunders, St. Louis

DiBartola SP, Rutgers HC, Zack PM and Tarr MJ (1987) Clinicopathologic findings associated with chronic renal disease in cats: 74 cases (1973–1984). *Journal of the American Veterinary Medical Association* **190**, 1196–1202

Dow SW, LeCouteur RA, Fettman MJ and Spurgeon TL (1987) Potassium depletion in cats: hypokalemic polymyopathy. *Journal of the American Veterinary Medical Association* **191**, 1563–1568

Elliott J and Barber PJ (1998) Feline chronic renal failure: clinical findings in 80 cases diagnosed between 1992 and 1995. *Journal of Small Animal Practice* **39**, 78–85

Fischer JR, Pantaleo V, Francey T and Cowgill LD (2004) Veterinary hemodialysis: advances in management and technology. *Veterinary Clinics of North America: Small Animal Practice* **34**, 935–967, vi–vii

Gerber B, Glaus TM, Unterer S and Reusch CE (2004) Evaluation of parameters for the differentiation of acute from chronic renal failure in the dog. *SAT, Schweizer Archiv fur Tierheilkunde* **146**, 365–373

Gwaltney-Brant S, Holding JK, Donaldson CW, Eubig PA and Khan SA (2001) Renal failure associated with ingestion of grapes or raisins in dogs. *Journal of the American Veterinary Medical Association* **218**, 1555–1556

Hadley RM, Richardson JA and Gwaltney-Brant SM (2003) A retrospective study of daylily toxicosis in cats. *Veterinary and Human Toxicology* **45**, 38–39

Jacob F, Polzin DJ, Osborne CA *et al.* (2003) Association between initial systolic blood pressure and risk of developing a uremic crisis or of dying in dogs with chronic renal failure. *Journal of the American Veterinary Medical Association* **222**, 322–329

King LG, Giger U, Diserens D and Nagode LA (1992) Anemia of chronic renal failure in dogs. *Journal of Veterinary Internal Medicine* **6**, 264–270

Krawiec DR (1996) Managing gastrointestinal complications of uremia. *Veterinary Clinics of North America: Small Animal Practice* **26**, 1287–1292

Kyles AE, Hardie EM, Wooden BG *et al.* (2005a) Clinical, clinicopathologic, radiographic, and ultrasonographic abnormalities in cats with ureteral calculi: 163 cases (1984–2002). *Journal of the American Veterinary Medical Association* **226**, 932–936

Kyles AE, Hardie EM, Wooden BG *et al.* (2005b) Management and outcome of cats with ureteral calculi: 153 cases (1984–2002). *Journal of the American Veterinary Medical Association* **226**, 937–944

Lane IF (2005) Nutritional management of urinary tract conditions. In: *Textbook of Veterinary Internal Medicine, 6th edn,* ed. SJ Ettinger and EC Feldman, pp. 584–586. Elsevier Saunders, St. Louis

Langston CE and Ludwig LL (2005) Renal transplantation. In: *Textbook of Veterinary Internal Medicine, 6th edn,* ed. SJ Ettinger and EC Feldman, pp. 1752–1756. Elsevier Saunders, St. Louis

Michell AR (2004) Physiology and pathophysiology of the internal environment. In: *Veterinary Pathophysiology,* ed. RH Dunlop and C-H Malbert, pp. 3–23. Blackwell Publishing, Ames

Michell AR, Bodey AR and Gleadhill A (1997) Absence of hypertension in dogs with renal insufficiency. *Renal Failure* **19**, 61–68

Nagode LA, Chew DJ and Podell M (1996) Benefits of calcitriol therapy and serum phosphorus control in dogs and cats with chronic renal failure. Both are essential to prevent or suppress toxic hyperparathyroidism. *Veterinary Clinics of North America: Small Animal Practice* **26**, 1293–1330

Poli A, Abramo F, Matteucci D *et al.* (1995a) Renal involvement in feline immunodeficiency virus infection: p24 antigen detection, virus isolation and PCR analysis. *Veterinary Immunology and Immunopathology* **46**, 13–20

Poli A, Falcone ML, Bigalli L *et al.* (1995b) Circulating immune complexes and analysis of renal immune deposits in feline immunodeficiency virus-infected cats. *Clinical and Experimental Immunology* **101**, 254–258

Polzin DJ, Osborne CA and Ross S (2005) Chronic kidney disease. In: *Textbook of Veterinary Internal Medicine, 6th edn,* ed. SJ Ettinger and EC Feldman, pp. 1756–1785. Elsevier Saunders, St. Louis

Reusch CE, Tomsa K, Zimmer C *et al.* (2000) Ultrasonography of the parathyroid glands as an aid in differentiation of acute and chronic renal failure in dogs. *Journal of the American Veterinary Medical Association* **217**, 1849–1852

Schwartz EJ and Klotman PE (1998) Pathogenesis of human immunodeficiency virus (HIV)-associated nephropathy. *Seminars in Nephrology* **18**, 436–445

Stokes JE and Forrester SD (2004) New and unusual causes of acute renal failure in dogs and cats. *Veterinary Clinics of North America: Small Animal Practice* **34**, 909–922, vi

Syme HM, Barber PJ, Markwell PJ and Elliott J (2002) Prevalence of systolic hypertension in cats with chronic renal failure at initial evaluation. *Journal of the American Veterinary Medical Association* **220**, 1799–1804

Ward MP, Guptill LF, Prahl A and Wu CC (2004a) Serovar-specific prevalence and risk factors for leptospirosis among dogs: 90 cases (1997–2002). *Journal of the American Veterinary Medical Association* **224**, 1958–1963

Ward MP, Guptill LF and Wu CC (2004b) Evaluation of environmental risk factors for leptospirosis in dogs: 36 cases (1997–2002). *Journal of the American Veterinary Medical Association* **225**, 72–77

Proteinuria

Jonathan Elliott and Gregory F. Grauer

Introduction

Persistent proteinuria with an inactive urine sediment has long been the clinicopathological hallmark of chronic kidney disease in dogs and, more recently, cats. Beyond this diagnostic utility, potential pathophysiological consequences of persistent proteinuria in dogs and cats include decreased plasma oncotic pressure, hypercholesterolaemia, systemic hypertension, hypercoagulability, muscle wasting and weight loss. The importance of proteinuria in canine and feline chronic kidney disease as a prognostic indicator and therapeutic target has only recently been recognized, stimulating a discussion about what level of protein in the urine is normal. Development of species-specific albumin enzyme-linked immunosorbent assay (ELISA) technology, which enables detection of low concentrations of canine and feline albuminuria, has helped drive this re-evaluation process. This chapter discusses the importance of assessing and classifying proteinuria in the patient with kidney disease, the diseases which may cause proteinuria in the dog and cat and the mechanisms by which it may cause progressive renal injury. The therapeutic approaches that might be used to treat significant proteinuria in dogs and cats are considered in Chapters 17 and 18.

Physiology of urine formation

The glomerular filter consists of fenestrated endothelium of the glomerular capillary, the basement membrane and the tubular epithelium lining the visceral aspect of the glomerular capillary wall (Figure 6.1). The functions of these structures are as follows:

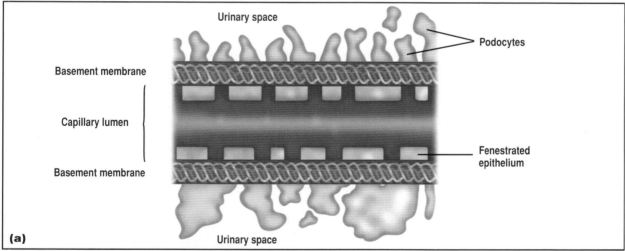

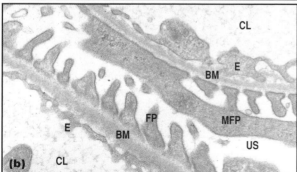

6.1 (a) Schematic diagram of the structure of the glomerular filter, showing the three components that the fluid elements of the blood have to transverse to move from the capillary to the urinary space. These consist of the capillary wall (fenestrated epithelium), the glomerular basement membrane and the visceral epithelium (podocytes with slit pores). (b) Transverse electron micrograph of a normal glomerulus. BM = Basement membrane; CL = Capillary lumen; E = Endothelial cell; FP = Foot process; MFP = Major foot process; US = Urinary space.

- The endothelium prevents passage of cells into the glomerular filter
- The basement membrane provides structural stability of the filter, anchoring cells in the correct position
- The transmembrane proteins of the podocytes (tubular epithelium), which form the slit diaphragm, act as the charge- and size-selective filtration barrier (D'Amico and Bazzi, 2003).

The most abundant plasma protein, albumin, appears in the ultrafiltrate at low concentrations, despite being present in the plasma at about 35 g/l (3.5 g/dl) (0.5 mM). This is because, with a molecular weight of 69,000 Daltons, it is close to the limit for filtration in terms of size. In addition, albumin is predominantly negatively charged and is repelled by the negatively charged proteins within the slit diaphragm. Nevertheless, recent data suggest that there is a significant transglomerular flux of albumin, such that more of this protein appears in the glomerular filtrate of normal kidneys than was once recognized (Greive *et al.*, 2001).

Proteins of molecular weight less than 7,000 Daltons are freely filtered at the glomerulus but most of this filtered protein is removed from the glomerular filtrate as it passes through the proximal convoluted tubule. The process used to achieve this is termed pinocytosis and the tubular cells breakdown the protein they take up in this way into its constitutive amino acids. The albumin that passes across the glomerular filter is inefficiently dealt with by such a process and, thus, is usually, the major urinary protein in normal healthy animals. Loss of protein in the urine in normal healthy dogs and cats usually does not exceed 10–20 mg/kg/ day (Grauer *et al.*, 1985) and 30 mg/kg/day (Monroe *et al.*, 1989), respectively. In addition to small amounts of albumin, urine protein excretion also results from the secretion of enzymes, mucoproteins and immunoglobulins by tubular and lower urinary and genital tract epithelial cells. These secreted proteins may account for as much as 50% of the proteins that are normally present in urine.

Detection of protein in the urine

Screening tests

Screening tests for proteinuria usually involve some form of dipstick test. These tests are semiquantitative, depending on the ability of amino groups of proteins to combine with indicator dyes (e.g. tetrabromophenol blue) which then change colour (Figure 6.2). The degree of binding depends on the number of free amino groups in the protein and, as albumin has more free amino groups than globulins or haemoglobin, the tests are usually two to three times more sensitive to albumin in the urine. The individual tests vary in their limits of detection but usually produce a positive reaction only if protein is present at a concentration above 0.3 g/l (30mg/dl).

False-positive results (decreased specificity) may be obtained if the urine is alkaline, the urine sediment is active (pyuria, haematuria and/or bacteriuria), the

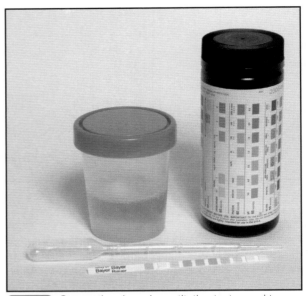

6.2 Conventional semiquantitative tests used to screen for protein in the urine.

urine has been contaminated with quaternary ammonium compounds, or the dipstick is left in contact with the urine long enough to leach out the citrate buffer that is incorporated in the filter paper pad. False-positive results with the dipstick occur more frequently in cats compared with dogs but are common in both species (Grauer *et al.*, 2004). False-negative results (decreased sensitivity) may occur in the setting of Bence Jones proteinuria, low concentrations of albuminuria and/or dilute or acidic urine.

An alternative screening test is the sulphosalicylic acid (SSA) turbometric test. This involves addition of an equal volume of 3–5% SSA to the urine sample and subjective assessment of the turbidity of the sample (0 to 4+) (Figure 6.3). In addition to albumin, the SSA test can detect globulins and Bence Jones proteins. False-positive results may occur if the urine contains radiographic contrast agents, penicillins, cephalosporins, sulfisoxazole or the urine preservative thymol. The protein content may also be overestimated with the SSA test if uncentrifuged, turbid urine is tested. False-negative results are less common in comparison with the conventional dipstick test due to the increased sensitivity of the SSA test. Because the varying de-

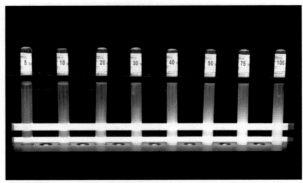

6.3 A set of standards demonstrating the increasing turbidity that develops when 5% SSA is mixed with urine containing increasing protein concentrations.

grees of precipitation turbidity are usually not standardized and interpretation is subjective, results may vary between individuals and laboratories.

Proteinuria detected by these semiquantitative screening methods has historically been interpreted in light of the urine specific gravity (SG) and urine sediment. For example, a positive dipstick reading of trace or 1+ proteinuria in hypersthenuric urine has often been attributed to urine concentration rather than abnormal proteinuria. In addition, a positive dipstick reading for protein in the presence of haematuria or pyuria was often attributed to urinary tract haemorrhage or inflammation. In both examples, the interpretation may not be correct. Given the limits of conventional dipstick test sensitivity, any positive result for protein, regardless of urine concentration, may be abnormal (except in the case of false-positive results). Likewise, haematuria and pyuria have an inconsistent effect on urine albumin concentrations; not all dogs with haematuria and pyuria have albuminuria.

The final screening test available is the Early Renal Damage (ERD®, Heska Ltd.) test. This is a very sensitive immunological test employing antibodies that are specific for canine and feline albumin. The test kit provides a method of diluting the urine sample to a SG of 1.010 to control for urine concentration and therefore urinary volume. The cut-off between negative and weakly positive has been set for an albumin concentration of 0.01 g/l (1.0 mg/dl) (i.e. some 30 times lower than the sensitivity of most standard dipstick tests) although samples may be diluted several fold before testing. Thus, this test detects microalbuminuria (see below), and samples with overt proteinuria (see below) are likely to give readings in the high to very high positive range. Animals that have negative urine samples on this test are likely to be truly non-proteinuric, whereas those with weakly or moderately positive results are likely to have microalbuminuria, and strongly positive results are likely to be overtly proteinuric (Syme and Elliott, 2005).

Quantitative tests to confirm the significance of proteinuria

If the results of the screening tests show persistent proteinuria, urine protein excretion should be quantified. This helps to evaluate the severity of renal lesions and to assess the response to treatment or the progression of disease. Renal proteinuria occurs primarily as a result of lesions involving the glomerular capillary wall or, in some cases, tubular disease.

The gold standard for assessing urinary protein loss would be to collect all the urine passed by the animal for a 24-hour period, measure its volume and protein concentration accurately and calculate the amount of protein lost (in mg protein in urine/kg body weight) in the 24-hour period. This technique is only used in the research setting because facilities that allow 24-hour urine collection are not usually available in clinical practices.

Measurement of the urine protein:creatinine ratio (UPC) is used in veterinary practice as an alternative to measurement of 24-hour urine protein excretion. Even in the presence of altered glomerular capillary wall

permeability or tubular disease, the quantity of proteinuria does not change significantly from day to day. What does change on a daily basis is the 24-hour urine volume. Similarly, the production of creatinine is constant (muscle mass is constant on a day-to-day basis) and it is freely filtered by the glomeruli without significant secretion or reabsorption by the renal tubules, so the concentration of creatinine in urine correlates with urine volume and concentration. By dividing the urine protein concentration (in mg/dl) by the urine creatinine concentration (in mg/dl), the effect of urine volume and concentration on the urine protein concentration is negated:

$$\text{Urine protein:creatinine ratio} = \frac{\text{Urine protein (mg/dl)}}{\text{Urine creatinine (mg/dl)}}$$

Units may need to be converted from SI units to perform the calculation:

Protein g/l x 100 = protein mg/dl
Creatinine µmol/l x 0.0113 = creatinine mg/dl

This ratio can be measured/calculated on a spot urine sample. It may be best performed after a period of confinement (overnight), so that the volume of urine upon which it is based is as large as possible.

Laboratories offering this test will measure creatinine and protein by quantitative analyses, express the concentration of both analytes in mg/dl (or g/l) and calculate the ratio of analyte concentrations. Such an approach has been shown to give results in cats and dogs which correlate well with 24-hour urine protein excretion measured under research conditions (Grauer et al., 1985; Monroe et al., 1989; Adams et al., 1992). It is not possible to use most standard practice chemistry analysers to make measurements of urine protein and creatinine. One manufacturer of a bench-top analyser has recently introduced a cartridge to allow UPC to be measured within the practice. Quality control standards should be run to ensure accuracy in the practice environment. Only test cartridges and in-house chemistry machines that have been specifically validated for use on urine should be used to measure urine protein and creatinine in practice. Reference ranges for cats indicating mild and severe proteinuria are presented in Figure 6.4.

A similar approach can be adopted for quantifying albumin concentration in canine and feline urine. Dog- and cat-specific ELISA assays have been produced and are commercially available. In human medicine, albumin is quantified in mg/l and creatinine in g/l so the result of the ratio has units of mg albumin per g of creatinine. There are few published data for the cat to define microalbuminuria. The cut-off points for human urine are 30 mg/g dividing between normal and microalbuminuric patients, and 300 mg/g dividing between microalbuminuria and overt proteinuria. Preliminary observations made in the authors' laboratory using a polyclonal sandwich ELISA test that has been devised and validated for the cat (Syme and Elliott, 2000) are presented in Figure 6.4.

Parameter	Cut-off levels	Interpretation	Comments
UPC	<0.2	Normal in humans	Would expect values <0.2 in young healthy cats
	<0.4	Normal in cats. Entire male cats can have UPC of up to 0.6	Based on 28 aged healthy cats
	0.4–2.0	Proteinuric (mild to moderate). Entire male cats can have UPC of up to 0.6	Could be indicative of glomerular or tubular dysfunction
	>2.0	Proteinuric (severe)	Likely to involve primary glomerular pathology
Albuminuria (mg/g)	<30	Normal in humans	Probably suitable cut-off point for cats
	<82	Normal in cats	Based on 28 aged healthy cats
	82–300	Microalbuminuric in cats	Many possible causes of microalbuminuria – see text
	>300	Proteinuric	Use UPC to quantify further

6.4 Interpretation of protein and albumin measurements in feline urine. Note that UPC does not have units, provided protein and creatinine concentrations have been expressed in the same mass per volume concentration. Units for albuminuria are mg of albumin per g of creatinine.

Most studies have shown that normal urine protein excretion in dogs is approximately 10 mg/kg over 24 hours and that normal UPCs are ≤0.2–0.3 (Grauer *et al.*, 1985). Initially recommended normal values for canine UPCs of <1.0 were probably conservative and have more recently been lowered. Today, UPCs <0.5 are considered to be normal (Lees *et al.*, 2005). It is likely however that this definition will continue to change with time and additional research. For example, even the ultra-low level, single nephron proteinuria that occurs secondary to intraglomerular hypertension in hypertrophied nephrons in chronic renal disease is abnormal in the face of what may be considered normal whole-body or whole-kidney proteinuria.

Microalbuminuria

Microalbuminuria is defined as a concentration of albumin in urine that is greater than normal but below the limit of detection using conventional semiquantitative urine protein screening methodology (see above). Due to the sensitivity of the conventional dipstick test, the upper end of urine albumin concentration that is considered to be microalbuminuria is 300 mg/l (30 mg/dl) or 300 mg/g (albumin:creatinine; see Figure 6.3). Urine albumin concentrations above this limit are called overt albuminuria and can often be detected using the UPC. The lower end of the microalbuminuria range has been less easily defined because of the requirement that this concentration is greater than 'normal' and the necessity that this concentration be reliably detected. In the dog and cat, the lower limit was defined based on the log mean + 2 standard deviations of populations of apparently healthy dogs and cats as >10 mg/l (1.0 mg/dl) in urine. Urine albumin concentrations can be adjusted for differences in urine concentration by dividing by urine creatinine concentrations. For example, a urine albumin:creatinine ratio >30 mg/g is considered abnormal in people. Alternatively, urine can be diluted to a standard concentration, such as 1.010, prior to assay. In one study of dogs, normalizing urine albumin concentrations to an SG of 1.010 yielded similar results to the urine albumin:creatinine ratio (Lees *et al.*, 2002).

The prevalence of microalbuminuria in dogs has been evaluated in several studies. In 86 dogs whose owners were not seeking veterinary care, the prevalence of microalbuminuria was 19% (Jensen *et al.*, 2001). However, the prevalence was higher (36%) in 159 dogs whose owners were seeking veterinary care for routine health screening, elective procedures and evaluation of health problems at a veterinary teaching hospital (Jensen *et al.*, 2001). In dogs evaluated at another veterinary teaching hospital for health problems, the prevalence of microalbuminuria was 30%, although microalbuminuria was more rigidly defined (20–200 mg/l) (Pressler *et al.*, 2001). In 3,041 dogs owned by the staff from over 350 veterinary clinics, the prevalence of microalbuminuria was 25% (Radecki *et al.*, 2003). Although the health status of these 3,041 dogs was not reported, a statistically significant correlation was found between increasing age and microalbuminuria in this study. The increasing prevalence of glomerular lesions in dogs as they age tends to corroborate the age-related prevalence of microalbuminuria (Rouse and Lewis, 1975; Muller-Peddinghaus and Trautwein, 1977).

The prevalence of microalbuminuria in apparently healthy cats appears to be approximately 15% and, similar to dogs, it is correlated with increasing age (Heska Ltd., 2003; Grauer *et al.*, 2004). Interestingly, when cats with medical conditions were evaluated, the overall prevalence increased to >40% and the correlation with age was less apparent (Heska Ltd., 2003).

Aetiopathogenesis of proteinuria

Having performed a screening test and found evidence suggestive of proteinuria, it is important to go on and characterize the likely site of the problem in the urinary system that is giving rise to an abnormal amount of protein appearing in the urine. Proteinuria can be classified as physiological or pathological (prerenal, renal or postrenal) in origin.

Physiological proteinuria

Physiological or benign proteinuria is often transient and abates when the underlying cause is corrected. Strenuous exercise, seizure, fever, stress and exposure to extreme heat or cold are examples of conditions that may cause physiological proteinuria. The mechanism of physiological proteinuria is not completely understood; however, relative renal vasoconstriction, ischaemia and congestion are thought to be involved. Decreased physical activity may also affect urine protein excretion in dogs; one study showed that urinary protein excretion is higher in dogs confined to cages than in dogs with normal activity levels (McCaw *et al.*, 1985).

Prerenal proteinuria

Prerenal proteinuria implies that abnormal concentrations of protein are being presented to the kidney in the plasma. If these proteins are of low molecular weight they will be filtered and may overwhelm the tubular reabsorptive process. Examples of proteins that are readily filtered include immunoglobulin light chains and haemoglobin and myoglobin that are not bound to haptoglobin. The detection of these proteins and their identification in the urine, in combination with other clinical signs of the diseases that give rise to these proteins appearing in excess in the plasma, will aid in the diagnosis of the underlying condition.

Postrenal proteinuria

Postrenal proteinuria implies protein is added to the urine in the urinary tract after the kidney (ureter, bladder or urethra). Inflammation of these parts of the urinary tract, most commonly due to bacterial infection, should be considered as a possible cause of proteinuria. Other causes of inflammation include the presence of nephroliths and tumours, both of which may be associated with bacterial infection. In many cases, the cat or dog will be showing signs of lower urinary tract disease, such as dysuria and pollakiuria. Microscopic examination of the urine sediment is likely to show it to be active, with evidence of haematuria, inflammatory cells and possibly bacteria (Figure 6.5). Some authors suggest that samples of relatively dilute urine (SG <1.030) should be routinely submitted for bacterial culture (even in the absence of lower urinary tract signs and microscopic evidence of inflammation) to rule out subclinical urinary tract infections.

Renal proteinuria

Renal proteinuria implies that defective renal function and/or inflammation of parenchymal kidney tissue is the cause of the appearance of protein in the urine. Active (acute) renal parenchymal inflammation is likely to be associated with acute kidney diseases (pyelonephritis, acute tubular necrosis), and this will be reflected in the history at presentation and the active microscopic urine sediment findings. Localization of the disease to the kidney may be possible on physical examination (painful swollen kidneys on palpation) or on the presence of tubular casts on urine microscopy. However, in some instances (e.g. chronic disease) these signs may be very subtle and localization of the

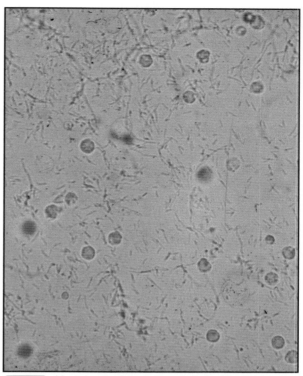

6.5 Unstained urine sediment viewed by light microscopy (magnification X400). The field of view shows >20 leucocytes and numerous chains of rod-shaped bacteria, suggesting urinary tract inflammation secondary to a bacterial urinary tract infection.

disease to the kidney can be difficult, even when advanced imaging techniques are used. In addition to renal inflammation, defective renal function may result in renal proteinuria, e.g. increased glomerular permeability (glomerular proteinuria) and decreased tubular reabsorption (tubular proteinuria).

If prerenal and postrenal causes of proteinuria have been ruled out, and there are no signs of active inflammation on urine sediment examination in an animal, renal proteinuria is likely to be of either glomerular or tubular origin (see below). This being the case, it is worthwhile quantifying the proteinuria more accurately.

Glomerular proteinuria can occur because of primary glomerular pathology leading to a defective filtration process. Examples of primary glomerular diseases include:

* Glomerulopathies due to developmental abnormalities in the components of the basement membrane and slit diaphragm (well recognized in human patients and a number of breeds of dog (see Chapter 7) but not reported in cats)
* Idiopathic membranoproliferative glomerulonephritis with immune complex deposition in the glomerulus. This form of primary glomerular disease is much more common in dogs than cats
* Amyloid deposition in the glomerulus.

A feature of primary glomerular diseases that may be helpful in distinguishing these from other causes of renal proteinuria is that the degree of proteinuria, particularly once the disease has become established, tends to be high (UPC >2.0 and often above 5–10). Really high levels (>10) may well be associated with the nephrotic syndrome. Dogs and cats with severe proteinuria are not always azotaemic when their kidney disease is diagnosed. Many will become azotaemic if they remain proteinuric, as persistent proteinuria of this severity undoubtedly leads to progressive renal injury (see below).

Lower level proteinuria (UPC 0.4–2.0 in cats and 0.5–2.0 in dogs) and microalbuminuria could be caused by an inability of the tubules to reabsorb the filtered protein (indicating tubular disease/dysfunction) as well as by an increased protein flux across the glomerulus. Increased transglomerular flux of proteins (particularly albumin) could occur because of:

- Increased glomerular capillary pressure (glomerular capillary hypertension) secondary to loss of functioning nephrons (adaptive response in chronic kidney disease)
- Early or late immune-complex disease involving the glomerulus.

In azotaemic dogs or cats with chronic kidney disease, assessment of the degree of proteinuria is an important part of classifying the disease and appears to provide information of prognostic value (see below). Moderate to severe proteinuria (UPC >1.0) appears to be predictive of progressive renal injury in dogs. However, the majority of cats with azotaemic chronic kidney disease appear to have either normal levels of protein in their urine, are microabuminuric or have mild proteinuria (UPC 0.4–1.0). The significance of micro-albuminuria or mild proteinuria in non-azotaemic dogs and cats is that it can act as a marker for a number of systemic diseases (see below). In non-azotaemic dogs and cats, whether persistent low-level proteinuria is damaging to the feline kidney or is a marker of progressive renal pathology remains to be determined.

Pathological processes of chronic kidney disease in the absence of primary glomerular disease

The most common pathological pattern of disease in the aging feline kidney is chronic interstitial fibrosis with a mild inflammatory interstitial infiltrate (Lucke, 1968; DiBartola et al., 1987; Elliott and Barber, 1998). This pattern of pathology is also common in dogs, accounting for approximately 50% of chronic kidney disease in one study involving 76 dogs (MacDougall et al., 1986).

Glomerular lesions (glomerulosclerosis) are thought to occur secondary to loss of functioning nephrons, which are replaced by fibrous tissue. Evidence of active primary glomerular disease is usually absent. In the aging dog and cat with chronic kidney disease, following loss of a critical amount of renal mass due to primary extrinsic damage (cause often not known), the remaining functioning nephrons are thought to adapt in response to local changes within the kidney. These adaptive changes lead to hyperfiltration secondary to glomerular capillary hypertension, possibly as a result of local activation of the renin–angiotensin system (RAS). Angiotensin II drives the hyperfiltration process by selective constriction of the efferent arteriole. In addition, angiotensin II stimulates nephron hypertrophy. Ultimately, these adaptive changes are detrimental and are thought to lead to further interstitial fibrosis and inflammation with further nephron loss occurring, even in the absence of any extrinsic factors which damage the kidney (the so-called intact nephron hypothesis leading to intrinsic progressive nephron loss; Hostetter et al., 1981).

One would predict, from the above discussion, that dogs and cats with chronic kidney disease where intrinsic progression was occurring would have higher levels of protein in their urine than dogs and cats where the kidney disease was stable and non-progressive. This is because the severity of the proteinuria might be indicative either of the degree of glomerular hypertension and hyperfiltration (increasing transglomerular protein flux per nephron) or of the degree of tubular dysfunction (leading to reduced tubular uptake of filtered protein).

Evidence that maladaptive glomerular capillary hypertension occurs in the canine and feline kidney has been documented in remnant kidney models (Brown et al., 1993; Brown and Brown, 1995). It was associated with an increase in protein excretion as assessed by measurement of UPC. This form of secondary (maladaptive) glomerular dysfunction is usually associated with low-level proteinuria. For example, in the remnant kidney model referred to above, prior to removal of kidney tissue the cats had UPCs of 0.07 ± 0.01 on average and after subtotal nephrectomy, this increased to an average of 0.31 ± 0.06. This change in protein excretion was associated with approximately a 10% rise in glomerular capillary pressure measured by micropuncture techniques. Over the course of 6–12 months, this model is associated with development of interstitial fibrosis, moderate inflammatory infiltrate of the interstitium and glomerulosclerosis.

Association between proteinuria and progressive renal injury – cellular mechanisms

Plasma proteins that have crossed the glomerular capillary wall can accumulate within the glomerular tuft and stimulate mesangial cell proliferation and increased production of mesangial matrix (Jerums et al., 1997). In addition, excessive amounts of protein in the glomerular filtrate can be toxic to human tubular epithelial cells and can lead to interstitial inflammation and fibrosis and cell death (Tang et al., 1999). Proximal tubular cells normally reabsorb protein from the glomerular filtrate by endocytosis. Albumin and other proteins accumulate in lysosomes and are then degraded into amino acids. In proteinuric conditions, excessive lysosomal processing can result in swelling and rupture of lysosomes causing enzymatic damage to the cytoplasm (Olbricht et al., 1986). Tubular injury may also occur as a consequence of tubular obstruction with proteinaceous casts (Bertani et al., 1986). Increased glomerular permeability to plasma proteins allows tubular cell contact with transferrin, complement and lipoproteins. Transferrin increases iron uptake by epithelial cells. Once inside the cell, the iron ions catalyse the formation of reactive oxygen species that can cause peroxidative injury (Alfrey *et al.*, 1989). Complement proteins can be activated on the brush border of proximal tubular cells, resulting in the insertion of a membrane attack complex followed by cytoskeletal damage and cytolysis (Camussi, 1994). Reabsorbed lipoproteins can release lipid moieties that can accumulate into lipid droplets or be oxidized to toxic radicals (Ong and Moorhead, 1994). All of these processes can irreversibly damage the proximal tubule and interstitium and result in nephron loss.

It is clear from studies in human medicine and in laboratory animals that moderate to severe urinary protein loss is associated with progressive renal injury and may in fact be a contributory cause of intrinsic progression (Remuzzi and Bertani, 1998). This conclusion stems from the fact that a number of therapeutic interventions, which by different mechanisms reduce proteinuria, also slow progressive renal injury.

Association between proteinuria and progressive renal injury – molecular mechanisms

In vitro studies have been carried out where proximal tubular cells, grown in cell culture, are exposed to albumin and transferrin in concentrations which overwhelm the ability of these cells to digest the proteins within their lysosomes. This leads to activation of nuclear factor κB (NF-κB), which turns on the expression of genes in these cells and causes them to secrete mediators from their basolateral cell surfaces (i.e.

towards the interstitium) (Benigni and Remuzzi, 2001). These mediators include endothelin-1 (ET-1), monocyte chemotractant protein-1 (MCP-1) and the immunoregulatory cytokine, regulated on activation, normal T expressed and secreted (RANTES). Expression and secretion of these proteins can be demonstrated *in vivo* in animal models of proteinuric renal disease (Donadelli *et al.*, 2000). Interventions that reduce proteinuria in these models also reduce the expression of these and other cytokines involved in progressive interstitial fibrosis. These molecular details may explain why proteinuria is an independent risk factor for progression of kidney disease in human medicine and why drugs such as ACE inhibitors successfully slow progression in proteinuric kidney diseases, independent of their effects on systemic arterial blood pressure. Figure 6.6 presents these concepts in a schematic diagram.

Risk factors for proteinuria in chronic kidney disease

In the authors' clinical practice, cats with renal disease which are mildly or moderately azotaemic (serum creatinine 140–400 μmol/l; 1.6–4.5 mg/dl), will be non-proteinuric (UPC <0.2) borderline proteinuric (UPC 0.2–0.4) or mildly proteinuric (UPC 0.4–1.0). In a large cross-sectional epidemiological study, risk factors associated with proteinuria were identified and included serum creatinine concentration (the higher the creatinine the more likely the cat is to be proteinuric) and systolic arterial blood pressure (the higher the blood pressure the more likely the cat is to be proteinuric)

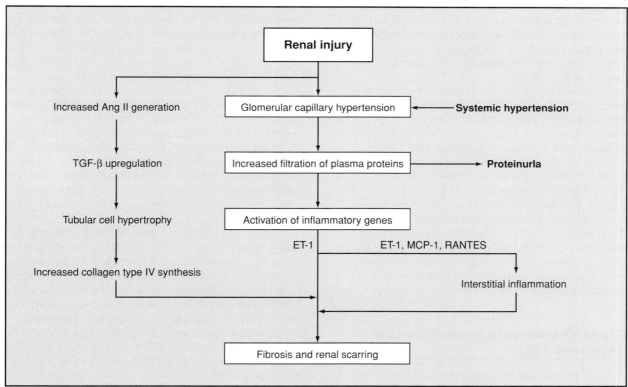

6.6 Schematic diagram showing the mechanisms involved in progressive renal injury caused by proteinuria. Ang II = Angiotensin II; ET-1 = Endothelin-1; MCP-1 = Monocyte chemotractant protein-1; RANTES = Immunoregulatory cytokine regulated on activation, normal T expressed and secreted; TGF-β = Tissue growth factor beta. (Adapted from Remuzzi and Bertani (1998))

(Syme *et al.*, 2006). These observations provide circumstantial evidence to support the hypothesis that cats with naturally occurring chronic kidney disease hyperfiltrate, particularly as they lose more functioning nephrons. If they have systemic hypertension the protein loss is greater, presumably because of the inability of diseased kidneys to autoregulate.

The cats included in the cross-sectional epidemiology study referred to above were also enrolled in a longitudinal survival study (Syme *et al.*, 2006). Cox's proportional hazards model was used to determine the predictive values of age, gender, plasma creatinine concentration, systolic arterial blood pressure and UPC ratio on all-cause mortality. In this study, log UPC as a continuous variable proved to be significantly and independently associated with survival (all-cause mortality) as were age and plasma creatinine concentration. No association was found between gender or systolic blood pressure and survival.

This observation suggests that measurement of UPC could be used as a prognostic indicator in cats with naturally occurring kidney disease, for all-cause mortality. About 50% of the deaths occurring in the authors' clinic population of cats suffering from chronic kidney disease are because of progressive kidney disease or acute decompensation of their azotaemia (uraemic crisis). In this study, the reference range for UPC derived from the non-azotaemic healthy cats had an upper limit of 0.43. In dogs with naturally occurring chronic kidney disease, proteinuria resulting in a UPC ≥1.0 was associated with a threefold greater risk of development of uraemic crises and death compared with dogs with UPC <1.0. The relative risk of adverse outcome was approximately 1.5 times higher for every 1 unit increase in UPC. In addition, dogs with UPC ≥1.0 had a decrease in renal function that was greater in magnitude than observed in dogs with UPCs <1.0 (Jacob *et al.*, 2005).

One might conclude from these studies that interventions designed to reduce urinary protein excretion would slow progressive renal injury and, therefore, improve survival in dogs and cats with chronic kidney disease. This conclusion assumes that protein in the urine in these animals is damaging to the remaining functioning nephrons and so leads to progressive renal injury. Another interpretation of these findings, however, is that the appearance of protein in the urine is merely a marker that progressive renal injury is occurring (Fine *et al.*, 2000). In this case, whilst renoprotective interventions might be expected to reduce protein excretion because they slow progressive renal injury, reducing urine protein excretion by any method will not necessarily prove to be renoprotective.

Microalbuminuria in non-azotaemic dogs and cats

There is a good deal of interest as to whether low-level proteinuria or microalbuminuria might be used as a test to identify kidney disease at an early stage (i.e. before the dog or cat has become azotaemic). This is one of the concepts behind the ERD® test produced by Heska

Ltd. There are, however, many systemic disease states that are associated with microalbuminuria, including chronic inflammatory disease (e.g. chronic stomatitis/gingivitis) and neoplastic conditions, and microalbuminuria may also be an indicator of early systemic disease. In human medicine, microalbuminuria is a risk factor for death from cardiovascular diseases, including heart failure, and may reflect a state of endothelial cell dysfunction which allows more transglomerular albumin flux (Yudkin *et al.*, 1988). It may be that persistent microalbuminuria gradually damages the kidney, but, in aging dogs and cats, many of the diseases that are linked with microalbuminuria probably lead to the death of the animal before the kidney damage is of clinical consequence. It does appear that albumin excretion in the urine increases with age in outwardly healthy dogs and cats. Furthermore, microalbuminuria was predictive of all-cause mortality in non-azotaemic apparently healthy cats studied at the Royal Veterinary College in London (Walker *et al.*, 2004). This study involved 59 cats, 15 of which died during the follow-up period. The survivors had significantly lower UPCs (median value 0.16) compared to the non-survivors (median value 0.3). This study included all-cause mortality, so does not answer the question as to whether microalbuminuria is predictive of kidney disease and its progression to the clinical phase.

One important disease that gives rise to microalbuminuria and mild but overt proteinuria in the cat, which deserves special mention, is hyperthyroidism. It is clear that the hyperthyroid state leads to glomerular hyperfiltration and probably glomerular capillary hypertension, due to inappropriate activation of the RAS in this disease. Approximately 50% of untreated non-azotaemic hyperthyroid cats had UPCs on initial diagnosis of >0.5 (Syme and Elliott, 2001). Management of the hyperthyroid state does lead to a reduction in UPC in the majority of cats, further supporting the conclusion that this was caused by the renal haemodynamic effects of thyroid hormones. In addition, it seems likely that if hyperthyroidism remains untreated for prolonged periods of time, this will be damaging to the cat's kidneys. However, the degree of proteinuria identified at diagnosis of hyperthyroidism does not appear to be predictive of the occurrence of azotaemia once the animal is stabilized in a euthyroid state (unpublished data).

Based on recent studies, microalbuminuria appears to be a good indicator of early renal disease in dogs, particularly those diseases that involve the glomerulus. Albuminuria was evaluated in 36 male dogs with X-linked hereditary nephropathy, a rapidly progressive glomerular disease that is secondary to a defect in type IV collagen, a structural component of the glomerular basement membrane (Lees *et al.*, 2002). In these dogs, lesions in the glomerular basement membrane become apparent by 8 weeks of age. Persistent microalbuminuria was detected between 8 and 23 weeks of age, 0–16 weeks before the onset of overt proteinuria, which occurred at 14–30 weeks of age. It was concluded that microalbuminuria was a reliable early marker of developing nephropathy.

In 12 healthy dogs that were experimentally infected with *Dirofilaria immitis* L3 larvae and longitudinally evaluated, all developed microalbuminuria. During a period of 14–23 months following infection, 82% of all samples collected were positive for microalbuminuria (Grauer *et al.*, 2002). The onset of microalbuminuria corresponded to the onset of antigenaemia. The magnitude of microalbuminuria increased over time and microalbuminuria preceded the development of overt proteinuria, as measured by UPC. At the end of the study, the dogs had histological evidence of glomerular disease by light (*n* = 11) or electron (*n* = 12) microscopy.

Lastly, the prevalence of microalbuminuria in 20 Soft-Coated Wheaten Terriers that were genetically at risk for the development of protein-losing enteropathy and nephropathy was 76% (Vaden *et al.*, 2001). The magnitude of microalbuminuria increased over time and 43% of the dogs with microalbuminuria eventually developed abnormal UPCs. Of interest is the observation that persistent microalbuminuria develops in dogs with this type of protein-losing nephropathy at approximately the same time that mesangial hypercellularity and segmental glomerular sclerosis occur. Concurrent inflammatory bowel disease may account for microalbuminuria in some of the dogs that have not progressed to overt proteinuria.

Other conditions have been reported in dogs with microalbuminuria, including infectious, inflammatory, neoplastic, metabolic and cardiovascular disease (Pressler *et al.*, 2001; Whittemore *et al.*, 2003). Results of an ongoing study of microalbuminuria in dogs with lymphosarcoma and osteosarcoma demonstrated that urine albumin concentrations were significantly increased in dogs with these tumours, even though UPC may not be increased above the reference range (Pressler *et al.*, 2003). Urine albumin concentrations did not, however, consistently decrease with decreased tumour burden.

The prevalence of microalbuminuria in dogs admitted to intensive care units is higher than in other reported patient populations and appears to vary with different classifications of disease (Pressler *et al.*, 2001; Whittemore *et al.*, 2003). As reported in people with acute inflammatory conditions, transient microalbuminuria occurred in some of these dogs. A large percentage of patients that were euthanased or died had microalbuminuria, suggesting that, as in people, the presence of microalbuminuria may be a negative prognostic indicator.

Further study is necessary to determine if microalbuminuria is an accurate predictor of overt proteinuria and various additional types of renal disease in dogs. If microalbuminuria does predict overt proteinuria and/or renal disease, this early detection tool should increase our ability to alter the disease progression. In addition, microalbuminuria may prove to be a valuable, early indicator of systemic disease that results in vascular inflammation.

Summary

Proteinuria is a common disorder in the dog, and to a lesser extent in the cat, that can indicate the presence of renal disease prior to the onset of azotaemia. Proteinuria is a marker for renal disease in both the dog and cat. Although a direct pathogenic link between glomerular disease, proteinuria and progressive renal damage has not been established in the dog or cat, attenuation of proteinuria has been associated with decreased renal functional decline in several studies. There is a need to continue to increase our understanding of the effects of proteinuria on the glomerulus, the tubule and the interstitium in dogs and cats. In addition to being a diagnostic marker of renal disease, proteinuria may also contribute to the progressive nature of canine renal disease and possibly in the cat, making it an important therapeutic target. Proteinuria is commonly associated with primary glomerular diseases; the loss of renal autoregulation that occurs secondary to nephron loss due to any cause (e.g. vascular, tubular, interstitial, as well as glomerular) can, however, also result in intraglomerular hypertension and proteinuria. Treatments shown to reduce proteinuria are discussed in Chapters 18 and 19.

References and further reading

Adams LG, Polzin DJ, Osborne CA and O'Brien TD (1992) Correlation of urine protein/creatinine ratio and twenty-four hour urinary protein excretion in normal cats and cats with induced chronic renal failure. *Journal of Veterinary Internal Medicine* **6**, 36–40

Alfrey AC, Froment DH and Hammond WS (1989) Role of iron in tubulointerstitial injury in nephrotoxic serum nephritis. *Kidney International* **36**, 753–759

Benigni A and Remuzzi G (2001) How renal cytokines and growth factors contribute to renal disease progression. *American Journal of Kidney Diseases* **37(Suppl 2)**, S21–S24

Bertani T, Cutillo F, Zoja C *et al.* (1986) Tubulointerstitial lesions mediate renal damage in adriamycin glomerulopathy. *Kidney International* **30**, 488–496

Brown SA and Brown CA (1995) Single-nephron adaptations to partial renal ablation in cats. *American Journal of Physiology* **269**, R1002–R1008

Brown SA, Walton CL, Crawford P and Bakris GL (1993) Long-term effects of antihypertensive regimens on renal hemodynamics and proteinuria. *Kidney International* **43**, 1210–1218

Camussi G (1994) Alternative pathway activation of complement by cultured human proximal tubular epithelial cells. *Kidney International* **45**, 451–460

D'Amico G and Bazzi C (2003) Pathophysiology of proteinuria. *Kidney International* **63**, 809–825

DiBartola SP, Rutgers HC, Zack PM and Tarr MJ (1987) Clinicopathologic findings associated with chronic renal disease in cats: 74 cases (1973–1984). *Journal of the American Veterinary Medical Association* **190**, 1196–1202

Donadelli R, Abbate M, Zanchi C *et al.* (2000) Protein traffic activates NF-kB gene signaling and promotes MCP-1-dependent interstitial inflammation. *American Journal of Kidney Diseases* **36**, 1226–1241

Elliott J and Barber PJ (1998) Feline chronic renal failure: clinical findings in 80 cases diagnosed between 1992 and 1995. *Journal of Small Animal Practice* **39**, 78–85

Fine LG, Bandyopadhay D and Norman JT (2000) Is there a common mechanism for the progression of different types of renal diseases other than proteinuria? Towards the unifying theme of chronic hypoxia. *Kidney International* **57(Suppl. 75)**, S22–S26

Grauer GF (in press) Measurement, interpretation and implications of proteinurea and albuminurea. *Veterinary Clinics of America: Small Animal Practice*

Grauer GF, Moore LE, Smith AR and Jensen WA (2004) Comparison of conventional urine protein test strip method and a quantitative ELISA for the detection of canine and feline albuminuria. *Journal of Veterinary Internal Medicine* **18**, 418–419 (abstract)

Grauer GF, Oberhauser EB, Basaraba RJ *et al.* (2002) Development of microalbuminuria in dogs with heartworm disease. *Journal of Veterinary Internal Medicine* **16**, 352 (abstract)

Grauer GF, Thomas CB and Eicker SW (1985) Estimation of quantitative proteinuria in the dog, using the urine protein-to-creatinine ratio from a random, voided sample. *American Journal* of Veterinary Research **46**, 2116–2119

Greive KA, Balazs ND and Comper WD (2001) Protein fragments in urine have been considerably underestimated by various protein assays. *Clinical Chemistry* **47**, 1717–1719

Gunn-Moore D (2003) Influence of proteinuria on survival time in cats with chronic renal insufficiency. *Journal of Veterinary Internal Medicine* **17**, 404 (abstract)

Heska Ltd (2003) Unpublished data

Hostetter TH, Olsen JL, Rennke HG, Venkatachalam MA and Brenner BM (1981) Hyperfiltration in remnant nephrons: a potentially adverse response to renal ablation. *American Journal of Physiology* **241**, F85–F93

Jacob F, Polzin DJ, Osborne CA *et al.* (2005) Evaluation of the association between initial proteinuria and morbidity rate or death in dogs with naturally occurring chronic renal failure. *Journal of the American Veterinary Medical Association* **226**, 393–400

Jensen WA, Grauer GF, Andrews J and Simpson D (2001) Prevalence of microalbuminuria in dogs. *Journal of Veterinary Internal Medicine* **15**, 300 (abstract)

Jerums G, Panagiotopoulos S, Tsalamandris C *et al.* (1997) Why is proteinuria such an important risk factor for progression in clinical trials? *Kidney International* **52**, S87–S92

Lees GE, Brown SA, Elliott J *et al.* (2005) Assessment and management of proteinuria in dogs and cats; 2004 ACVIM Forum Consensus Statement (Small Animal). *Journal of Veterinary Internal Medicine* **19**, 377–385

Lees GE, Jensen WA, Simpson DF and Kashtan CE (2002) Persistent albuminuria precedes onset of overt proteinuria in male dogs with X-linked hereditary nephropathy. *Journal of Veterinary Internal Medicine* **16**, 353 (abstract)

Loutzenhiser R and Epstein M (1989) Renal hemodynamic effects of calcium antagonists. In: *Calcium Channel Antagonists and the Kidney,* ed. M Epstein and R Loutzenhiser, pp. 33–74. Hanley & Belfus, Philadelphia

Lucke VM (1968) Renal disease in the domestic cat. *Journal of Pathology and Bacteriology* **95**, 67–91

Lulich JP, Osborne CA, O'Brien TD and Polzin DJ (1992) Feline renal failure: questions, answers, questions. *Compendium on Continuing Education for the Practicing Veterinarian* **14**, 127–152

MacDougall DF, Cook T, Steward AP *et al.* (1986) Canine chronic renal disease: prevalence and types of glomerulonephritis in the dog. *Kidney International* **29**, 1144–1151

McCaw DL, Knapp DW and Hewett JE (1985) Effect of collection time and exercise restriction on the prevention of urine protein excretion, using urine protein/creatinine ratio in dogs. *American Journal of Veterinary Research* **46**, 1665–1669

Monroe WE, Davenport DJ and Saunders GK (1989) Twenty-four hour urinary protein loss in healthy cats and the urinary protein to creatinine ratio as an estimate. *American Journal of Veterinary Research* **50**, 1906–1909

Muller-Peddinghaus R and Trautwein G (1977) Spontaneous GN in dogs 1. Classification and immunopathology. *Veterinary Pathology* **14**, 1–13

Nash AS, Wright NG, Spencer AJ, Thompson H and Fisher EW (1979) Membranous nephropathy in the cat: a clinical and pathological study. *Veterinary Record* **105**, 71–77

Olbricht CJ, Cannon JK, Garg LC and Tisher CC (1986) Activities of cathepsin B and L in isolated nephron segments from proteinuric

and nonproteinuric rats. *American Journal of Physiology* **250**, F1055–F1062

Ong A and Moorhead J (1994) Tubular lipidosis: epiphenomenon or pathogenetic lesion in human renal disease. *Kidney International* **45**, 753–762

Peterson JC, Alder S, Burkart JM *et al.* (1995) Blood pressure control, proteinuria, and the progression of renal disease. The modification of diet in renal disease study. *Annals of Internal Medicine* **123**, 754–762

Pressler BM, Proulx DA, Williams LE *et al.* (2003) Urine albumin concentration is increased in dogs with lymphoma or osteosarcoma. *Journal of Veterinary Internal Medicine* **17**, 404 (abstract)

Pressler BM, Vaden SL and Jensen WA (2001) Prevalence of microalbuminuria in dogs evaluated at a referral veterinary hospital. *Journal of Veterinary Internal Medicine* **15**, 300 (abstract)

Radecki S, Donnelly R, Jensen WA and Stinchcomb DT (2003) Effect of age and breed on the prevalence of microalbuminuria in dogs. *Journal of Veterinary Internal Medicine* **17**, 406 (abstract)

Remuzzi G and Bertani T (1998) Pathophysiology of progressive nephropathies. *New England Journal of Medicine* **339**, 1448–1456

Rouse BT and Lewis RJ (1975) Canine glomerulonephritis: prevalence in dogs submitted at random for euthanasia. *Canadian Journal of Comparative Medicine* **39**, 365–370

Syme HM and Elliott J (2000) Development and validation of an enzyme linked immunosorbent assay for the measurement of albumin in feline urine. *Journal of Veterinary Internal Medicine* **14**, 352 (abstract)

Syme HM and Elliott J (2001) Evaluation of proteinuria as a predictive indicator of sub-clinical renal failure in untreated hyperthyroid cats. *Journal of Veterinary Internal Medicine* **15**, 299 (abstract)

Syme HM and Elliott J (2005) Semiquantitative evaluation of protein in feline urine. *Journal of Veterinary Internal Medicine* **19**, 432 (abstract)

Syme HM, Markwell PJ, Pfeiffer DU and Elliott J (2006) Survival of cats with naturally occurring chronic renal failure is related to severity of proteinuria. *Journal of Veterinary Internal Medicine* **20**, 528–535

Tang S, Sheerin NS, Zhou W *et al.* (1999) Apical proteins stimulate complement synthesis by cultured human proximal tubular epithelial cells. *Journal of the American Society of Nephrology* **10**, 69–76

Vaden SL, Jensen WA, Longhofer SL and Simpson DF (2001) Longitudinal study of microalbuminuria in soft-coated wheaten terriers. *Journal of Veterinary Internal Medicine* **15**, 300 (abstract)

Walker D, Syme HM, Markwell PJ and Elliott J (2004) Proteinuria predicts survival of healthy non-azotaemic cats. *Journal of Veterinary Internal Medicine* **18**, 417 (abstract)

Whittemore JC, Jensen WA, Prause L and Radecki S (2003) Comparison of microalbuminuria, urine dipstick, and urine protein creatinine ratio results in clinically ill dogs. *Journal of Veterinary Internal Medicine* **17**, 437 (abstract)

Wright NG, Nash AS, Thompson H and Fisher EW (1981) Membranous nephropathy in the cat and dog: a renal biopsy and follow-up study of sixteen cases. *Laboratory Investigation* **45**, 269–277

Yudkin JS, Forrest RD and Jackson CA (1988) Microalbuminuria as a predictor of vascular disease in non-diabetic subjects. Islington Diabetes Survey. *Lancet* **2**, 530–533

7

Juvenile and familial nephropathies

George E. Lees

Introduction

Hereditary renal diseases have been recognized in several breeds or kindreds of dogs and cats (Lees, 1996; DiBartola, 2005), and more examples of such conditions are likely to be identified as renal diseases that occur in a familial pattern are investigated thoroughly. In affected breeds, accurate diagnosis of familial nephropathies is especially important because of the potential health and selective breeding implications for related animals. Juvenile onset of chronic kidney disease is the most common consequence of familial renal disease. Discovery of kidney disease in a young dog or cat often evokes concern, therefore, about whether the condition is congenital or acquired, and, if it is congenital, whether or not it is inherited.

The number and diversity of familial renal diseases that have been described in dogs are greater than those described in cats, but polycystic kidney disease in cats probably is the single most common inherited nephropathy that occurs in these two companion animal species worldwide. The main categories of familial nephropathies are renal dysplasia, primary glomerulopathies, polycystic kidney disease, amyloidosis, glomerulonephritis and a miscellany of other diseases that are notable for occurrence in a particular breed (Figure 7.1). The specific pathogenesis and underlying gene defect have been determined for only a few of the familial nephropathies that have been identified in dogs and cats to date. However, the pace of progress in this field is accelerating rapidly because of advancing technology and increasing availability of genetic information for these species.

Dogs
Renal dysplasia
Lhasa Apso
Shih Tzu
Standard Poodle
Soft-Coated Wheaten Terrier
Chow Chow
Alaskan Malamute
Miniature Schnauzer
Dutch Kooiker (Dutch Decoy)
Golden Retreiver

7.1 Familial nephropathies in dogs and cats, with the mode of inheritance if known. (continues) ▶

Dogs
Primary glomerulopathies
Samoyed kindred and Navasota kindred (X-linked)
English Cocker Spaniel (autosomal recessive)
Bull Terrier (autosomal dominant)
Dalmatian (autosomal dominant)
Dobermann
Bull Mastiff
Newfoundland
Rottweiler
Pembroke Welsh Corgi
Beagle
Polycystic kidney disease
Bull Terrier (autosomal dominant)
Cairn Terrier and West Highland White Terrier (autosomal recessive)
Amyloidosis
Shar Pei
English Foxhound
Beagle
Immune-mediated glomerulonephritis
Soft-Coated Wheaten Terrier
Bernese Mountain Dog (autosomal recessive, suspected)
Brittany Spaniel (autosomal recessive)
Miscellaneous
Basenji – Fanconi syndrome
German Shepherd – multifocal cystadenocarcinoma (autosomal dominant)
Pembroke Welsh Corgi – telangiectasia
Cats
Polycystic kidney disease
Persian (autosomal dominant)
Amyloidosis
Abyssinian (autosomal dominant with incomplete penetrance, suspected)
Siamese and Oriental

7.1 (continued) Familial nephropathies in dogs and cats, with the mode of inheritance if known.

Most familial renal diseases are progressive and ultimately fatal, although the rate of progression often varies considerably among individuals with the same disorder. Therapeutic efforts generally are focused on combating complications (e.g. hypertension, urinary tract infection) as they arise and using conventional strategies for the medical management of chronic kidney disease to minimize disease progression and uraemia (see Chapter 18).

Clinical findings

The clinical syndrome produced by most familial nephropathies that come to veterinary attention is chronic kidney disease, which often develops while the animals are adolescents or young adults. In dogs with renal dysplasia and some primary glomerulopathies, onset of renal failure usually occurs at 3 months to 3 years of age, with peak occurrence at about 1 year of age. However, many familial nephropathies often produce renal failure somewhat later in life. For polycystic kidney disease, some primary glomerulopathies, amyloidosis and glomerulonephritis, onset of renal failure is often at 3–7 years of age, depending on the condition.

Reduced appetite or anorexia, stunted growth or weight loss, polyuria, polydipsia and vomiting are the most common clinical signs reported by the owners of dogs and cats with renal failure due to a familial nephropathy. Other signs that are often reported include poor hair coat, halitosis and diarrhoea. Haematuria, dysuria and abdominal pain are the clinical signs associated with renal telangiectasia in Pembroke Welsh Corgis, and haematuria also occurs in German Shepherd Dogs with multifocal renal cystadenocarcinoma.

Physical examination findings often include thin body condition, dehydration, mucous membrane pallor, uraemic breath odour and oral ulceration. Fibrous osteodystrophy or rubber jaw is occasionally observed, mainly in dogs that develop renal failure before 6 months of age. The kidneys of animals, especially cats, with polycystic kidney disease are often palpably enlarged. Otherwise, the kidneys are usually normal or reduced in size. Dogs with severe renal dysplasia often have especially small kidneys.

Diagnosis

Laboratory testing most often reveals the expected abnormalities associated with chronic kidney disease and renal failure:

- Impaired urine-concentrating ability
- Azotaemia
- Hyperphosphataemia
- Non-regenerative anaemia.

These findings usually reflect the severity of the animal's renal failure, independent of its cause.

Urinalysis findings, however, frequently help discriminate among the common causes of juvenile or familial nephropathy:

- Dogs with primary glomerulopathies and familial glomerulonephritis consistently have persistent renal proteinuria that emerges early in the course of disease and typically is of high magnitude (urinary protein:creatinine ratio (UPC) ≥ 2)
- Dogs with renal dysplasia and dogs and cats with polycystic kidney disease usually exhibit little or no proteinuria
- Proteinuria is an inconsistent finding that depends on the extent of glomerular involvement in dogs and cats with familial amyloidosis
- Renal glucosuria is a consistent feature of the Fanconi syndrome in Basenjis but occasionally is observed in dogs with renal dysplasia or primary glomerulopathies
- Haematuria is the cardinal feature of telangiectasia in Pembroke Welsh Corgis, which may develop anaemia due to blood loss in the urine
- Bacterial urinary tract infection also sometimes develops as a secondary complication in dogs and cats with juvenile or familial nephropathies.

Diagnostic renal imaging is most helpful for animals with polycystic kidney disease in which a definitive diagnosis can be made by finding multiple cysts distributed in both kidneys using ultrasonography. In dogs with renal dysplasia, ultrasonography can demonstrate abnormal size, shape and sonic architecture of the kidneys, but it cannot distinguish renal dysplasia from other possible causes of small, fibrotic end-stage kidneys in affected dogs.

For specific nephropathies, known or suspected to be inherited in particular breeds, diagnosis of the condition generally rests on recognition of the expected clinical features, exclusion of other conditions that might produce similar signs, and ultimately upon identification of characteristic renal lesions. The exclusion of other disorders (especially those that are potentially treatable) is an important step, because a variety of acquired diseases may occur in the same breeds and age groups of animals that might have familial nephropathies. Careful interpretation of the results obtained from a thorough clinical investigation (history, physical examination, blood pressure determination, complete urinalysis, urine culture and appropriate diagnostic imaging) is often adequate for a presumptive diagnosis of familial nephropathy. Even when the diagnosis remains uncertain, however, such an investigation is generally sufficient to guide the animal's medical care.

Nonetheless, definitive diagnosis of many familial nephropathies ultimately rests upon detection of characteristic lesions in kidney specimens obtained at necropsy or by biopsy. Light microscope examination is sufficient for many disorders, but, especially for glomerular diseases, transmission electron microscope and immunopathological studies are often needed as well. Special materials and procedures are required for these evaluations, so prior planning is needed to ensure that specimens that will be suitable are obtained when the tissue is collected. Centres that perform such studies should be contacted for guidance.

In breeds or families known to be at risk for certain familial nephropathies, apparently healthy animals can be screened with tests to enable early identification of affected individuals. The foremost examples of such screening are the use of ultrasonography to identify polycystic kidney disease and urinalysis to detect persistent renal proteinuria in animals that are at risk for glomerular disorders.

When a juvenile nephropathy is identified, questions about inheritance of the condition frequently arise. For breeds in which the specific nephropathy that has been diagnosed is known to be inherited, genetic counselling can be provided. In most other circumstances, heritability of the condition remains unknown unless, or until, studies of related animals show a familial pattern of disease occurrence.

Specific disorders

Renal dysplasia

Renal dysplasia is defined as disorganized development of renal parenchyma that is due to abnormal differentiation. Definitive diagnosis of this category of conditions is by microscopic observation of structures in the kidney that are inappropriate for the stage of development of the animal. Findings include:

- The presence of immature glomeruli and tubules, usually within radial bands adjacent to more normally developed tissue (i.e. asynchronous differentiation of nephrons): the most consistent feature (Picut and Lewis, 1987b)
- Persistent immature mesenchyme
- Persistent metanephric ducts
- Atypical tubular epithelial proliferation
- Dysontogenic metaplasia: rare in dogs.

Secondary changes that are commonly observed include:

- Compensatory hypertrophy and hyperplasia of glomerular tufts and tubules
- Interstitial fibrosis
- Tubulointerstitial nephritis
- Pyelonephritis
- Dystrophic mineralization
- Cystic glomerular atrophy
- Microcystic tubules
- Retention cysts
- Glomerular lipidosis.

Renal dysplasia is most extensively reported and presumed to be familial in the Lhasa Apso and Shih Tzu (O'Brien et al., 1982; Picut and Lewis, 1987b). Other breeds in which published reports have suggested that renal dysplasia occurs in a familial pattern include the Soft-Coated Wheaten Terrier (Eriksen and Gröndalen, 1984; Nash et al., 1984), Standard Poodle (DiBartola et al., 1983), Alaskan Malamute (Vilafranca and Ferrer, 1994), Golden Retriever (Kerlin and Van Winkle, 1995; de Morais et al., 1996), Chow Chow (Brown et al., 1990), Miniature Schnauzer (Morton et al., 1990) and the Dutch Kooiker (Dutch Decoy) (Schulze et al., 1998). Additionally, juvenile nephropathies with microscopic features of renal dysplasia have been reported

in one or more unrelated dogs of so many different breeds that it seems likely that the disorder occurs at least sporadically in all breeds.

The causes and pathogenesis of canine renal dysplasia are unknown. Renal dysplasia is widely accepted to be the same disease entity in both Lhasa Apsos and Shih Tzus, but whether the other familial or sporadic forms of renal dysplasia are fundamentally the same disease or different diseases having similar adverse effects on development of the kidneys in affected dogs is uncertain. To date, evidence documenting the validity of genetic testing for renal dysplasia has not been published for any breed.

Primary glomerulopathies

Several primary glomerulopathies have been described, including a number of the most well characterized inherited renal diseases of dogs. An abnormality of the type IV collagen in the glomerular basement membrane (GBM) is known or suspected to cause the disease in many of these conditions. All basement membranes contain collagen IV, but in the GBM a special collagen network containing the $\alpha3$, $\alpha4$ and $\alpha5$ chains of type IV collagen is crucial for long-term maintenance of normal structure and function of the glomerular capillary wall. When this $\alpha3-\alpha4-\alpha5(IV)$ network is not formed properly, distinctive ultrastructural changes develop in the GBM and initiate progressive renal disease, leading to chronic kidney disease. The changes can be identified only by transmission electron microscopy. These conditions are analogous to the nephropathy that occurs in human Alport syndrome, which is a genetically and clinically heterogeneous group of diseases because the functional integrity of the GBM $\alpha3-\alpha4-\alpha5(IV)$ network can be disrupted in diverse ways. In dogs, as in people, the mode of inheritance can be X-linked, autosomal recessive or autosomal dominant.

Samoyed kindred and Navasota kindred

X-linked hereditary nephropathies caused by mutations in the gene (*COL4A5*) encoding the $\alpha5(IV)$ collagen chain have been described in two canine families (Jansen et al., 1984, 1987; Lees et al., 1999). In the Samoyed kindred, which was described first, a single nucleotide substitution in exon 35 (of 51) converts a glycine codon to a stop codon (Zheng et al., 1994). In the Navasota kindred, a 10-base pair deletion in exon 9 creates a frame-shift and a stop codon in exon 10 (Cox et al., 2003). Thus, although unique within each kindred, both mutations cause *COL4A5* to encode truncated $\alpha5$ chains incapable of combining with $\alpha3$ and $\alpha4$ chains to form $\alpha3-\alpha4-\alpha5$ heterotrimers, which are required for assembly of the normal collagen IV network in the GBM. Consequently, the molecular, pathological and clinical expressions of renal disease in both kindreds are similar. In affected males, GBM expression of collagen IV $\alpha5$ chains, as well as that of $\alpha3$ and $\alpha4$ chains, is totally absent, as indicated by immunostaining with chain-specific antibodies (Harvey et al., 1998; Lees et al., 1999). Focal GBM splitting can be detected by electron microscopy beginning at about 1 month of age (Harvey et al., 1998). These changes subsequently progress in extent and severity, eventually producing the global severe GBM thickening and multilaminar splitting that is the characteristic structural feature of this nephropathy.

Persistent proteinuria, which is the first clinical manifestation of the disease, begins at 3–6 months of age, and renal function subsequently deteriorates progressively, usually causing azotaemia by 6–9 months of age and death from renal failure by 9–15 months of age (Jansen *et al.*, 1987; Lees *et al.*, 1999). The light microscopic features of the nephropathy are non-specific, having the morphological features of a membranoproliferative glomerulonephropathy accompanied by secondary changes in the tubulo-interstitium. Carrier females have mosaic expression of the α3–α4–α5(IV) network in their GBM. They develop persistent proteinuria at about the same age as their affected brothers, but their nephropathy rarely progresses to renal failure until they are older than 5 years (Baumal *et al.*, 1991).

Cocker Spaniels

An autosomal recessive hereditary glomerulopathy occurs in Cocker Spaniels (known in North America as English Cocker Spaniels) worldwide (Steward and Macdougall, 1984; Robinson *et al.*, 1985; Lees *et al.*, 1997). Immunostaining of kidney from affected dogs indicates that they also lack the normal α3–α4–α5(IV) network in their GBM, but expression of α5 chains is present in basement membranes where they are co-expressed with α6 chains (Lees *et al.*, 1998b). This pattern of collagen IV expression implicates *COL4A3*

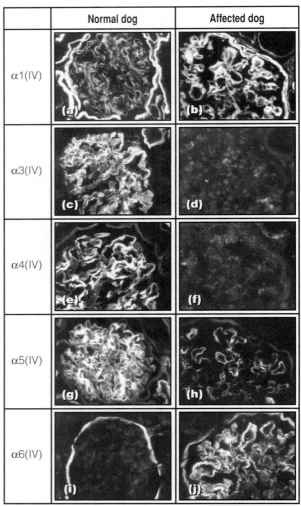

	Normal dog	Affected dog
α1(IV)	(a)	(b)
α3(IV)	(c)	(d)
α4(IV)	(e)	(f)
α5(IV)	(g)	(h)
α6(IV)	(i)	(j)

7.3 Immunofluorescence staining for collagen IV chains in the glomeruli of English Cocker Spaniels. The panels on the left side (a, c, e, g and i) are from normal dogs. The panels on the right side (b, d, f, h and j) are from dogs with the autosomal recessive form of hereditary glomerulopathy that occurs in this breed, and illustrate the distinctive pattern of abnormal collagen IV α-chain expression in renal basement membranes that characterizes this disorder. **(a and b)** Staining specific for α1(IV) chains, which are overexpressed in the GBM of affected dogs. **(c and d)** Staining specific for α3(IV) chains, which are completely absent from the GBM of affected dogs. **(e and f)** Staining specific for α4(IV) chains, which are completely absent from the GBM of affected dogs. **(g and h)** Staining specific for α5(IV) chains, which are present but reduced in the GBM of affected dogs. **(i and j)** Staining specific for α6(IV) chains, which are normally absent from the GBM of juvenile and young adult dogs and are overexpressed in the GBM of affected dogs. (Reproduced from Lees *et al.*, 1998b, with permission from *Kidney International*.)

7.2 Electron micrographs of glomerular basement membranes (GBMs) in the glomerular capillary walls of English Cocker Spaniels. **(a)** Normal GBM thickness and ultrastructure in a healthy 6-month-old dog. **(b)** Thickened GBM that has bilaminar splitting of the lamina densa and an irregular contour of its subepithelial aspect (subepithelial frilling) from a 6-month-old dog with an autosomal recessive hereditary glomerulopathy, causing proteinuria but not azotaemia. **(c)** Greatly thickened GBM that has multilaminar splitting of the lamina densa from a 22-month-old dog with the same disease, causing renal failure that had advanced to end-stage. CL = Capillary lumen; US = Urinary space. (Multiplication X15,000.) (Reproduced from Lees *et al.*, 1998b, with permission from *Kidney International*.)

and *COL4A4*, which encode the α3 and α4 chains, as candidate genes for the disorder, but the causative mutation has not yet been identified. Except that males and females are affected equally, the inherited nephropathy in Cocker Spaniels is clinically and pathologically similar to the X-linked disorders. Persistent proteinuria develops at 5–8 months of age, and renal function subsequently declines progressively leading to death from renal failure at 10–27 months of age (Lees *et al.*, 1998a,b).

Because light microscopy findings are non-specific, definitive pathological diagnosis requires electron microscopy to demonstrate the characteristic multilaminar splitting and thickening of the GBM (Figure 7.2). Immunostaining that shows the distinctively abnormal pattern of type IV collagen α-chain expression in renal basement membranes is also diagnostic when available (Figure 7.3). The disease is truly recessive; obligate carriers (parents of affected dogs) are clinically and pathologically indistinguishable from normal dogs, even using electron microscopy and immunostaining to examine their renal basement membranes (Lees *et al.*, 1998b).

Bull Terriers and Dalmatians

Autosomal dominant inherited glomerulopathies have been described in Bull Terriers and Dalmatians, mainly from Australia (Robinson *et al.*, 1989; Hood *et al.*, 1991, 1995, 2000, 2002a,b). The nephropathy in Bull Terriers has been studied more than the one in Dalmatians, but the two conditions are reported to have similar clinical and pathological features. These disorders are characterized by ultrastructural abnormalities in the GBM that can be definitively diagnosed only by electron microscopy (Hood *et al.*, 1995, 2000, 2002b). The GBM changes are similar to those that characterize the X-linked and autosomal recessive conditions described above. In contrast, however, immunostaining of kidney from affected Bull Terriers and Dalmatians shows a normal pattern of type IV collagen α-chain expression in their basement membranes (Hood *et al.*, 2000, 2002b). These findings are consistent with possible existence of a functionally defective α3–α4–α5 network due to mutations in *COL4A3* or *COL4A4*, such as have been reported in the rare human forms of Alport syndrome that have autosomal dominant inheritance. However, gene defects that cause these nephropathies in Bull Terriers and Dalmatians have not been identified, and a few autosomal dominant human diseases with some features resembling Alport syndrome are caused by mutations in other genes (e.g. *MYH9*, *LMX1*).

Clinical expression of canine autosomal dominant glomerulopathy is somewhat variable. All affected dogs have proteinuria (defined as UPC ≥0.3 by the investigators who studied these disorders), but the onset of renal failure occurs at 11 months to 8 years of age in Bull Terriers (Robinson *et al.*, 1989) and at 8 months to 7 years of age in Dalmatians (Hood *et al.*, 2002b). As is the case for the glomerulopathies described above, progression of these nephropathies to renal failure is associated with extensive secondary tubulointerstitial changes (Hood *et al.*, 2002a,b).

Other breeds

Other breeds, in which a renal disease having the clinicopathological features of a primary glomerulopathy has been described in related dogs, include the Dobermann (Wilcock and Patterson, 1979; Chew *et al.*, 1983; Picut and Lewis, 1987a), Bull Mastiff (Casal *et al.*, 2004), Beagle (Rha *et al.*, 2000), Rottweiler (Cook *et al.*, 1993), Pembroke Welsh Corgi (McKay *et al.*, 2004) and Newfoundland (Koeman *et al.*, 1994). The causes and pathogenesis of these conditions are uncertain, although the glomerular lesions sometimes have been examined at the ultrastructural as well as light microscopic levels.

Polycystic kidney disease

Autosomal dominant polycystic kidney disease is prevalent in Persian and Persian-cross cats, affecting approximately 38% of Persian cats worldwide (Barrs *et al.*, 2001; Beck and Lavelle, 2001; Cannon *et al.*, 2001; Barthez *et al.*, 2003). Recently, a single mutation in the feline *PKD1* gene has been incriminated as the cause of this disorder in many if not all affected cats (Lyons *et al.*, 2004). A stop mutation caused by a single nucleotide transversion in exon 29 (of 46) was found in the heterozygous state in each of 48 affected cats (41 Persians and one cat in each of seven other breeds) from the United States. Because the mutation is likely to be identical by descent within the breed, a DNA test is now possible to identify Persian and Persian-cross cats that have or will develop polycystic kidney disease, although the expectation that this single mutation causes the disease worldwide remains to be verified by further studies.

In affected cats, multiple cysts form in both kidneys and occasionally in the liver. Renal cysts arise from tubules and occur in both the cortex and the medulla (Eaton *et al.*, 1997). They form early in life and gradually become more numerous and larger in size as the cat ages. Detection of multiple cysts distributed in both kidneys using ultrasonography is diagnostic. Cysts can sometimes be detected in kittens as young as 6–8 weeks of age; however, because the number and size of cysts increase with time, sensitivity of ultrasonography as a diagnostic test for polycystic kidney disease increased from 75% at 16 weeks of age to 91% at 36 weeks of age in one study (Biller *et al.*, 1996). Cyst growth eventually causes renomegaly, which can be an incidental finding during physical examination of seemingly healthy cats, and renal failure ensues later in adult life (at 3–10 years of age, average 7 years).

Autosomal dominant polycystic kidney disease has also been described in Bull Terriers, mainly in Australia (Burrows *et al.*, 1994; O'Leary *et al.*, 1999). Affected dogs are identified by ultrasonography when multiple (three or more) cysts distributed in both kidneys are detected in dogs with a family history of the disease. The gene mutation that causes this disease has not been identified (O'Leary *et al.*, 2003), but dogs at risk for the disease can be screened with ultrasonography prior to breeding to minimize production of additional affected animals (O'Leary *et al.*, 1999). Bull Terriers with polycystic kidney disease that develop renal failure do so as adults, and hepatic cysts have not been described in affected dogs. Some Bull Terriers have renal lesions consistent with concurrent existence of both polycystic kidney disease and the hereditary GBM nephropathy (O'Leary et al., 2002).

Autosomal recessive polycystic kidney and liver disease has been described in the Cairn Terrier and the West Highland White Terrier (McKenna and Carpenter, 1980; McAloose et al., 1998). Affected puppies become clinically ill before 2 months of age and have marked enlargement of their livers and kidneys caused by the presence of numerous cysts.

Amyloidosis

Familial forms of reactive systemic amyloidosis with predilection for renal involvement occur in both dogs and cats. In dogs, familial renal amyloidosis has been described most often in the Shar Pei (DiBartola et al., 1990; Rivas et al., 1993), but also in the Beagle (Bowles and Mosier, 1992) and English Foxhound (Mason and Day, 1996). In cats, this condition occurs mainly in Abyssinians (Chew et al., 1982; Boyce et al., 1984; DiBartola et al., 1986), but has also been reported in the Siamese and Oriental (a colour variant of Siamese) breeds (Zuber, 1993; Godfrey and Day, 1998).

In Shar Pei dogs, familial amyloidosis usually causes renal failure at 1–6 years of age (average 4 years) (DiBartola et al., 1990). Some dogs have a history of previous episodes of high fever and joint swelling, and this disease in Shar Peis may be analogous to familial Mediterranean fever in humans (May et al., 1992; Rivas et al., 1992). Some evidence suggests that amyloidosis in Shar Peis is inherited in an autosomal recessive fashion (Rivas et al., 1993). Affected Shar Peis invariably have moderate to severe medullary interstitial amyloid deposits, but only two thirds have glomerular deposits. Proteinuria and other elements of the nephrotic syndrome, which reflect the severity of glomerular involvement, occur in some dogs. Amyloid is also frequently deposited in many other organs. Severe amyloid deposition in the liver may cause hepatomegaly, jaundice or hepatic rupture (Loeven, 1994a,b).

In Abyssinian cats, familial amyloidosis is probably inherited as an autosomal dominant trait with variable penetrance (DiBartola, 2005). Renal amyloid deposits first appear between 9 and 24 months of age, mainly in the medullary interstitium. Glomerular deposits are usually mild but are occasionally severe, so proteinuria is a variable feature. Affected cats usually develop chronic kidney disease at 1–5 years of age (average 3 years), but cats with mild deposits can live to be much older. Additionally, cats with severe medullary involvement sometimes develop papillary necrosis. Amyloid deposits are also often found in other organs, but in Abyssinian cats, extrarenal amyloid deposition is usually of little clinical consequence. In Siamese and Oriental cats with familial amyloidosis, however, severe amyloid deposition occurs predominantly in the liver and mainly causes intra-abdominal haemorrhage from hepatic rupture (Zuber, 1993; Godfrey and Day, 1998). Nonetheless, amyloid deposition also occurs in the kidneys and leads to renal failure in some affected cats. Amino acid sequences of amyloid AA proteins isolated from Siamese cats are slightly different from those of AA proteins from Abyssinian cats, possibly accounting for the difference in the predominant site of amyloid deposition between the two breeds (Niewold et al., 1999).

Immune-mediated glomerulonephritis

A familial disorder that causes protein-losing enteropathy, protein-losing nephropathy, or both, has been described in Soft-Coated Wheaten Terriers (Littman et al., 2000). Although the pathogenesis of the disorder is incompletely understood, evidence suggests that food hypersensitivity and altered intestinal permeability develop first and that immune complex glomerulonephritis develops subsequently (Vaden et al., 2000a,b). The mode of inheritance has not been defined, but the disorder is common among Soft-Coated Wheaten Terriers, particularly in the United States, where the condition is estimated to affect as many as 10–15% of the dogs of this breed.

Females are affected slightly more often than males, and the average age when renal disease is diagnosed in affected dogs is 6 years of age. Clinical signs associated with the nephropathy include polyuria, polydipsia, vomiting and weight loss. Laboratory findings include proteinuria, hypoalbuminaemia and hypercholesterolaemia, often associated with abnormalities attributable to renal failure (azotaemia, hyperphosphataemia and non-regenerative anaemia). The disease is complicated by thromboembolism in about 12% of cases, and hypertension occurs occasionally (Littman et al., 2000).

Under light microscopy, renal lesions are seen as a membranous to membranoproliferative glomerulonephritis progressing to glomerular sclerosis accompanied by periglomerular fibrosis and secondary tubulointerstitial changes. Evidence of mesangial deposition of immunoglobulin A (IgA), IgM and complement has been detected in the glomeruli of affected dogs using immunofluorescent labelling and electron microscopy (Afrouzian et al., 2001).

Membranoproliferative glomerulonephritis has also been described in 2–7-year-old Bernese Mountain Dogs (Minkus et al., 1994; Reusch et al., 1994). Pedigree analysis suggested autosomal recessive inheritance of the disorder. Laboratory findings were those of renal failure accompanied by marked proteinuria, hypoalbuminaemia and hypercholesterolaemia. Glomerular ultrastructural lesions resembled those of human membranoproliferative glomerulonephritis type I, with electron-dense immune deposits, mainly in subendothelial locations, and reduplication of the GBM. Immunolabelling consistently demonstrated glomerular IgM and complement deposition, with labelling for IgA or IgG detected only occasionally. Most of the affected dogs had high serum titres against Borrelia burgdorferi, but the organism could not be detected immunohistochemically in the tissues of affected dogs.

Membranoproliferative glomerulonephritis has also been reported in Brittany Spaniels with a genetically determined deficiency of the third component of complement (Cork et al., 1991).

Miscellaneous conditions

Fanconi syndrome
An inherited form of Fanconi syndrome, which is caused by generalized impairment of the reabsorptive functions of proximal renal tubules and results in excessive urinary losses of multiple solutes and water, occurs in Basenjis (Bovee et al., 1979; Noonan and Kay, 1990). Most affected dogs are 4–7 years of age at onset, but substantial diversity in the spectrum and severity of reabsorptive defects exists among affected dogs. Polyuria, polydipsia, renal glucosuria, mild proteinuria and aminoaciduria are consistent findings. Some dogs maintain normal serum biochemical profiles, but others may develop various derangements, most notably hyperchloraemic metabolic acidosis or hypokalaemia.

Treatment is generally focused on minimizing the systemic effects of urinary losses of important solutes by supplementing their intake. A medical management protocol that espouses an aggressive approach to bicarbonate treatment as well as routine supplementation of amino acids, vitamins and minerals has been promoted (Gonto, 2003) and is widely used but has not been directly compared with any other management protocol.

Some affected dogs develop renal failure, but a recent study found that the expected lifespan for affected dogs was similar to that for unaffected dogs and that affected dogs generally had a good or excellent quality of life as judged by their owners (Yearley et al., 2004). Notably, most of the dogs in the study were managed using the aggressive protocol. In addition, owner tolerance of polydipsia and polyuria is likely to be an important factor that influences life expectancy of dogs with Fanconi syndrome. Sporadic cases of persistent Fanconi syndrome also have been described in dogs of a number of other breeds, but evidence of familial occurrence of the condition in breeds other than the Basenji has not been reported.

Hereditary multifocal renal cystadenocarcinoma and nodular dermatofibrosis
Hereditary multifocal renal cystadenocarcinoma and nodular dermatofibrosis is a canine cancer syndrome originally described in German Shepherd Dogs. The condition is inherited as an autosomal dominant trait, and a mutation in the canine *BHD* gene recently has been incriminated as the cause of the disorder (Lingaas et al., 2003). The disease is characterized by development of bilateral, multifocal tumours in the kidneys, numerous firm nodules in the skin and subcutis and uterine leiomyomas. Affected dogs are usually diagnosed at 5–11 years of age (average, 8 years) when they are examined, because of the skin lesions or a variety of non-specific signs (Moe and Lium, 1997).

Telangiectasia
Pembroke Welsh Corgis with telangiectasia have episodes of gross haematuria beginning at 2–8 years of age (Moore and Thornton, 1983). Signs of abdominal distress or dysuria may occur as well. Several months often elapse between episodes, but urinary bleeding can be sufficiently severe to cause anaemia or formation of blood clots in the urine. Affected dogs may develop nephrocalcinosis or calculi, and hydronephrosis may develop if a calculus or blood clot obstructs the ureter.

References and further reading

Afrouzian M, Vaden SL, Harris T et al. (2001) Immune complex mediated proliferative and sclerosing glomerulonephritis in Soft Coated Wheaten Terriers (SCWT): Is this an animal model of IgA nephropathy or IgM mesangial nephropathy? *Journal of the American Society of Nephrology* **12**, 670A [abstract]

Barrs VR, Gunew M, Foster SF, Beatty JA and Malik R (2001) Prevalence of autosomal dominant polycystic kidney disease in Persian cats and related-breeds in Sydney and Brisbane. *Australian Veterinary Journal* **79**, 257–259

Barthez PY, Rivier P and Begon D (2003) Prevalence of polycystic kidney disease in Persian and Persian related cats in France. *Journal of Feline Medicine and Surgery* **5**, 345–347

Baumal R, Thorner P, Valli VE et al. (1991) Renal disease in carrier female dogs with X-linked hereditary nephritis; implications for female patients with this disease. *American Journal of Pathology* **139**, 751–764

Beck C and Lavelle RB (2001) Feline polycystic kidney disease in Persian and other cats: a prospective study using ultrasonography. *Australian Veterinary Journal* **79**, 181–184

Biller DS, DiBartola SP, Eaton KA (1996) Inheritance of polycystic kidney disease in Persian cats. *Journal of Heredity* **87**, 1–5

Bovee KC, Joyce T, Blazer-Yost B, Goldschmidt MS and Segal S (1979) Characterization of renal defects in dogs with a syndrome similar to the Fanconi syndrome in man. *Journal of the American Veterinary Medical Association* **174**, 1094–1099

Bowles MH and Mosier DA (1992) Renal amyloidosis in a family of beagles. *Journal of the American Veterinary Medical Association* **201**, 569–574

Boyce JT, DiBartola SP, Chew DJ and Gasper PW (1984) Familial renal amyloidosis in Abyssinian cats. *Veterinary Pathology* **21**, 33–38

Brown CA, Crowell WA, Brown SA, Barsanti JA and Finco DR (1990) Suspected familial renal disease in chow chows. *Journal of the American Veterinary Medical Association* **196**, 1279–1284

Burrows AK, Malik R, Hunt GB et al. (1994) Familial polycystic kidney disease in bull terriers. *Journal of Small Animal Practice* **35**, 364–369

Cannon MJ, MacKay AD, Barr FJ et al. (2001) Prevalence of polycystic kidney disease in Persian cats in the United Kingdom. *Veterinary Record* **149**, 409–411

Casal ML, Dambach DM, Meister T et al. (2004) Familial glomerulonephropathy in the Bullmastiff. *Veterinary Pathology* **41**, 319–325

Chew DJ, DiBartola SP, Boyce JT and Gasper PW (1982) Renal amyloidosis in related Abyssinian cats. *Journal of the American Veterinary Medical Association* **181**, 139–142

Chew DJ, DiBartola SP, Boyce JT, Hayes HM Jr and Brace JJ (1983) Juvenile renal disease in Doberman Pinscher dogs. *Journal of the American Veterinary Medical Association* **182**, 481–485

Cook SM, Dean DF, Golden DL, Wilkinson JE and Means TL (1993) Renal failure attributable to atrophic glomerulopathy in four related rottweilers. *Journal of the American Veterinary Medical Association* **202**, 107–109

Cork LC, Morris JM, Olson JL et al. (1991) Membranoproliferative glomerulonephritis in dogs with a genetically determined deficiency of the third component of complement. *Clinical Immunology and Immunopathology* **60**, 455–470

Cox ML, Lees GE, Kashtan CE and Murphy KE (2003) Genetic cause of X-linked Alport syndrome in a family of domestic dogs. *Mammalian Genome* **14**, 396–403

de Morais HS, DiBartola SP and Chew DJ (1996) Juvenile renal disease in golden retrievers: 12 cases (1984–1994). *Journal of the American Veterinary Medical Association* **209**, 792–797

DiBartola SP (2005) Familial renal disease in dogs and cats. In: *Textbook of Veterinary Internal Medicine, 6th edn*, ed. SJ Ettinger and EC Feldman, pp. 1819–1824. Elsevier Saunders, St. Louis

DiBartola SP, Chew DJ and Boyce JT (1983) Juvenile renal disease in related Standard Poodles. *Journal of the American Veterinary Medical Association* **183**, 693–696

DiBartola SP, Tarr MJ and Benson MD (1986) Tissue distribution of amyloid deposits in Abyssinian cats with familial amyloidosis. *Journal of Comparative Pathology* **96**, 387–398

DiBartola SP, Tarr MJ, Webb DM and Giger U (1990) Familial renal amyloidosis in Chinese shar pei dogs. *Journal of the American Veterinary Medical Association* **197**, 483–487

Eaton KA, Biller DS, DiBartola SP, Radin MJ and Wellman ML (1997) Autosomal dominant polycystic kidney disease in Persian and Persian-cross cats. *Veterinary Pathology* **34**, 117–126

Eriksen K and Gröndalen J (1984) Familial renal disease in soft-coated Wheaten terriers. *Journal of Small Animal Practice* **25**, 489–500

Godfrey DR and Day MJ (1998) Generalised amyloidosis in two Siamese cats: spontaneous liver haemorrhage and chronic renal failure. *Journal of Small Animal Practice* **39**, 442–447

Gonto S (2003) Fanconi disease management protocol for veterinarians. Available at: www.basenji.org/fanconiprotocol2003.pdf (Accessed 6 May 2005)

Harvey SJ, Zheng K, Sado Y *et al.* (1998) Role of distinct type IV collagen networks in glomerular development and function. *Kidney International* **54**, 1857–1866

Hood JC, Dowling J, Bertram JF *et al.* (2002a) Correlation of histopathological features and renal impairment in autosomal dominant Alport syndrome in Bull terriers. *Nephrology, Dialysis and Transplantation* **17**, 1897–1908

Hood JC, Huxtable C, Naito I, Smith C, Sinclair R and Savige J (2002b) A novel model of autosomal dominant Alport syndrome in Dalmatian dogs. *Nephrology, Dialysis and Transplantation* **17**, 2094–2098

Hood JC, Robinson WF, Clark WT *et al.* (1991) Proteinuria as an indicator of early renal disease in Bull terriers with hereditary nephritis. *Journal of Small Animal Practice* **32**, 241–248

Hood JC, Savige J, Hendtlass A *et al.* (1995) Bull terrier hereditary nephritis: a model for autosomal dominant Alport syndrome. *Kidney International* **47**, 758–765

Hood JC, Savige J, Seymour AE *et al.* (2000) Ultrastructural appearance of renal and other basement membranes in the Bull terrier model of autosomal dominant hereditary nephritis. *American Journal of Kidney Disease* **36**, 378–391

Jansen B, Thorner PS, Singh A *et al.* (1984) Animal model of human disease: hereditary nephritis in Samoyed dogs. *American Journal of Pathology* **116**, 175–178

Jansen B, Valli VE, Thorner P, Baumal R and Lumsden JH (1987) Samoyed hereditary glomerulopathy: serial, clinical and laboratory (urine, serum biochemistry and hematology) studies. *Canadian Journal of Veterinary Research* **51**, 387–393

Kerlin RL and Van Winkle TJ (1995) Renal dysplasia in golden retrievers. *Veterinary Pathology* **32**, 327–329

Koeman JP, Biewenga WJ and Gruys E (1994) Proteinuria associated with glomerulosclerosis and glomerular collagen formation in three Newfoundland dog littermates. *Veterinary Pathology* **31**, 188–193

Lees GE (1996) Congenital renal diseases. *Veterinary Clinics of North America: Small Animal Practice* **26**, 1379–1399

Lees GE, Helman RG, Homco LD *et al.* (1998a) Early diagnosis of familial nephropathy in English cocker spaniels. *Journal of the American Animal Hospital Association* **34**, 189–195

Lees GE, Helman RG, Kashtan CE *et al.* (1998b) A model of autosomal recessive Alport syndrome in English cocker spaniel dogs. *Kidney International* **54**, 706–719

Lees GE, Helman RG, Kashtan CE *et al.* (1999) New form of X-linked dominant hereditary nephritis in dogs. *American Journal of Veterinary Research* **60**, 373–383

Lees GE, Wilson PD, Helman RG, Homco LD and Frey MS (1997) Glomerular ultrastructural findings similar to hereditary nephritis in 4 English cocker spaniels. *Journal of Veterinary Internal Medicine* **11**, 80–85

Lingaas F, Comstock KE, Kirkness EF *et al.* (2003) A mutation in the canine BHD gene is associated with hereditary multifocal renal cystadenocarcinoma and nodular dermatofibrosis in the German Shepherd dog. *Human Molecular Genetics* **12**, 3043–3053

Littman MP, Dambach DM, Vaden SL and Giger U (2000) Familial protein-losing enteropathy and protein-losing nephropathy in Soft Coated Wheaten Terriers: 222 cases (1983–1997). *Journal of Veterinary Internal Medicine* **14**, 68–80

Loeven KO (1994a) Hepatic amyloidosis in two Chinese Shar Pei dogs. *Journal of the American Veterinary Medical Association* **204**, 1212–1216

Loeven KO (1994b) Spontaneous hepatic rupture secondary to amyloidosis in a Chinese Shar Pei. *Journal of the American Animal Hospital Association* **30**, 577–579

Lyons LA, Biller DS, Erdman CA *et al.* (2004) Feline polycystic kidney disease mutation identified in PKD1. *Journal of the American Society of Nephrology* **15**, 2548–2555

Mason NJ and Day MJ (1996) Renal amyloidosis in related English foxhounds. *Journal of Small Animal Practice* **37**, 255–260

May C, Hammill J and Bennett D (1992) Chinese shar pei fever syndrome: a preliminary report. *Veterinary Record* **131**, 586–587

McAloose D, Casal M, Patterson DF and Dambach DM (1998) Polycystic kidney and liver disease in two related West Highland White Terrier litters. *Veterinary Pathology* **35**, 77–81

McKay LW, Seguin MA, Ritchey JW and Levy JK (2004) Juvenile nephropathy in two related Pembroke Welsh corgi puppies. *Journal of Small Animal Practice* **45**, 568–571

McKenna SC and Carpenter JL (1980) Polycystic disease of the kidney and liver in the Cairn Terrier. *Veterinary Pathology* **17**, 436–442

Minkus G, Breuer W, Wanke R *et al.* (1994) Familial nephropathy in Bernese mountain dogs. *Veterinary Pathology* **31**, 421–428

Moe L and Lium B (1997) Hereditary multifocal renal cystadenocarcinomas and nodular dermatofibrosis in 51 German shepherd dogs. *Journal of Small Animal Practice* **38**, 498–505

Moore FM and Thornton GW (1983) Telangiectasia of Pembroke Welsh Corgi dogs. *Veterinary Pathology* **20**, 203–208

Morton LD, Sanecki RK, Gordon DE *et al.* (1990) Juvenile renal disease in miniature schnauzer dogs. *Veterinary Pathology* **27**, 455–458

Nash AS, Kelly DF and Gaskell CJ (1984) Progressive renal disease in soft-coated Wheaten terriers: possible familial nephropathy. *Journal of Small Animal Practice* **25**, 479–487

Niewold TA, van der Linde-Sipman JS, Murphy C, Tooten PC and Gruys E (1999) Familial amyloidosis in cats: Siamese and Abyssinian AA proteins differ in primary sequence and pattern of deposition. *Amyloid* **6**, 205–209

Noonan CHB and Kay JM (1990) Prevalence and geographic distribution of Fanconi syndrome in Basenjis in the United States. *Journal of the American Veterinary Medical Association* **197**, 345–349

O'Brien TD, Osborne CA, Yano BL and Barnes DM (1982) Clinicopathologic manifestations of progressive renal disease in Lhasa Apso and Shih Tzu dogs. *Journal of the American Veterinary Medical Association* **180**, 658–664

O'Leary CA, Atwell RB, and Laing NG (2003) No disease-associated mutations found in the coding sequence of the canine polycystic kidney disease gene 1 in Bull Terriers with polycystic kidney disease. *Animal Genetics* **34**, 358–361

O'Leary CA, Ghoddusi M and Huxtable CR (2002) Renal pathology of polycystic kidney disease and concurrent hereditary nephritis in Bull Terriers. *Australian Veterinary Journal* **80**, 353–361

O'Leary CA, Mackay BM, Malik R *et al.* (1999) Polycystic kidney disease in bull terriers: an autosomal dominant inherited disorder. *Australian Veterinary Journal* **77**, 361–366

Picut CA and Lewis RM (1987a) Juvenile renal disease in the Doberman Pinscher: ultrastructural changes of the glomerular basement membrane. *Journal of Comparative Pathology* **97**, 587–596

Picut CA and Lewis RM (1987b) Microscopic features of canine renal dysplasia. *Veterinary Pathology* **24**, 156–163

Reusch C, Hoerauf A, Lechner J *et al.* (1994) A new familial glomerulonephropathy in Bernese mountain dogs. *Veterinary Record* **134**, 411–415

Rha JY, Labato MA, Ross LA, Breitschwerdt E and Alroy J (2000) Familial glomerulonephropathy in a litter of beagles. *Journal of the American Veterinary Medical Association* **216**, 46–50

Rivas AL, Tintle L, Kimball ES, Scarlett J and Quimby FW (1992) A canine febrile disorder associated with elevated interleukin-6. *Clinical Immunology and Immunopathology* **64**, 36–45

Rivas AL, Tintle L, Meyers-Wallen V *et al.* (1993) Inheritance of renal amyloidosis in Chinese Shar-pei dogs. *Journal of Heredity* **84**, 438–442

Robinson WF, Huxtable CR and Gooding JP (1985) Familial nephropathy in cocker spaniels. *Australian Veterinary Journal* **62**, 109–112

Robinson WF, Shaw SE, Stanley B *et al.* (1989) Chronic renal disease in bull terriers. *Australian Veterinary Journal* **66**, 193–195

Schulze C, Meyer HP, Blok AL, Schipper K and van den Ingh TS (1998) Renal dysplasia in three young adult Dutch kooiker dogs. *Veterinary Quarterly* **20**, 146–148

Steward AP and Macdougall DF (1984) Familial nephropathy in the cocker spaniel. *Journal of Small Animal Practice* **25**, 15–24

Vaden SL, Hammerberg B, Davenport DJ *et al.* (2000a) Food hypersensitivity reactions in Soft Coated Wheaten Terriers with protein-losing enteropathy or protein-losing nephropathy or both: gastroscopic food sensitivity testing, dietary provocation, and fecal immunoglobulin E. *Journal of Veterinary Internal Medicine* **14**, 60–67

Vaden SL, Sellon RK, Melgarejo LT *et al.* (2000b) Evaluation of intestinal permeability and gluten sensitivity in Soft-Coated Wheaten Terriers with familial protein-losing enteropathy, protein-losing nephropathy, or both. *American Journal of Veterinary Research* **61**, 518–524

Vilafranca M and Ferrer L (1994) Juvenile nephropathy in Alaskan Malamute littermates. *Veterinary Pathology* **31**, 375–377

Wilcock BP and Patterson JM (1979) Familial glomerulonephritis in Doberman pinscher dogs. *Canadian Veterinary Journal* **20**, 244–249

Yearley JH, Hancock DD and Mealey KL (2004) Survival time, lifespan, and quality of life in dogs with idiopathic Fanconi syndrome. *Journal of the American Veterinary Medical Association* **225**, 377–383

Zheng K, Thorner PS, Marrano P, Baumal R and McInnes RR (1994) Canine X chromosome-linked hereditary nephritis: a genetic model for human X-linked hereditary nephritis resulting from a single base mutation in the gene encoding the alpha 5 chain of collagen type IV. *Proceedings of the National Academy of Science USA* **91**, 3989–3993

Zuber RM (1993) Systemic amyloidosis in Oriental and Siamese cats. *Australian Veterinary Practice* **23**, 66–70

8

Complete urinalysis

Heather Wamsley and Rick Alleman

Introduction

Complete urinalysis (Figure 8.1) includes assessment of several physical and chemical characteristics of urine. It is a simple, economical test that requires minimal specialized equipment and can be routinely performed by trained individuals in general veterinary practice. With proper sample handling and testing, data generated by urinalysis rapidly disclose vital information about the urinary tract and also provide a general screen of other body systems (e.g. endocrine, hepatic). There are several potential indications for urinalysis (Figure 8.2); however, complete urinalysis is an essential component in the diagnostic evaluation of a patient with clinical signs of disease which localize to the urinary tract or to other body systems.

To gain the full benefit of urinalysis and to avoid potential misinterpretation of laboratory results, all components of a complete urinalysis should ideally be performed. For example, knowledge of the urine specific gravity (SG) is necessary for effective interpretation of the serum urea, serum creatinine, urine protein and urine bilirubin concentrations. Also, microscopic examination of the urine sediment for signs of active inflammation or infection is required to determine the significance of proteinuria by aiding in its localization (e.g. glomerular *versus* lower urinary tract).

Urine sample collection method, timing and handling prior to analysis

In addition to biological variability of the patient, urinalysis results are influenced by the urine collection method, the timing of urine collection, administration of therapeutic or diagnostic agents prior to collection and how the sample is handled prior to analysis. There are several methods of urine collection, each with their own advantages and disadvantages (Figures 8.3 and 8.4). Ideally at least 6 ml of urine should be collected prior to the administration of therapeutic or diagnostic agents so that baseline information can be established. In most situations, either naturally voided urine collected midstream into a sterile container or urine obtained by

| Gross inspection of the urine |
| Specific chemical testing of the urine |
| Microscopic examination of the urine sediment |

8.1 Components of complete urinalysis.

| **Aids in interpretation of elevated serum urea nitrogen and creatinine concentrations** |
| **Screen for occult disease in clinically normal patients** |
| Pre-anaesthetic |
| Geriatric |
| **Minimum laboratory database for diseased patients** |
| Clinical signs referable to the urinary system |
| Clinical signs referable to other body systems, for example: |
| Endocrine (e.g. detect glucosuria or urinary tract infection) |
| Hepatic (e.g. detect bilirubinuria or ammonium biurate crystals) |
| Haematological (e.g. help localize haemolysis as intravascular by detecting haemoglobinuria) |
| Neurological (e.g. detect bacteriuria associated with discospondylitis) |
| **Tool for monitoring** |
| Progression of renal disease |
| Response to therapy for urinary tract disease |
| Safety of potentially nephrotoxic drugs |

8.2 Indications for and uses of complete urinalysis.

| **General** |
| Sterile, sealable, opaque, plastic sample cup |
| 6 ml sterile syringe |
| **Natural voiding (feline)** |
| Non-absorbent, plastic granular litter |
| **Catheterization** |
| Sterile urinary catheter in good condition |
| Sterile gloves |
| Sterile lubricant |
| **Cystocentesis** |
| Dogs: 22-gauge sterile needle, 38 mm (1.5 inch) to 76 mm (3 inch), depending on patient size |
| Cats: 23-gauge sterile needle, 16 mm (5/8 inch) to 25 mm (1 inch), depending on patient size |
| **If intended for urine culture** |
| Culture tube |

8.3 Materials that may be used during urine collection.

Collection method	Advantages	Disadvantages/precautions
Midstream, naturally voided	Non-invasive, relatively easy technique (in dogs) Can be performed by clients and is therefore useful to collect first morning, maximally concentrated urine samples from out-patients Unlike cystocentesis or catheterization, is not associated with iatrogenic haematuria Although not ideal, a freshly voided sample can be used for urine culture, as long as a quantitative urine culture is performed	Likely to be contaminated by a variable amount of material from the lower genitourinary tract (e.g. bacteria, epithelial cells, blood, sperm, debris), perineum (e.g. *Trichuris* ova) or environment (e.g. pollen), which may be observed during microscopic examination of the urine sediment Cleanser residues or microorganisms within the collection vessel may affect results. Urine should be collected into a sterile, single-use urine collection cup rather than a reusable container provided by the client or veterinary practice Avoid manual bladder compression to induce micturition, which may cause reflux of urine into other organs (e.g. kidneys, prostate) or iatrogenic haematuria
Transurethral catheterization	Useful collection method when an indwelling urinary catheter is already present for another reason Although not ideal, sample can be used for urine culture, as long as a quantitative urine culture is performed	Risk of traumatic catheterization, which may injure the patient and contaminate the sample with blood Risk of iatrogenic infection, especially in patients predisposed to urinary tract infection (e.g. lower urinary tract disease, renal failure, diabetes mellitus, hyperadrenocorticism) Should be performed aseptically and atraumatically by a trained, experienced individual Urine sample may be contaminated by variable numbers of epithelial cells, bacteria and debris from the lower genitourinary tract, which may be observed during microscopic examination of the urine sediment Catheters that are chemically sterilized may contain residue of the antiseptic solution, which can irritate mucosal linings and affect results of urinalysis and urine culture Catheterization may be technically challenging in female patients. Use of a vaginal endoscope may facilitate collection
Antepubic cystocentesis	Avoids lower genitourinary tract contamination of urine sample Ideal sample for urine culture Less risk of iatrogenic infection compared with transurethral catheterization Easier than collection of a voided sample from cats Better tolerated than catheterization, especially by cats and bitches	Contraindicated in patients with a bleeding diathesis (e.g. thrombocytopenia), may be performed with great caution after cystotomy An adequate volume of urine within the bladder is required Blind cystocentesis without at least manual localization and immobilization of the bladder is not recommended. Ultrasound-guided needle placement is helpful, though not mandatory Misdirection of the needle can lead to a non-diagnostic or contaminated sample (e.g. enterocentesis) A variable degree of iatrogenic microscopic haematuria, which cannot be readily distinguished from pathological, disease-induced haematuria, may be caused by this collection method. This type of contamination can be particularly pronounced when the bladder wall is inflamed or congested. Iatrogenic haematuria may limit the utility of this collection method when monitoring the progression of disease in a patient that has pathological haematuria

8.4 The advantages and disadvantages of methods of urine collection.

cystocentesis is preferred. Factors which may be useful to consider when selecting a urine collection method include the patient's clinical status, the logistics of the collection method and the intended use of the sample. For example, cystocentesis is the ideal collection method when a bacterial culture is desired. However, patients with cystitis may exhibit urge incontinence, making cystocentesis virtually impossible. In this situation, a voided sample collected from the examination room tabletop may be all that is available for analysis. A urine sample collected by this method will probably be contaminated by material from the tabletop, such as disinfectant cleanser residues or microorganisms. If

analysed with minimal delay, to prevent overgrowth of contaminating microorganisms, such a sample may yield useful initial information (e.g. detection of pyuria). Some chemical tests (e.g. glucose, haem, pH, protein) may, however, be affected by the presence of disinfectant residues.

Since urine collection method can have a significant effect upon urinalysis results, it is important to record the collection method in medical records and on submission forms if a referral diagnostic laboratory is used. It should also be indicated whether or not therapeutic or diagnostic agents (e.g. parenteral fluids, antimicrobials, glucocorticoids, diuretics, anti-

Analgesics

May interfere with biochemical tests:
  Etodolac metabolites – bilirubin
  Phenazopyridine – bilirubin, ketones, nitrite, protein, urobilinogen

Anticonvulsants, diuretics, glucocorticoids and parenteral fluids

Cause production of dilute urine:
  Lowers specific gravity
  Dilutes concentration of material in the urine sediment
  Cell lysis may occur if urine is hyposthenuric (specific gravity <1.008)
Some diuretics directly alter urine pH

Antihypertensives (e.g. captopril) and other drugs with free sulphydryl groups (e.g. D-penicillamine, methionine)

May interfere with biochemical tests: haem; ketones

Antimicrobials

May interfere with biochemical tests:
  Specific gravity (high doses)
  Glucose (by Chemstrips 10 SG or Clinitest tablet method)
  Haem
  Urobilinogen
  Sulphosalicylic acid protein precipitation (high doses)
May cause false-negative urine cultures

Radiographic contrast media

May interfere with biochemical tests:
  Specific gravity
  Glucose (by Clinitest tablet method)
  Sulphosalicylic acid protein precipitation
May cause crystalluria

Urine pH modulators (e.g. methionine, ascorbic acid)

Alteration of pH may affect other biochemical tests (e.g. protein) and sediment evaluation (very alkaline urine may cause degeneration of cells and casts)
Therapeutic agents may directly interfere with biochemical tests:
  Methionine – haem, ketones
  Ascorbic acid – bilirubin, glucose, haem, nitrite

8.5 General categories of diagnostic and therapeutic agents that may affect urinalysis results (list may not be all inclusive).

hypertensives, radiographic contrast) have been administered prior to urine collection (Figure 8.5). If so, the type of agent and timing and duration of administration relative to urine collection should be recorded.

Urinalysis results are also affected by the timing of urine collection relative to ingestion of water or a meal or relative to when the urine accumulated within the bladder (Figure 8.6). As with collection method, the intended purpose of the sample is a useful factor to consider when selecting the timing of urine collection. For example, culture of a randomly collected urine sample may be more useful than culture of the first morning urine. First morning urine typically is held within the bladder overnight for several hours, which may decrease the viability of fastidious microorganisms and cause a false-negative urine culture. Similarly, cellular morphology may be better preserved in a randomly collected urine sample, rather than in urine which has been held overnight within the bladder, since urine pH and nitrogenous waste materials may cause cells to degenerate.

A key goal of urine sample collection is to obtain and analyse a sample that most closely represents urine as it exists in the body. One step in achieving this goal is to handle urine samples in a way which minimizes the effects of post-collection *in vitro* artefacts (Figure 8.7). Ideally, urine should be collected into a sterile, opaque, sealable, labelled container and analysed within 60 minutes of collection. If it is not possible to analyse the sample within 60 minutes or if it must be shipped to a diagnostic laboratory, the sample should be preserved by refrigeration soon after collection for up to approximately 12 hours (i.e. overnight). Samples intended for routine urinalysis should not be frozen. Also, although numerous chemical preservatives of urine exist (e.g. boric acid, formalin, Mucolexx™), routine use of these preservatives is not recommended, since each may affect different components of the urinalysis.

Refrigeration is considered the optimal preservation method since it prevents bacterial overgrowth, preserves cellular and cast morphology and does not

Collection time	Advantages	Disadvantages
First morning urine – urine is formed after a period of several hours of nil by mouth	Represents the patient's maximally concentrated urine and is therefore ideal for assessing the ability of the renal tubules to concentrate urine Microscopic sediment will be more concentrated Postprandial alterations unlikely (e.g. postprandial alkalinuria) Urine more likely to be acidic, so casts may be better preserved (proteinaceous structures dissolve in alkaline urine)	Urine present within bladder for a relatively prolonged period: May alter cellular morphology observed during microscopic examination May decrease viability of fastidious microorganisms, resulting in false-negative culture results
Postprandially	Useful to assess the effect of diets intended to modulate urinary pH when collected 3–6 hours postprandially More likely to detect hyperglycaemic glucosuria when collected 3–4 hours postprandially	pH may be elevated by postprandial alkaline tide when collected within 1 hour postprandially
Randomly timed urine sample – represents urine that has accumulated within the bladder for minutes to hours or urine that has been diluted by recent ingestion of water	Microscopic cellular morphology and viability of fastidious microorganisms may be better preserved since urine is stored within the bladder for relatively less time	If the urine is isosthenuric or minimally concentrated, no conclusion can be drawn about renal tubular concentrating ability

8.6 Timing of urine sample collection, indications and potential effects upon urinalysis results.

affect chemical testing as long as the sample is returned to room temperature prior to analysis. However, refrigeration can cause artefactual changes, particularly crystal formation (i.e. calcium oxalate dihydrate, magnesium ammonium phosphate) that becomes worse as the duration of storage increases (Albasan *et al.*, 2003). To minimize refrigeration artefacts, samples should be allowed to warm to room temperature prior to urinalysis. Also, if crystalluria is observed in a sample that has been refrigerated or that has been stored for more than 6 hours regardless of the storage temperature, the finding should be confirmed with a freshly obtained, non-refrigerated urine sample that will be analysed within 30–60 minutes of collection.

Ideal urine sample handling

Urine should be collected in a sterile, opaque, airtight, labelled container

Either analysis should occur within 60 minutes of collection or the sample should be refrigerated until the time for analysis (for up to approximately 12 hours)

If the sample has been refrigerated, it should be warmed to room temperature prior to analysis to minimize artefacts caused by cooling of the sample

Potential artefacts associated with refrigeration

In vitro crystal formation (especially calcium oxalate dihydrate) increases with the duration of storage. When clinically significant crystalluria is suspected, it is best to confirm the finding with a freshly collected urine sample that has not been refrigerated and which is analysed within 60 minutes of collection

A cold urine sample may inhibit enzymatic reactions in the dipstick (e.g. glucose), leading to falsely decreased results

The specific gravity of cold urine may be falsely increased, because cold urine is denser than room temperature urine

Potential artefacts associated with prolonged storage at room temperature

Bacterial overgrowth can cause:
  Increased urine turbidity
  Altered pH
  Increased pH, if urease-producing bacteria are present
  Decreased pH, if bacteria use glucose to form acidic metabolites
  Decreased concentration of chemicals that may be metabolized by bacteria (e.g. glucose, ketones)
  Increased number of bacteria in urine sediment
  Altered urine culture results

Increased urine pH, which may occur due to loss of carbon dioxide from the sample or bacterial overgrowth, can cause:
  False-positive dipstick protein reaction
  Degeneration of cells and casts
  Alteration of the type and amount of crystals present

Other potential artefacts

Evaporative loss of volatile substances (e.g. carbon dioxide, ketones, urine water). Avoid this artefact by using an airtight sample container

Photodegradation of light-sensitive chemicals (e.g. bilirubin, urobilinogen). Avoid this artefact by using a sample container that does not transmit light (i.e. an opaque sample container)

8.7 Ideal conditions for urine sample handling and potential *in vitro* artefacts associated with urine storage.

Urinalysis method

During complete urinalysis several physical and chemical characteristics of urine are evaluated (see Figure 8.1). A list of the materials needed and a detailed method of routine urinalysis are provided in Figures 8.8 and 8.9. Urinalysis may yield erroneous results if laboratory materials are used incorrectly, if materials have been stored improperly or if materials are used that have not been validated in veterinary species.

Sterile, single-use, translucent, 15 ml polystyrene conical centrifuge tubes with lids

Translucent test tubes

Test tube rack

Disposable transfer pipettes

Clean, glass microscope slides

Clean, 22 × 22 mm glass coverslips

Temperature-compensated veterinary refractometer, ideally one with a feline urine specific gravity scale

Timer that indicates seconds

Urine dipstick multiple chemical test strip

Centrifuge

Microscope with X10 and X40 objectives

Optional items:
  Portable pH meter
  5% sulphosalicylic acid
  Rapid aqueous stain (e.g. new methylene blue, Sedi-Stain™)
  Diff Quik® or other aqueous-based modified Wright stain

8.8 Materials needed for complete urinalysis.

Urine dipsticks

Urine dipstick multiple chemical test strips have various reagents impregnated within each test pad. Guidelines for appropriate use and storage of urine dipsticks are provided (Figure 8.10). Many of the dipstick reagents will be damaged by exposure to light or to disinfectant cleansers, which can cause false-positive or false-negative results, depending upon the test. To prevent inactivation of the reagents, urine dipsticks should be stored with the lid tightly sealed, in the container provided by the manufacturer or another airtight container that completely obstructs light. If urine dipsticks are desired at more than one workstation, empty used containers provided by the manufacturer may be refilled and placed at each workstation, as long as the same type of dipstick is used to refill the container (i.e. the urine dipstick *must* correspond to the interpretation key printed on the outside of the container).

Over-saturation of test pads with urine can dilute the reagents and cause false results (e.g. false-positive dipstick protein). Also, urine should not be allowed to flow from one test pad to another. This can cause reagents in one test pad to intermingle with those in the adjacent pad, invalidating results. For example, on the Multistix® dipstick, the pH test pad is immediately adjacent to the protein test pad, which contains an acidic buffer. If the acidic buffer from the protein test pad contaminates the pH test pad, the measured pH

1. Ideally collect at least 6 ml of urine by cystocentesis or midstream during natural micturition into a sterile, opaque, sealable container.

2. Record the following in the medical record and on the sample submission form, if a referral laboratory will be used:
   - Urine collection method
   - Time of urine collection
   - Volume of urine collected
   - Method of preservation, if applicable (e.g. refrigeration, chemical)
   - Medications (e.g. antibiotics, diuretics, glucocorticoids), prescription diet or diagnostic agents administered (e.g. radiographic contrast medium)
   - Whether or not the patient was fasted.

3. Ensure that the container holding the urine, not just the lid, is adequately labelled (e.g. patient identification, date, collection method).

4. If the sample has been refrigerated, allow it to warm to room temperature before performing the urinalysis.

5. Mix the sample well and then transfer 5 ml of urine into a labelled conical centrifuge tube. Save the remaining urine in the refrigerator for additional or confirmatory tests, if indicated.

6. In a well lit area, against a white background, perform a gross inspection of the urine in the conical tube:
   - Record the urine colour (e.g. light yellow, yellow, dark yellow, red–brown)
   - Record the clarity of the urine (e.g. cloudy, slightly cloudy, clear).

7. Perform biochemical evaluation using a urine dipstick multiple chemical test strip and a timer that indicates seconds:
   - Wet each pad of the test strip either by briefly immersing the strip in the urine sample or by using a pipette to place individual drops of urine on each test pad and then start the timer. Avoid over-saturation or prolonged contact of the test pads with urine. Dab excess urine from the test pads. Do not allow urine from adjacent test pads to mix
   - Observe colour changes *at the times indicated on the bottle*, compare to the coloured squares on the bottle and record the results.

8. Centrifuge the sample to prepare for additional biochemical tests and microscopic examination of the sediment:
   - Centrifuge the 5 ml aliquot of urine in the conical tube (from Step 5) for 5 minutes at 400 *G* (1500 rpm)
   - After centrifugation, observe the tube for the presence of a lipid layer floating at the top of the supernatant. If lipid is present, record its approximate volume, remove it from the supernatant and discard it
   - Remove and save in a separate tube 4 ml of the supernatant (or 80% of the original volume, if the initial aliquot volume was less than 5 ml (at Step 5)) for additional biochemical tests. Save the sediment and remaining 1 ml (i.e. 20%) of supernatant for microscopic examination.

9. Perform additional biochemical tests on the 4 ml aliquot of supernatant:
   - Determine the urine specific gravity using a refractometer. Place one or two drops of urine supernatant on the refractometer and determine the specific gravity using the appropriate scale. If the indicated specific gravity is greater than the upper limit of the refractometer scale (usually 1.050 or 1.060), the sample should be diluted and re-read to obtain a more precise measurement if one is desired:
     – Dilute the sample 1-to-1 with distilled water and mix well
     – Place one or two drops of diluted urine on the refractometer and determine the specific gravity using the appropriate scale. This value must be adjusted for the dilution factor before it is reported
     – Adjust the indicated specific gravity for the dilution by multiplying the last two digits by two and report the adjusted value (e.g. if the specific gravity of the diluted sample is 1.035, report the specific gravity as 1.070).
   - (Optional) Perform the 5% sulphosalicylic acid precipitation test for protein:
     – Completely mix equal parts (approximately 0.5 ml each) of urine supernatant and 5% sulphosalicylic acid in a translucent test tube
     – In a well lit area, against a dark background, inspect the tube for the formation of white precipitate (e.g. cloudy white with or without flocculation) and interpret according to a standard scale.

10. Prepare the sediment for microscopic examination:
    - Resuspend the sediment pellet in the remaining 1 ml of supernatant that was left in the conical tube (at Step 8) (or resuspend the pellet in the remaining 20% of the original volume, if the initial aliquot volume was less than 5 ml (at Step 5))
    - Mix the solution by gentle agitation of the conical tube (e.g. by finger-flicking the bottom) or by aspirating the remaining 1 ml of fluid and gently expressing it back into the tube a few times using a transfer pipette. Casts are fragile, so it is imperative to mix the solution well, while avoiding overly aggressive agitation (e.g. vortexing)
    - Prepare a wet mount of the sediment solution. Pipette a single drop of the sediment solution on to one end of a clean, glass microscope slide and coverslip. The slide is ready for examination. If the slide will not be examined immediately, the slide should be stored in a humidified Petri dish, as described below
    - (Optional) Stain the sediment solution and prepare a wet mount of the stained solution. Mix 2 drops of the sediment solution and 1 drop of new methylene blue (or other rapid aqueous stain) in a separate test tube and gently mix. Pipette a single drop of this solution on to the other end of the clean, glass microscope slide. The slide, which now holds two wet mounts, is ready for examination
    - If there will be a delay between the time that the sediment wet mount is prepared and the time that it is examined, the wet mount should be stored in a humidified Petri dish to prevent evaporation of the sample:
      – Place a dampened, thin piece of absorbent material (e.g. paper towel, gauze, filter paper) in the bottom portion of a Petri dish
      – Place wooden sticks prepared from the broken handle of a cotton-tipped applicator on top of the moist, absorbent material
      – Place the microscope slide with the sediment wet mount on top of the wooden sticks
      – Cover the Petri dish with the provided lid. The wet mount will be stable for up to an hour. Multiple sediments can be prepared and examined in a batch if this procedure is followed.

8.9 Method for routine urinalysis. (continues) ▶

11. Perform systematic microscopic examination of sediment using reduced illumination:
    * Reduce the illumination of the microscope slide *either* by lowering the microscope's condenser to a couple of centimetres below the stage *or* by partially closing the aperture of the iris diaphragm within the condenser. (Both lowering the condenser and closing the iris diaphragm will excessively reduce the light and should not be done)
    * Examine 10 microscopic fields of the slide under low power using the X10 objective for the presence of the following things and provide an assessment of their amounts in the unstained wet mount:
        – Crystals: record type(s) present, and qualitative impression of the amount of each type of crystal (none, few, moderate number, many)
        – Cast: may be better visualized at the margins of the coverslip. Record type(s) present (e.g. hyaline, cellular, granular, waxy, lipid, haemoglobin) and record the number of each type of cast per X10 low power field (lpf) as a range (e.g. 0–2/lpf)
        – Epithelial cells: record type(s) present and the number of each type of epithelial cell per X10 lpf as a range (e.g. 0–4/lpf). Observe cellular morphology for the presence of dysplastic or neoplastic morphological changes
        – Mucus threads: record qualitative impression of the number of mucus threads (none, few, moderate number, many)
        – Helminth ova, larva, adult worms or other parasites: record qualitative impression of the number of parasite structures (none, few, moderate number, many)
    * Examine 10 microscopic fields of the slide under higher power using the X40 objective. Scrutinize the morphology of structures observed at low power. Confirm the identification of the structures observed at low power. Again, inspect epithelial cells for dysplastic or neoplastic morphological changes. Inspect the slide for the presence of the following things and provide an assessment of their amounts in the unstained wet mount:
        – Erythrocytes: record the number of erythrocytes per X40 high power field (hpf) as a range (e.g. 2–4/hpf)
        – Leucocytes: record the number of leucocytes per X40 hpf as a range (e.g. 0–3/hpf)
        – Microorganisms (e.g. bacteria, yeast, fungi, algae): record morphology of bacteria (e.g. cocci, bacilli, filamentous, spore-forming) and qualitative impression of the number of each type of microorganism (none, few, moderate number, many)
        – Lipid droplets: lipid droplets need to be distinguished from erythrocytes. They are variably sized, refractile and often float above the focal plane. Record qualitative impression of the number of lipid droplets (none, few, moderate number, many)
        – Sperm: record qualitative impression of the number of sperm (none, few, moderate number, many)
        – Other structures or unidentified structures: identify the structures or describe their morphology and record qualitative impression of the number of these structures (none, few, moderate number, many).

8.9   (continued) Method for routine urinalysis.

will be falsely decreased. Suggested ways to avoid over-saturation and cross-contamination of test pads are provided (Figures 8.10 and 8.11).

---

* Store urine dipsticks sealed in the container provided by the manufacturer
* If the urine sample has been refrigerated, allow the aliquot of the sample that will be tested to warm to room temperature before urinalysis
* Mix the sample well so that materials (e.g. erythrocytes) which may have sedimented due to gravity are in solution
* Avoid over-saturating the dipstick test pads with urine and do not allow urine to mix between dipstick test pads (Figure 8.11):
    Wet each pad of the test strip either by briefly immersing the strip in the urine sample or by using a pipette to place individual drops of urine on each test pad and then start the timer. If a pipette is used, make sure that the surface tension of the urine drops is disrupted so that the urine soaks completely into the test pad
    Dab excess urine from the test pads by laying the dipstick horizontally on a paper towel and gently elevating one edge of the dipstick along its long axis so that excess urine is pulled by gravity and capillary action into the paper towel
* Observe test pad colour changes at the interpretation times designated by the manufacturer on the label, not before or after
* The following dipstick reactions are not valid or useful in dogs and cats and should be ignored if they are present on the dipstick:
    Leucocytes: specific, but insensitive in dogs; invalid in cats
    Nitrite
    Specific gravity
    Urobilinogen

8.10   Guidelines for appropriate use and storage of urine dipstick multiple chemical test strips.

Interpretation of urine dipsticks is based upon the colour change that occurs within a specific time after urine is applied to the test pad (Figure 8.12). Colour will continue to develop beyond the indicated interpretation time, therefore results observed after the designated interpretation times are invalid. Cold urine will slow enzymatic reactions that occur in some of the test pads on the dipstick (e.g. glucose) and cause falsely decreased results. To avoid this artefact of refrigeration, allow the sample to warm to room temperature before urinalysis. Abnormally coloured urine will also affect interpretation of some tests (e.g. bilirubin, ketones).

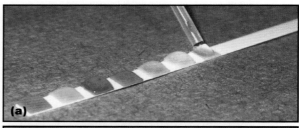
(a)

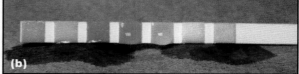
(b)

8.11   Application of urine to the urine dipstick pad. **(a)** Placement of individual drops of urine on to each test pad, breaking the surface tension of each drop after placement. **(b)** Careful removal of excess urine to avoid over-saturation of the test pads and intermingling of reagents between test pats.

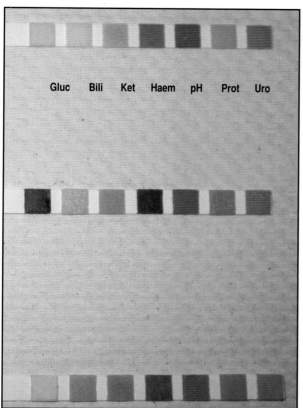

8.12 Interpretation of urine dipstick test reactions is based upon the colour change that develops within the specific amount of time designated by the manufacturer. Distilled water was placed on the top dipstick for comparison with the lower two dipsticks, to which urine from two different patients was applied. The middle dipstick exhibits a strongly positive reaction for glucose and haem and moderate reaction for protein. The bottom dipstick reveals a weakly positive reaction for haem and protein.

Refractometer

Guidelines for appropriate use and storage of refractometers are provided in Figure 8.13. Refractometers are used to estimate the urine SG, which is an indication of how much solute is dissolved in the urine (i.e. the concentration of the urine). Refractometric estimation of urine SG is performed to determine the ability of the renal tubules to conserve water and produce well concentrated urine. Refractometers take advantage of the fact that a beam of light is bent when it passes from air into water. The degree to which the beam of light is bent is directly proportional to the number of molecules that are dissolved in solution. However, the light beam is also bent by other materials (e.g. cells, crystals, mucus, bacteria) that are present within the urine. The presence of these other materials causes overestimation of the urine SG determined by refractometry and, therefore, overestimation of the renal tubular ability to conserve water and produce concentrated urine. This potential inaccuracy can be avoided by measuring the SG of the supernatant after centrifugation of the urine, which causes cells, crystals, etc. to collect in the sediment pellet (see Figure 8.9).

- Store refractometers away from heating and cooling vents
- If the urine sample has been refrigerated, allow the aliquot of the sample that will be tested to warm to room temperature before urinalysis
- Measure the urine specific gravity of the supernatant formed after centrifugation
- Use a veterinary refractometer with canine and feline scales. Alternatively, for feline urine samples, use the formula to convert human urine specific gravity values to the corresponding feline value: feline specific gravity = (0.846 × human specific gravity) + 0.154

8.13 Guidelines for use and storage of refractometers.

Most newer refractometers are temperature-compensated and are designed to be used at ambient temperatures. Refractometers should be stored away from heating and cooling vents, as this may cause spurious results. Also, cold fluids are denser than warm fluids. Therefore, the urine SG determined by refractometry is falsely increased in urine that is cold. To avoid this artefact of refrigeration, allow the sample to warm to room temperature before urinalysis.

Feline urine is naturally more refractive than canine and human urine. Consequently, feline urine SG will be slightly overestimated to a variable degree when a refractometer designed for humans is used (i.e. by approximately 0.002–0.005 units). There are two possible ways to prevent this inaccuracy. Feline urine SG can be measured using a veterinary refractometer that has separate scales for canine and feline samples. Alternatively, feline urine SG can be calculated using a formula to convert the SG indicated by a human refractometer to the equivalent feline value (George, 2001). The conversion formula for feline SG is as follows:

$$\text{Feline SG} = (0.846 \times \text{human SG}) + 0.154$$

Urine sediment evaluation

Guidelines for urine sediment preparation and evaluation are provided in Figure 8.14. Because increased concentrations of cells, casts, microorganisms or crystals may indicate underlying urinary tract disease, one goal of urine sediment evaluation is to determine semiquantitatively the concentration of these materials within the urine. In addition to the patient's urinary tract health, the concentrations of these materials are directly affected by how the sediment is prepared.

Since cells, crystals, etc. will spontaneously sediment due to gravity, it is necessary to mix the urine sample well before removing an aliquot for centrifugation to ensure that the urine sediment wet mount is fully representative of the whole urine sample. Also, the concentration of the sediment is affected by the starting urine aliquot volume that is centrifuged to form the sediment pellet and the volume of supernatant urine that is used to resuspend the sediment pellet prior to wet mounting. For example, if two aliquots of urine, one containing 10 ml and one containing 5 ml, were centrifuged, there would be twice as much material in the sediment formed from the 10 ml urine aliquot compared with the sediment formed from the 5 ml urine aliquot. If

1. Since cells, crystals, casts, etc. will spontaneously sediment due to gravity, mix the whole urine sample well before removing an aliquot for centrifugation to ensure that the urine sediment wet mount is representative of the whole urine sample.

2. Use a standard volume aliquot of urine for centrifugation (e.g. 5 ml).

3. Use a standard volume of urine supernatant to resuspend the sediment pellet (i.e. 20% of the original aliquot volume):

   If centrifuged 5 ml of urine, remove 4 ml of supernatant and resuspend the pellet in the remaining 1 ml

   If centrifuged 4 ml of urine, remove 3.2 ml of supernatant and resuspend the pellet in the remaining 0.8 ml

   If centrifuged 3 ml of urine, remove 2.4 ml of supernatant and resuspend the pellet in the remaining 0.6 ml

   If centrifuged 2 ml of urine, remove 1.6 ml of supernatant and resuspend the pellet in the remaining 0.4 ml.

4. Examine a standard number of microscopic fields (i.e. 10 fields) using both the 10X and 40X objectives.

5. Determine the concentration of materials within the sediment in the *unstained* wet mount (e.g. cells per high power field as a range, i.e. 0–2), since the addition of stain dilutes the sediment.

6. Stain (e.g. new methylene blue) is helpful for identification of nucleated structures, but may form crystals or may be contaminated with microorganisms. If crystals or microorganisms are observed in a stained sediment wet mount, confirm their presence in an unstained wet mount of the sediment.

8.14 Guidelines for urine sediment preparation and evaluation.

the sediment pellets of both urine aliquots were resuspended in an equal volume of supernatant (e.g. 1 ml), then the sediment prepared from the 10 ml urine aliquot would give the false impression of increased concentrations of cells, microorganisms, etc. and may lead one to conclude wrongly that urinary tract disease exists. To avoid this type of error, a standard urine volume should be used as an aliquot for centrifugation and the resultant pellet should be resuspended in a standard volume of supernatant. Reference values for interpretation of urine sediment concentrations of cells and casts are based upon sediment pellets that were resuspended in 20% of the original urine aliquot volume. 5 ml is generally recommended as a reasonable urine aliquot volume for centrifugation, and it is generally recommended that a pellet formed by centrifugation of 5 ml of urine be resuspended in 1 ml of supernatant, which represents 20% of the original volume.

Unfortunately, a full 5 ml of urine is not always available for urinalysis. In these instances, the volume of supernatant used to resuspend the pellet will need to be adjusted down to account for the smaller volume of urine available for centrifugation. The volume of supernatant used should be adjusted down to 20% of whatever the original urine aliquot volume is (e.g. resuspend the pellet formed from a 4 ml urine aliquot in 0.8 ml of supernatant, rather than 1 ml) (Figure 8.14). There are commercial urinalysis centrifugation systems (e.g. StatSpin® Urine Sediment Analysis System) that use smaller urine volumes to prepare urine sediments for microscopic examination. Follow the manufacturer's usage and maintenance guidelines to ensure uniform, standardized results.

Since the concentration of materials observed in urine are reported as a range per microscopic field (e.g. 0–2 leucocytes per high power field), a standard number of microscopic fields (i.e. 10 fields) using both the X10 and X40 objectives should be evaluated for each urine sample. A stained wet mount (e.g. new methylene blue) may be helpful to identify nucleated cells; however, addition of stain will dilute the concentration of the sediment. If necessary, nucleated cells can be identified in a stained wet mount, but they should be counted in the unstained wet mount (Figure 8.15). Also, if there will be a delay between when the urine sediment is prepared and when it will be examined, the slide can be stored in a humidified Petri dish (Figure 8.16)

Stain may form crystals or may be contaminated by microorganisms (Figures 8.17). To avoid false urinalysis results, any crystals or microorganisms that are identified in a stained wet mount should be confirmed in the unstained wet mount, which will not contain contaminants that may be present in the stain. Cytological examination of the urine sediment pellet that has been aspirated from the conical centrifuge tube, smeared on to a microscope slide and stained, similarly to the process for a fine needle aspirate, is also useful for verification, detection and identification of microorganisms (Swenson *et al.*, 2004). The method for preparing direct smears of the urine sediment pellet is described later in the Chapter.

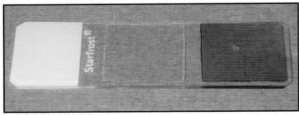

8.15 Unstained and new methylene blue-stained urine sediment wet mounts. If desired, both the unstained and stained wet mounts can be prepared on a single microscope slide.

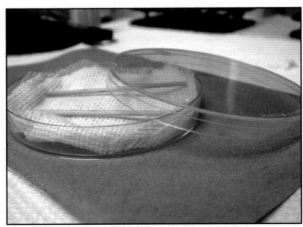

8.16 Humidified Petri dish to preserve wet mounts. If there is to be a significant delay between the time that the sediment wet mount is prepared and the time that it is examined, it can be preserved in a humidified Petri dish created by moistening absorbent material at the bottom of the dish. Details on its construction are provided in Figure 8.9 (Step 10).

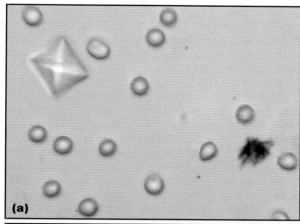

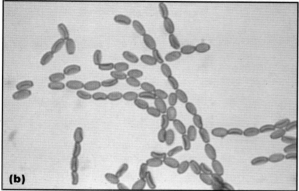

8.17 New methylene blue-stained urine sediment wet mount. **(a)** Two crystals are present: a calcium oxalate dihydrate crystal (left) and a contaminating crystal from the new methylene blue (right). When crystals are observed in a stained wet mount, they should be verified in the unstained preparation. Note the numerous pale orange erythrocytes in the background, which are swollen by water uptake within relatively hypotonic, dilute urine. (New methylene blue stain; original magnification X500) **(b)** Numerous budding yeasts are observed as contaminants in a new methylene blue-stained wet mount. When microorganisms are observed in a stained wet mount, they should be verified in the unstained preparation. (New methylene blue stain; original magnification X400)

Urinalysis interpretation

Gross inspection of the urine

Normal urine may be various shades of yellow due to the presence of natural urine pigments, referred to as *urochromes*. Well concentrated urine may be a darker shade of yellow, but this is not always true. If present, bilirubinuria may impart a dark yellow–orange colour and give the false impression of concentrated urine. Also, urine may become darker yellow with exposure to light, which causes urochrome degradation. Therefore, urine colour should not be used to assess renal tubular ability to produce well concentrated urine. Urine colour may also be altered by the presence of substances that are not normally found in urine, such as haemoglobin or myoglobin (Figure 8.18).

Normal urine is clear (i.e. transparent) or slightly cloudy due to the presence of epithelial cells or crystals. In fresh, well mixed urine of dogs and cats,

Finding	Cause
Colour	
Pale yellow Yellow	Normal Highly concentrated urine
Dark yellow	Highly concentrated urine Bilirubinuria Photodegradation of urine pigments
Orange–yellow	Highly concentrated urine Bilirubinuria
Red–orange Red Dark red–brown	Haematuria Haemoglobinuria Myoglobinuria
Pink	Haematuria Haemoglobinuria Porphyrinuria (rare)
Brown to black	Methaemoglobin from haemoglobin or myoglobin breakdown Bile pigments
Green	Biliverdin (green) – can form due to *in vitro* degradation of bilirubin Urobilin (green) – can form due to oxidation of urobilinogen in acidic urine
Blue	Various drugs and drug metabolites
Clarity	
Clear Slightly cloudy	Normal
Cloudy	Cells Crystals Casts Microorganisms Lipid Mucus Semen

8.18 Potential findings during gross inspection of urine and their common causes.

increased cloudiness is an abnormal, but non-specific finding that can occur due to the presence of cells, crystals, casts, microorganisms, lipid, mucus or semen. Even if urine is not cloudy, abnormalities may still be detected during microscopic evaluation of the sediment. Therefore, urine clarity should not be used as the sole method to detect cells, crystals, etc. However, some individuals suggest that if the urine is grossly normal (i.e. yellow and clear) *and* the urine dipstick tests are *all* normal, then microscopic examination, which in most instances will also be normal, is an unnecessary expenditure of resources; it could be omitted in this specific situation with the knowledge that the small percentage of animals with microscopic abnormalities will go undetected.

Specific chemical testing of the urine

Urine specific gravity

Urine SG primarily reflects renal tubular ability to respond to antidiuretic hormone stimulation and conserve water by producing well concentrated urine.

Urine SG values may be classified into four categories based upon the value relative to the SG of glomerular filtrate, which ranges from 1.008–1.012 and represents urinary filtrate that has not yet been modified by the renal tubules (Figure 8.19). To determine the clinical significance of a given urine SG measurement, the value must be interpreted in light of the patient's age, hydration status, concurrent diseases, serum urea nitrogen and creatinine concentrations, urine glucose and protein concentrations, and recent administration of therapeutic agents (e.g. parenteral fluids, glucose, diuretics, anticonvulsants). For example, a urine SG of 1.020 in a euhydrated dog would probably represent a normal physiological variation in response to recent water ingestion; however, the same value in a dehydrated, azotaemic dog would indicate renal tubular concentrating dysfunction that could indicate renal dysfunction. Severe proteinuria or glucosuria both increase measured urine SG; therefore, the value will not be entirely representative of renal tubular concentrating function (Figure 8.19).

Urine SG is relatively insensitive for the detection of renal failure, since kidney function must be compromised by at least two thirds (67%) before renal tubular concentrating dysfunction lowers the urine SG. Reduction in urine SG due to decreased conservation of water by the renal tubules typically occurs before glomerular dysfunction manifests as azotaemia, which is observed when kidney function has been reduced by three quarters (75%). In an azotaemic patient, urine SG should be used to help localize the cause of azotaemia as prerenal, renal or postrenal (Figure 8.20).

Classification	Dog	Cat	Significance
Well concentrated	>1.030	>1.035	Renal tubules can produce well concentrated urine Urine may be less concentrated in clinically normal juvenile animals
Range of minimal concentration	1.013–1.029	1.013–1.034	Could represent an appropriate variation due to recent ingestion of water or administration of fluids Inappropriate value in dehydrated or azotaemic patients Can be observed in patients with renal failure
Isosthenuria	1.008–1.012	1.008–1.012	Could represent an appropriate variation due to recent ingestion of water or administration of fluids Inappropriate value in dehydrated or azotaemic patients Can be observed in patients with renal failure
Hyposthenuria	<1.008	<1.008	Indicates that renal tubules can produce dilute urine, reduces the likelihood of renal failure Inappropriate value in dehydrated or azotaemic patients Can be observed with various conditions: • Polyuria due to various aetiologies, causing loss of renal medullary solute concentration gradient • Hyperadrenocorticism/hypercortisolaemia • Hypercalcaemia • Hepatic disease • Pyometra due to endotoxin exposure • Psychogenic polydipsia • Diabetes insipidus (central or primary renal) • Therapeutic agent administration: Anticonvulsants Diuretics Fluid therapy Glucocorticoids Excessive thyroxine supplementation

8.19 Classification of urine specific gravity measurements and clinical significance. Note that for each 55.5 mmol/l (1000 mg/dl) of glucose, the specific gravity is increased by 0.0004–0.0005, and for each 10 g/l (1000 mg/dl) of protein, the specific gravity is increased by 0.0003–0.0005.

Localization of azotaemia	Urine specific gravity		Causes of azotaemia
	Dogs	Cats	
Prerenal	>1.035	>1.045	Decreased delivery of nitrogenous waste to the kidneys due to renal hypoperfusion Increased generation of nitrogenous waste
Renal	1.008–1.029	1.008–1.035 occasionally >1.045	Decreased removal of nitrogenous waste from circulation due to primary renal dysfunction
Postrenal	Variable		Decreased elimination of nitrogenous waste due to urethral obstruction or bladder rupture

8.20 Use of urine specific gravity to aid in anatomical localization and causes of azotaemia.

With prerenal azotaemia, adequately functioning kidneys respond to decreased perfusion by conserving water and producing concentrated urine that has a high SG. Renal azotaemia is typically associated with inadequate renal tubular water conservation and production of dilute urine that has a low urine SG. However, some cats with renal azotaemia, which indicates that kidney function is at 25% of optimum, maintain their ability to conserve water and can have concentrated urine with a SG ≥1.035. The urine SG associated with postrenal azotaemia is variable. Other clinical findings, such as oliguria or anuria with a firm, possibly distended bladder, can be used to diagnose this cause of azotaemia.

Bilirubin

Normal metabolism of haemoglobin from senescent erythrocytes results in hepatic formation of conjugated bilirubin, which is removed from the body primarily in bile via the gastrointestinal tract and, to a lesser extent, in urine via the kidneys. Chemical testing of urine for the presence of bilirubin is performed as a screen to detect haemolytic or hepatobiliary diseases (i.e. intrahepatic or posthepatic cholestasis) (Figure 8.21). However, this screening test has reduced utility in dogs. Clinically normal dogs, especially intact male dogs, form conjugated bilirubin in renal tubular epithelial cells and excrete a small amount into concentrated urine (SG >1.030) in the absence of diseases associated with icterus. To determine the clinical significance of bilirubinuria in dogs, the bilirubin concentration must be interpreted in the context of the urine SG. More concentrated urine with a higher SG may have a greater amount of bilirubin, whereas less concentrated urine should have a lower amount of bilirubin. For example, a 2+ urine bilirubin in a dog that has a urine SG of 1.040 is unlikely to be clinically significant. The same urine bilirubin concentration in a dog that has a urine SG of 1.020 should raise concern for diseases associated with icterus.

In cats, the renal threshold for bilirubin excretion is nine times greater than it is in dogs. Therefore, any amount of bilirubinuria is clinically significant in cats and should raise concern for diseases associated with icterus. In both species, it is generally accepted that with diseases that cause jaundice, excess bilirubin first accumulates within urine, subsequently increases in plasma and ultimately is visible at mucous membranes. However, due to a relatively high rate of false-negative bilirubin reactions, the absence of bilirubinuria should not be used to exclude the possibility of diseases associated with icterus (i.e. haemolytic or hepatobiliary), and other tests, such as serum biochemistry, should also be performed.

Glucose

Glucose is a small molecule that freely passes through the glomerulus into the urine; however, virtually all of the glucose that is present within the initial glomerular filtrate is efficiently removed from the urine and conserved by properly functioning renal tubules. Screening urine for the presence of glucose is done to detect diseases that cause an excess amount of glucose to be present in the glomerular filtrate (i.e. hyperglycaemia) or to detect diseases that cause proximal renal tubular dysfunction with failure to remove glucose from the glomerular filtrate.

There are several potential causes of glucosuria (see Figure 8.21), however diabetes mellitus and stress-induced transient hyperglycaemia in cats are the most common causes. Serum biochemistry, potentially with evaluation of serum fructosamine, is indicated in the diagnosis and management of patients with diabetes mellitus. Fructosamine is a glycosylated protein, whose serum concentration is directly proportional to the serum glucose concentration over the preceding 2–3 weeks. Fructosamine evaluation is useful in cats to distinguish diabetic hyperglycaemia from transient, stress hyperglycaemia (Plier *et al.*, 1998) and can be used as an indicator of glycaemic control during the medical management of diabetic dogs and cats.

Persistent glucosuria, as is seen with diabetes mellitus, predisposes patients to urinary tract infections that may not be apparent during urine sediment evaluation, and urine culture is necessary in patients

Urine biochemical finding	Causes of urine biochemical finding	Causes of false-negative results or decreases	Causes of false-positive results or increases
Bilirubinuria	• Normal in concentrated urine of dogs (specific gravity >1.030) • Haemolytic disease • Cholestatic diseases (hepatic or posthepatic) • Mild increase with prolonged anorexia or fever • Test is sensitive to conjugated bilirubin, but not unconjugated bilirubin (i.e. bilirubin bound to albumin); therefore, albuminuria caused by glomerular disease is *not* a cause of detectable bilirubinuria	• Photodegradation of bilirubin due to exposure of the urine sample to light for more than 30 minutes • Oxidation of bilirubin to biliverdin, which is green. Oxidation occurs spontaneously and is accelerated by exposure of the urine sample to air • Discoloured urine may mask test pad colour change • Centrifugation of the urine sample prior to bilirubin test may cause bilirubin to precipitate • Drugs: ascorbic acid	• Drugs: etodolac metabolites; phenothiazines (large doses, reported in humans); phenazopyridine (makes urine red)

8.21 Interpretation of urine biochemistry results determined by urine dipstick. Causes of false-positive or false-negative results vary with different test methods; consult product documentation for specific details. (continues) ▶

Urine biochemical finding	Causes of urine biochemical finding	Causes of false-negative results or decreases	Causes of false-positive results or increases
Glucosuria	***Persistent or transient hyperglycaemia:*** • Diabetes mellitus • Extreme stress in cats (glucosuria may temporarily persist after resolution of hyperglycaemia) • Hyperadrenocorticism (<10% of cases) • Acute pancreatitis • Rare causes: acromegaly; dioestrus; hyperglucagonaemia; hyperthyroidism; phaeochromocytoma • Drugs or toxins: dextrose-containing fluids; adrenocorticotropic hormone; adrenaline; glucocorticoids; ethylene glycol; megestrol acetate; morphine; phenothiazines; progesterone; thiazide diuretics; potentially other drugs that cause hyperglycaemia (e.g. detomidine, ketamine, propanolol, xylazine) ***Acquired or congenital proximal renal tubular disease:*** • Fanconi syndrome • Primary renal glucosuria • Aminoglycoside toxicity • Acute renal failure with severe tubular pathology (e.g. infection, ischaemia, toxicosis)	• Cold urine sample applied to test pad • Outdated dipsticks • Dipsticks exposed to sunlight • Discoloured urine may mask test pad colour change • *In vitro* bacterial overgrowth may decrease glucose; numerous bacteria will be present in the sediment • In samples with low glucose concentration, moderate ketonuria (2+ (0.4 g/l)) will cause a false-negative • Very high specific gravity • Drugs: in samples with low glucose concentration, ascorbic acid will cause a false-negative; tetracyclines due to ascorbic acid formation (above); formaldehyde formed from methenamine (hexamine)	• Contamination of dipsticks or urine sample with oxidizing chemicals (e.g. bleach, hydrogen peroxide) • Prolonged exposure of dipsticks to air (days) • Urinary haemorrhage in a patient with mild hyperglycaemia (i.e. <10.0 mmol/l (180 mg/dl) in dogs; <15.5 mmol/l (280 mg/dl) in cats) • One report observed 'pseudoglucose' in cats with urethral obstruction • Drugs: cefalexin (Chemstrips 10 SG) (Rees and Boothe, 2004)
Haem reaction	• Pathological or iatrogenic haematuria (erythrocytes may not be observed in urine sediment due to lysis in dilute urine (specific gravity <1.008), very alkaline urine (pH >9) or moderately alkaline (pH >7.5) very concentrated urine (specific gravity >1.035)) • Haemoglobinuria due to destruction of erythrocytes that occurs either outside of or within the urinary tract • Myoglobinuria due to myocyte injury	• Failure to mix the urine sample well prior to testing in order to resuspend sedimented erythrocytes • Outdated dipsticks • Very high specific gravity • Possible but unlikely: large amount of nitrite from bacteria in urinary tract infection • Drugs: ascorbic acid; captopril; formaldehyde formed from methenamine (hexamine)	• In a voided sample, genital tract haemorrhage or oestrus are sources of intact erythrocytes • Contamination of dipsticks or urine sample with oxidizing chemicals (e.g. bleach, hydrogen peroxide) • Contamination of urine sample with digested haemoglobin in flea excrement ('flea dirt') • High urine bilirubin • Possible but unlikely: peroxidases from bacteria, leucocytes, epithelial cells or sperm; large amount of bromide or iodide (e.g. KBr administration)
Urobilinogen reaction	• This test has minimal clinical significance in veterinary medicine • A small amount (0.2 mg/l) is normal, though normal animals may have none due to diurnal variation ***Increased amount:*** • Usually spurious • May be seen with haemolytic or hepatobiliary disease ***Decreased amount:*** • Spurious • Diurnal variation • Bile duct obstruction	• Photodegradation of urobilinogen due to exposure of the urine sample to light • Oxidized by acidic urine to urobilin (green) • Drugs: formaldehyde formed from methenamine (hexamine)	• Outdated dipsticks • Improper storage of dipstick near a heat source • Drugs: aminosalicylic acid; aminobenzoic acid; phenazopyridine; sulphonamides

8.21 (continued) Interpretation of urine biochemistry results determined by urine dipstick. Causes of false-positive or false-negative results vary with different test methods; consult product documentation for specific details. (continues)

▶

Urine biochemical finding	Causes of urine biochemical finding	Causes of false-negative results or decreases	Causes of false-positive results or increases
Ketonuria	*Hyperglycaemic ketonuria:* • Uncontrolled diabetes mellitus (a common and important cause) *Normo- or hypoglycaemic ketonuria (most are uncommon causes):* • Prolonged anorexia/starvation (more likely cause in young animals) • Severe carbohydrate restriction • Strenuous exercise • Extreme cold • Fever • Hyperglucagonaemia due to liver disease causing reduced hepatic clearance of glucagon • Glycogen storage disease • Lactation • Methylmalonic acidaemia (reported in a family of Maltese Dogs) • Postpancreatectomy • Pregnancy • Renal glucosuria • Hyperthyroidism (ketonuria documented in humans) *Uncommon endocrinopathies with associated with variable blood glucose:* • Acromegaly • Adrenal tumours • Glucagonoma • Insulinoma • Pituitary adenomas • Drugs: aspirin intoxication; growth hormone administration; streptozotocin	• Predominant ketone is β-hydroxybutyrate, which is poorly detected by dipstick • Improper storage of dipsticks (exposure of reagent to light, heat, moisture) • Improper storage of urine sample which can allow evaporation of ketones • Ketones in the sample can be decreased by bacteria that are present due to urinary tract infection or *in vitro* contamination	• Discoloured urine • Low pH may cause trace reaction • High specific gravity may cause trace reaction • Presence of the amino acid, cystine, in urine due to proximal renal tubular disease • Presence of pyruvate in urine released due to mitochondrial myopathy • Drugs or diagnostic agents: *N*-acetylcysteine; bromosulphophthalein; captopril; dimercaprol; methionine; levodopa metabolites; mesna; D-penicillamine; phenazopyridine; tiopronin (2-MPG); valproic acid; others
pH	*High pH >7.5:* • Postprandial alkaline tide (1 hour postprandially) • Urinary tract infection caused by urease-producing bacteria (e.g. *Staphylococcus*, *Proteus*) that generate ammonium • High vegetable content diet • Alkalosis, usually metabolic (e.g. due to vomiting) • Renal tubular acidoses (rare). Early proximal renal tubular acidosis due to bicarbonate loss into urine; later develop aciduria once bicarbonate depleted. Distal renal tubular acidosis: pH is inappropriately high (>6) given the presence of concurrent metabolic acidosis caused by failure to excrete hydrogen ions • Alkalinizing therapy (see Figure 8.23)	• Overflow of urine between test pads, causing contamination of pH test pad by acid buffer from protein test pad • *In vitro* overgrowth of bacteria that use glucose to form acidic metabolites, numerous bacteria will be present in the sediment • Discoloured urine may interfere with interpretation of colour change • Dipstick pH measurements *estimate* pH within ± 1 pH unit of that determined by pH meter. Feline urine pH determined by dipstick is consistently lower than pH determined by meter	• Contamination of dipsticks or urine sample with cleanser residues (e.g. quaternary ammonium compounds) • Improper storage of urine sample which can allow loss of carbon dioxide, raising pH • *In vitro* overgrowth of urease-producing bacteria that generate ammonium, numerous bacteria will be present in the sediment • Discoloured urine may interfere with interpretation of colour change • Dipstick pH measurements *estimate* pH within ± 1 pH unit of that determined by pH meter

8.21 (continued) Interpretation of urine biochemistry results determined by urine dipstick. Causes of false-positive or false-negative results vary with different test methods; consult product documentation for specific details.(continues) ▶

Urine biochemical finding	Causes of urine biochemical finding	Causes of false-negative results or decreases	Causes of false-positive results or increases
pH (continued)	*Low pH <7:* • Normal in carnivores (usually between 5.5–7.5) • Urinary tract infection caused by acid-producing bacteria • High meat content diet • Increased protein catabolism (e.g. fever, anorexia) • Acidosis, usually metabolic (e.g. diabetic ketoacidosis, lactic acidosis, uraemic) • Hypokalaemia • Severe diarrhoea • Metabolic alkalosis with paradoxic aciduria associated with severe vomition, upper gastrointestinal obstruction, etc. • Proximal renal tubular acidosis (rare) once bicarbonate depleted • Acidifying therapy (see Figure 8.23)		
Proteinuria	*Preglomerular:* • Physiological proteinuria (transient): fever; seizures; stress; temperature extremes; venous congestion • Glomerular and tubular overload: severe hyperglobulinaemia (i.e. mono- or polyclonal gammopathy); Bence Jones proteinuria; haemoglobinuria [a]; myoglobinuria; excessive plasma administration *Glomerular:* • Primary glomerular proteinuria: immune-mediated destruction; glomerular haematuria [a]; inflammatory; neoplastic • Secondary glomerular proteinuria: amyloidosis (dogs); glomerular hyperfiltration; hyperadrenocorticism; immune complex deposition *Postglomerular:* • Urogenital tract disease: haemorrhagic [a]; inflammatory; ischaemic; neoplastic; traumatic • Normal genital secretions • Acquired or congenital proximal renal tubular disease uncommon) (e.g. Fanconi's syndrome, nephrotoxic drug administration (e.g. aminoglycoside))	• Low level albuminuria (microalbuminuria) or proteinuria associated with proteins other than albumin (e.g. haemoglobin, Bence Jones proteins)	• [a] In order to attribute proteinuria to haemorrhage alone, the dipstick haem reaction must be ≥ 3+, large and haematuria should be visible grossly • Elements in the sediment (cells, casts, microorganisms) may be the cause of a positive reaction • Moderately alkaline, well concentrated urine or extremely alkaline (pH >9) urine • Over-saturation of urine test pad which dilutes a necessary buffer from the test pad • Contamination of the urine sample or dipsticks with cleanser residues (e.g. quaternary ammonium, chlorhexidine) • Improper storage of dipsticks (exposure to moisture) • Drugs: phenazopyridine
Nitrite	Leucocytes Specific gravity These dipstick reactions are not valid or useful in dogs and cats and should be ignored if they are present on the dipstick	The dipstick leucocyte test is specific (93%), but insensitive (46%) in dogs (Vail *et al.*, 1986)	The dipstick leucocyte test is positive is many feline urine samples even if they do not contain leucocytes (34% specificity) and is therefore invalid in cats (Holan *et al.*, 1997)

8.21 (continued) Interpretation of urine biochemistry results determined by urine dipstick. Causes of false-positive or false-negative results vary with different test methods; consult product documentation for specific details.

with persistent glucosuria to exclude underlying urinary tract infection. Diabetic patients can be immunocompromised and may develop urinary tract infections, which are associated with diminished inflammatory response by leucocytes (see Figure 8.42). Consequently, the infections are referred to as *silent*, since pyuria may not be observed. Also, glucose is an osmotic diuretic, causing formation of large volumes of dilute urine. The dilution of cells and bacteria in the sediment may decrease their concentration to a level that is below the detection limit by light microscopy. Therefore, even if bacteriuria is not observed, urine culture is necessary to exclude urinary tract infection in patients with persistent glucosuria.

Haem reaction

The haem reaction is performed to screen urine for the presence of intact erythrocytes, free haemoglobin from lysed erythrocytes or free myoglobin from damaged myocytes (see Figure 8.21). A low number of erythrocytes (<5 per high power field) is a normal microscopic finding in urine and does not cause a positive haem reaction. An increased number of urine erythrocytes may be observed due to:

- Iatrogenic haematuria caused by collection
- Pathological haematuria due to urinary tract haemorrhage
- Genital sources of erythrocytes (e.g. oestrus) if the sample is voided.

Chapter 1 provides additional information about haematuria. Free haemoglobin and free myoglobin are not normally detected in urine. Free haemoglobin may be observed in urine during systemic haemolytic diseases or when previously intact erythrocytes are lysed within urine that is either dilute (SG <1.008) or very alkaline. Persistent haemoglobinuria in the absence of systemic haemolytic disease should prompt further evaluation of the patient for occult urinary tract haemorrhage (e.g. diagnostic imaging). Myoglobinuria due to myocyte injury (e.g. ischaemic, toxic, traumatic) occurs uncommonly in dogs and cats.

Positive haem reactions are most commonly due to haematuria. However, a positive haem reaction is a non-specific finding and additional information obtained from urinalysis and the peripheral blood is necessary to discriminate the cause of a positive reaction. With some urine dipsticks, intact erythrocytes will cause a stippled green colour change (Figure 8.22). Centrifugation and observation of urine colour facilitate identification of the source of a positive haem reaction. Urine that contains erythrocytes, haemoglobin or myoglobin may be various shades of red–brown. Centrifugation will cause red blood cells to sediment and the supernatant to become more yellow; if haemoglobin or myoglobin is present, the colour of the supernatant will be unchanged. Sediment evaluation can be used to detect intact erythrocytes, as long as the urine is not dilute or extremely alkaline (both can cause erythrocyte lysis). If erythrocytes are not observed in the sediment, the positive haem reaction is likely to be due to haemoglobinuria or myoglobinuria.

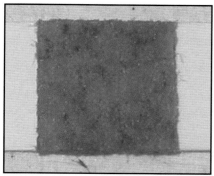

8.22 Positive haem reaction indicating the presence of intact erythrocytes. The positive haem reaction in this case indicates the presence of intact erythrocytes by its speckled green appearance. Compare this colour change to the diffusely green 3+ positive haem reaction of the middle dipstick in Figure 8.12, which could either be due to intact erythrocytes, free haemoglobin or free myoglobin.

Complete blood cell count (CBC) and serum biochemistry may be used to distinguish haemoglobinuria and myoglobinuria. Pink or red plasma colour can be observed with haemoglobinuria, but not with myoglobinuria. Methaemoglobinaemia, associated with Heinz body haemolytic anaemia, which is an uncommon cause of haemoglobinuria, will cause blood to be chocolate brown. CBC abnormalities that are suggestive of haemolytic disease include regenerative anaemia, abnormal erythrocyte morphology (e.g. spherocytes, schistocytes, erythrocyte ghosts) and leucocytosis. Concurrent with myoglobinuria, the serum creatine kinase concentration should be markedly elevated. Creatine kinase is muscle specific and will not be elevated with *in vivo* haemolysis. If necessary, additional specialized tests are available at referral laboratories to differentiate haemoglobinuria from myoglobinuria (e.g. ammonium sulphate precipitation, electrophoresis).

Ketones

Ketones are small organic acids that are normally produced in very small quantities when fatty acids are catabolized to produce energy. Ketones are not detected in the urine of healthy animals that are receiving adequate, balanced nutrition. In diseases or conditions associated with aberrant carbohydrate metabolism (e.g. diabetes mellitus, renal glucosuria, pregnancy), alternative sources of energy are required. A compensatory increase in the rate of fat catabolism (i.e. lipolysis), which generates additional ketone byproducts, occurs in an attempt to meet energy demands. Increased ketone production is usually first detected as ketonuria (see Figure 8.21), which typically precedes the development of ketonaemia, since ketones are readily removed from the circulation via the kidneys.

Ketonuria is uncommonly observed in dogs and cats (1.9% of dogs, 2.6% of cats) (Osborne and Stevens, 1999) and is most often detected in poorly regulated diabetic patients that are glucosuric and either ketotic or ketoacidotic. The latter is characterized by the concurrent presence of ketosis with ketonuria, increased anion gap metabolic acidosis, consistent clinical signs (e.g. dehydration, lethargy) and often disease of another organ (e.g. infection, pancreatitis, renal failure) in a patient with diabetes mellitus.

Urine screening for ketones is typically performed to aid in the diagnosis of diabetes mellitus and to regulate insulin therapy, even though commonly used dipstick reagents do not detect the ketone that is usually most abundant in dogs and cats, β-hydroxybutyrate. Other ketones (i.e. acetone and acetoacetic acid) are detected by the urine dipstick and are usually present in urine along with β-hydroxybutyrate.

Similar to glucosuria, ketonuria has a diuretic effect, causing formation of large volumes of dilute urine, which may dilute urine sediment constituents (e.g. cells, casts; see Glucose, above). Also, excretion of ketones into urine causes concurrent loss of sodium and potassium into the urine and predisposes the patient to hyponatraemia and hypokalaemia. Careful monitoring of serum electrolytes (e.g. magnesium, phosphorus, potassium, sodium) in patients with diabetic ketoacidosis is helpful to monitor for complications associated with the disease and its treatment.

pH

Urine pH measurement (see Figures 8.21 and 8.23) provides a rough assessment of systemic acid–base status and facilitates diagnosis of urinary tract infections and uncommon renal tubular diseases (i.e. renal tubular acidoses). Urine pH values are stable for up to 24 hours in urine that has been refrigerated (Raskin *et al.*, 2002; Albasan *et al.*, 2003). Urine dipsticks estimate pH to within 1 pH unit above or below that measured by the pH meter. In cats, urine pH is consistently underestimated by urine dipsticks; in dogs, there is no consistent direction of this error (Heuter *et al.*, 1998). Therefore, when more precise measurement of urine pH is required (e.g. during management of urolithiasis), measurement of pH using a properly calibrated and maintained pH meter is necessary. Hand-held, portable pH meters can be purchased for this purpose. However, electrodes may need to be replaced every 6 months (Raskin *et al.*, 2002), which would probably render their use impractical in general veterinary practice. If necessary, shipment of refrigerated urine within 24 hours of collection to a referral diagnostic laboratory that has a pH meter may be a more feasible option.

Effective interpretation of urine pH requires knowledge of the patient's acid–base status, therapeutic agent administration, timing of urine collection relative to ingestion of a meal and urine sediment findings. Inappropriate pH values may fall within the reference range (5.5–7.5); therefore, measurements of serum total carbon dioxide concentration or blood pH are helpful to determine if a given urine pH value is physiologically inappropriate. It is uncommon for pH measurements to exceed the limits of the reference range. Extreme pH values of undetermined cause should prompt investigation for an underlying abnormality (most commonly urinary tract infection) or artefact (e.g. contamination of the dipstick or sample container with cleanser residues).

Consideration of the urine pH is helpful when interpreting other components of the urinalysis (e.g. dipstick protein, sediment). Urine that is either markedly alkaline (pH >9) or moderately alkaline (pH >7.5) and highly concentrated (SG >1.035) will probably cause a false-positive dipstick protein reaction. Highly alkaline urine also causes cells and tubular casts to degenerate more rapidly, so they may be absent from the sediment. Acidic urine is inhospitable to leptospires, and may cause false-negative leptospire culture. Urine pH has a direct effect upon the type of crystals that may be observed in the sediment; and it can also be used to predict urolith mineral content while awaiting results of proper urolith analysis.

Protein

Urine dipstick protein testing is performed to screen for diseases that cause excess protein loss by the urinary tract (e.g. glomerular diseases) or that cause excess systemic production of protein with overflow into urine (e.g. multiple myeloma). However, since other non-pathological or pathological causes of proteinuria occur more commonly, a positive protein reaction should be interpreted judiciously. Figure 8.21 and Chapter 6 provide additional information about proteinuria.

The dipstick protein reaction is most sensitive to albumin. Other proteins (e.g. haemoglobin, immunoglobulin light chains (Bence Jones proteins)) must be present at very high concentrations to react with dipstick reagents and cause a positive reaction. The sulphosalicylic acid protein precipitation test is a simple method that screens for all types of protein and permits verification of dipstick results (see Figures 8.9 (Step 9), 8.24 and 8.25). The test is very easy to perform and the single reagent used in the test has a long shelf-life. All types of protein may be detected by this method, therefore Bence Jones proteinuria, which would most likely go undiagnosed by urine dipstick, can be identified.

Additional data from the urinalysis (i.e. SG, pH, sediment examination) are needed to determine the significance of proteinuria detected by the dipstick reaction. A positive protein reaction should be interpreted in the context of the urine SG, since a small amount of protein (trace to 1+, <0.30 g/l) can be a

Agents that increase pH
Carbonic anhydrase inhibitors (e.g. acetazolamide)
Alkalinizing prescription diet
Citrate salts (e.g. potassium citrate)
Sodium salts (e.g. acetate, bicarbonate, lactate)
Thiazide diuretics (e.g. chlorothiazide)

Agents that decrease pH
Ammonium chloride
Ascorbic acid
Acidifying prescription diet
Loop diuretics (e.g. furosemide)
Methenamine (hexamine)
Methionine
Phosphate salts (ammonium, potassium, sodium)

8.23 Therapeutic agents that may affect urine pH.

Interpretation	Amount of precipitate formed
Negative	No cloudiness
Trace	Cloudiness just perceptible against a dark background
1+	Cloudiness is distinct, but not granular
2+	Cloudiness is distinct and granular
3+	Cloudiness is heavy with distinct clumps
4+	Cloudiness is dense with large clumps
False-negative reactions	
Highly alkaline urine	
False-positive or increased reactions	
Testing uncentrifuged urine (the test should only be performed on the supernatant urine after centrifugation)	
Co-precipitation of crystals due to acid pH	
Administration of radiocontrast medium or massive doses of some antibiotics	

8.24 Standard scale for interpretation of sulphosalicylic acid protein precipitation and causes of spurious results.

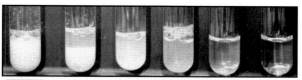

8.25 Sulphosalicylic acid precipitation of a serially diluted protein solution. Sulphosalicylic acid protein precipitation has been performed on solutions containing a known amount of protein, demonstrating the semiquantitative results obtained by sulphosalicylic acid protein precipitation. A white precipitate is formed in protein-containing solutions. The amount of precipitate formed is directly proportional to the protein concentration. Here, the amount of protein present in each tube is decreasing from 4+ in the leftmost tube to negative in the rightmost tune.

normal finding in a *single* well concentrated urine sample (SG >1.035); however, *persistent* trace or 1+ proteinuria should prompt further investigation (Lees *et al.*, 2005). A similar protein concentration in dilute urine or in an animal receiving potentially nephrotoxic drugs regardless of urine concentration would be abnormal.

Also, recent advances in our understanding of proteinuria have prompted re-evaluation of what protein concentration should be considered normal and have called into question the utility of the dipstick protein test, particularly in cats (see below and Chapter 6).

Consideration of the urine pH is necessary, since urine that is either markedly alkaline (pH >9) or moderately alkaline (pH 7.5) and well concentrated (SG >1.035) will be likely to cause a false-positive dipstick protein reaction. In one study, false-positive dipstick protein reactions were more common in cats than in dogs (Grauer *et al.*, 2004). The specificity of the dipstick protein reaction was 31% in cats and 69% in dogs when compared to a species-specific albumin ELISA. False-positive reactions may have occurred due to the

presence of non-albumin proteins or other interfering substances. Contamination of the urine sample with cleanser residues or improper dipstick usage or storage can also cause false-positive reactions (see Figure 8.21).

Knowledge of the urine sediment is requisite for accurate interpretation of urine dipstick protein. The most common pathological causes of increased urine protein concentration are urinary tract inflammation, infection, haemorrhage, or some combination of the three that most often arises from the lower urinary or genital tracts. In these instances, microscopic examination of the urine sediment will probably disclose pyuria, bacteriuria or haematuria. In order to attribute dipstick proteinuria entirely to haemorrhage, the haem reaction must be at least 3+ (large) and macroscopic haematuria should be present. If the haem reaction is less than 3+ and no other causes of a persistently positive protein reaction (e.g. pyuria, bacteriuria, spurious) are detected, then underlying disease (e.g. nephrotic syndrome, multiple myeloma, proximal renal tubular defect) may be present.

Urine protein: creatinine ratio: When significant dipstick proteinuria has been verified as persistent based upon a second urinalysis and when other sources of a positive protein reaction (e.g. pyuria with or without bacteriuria) have been excluded, measurement of the urine protein:creatinine ratio (UPC) is necessary to determine the severity of proteinuria more precisely. The UPC should be <1.0, although recent advances in canine and feline urine albumin testing have prompted re-evaluation of this reference value. Some investigators now favour use of <0.5 as the UPC reference value for non-azotaemic animals, <0.5 for azotaemic dogs and <0.4 for azotaemic cats (Lees *et al.*, 2005). A UPC >1.0 in a sample obtained by cystocentesis should arouse concern for glomerular disease (e.g. glomerulonephritis, glomerulosclerosis or canine amyloidosis), Bence Jones proteinuria or, much less commonly, tubular proteinuria. Serum biochemistry and serum or urine protein electrophoresis are useful initial tests that will help localize the cause of proteinuria to preglomerular *versus* renal causes, and these results may direct the course of future diagnostic testing (e.g. bone marrow biopsy *versus* renal biopsy). Chapter 6 provides additional detailed information on this topic.

Serial measurement of the UPC can be used to stage the progression of renal disease and to evaluate the response to therapy. Determination of the UPC may also be performed to help establish the prognosis for newly diagnosed cases of canine chronic kidney disease (Jacob *et al.*, 2005). A UPC >1.0 at the time of initial chronic kidney disease diagnosis is a negative prognostic indicator. Compared with patients with a UPC <1.0, canine chronic kidney disease patients with a UPC >1.0 experience more rapid progression of renal disease, greater likelihood of uraemic crisis and greater risk of death due to either renal or non-renal causes. The rate of disease progression and risk of complications were directly proportional to the magnitude of UPC elevation. Similarly, proteinuria predicts reduced survival times in healthy, non-azotaemic cats

(Walker *et al.*, 2004) and in cats with chronic kidney disease (Syme and Elliot, 2003). UPCs >0.3 in healthy non-azotaemic cats or >0.4 in cats with chronic kidney disease were significant predictors of reduced survival times in these two studies.

Microalbuminuria: An assay to detect micro-albuminuria is available (E.R.D.-Screen™ Urine Test). Microalbuminuria refers to increased urine albumin that remains beneath the detection limit of the urine dipstick protein reaction (i.e. urine albumin >0.01 g/l but <0.30 g/l). The prevalence of microalbuminuria has been reported as 15–19% in clinically normal dogs (Jensen *et al.*, 2001; Gary *et al.*, 2004) and 14% in clinically normal cats. Increased prevalence has been reported with older age or the presence of non-renal disease (Heska Corporation unpublished data, available at http://www.heska.com/erd).

In canine experimental models of progressive glomerular disease, the prevalence of microalbuminuria was 75–100% and persistent microalbuminuria preceded the development of overt proteinuria (Grauer *et al.*, 2002; Lees *et al.*, 2002). Controlled studies to establish reference ranges for clinically normal animals, animals with non-renal disease and animals with early glomerular disease, or controlled clinical studies to correlate identification of microalbuminuria in apparently healthy animals with the subsequent development of renal disease have not yet been published. However, these preliminary investigations suggest that, similar to humans, detection of persistent microalbuminuria in dogs may aid in early diagnosis of occult glomerular disease prior to the development of a positive dipstick protein reaction or increased UPC.

Microscopic examination of the urine sediment

Microscopic evaluation of the urine sediment is performed to detect increased concentrations of cells, casts, microorganisms or crystals, which may indicate underlying urinary tract disease. The concentration of the sediment and the preservation of cellular morphology are directly affected by the technique used to prepare and examine the sediment (see Figure 8.14), potential contaminants from stain (see Figure 8.17) and by urine biochemistry (Figure 8.26). Therefore, it is important to consider results of the urine dipstick tests when evaluating the sediment. For example, within dilute urine (SG <1.008) erythrocytes will probably be lysed. Highly alkaline urine may reduce the numbers of cells and casts observed in the sediment, and urine pH also strongly influences crystal formation (Figure 8.27).

Urine specific gravity

Very concentrated (>1.035)
  Shrinkage and crenation of erythrocytes
  Shrinkage of leucocytes
Hyposthenuric (<1.008)
  Erythrocyte and leucocyte swelling or lysis
  Usually associated with larger urine volumes so sediment constituents may be diluted

Bilirubinuria
Casts may be orange–yellow due to bilirubin The number of bilirubin crystals will be increased
Glucosuria
Has a diuretic effect so larger urine volumes are produced which dilutes sediment constituents Secondary urinary tract infection is common, therefore pyuria and bacteriuria may be observed
Ketonuria
Has a diuretic effect so larger urine volumes are produced which dilutes sediment constituents
Alkalinuria
Cell lysis Cast degeneration Promotes formation of crystals that form in alkaline urine
Aciduria
Casts may be better preserved Promotes formation of crystals that form in acidic urine

8.26   Effects of abnormal urine biochemistry on sediment evaluation.

Crystal	Acidic urine	Neutral urine	Alkaline urine
Ammonium biurate	✓	✓	
Bilirubin	✓		
Calcium carbonate (not reported in dogs and cats)			✓
Calcium oxalate dihydrate	✓	✓	✓ (in stored samples)
Calcium oxalate monohydrate	✓	✓	
Cystine	✓	✓	
Magnesium ammonium phosphate (struvite)		✓	✓
Amorphous phosphates			✓
Sulphonamide metabolites	✓		
Amorphous urates	✓		
Uric acid	✓		

8.27   pH influence on formation of commonly observed urine crystals.

Crystalluria

Crystalluria occurs when urine is saturated with dissolved minerals or other crystallogenic substances that precipitate out of solution to form crystals. Crystals may form *in vivo* for either pathological or non-pathological reasons, or crystals may precipitate in urine *ex vivo* due to cold temperature or prolonged storage, postcollection alterations of urine pH or evaporation of water from the sample (Figure 8.28). To increase the likelihood that crystals present in the urine sample represent those formed *in vivo*, fresh, non-refrigerated urine samples should be analysed within 1 hour of collection.

In most instances, crystalluria does not necessarily indicate the presence of uroliths or even a predisposition to form uroliths. For example, a small number of magnesium ammonium phosphate or amorphous phosphate crystals are frequently observed in clinically

Crystal	Causes
Magnesium ammonium phosphate (struvite)	Refrigerated storage for more than 1 hour Commonly seen in clinically normal animals Urinary tract bacterial infection by urease-producing bacteria Alkaline urine for reasons other than infection (e.g. diet, recent meal, renal tubular ammoniagenesis in cats, postcollection artefact) Sterile or infection-associated uroliths of potentially mixed mineral composition
Calcium oxalate dihydrate	Storage for more than 1 hour with or without refrigeration Acidic urine (e.g. diet, postcollection artefact) May be seen in clinically normal animals Calcium oxalate urolithiasis Hypercalciuria (e.g. due to hypercalcaemia or hypercortisolaemia) Hyperoxaluria (e.g. ingestion of oxalate-containing vegetation, ethylene glycol or chocolate)
Calcium oxalate monohydrate	Hyperoxaluria (e.g. ingestion of ethylene glycol or chocolate)
Calcium carbonate	Not reported in dogs and cats Sulphonamide crystals with similar morphology may be mistaken for calcium carbonate
Bilirubin	A low number commonly found in concentrated canine urine, especially males Altered bilirubin metabolism (e.g. haemolytic or hepatobiliary diseases)
Amorphous phosphates	Insignificant finding in clinically normal animals
Amorphous urates Uric acid Ammonium biurate	Portovascular malformation Severe hepatic disease Ammonium biurate urolithiasis Breed associated: Dalmatians, English Bulldogs, low number of crystals is an insignificant finding
Cystine	Defect in proximal renal tubular transport of amino acids
Iatrogenic	Sulphonamide crystals (sulpha-containing antibiotic administration) Xanthine crystals (allopurinol administration) Radiocontrast medium crystals Fluoroquinolone and other drug crystals (reported in humans)

8.28 Potential causes of commonly observed urine crystals.

normal dogs and cats. Detection of crystalluria may be diagnostically useful in the following situations:

- When abnormal crystal types are identified (e.g. ammonium biurate, calcium oxalate monohydrate, cystine)
- When large aggregates of magnesium ammonium phosphate or calcium oxalate dihydrate crystals are found
- When crystalluria is observed in a patient that has confirmed urolithiasis.

Evaluation of the type of crystals present may be useful to estimate the mineral component of the urolith(s), while awaiting results of complete urolith analysis. Uroliths are often heterogenous; therefore crystalluria is not a definitive indicator of urolith mineral content. Sequential evaluation of crystalluria may aid in monitoring a patient's response to therapy for urolith dissolution. Specific types of common urine crystals are discussed here. Further details, including uncommon types of crystalluria, can be found in texts devoted entirely to urinalysis (e.g. Osborne and Stevens, 1999).

Magnesium ammonium phosphate crystals: These are referred to as struvite crystals, triple phosphate crystals (a misnomer) or infection crystals (an older term) (Figure 8.29a). They are colourless and frequently form variably sized, casket cover-shaped crystals. They also form three- to eight-sided prisms, needles or flat crystals with oblique ends. Magnesium ammonium phosphate crystals most commonly form in alkaline urine, which often occurs in association with bacterial infection. They may develop after collection in refrigerated urine samples (Albasan *et al.*, 2003), or in those that become alkaline during storage due to bacterial overgrowth or contamination of the sample with cleanser residues, for example. When magnesium ammonium phosphate crystals are detected in a stored urine sample, the finding should be verified by prompt examination of a freshly obtained urine sample that has not been refrigerated.

Magnesium ammonium phosphate crystals are very commonly seen in dogs and occasionally in cats. When found in significant number, they are most frequently associated with bacterial infection by urease-producing bacteria, such as *Staphylococcus* spp. or *Proteus* spp. However, in cats, they can occur in the absence of infection, probably due to ammonia excretion by the renal tubules. Magnesium ammonium phosphate crystals may also be seen in clinically normal animals that have alkaline urine for reasons other than infection (e.g. diet, recent meal), animals that have sterile or infection-associated uroliths of potentially mixed mineral composition, or with urinary tract disease in the absence of urolithiasis.

Calcium oxalate crystals: These occur in two forms, dihydrate and monohydrate (see Figures 8.17a and 8.29b,c). Calcium oxalate dihydrate crystals occur much more commonly. They are colourless, variably sized octahedrons that resemble a small envelope or a Maltese cross and most commonly form in acidic urine.

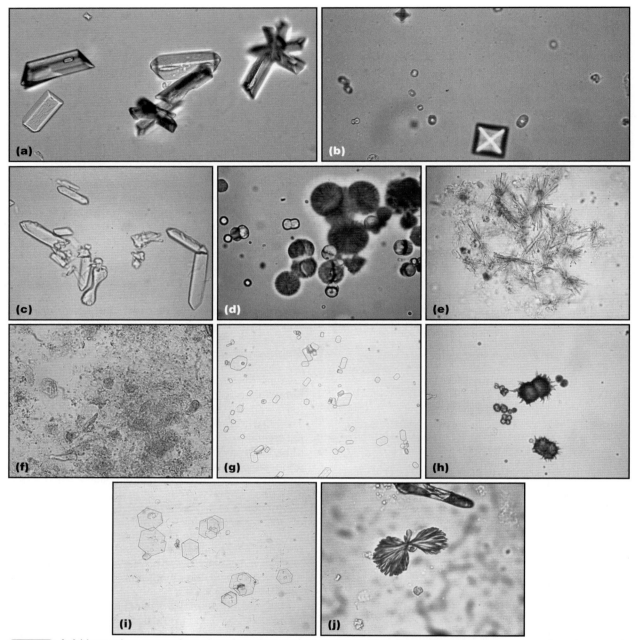

8.29 **(a)** Magnesium ammonium phosphate (struvite) crystals in feline urine sediment. A casket cover form is present (lower left). (Unstained, original magnification X500) **(b)** Calcium oxalate dihydrate crystals in canine urine sediment. **(c)** Calcium oxalate monohydrate in feline urine sediment. Two morphologies are present: most crystals resemble picket fence boards and a single dumbbell-shaped crystal is found near the centre of the field. The picket fence board morphology is highly suggestive of recent ethylene glycol ingestion. This form appears similar to magnesium ammonium phosphate crystals, but calcium oxalate monohydrate crystals are always flat, while magnesium ammonium phosphate crystals form three-dimensional prisms (a). (Unstained, original magnification X400) **(d)** Calcium carbonate crystals forming spheres with radial striations in equine urine sediment. These crystals have not been reported in dogs or cats. Sulphonamide crystals may form globules with radial striations and could be mistaken for calcium carbonate crystals.
(e) Bilirubin crystals in canine urine sediment. Copious sheaves of needle-like, dark orange bilirubin crystals are found clumped within urine sediment from a dog with hepatobiliary disease. **(f)** Amorphous phosphate crystals in urine sediment from alkaline urine from a clinically normal dog. Compare with amorphous urate crystals in Figure 8.41a.
(g) Uric acid crystals in canine urine sediment. Several flat, six-sided, diamond-to-rectangular shaped uric acid crystals are present in acidic urine from a clinically normal Dalmatian. **(h)** Ammonium biurate crystals. Dark golden-brown spheroids and sarcoptic mange-like ammonium biurate crystals are identified in urine sediment from a hepatoencephalopathic cat with portovascular malformation. **(i)** Cystine crystals in canine urine sediment. Cystine crystals, which are never a normal sediment finding, form flat hexagons with unequal sides in acidic urine. They most commonly occur in male dogs of certain breeds with proximal renal tubular disease and are a risk factor for cystine urolithiasis. Note the large number of sperm in the background. **(j)** Sulphonamide crystals in canine urine sediment after sulpha-containing antibiotic administration. A sheave of pale yellow, needle-like sulphonamide crystals are seen surrounded by a few yellow globular forms. ((b), (d), (e), (f), (g), (h), (i), (j) unstained; original magnification X100)

They may develop after collection in stored urine samples with or without refrigeration (Albasan *et al.*, 2003) or in those that become acidic during storage due to bacterial overgrowth, for example. When calcium oxalate dihydrate crystals are detected in a stored urine sample, the finding should be verified by prompt examination of freshly obtained urine that has not been refrigerated. Calcium oxalate dihydrate crystals may be seen in clinically normal animals. They also occur with calcium oxalate urolithiasis, hypercalciuria (e.g. due to hypercalcaemia or hypercortisolaemia) or hyperoxaluria (e.g. ingestion of vegetation high in oxalates (e.g. Brassica family), ethylene glycol or chocolate). They have been reported with increased frequency in cats as a complication of urine acidification to manage magnesium ammonium phosphate formation.

Calcium oxalate monohydrate crystals are colourless and variably sized. They may be flat with pointed ends and resemble picket fence boards. They may also form spindle- or dumbbell-shaped crystals. Although either calcium oxalate monohydrate or dihydrate crystals can be seen with acute ethylene glycol intoxication, the monohydrate form with picket fence board morphology is more diagnostic of intoxication, since this form is usually only seen during acute ethylene glycol toxicity. Formation of these crystals is time-dependent and occurs only during the early phase of intoxication. Crystalluria may be observed within 3 hours of ingestion in cats and within 6 hours in dogs and may last up to 18 hours after ingestion. Calcium oxalate monohydrate crystals with spindle or dumbbell morphology are uncommonly observed with other causes of hyperoxaluria (e.g. chocolate ingestion).

Calcium carbonate crystals: These are variably sized, yellow–brown or colourless, variably shaped crystals (tic-tac-shaped, dumbbell-shaped or spheres with radial striations) that are found individually or in clusters usually within alkaline urine (see Figure 8.29d). They are seen in clinically normal horses, elephants, goats, rabbits and guinea pigs. Anecdotally, they may very rarely be seen in dogs. Sulphonamide crystals, which can be seen in dogs and cats after sulpha-containing antibiotic administration, may form globules with radial striations and could be mistaken for calcium carbonate crystals.

Bilirubin crystals: These may precipitate as orange to reddish-brown granules or needle-like crystals (see Figure 8.29e). A low number of crystals are routinely observed in canine urine, especially in highly concentrated samples from male dogs. When bilirubin crystals are found in other species or in persistently large quantities in a canine patient, a disease associated with icterus (i.e. haemolytic or hepatobiliary disease) may be present.

Amorphous phosphate and amorphous urate crystals: These are similar in shape and may form amorphous debris or small spheroids (see Figure 8.29f). Amorphous phosphates are distinguished from amorphous urates in two ways: phosphates are colourless or light yellow and form in alkaline urine, while urates are yellow–brown to black and form in acidic urine. Amorphous phosphates are commonly observed in alkaline urine of clinically normal animals, and they are not clinically significant. Conversely, amorphous urates are an uncommon abnormal finding in most breeds. They may be seen in animals with portovascular malformation, severe hepatic disease or ammonium biurate urolithiasis. Amorphous urates are routinely found in Dalmatians and English Bulldogs and may represent a predisposition for urate urolithiasis in these breeds.

Compared with other breeds, Dalmatians excrete a larger amount of uric acid in their urine and are therefore prone to form *uric acid crystals* (Figure 8.29g). Uric acid crystals are colourless, flat, variably, but often diamond-shaped, six-sided crystals. Most other breeds convert uric acid to a water-soluble compound (i.e. allantoin) for excretion. Dalmatians have diminished hepatocellular uptake of uric acid, preventing this conversion, so that uric acid is excreted in its native form into the urine. Also, Dalmatians have decreased tubular reabsorption of uric acid compared with other breeds. Uric acid crystals can also occasionally be seen in English Bulldogs. They are rarely seen in other dog breeds or cats and, when observed, have the same significance as amorphous urate or ammonium biurate crystals.

Ammonium biurate crystals: These are golden-brown and spherical with irregular protrusions, giving a thorn-apple or sarcoptic mange-like appearance (see Figure 8.29h). In cats, they may form smooth aggregates of spheroids. Ammonium biurate crystals are seen in animals with portovascular malformation, severe hepatic disease, ammonium biurate urolithiasis and, uncommonly, in clinically normal Dalmatians and English Bulldogs.

Cystine crystals: These are colourless, flat hexagons that may have unequal sides (see Figure 8.29i). Cystine crystalluria is an abnormal finding seen in animals that are cystinuric due to an inherited defect in proximal renal tubular transport of several amino acids (i.e. arginine, cystine, lysine, ornithine). Crystals are prone to develop in cystinuric patients that have concentrated, acidic urine. Cystinuria is a predisposition for the development of cystine urolithiasis, though not all cystinuric individuals develop uroliths. Among dogs, male Dachshunds, Basset Hounds, English Bulldogs, Yorkshire Terriers, Irish Terriers, Chihuahuas, Mastiffs, Rottweilers and Newfoundlands are affected with increased frequency. Uroliths often lodge at the base of the os penis and may be missed on survey radiographs since they are relatively radiolucent. Bitches and other breeds may also be affected. In cats, this disease has been recognized in male and female Siamese and American domestic shorthairs.

Iatrogenic crystalluria: This can be seen with administration of some antibiotics, allopurinol and radio-contrast medium. Sulphonamide crystals (see Figure 8.29j) are pale yellow crystals and may form haystack-like bundles or globules with radial striations. The latter morphology may be mistaken for calcium carbonate crystals.

Renal tubular casts and pseudocasts

Renal tubular casts are formed by proteinaceous plugs of dense, mesh-like mucoprotein (Tamm–Horsfall mucoprotein) that accumulate within the distal portion of the nephron (i.e. Henlé's loop, distal tubule, collecting duct). A low number (fewer than two per high power field) of these proteinaceous hyaline casts can occasionally be observed in urine of normal animals (Figure 8.30). Diuresis of dehydrated animals or proteinuria of preglomerular or renal aetiology can cause an increased number of hyaline casts to be present in urine. Renal tubular epithelial cells that die and slough into the tubular lumen can be entrapped within the dense mucoprotein matrix (Figure 8.31). If present, inflammatory cells associated with renal tubulointerstitial inflammation may also be entrapped.

During microscopic sediment evaluation, cellular casts are further classified as either epithelial, leucocyte or erythrocyte casts, if the constituent cells can be discerned. Once locked within the proteinaceous matrix, cells continue to degenerate, progressing from intact cells, to granular cellular remnants, and finally to a waxy cholesterol-rich end-product. A cast may dislodge from a given renal tubular lumen at any time during this degenerative process and may be observed in the urine sediment. However, in clinically normal animals only granular casts are rarely found (fewer than two per high power field). Other material can lodge within the proteinaceous matrix, such as lipid from degenerated renal tubular epithelial cells, haemoglobin during haemolytic disease and bilirubin (Figure 8.32).

The number of casts observed in the sediment does not correlate with the severity of renal disease or its reversibility; and the absence of casts from urine sediment cannot be used to exclude the possibility of renal disease, especially since casts are fragile and prone to degeneration, particularly in alkaline urine. When hyaline or granular casts are present in increased numbers or when other cast types are observed, one can only conclude that the renal tubules are involved in an active pathological process of unknown severity or reversibility. When present, the type of cast observed may provide additional information. Leucocyte casts indicate active renal tubulointerstitial inflammation. Waxy

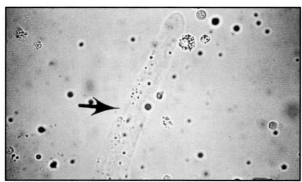

8.30 Translucent hyaline renal tubular cast in canine urine sediment. Note the evenly separated, parallel sides and rounded end of the cast, which allows this cast to be distinguished from a mucus thread (see Figure 8.33c). A transitional epithelial cell is touching the cast. A few smaller leucocytes are also seen in the background. (Unstained; original magnification X400)

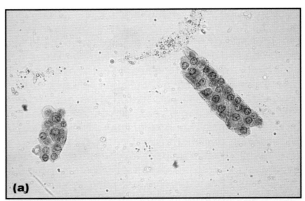

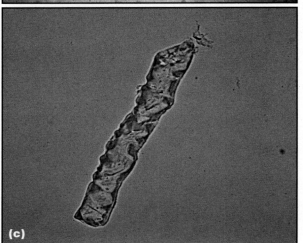

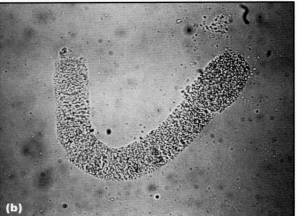

8.31 **(a)** Cellular renal tubular cast comprised of desquamated renal tubular epithelial cells in the urine sediment of a dog with acute renal failure. The cells within the cast are well preserved, suggesting that the cast recently formed and was dislodged from the renal tubule before appreciable cellular degeneration occurred. (New methylene blue stain; original magnification X400) **(b)** Granular renal tubular cast in feline urine sediment. Although the cast is curvilinear, note the evenly separated parallel sides. Falling between intact cellular casts and aged waxy casts, granular casts represent an intermediate stage of cellular degeneration. A low number of granular casts are occasionally seen in urine from clinically normal animals. **(c)** Cholesterol-rich waxy renal tubular cast in feline urine sediment, indicating that a chronic renal tubular lesion is present. These casts have characteristic sharply broken, blunt ends and are less translucent than hyaline casts. ((b) and (c) Unstained; original magnification X400)

casts reflect a chronic tubular lesion. To recognize the onset of nephrotoxicity in patients receiving amino-glycoside antibiotic therapy, it is useful to monitor urine sediment for the appearance of tubular epithelial cell casts, which should prompt withdrawal of the antibiotic. Other abnormalities seen with aminoglycoside-induced nephrotoxicity include isosthenuria, proteinuria, gluco-suria and aminoaciduria, all of which may precede the onset of azotaemia.

Structures such as mucus threads or fibres may resemble casts and should not be mistaken for them during microscopic examination (Figure 8.33). Mucus

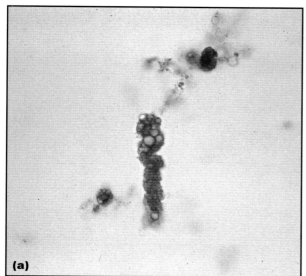

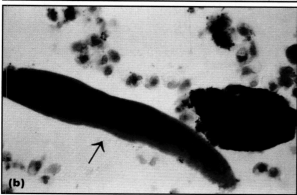

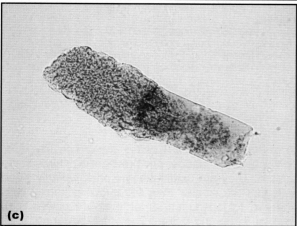

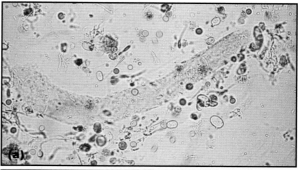

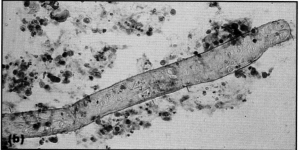

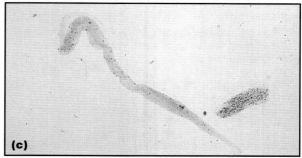

8.32 **(a)** Fatty renal tubular cast in feline urine sediment, consisting of granular cellular remnants admixed with non-staining, spherical lipid droplets. Feline renal tubular epithelial cells are relatively lipid-rich; therefore these casts are more commonly seen in cats. (New methylene blue stain; original magnification X100) **(b)** Haemoglobin renal tubular cast (arrowed) in canine urine sediment. The haemoglobin content of the cast imparts a dark reddish-brown colour. When observed in patients with haemolytic disease, this finding specifically indicates intravascular haemolysis, rather than extravascular haemolysis. **(c)** Bright orange bilirubin-containing, mixed granular and waxy renal tubular cast in canine urine sediment. The cellular material is more degenerated in the right portion of the cast. ((b) and (c) Unstained; original magnification X400)

8.33 **(a)** Curved hyaline renal tubular cast within an active canine urine sediment. The cast is surrounded by several pale orange erythrocytes and some leucocytes and transitional epithelial cells. There also several bacteria and sperm in the background. Note the size of the cast relative to the surrounding cells and the difference in magnification of this image compared with (b). (Unstained; original magnification X400) **(b)** Large, synthetic fibre within an active canine urine sediment. The fibre, which could be mistaken for a cast, is present surrounded by numerous cells that are relatively much smaller than the fibre. Note the uneven, irregular separation of the parallel sides, the repetitive internal structure and the dull blunt end of the fibre. (Unstained; original magnification X100) **(c)** Mucus thread in feline urine sediment. Mucus threads could be mistaken for hyaline casts, but are distinguished by their irregularly spaced, twisting parallel sides and pointed, wispy ends. (New methylene blue stain; original magnification X100)

threads are distinguished by their variable width and tapered ends. Fibres are typically much larger than the surrounding cells and may contain a repetitive internal structure, suggesting a synthetic origin.

Epithelial cells

Epithelial surfaces along the length of the genitourinary tract undergo constant turnover, therefore it is routine to see a low number of epithelial cells (fewer than five per low power field) in normal urine samples. Using wet-mount preparations, it can be challenging to distinguish the different types of epithelial cells, since transitional cells are highly pleomorphic and all epithelial cells will become rounded within a fluid milieu and degenerate when exposed to urine. Cell morphology is best appreciated in freshly formed and collected urine that is promptly analysed. When evaluation of cell morphology is critical, the sediment pellet can be evaluated by routine cytology, similar to that performed with a fine needle aspirate (Figure 8.34). A greater number of epithelial cells are seen in urine samples collected by catheterization or in patients with inflamed, hyperplastic or neoplastic mucosa. Methods to diagnose structural lesions within the urinary tract (e.g. ultrasonography, catheter biopsy) that are more reliable and conclusive than urinalysis are available.

---

1. Centrifuge the urine as is done for wet mounting (see Figure 8.9, Step 8).

2. Use a transfer pipette to aspirate the pellet from the bottom of the conical centrifuge tube.

3. Place a small drop of the aspirated material on to a clean, glass microscope slide.

4. Allow the slide to air-dry. Heat fixation is not necessary and will alter cell morphology.

5. Stain as a routine cytology using Diff Quik® or other similar stain. Alternatively, the slide can be stored in a covered container at room temperature and sent to a referral diagnostic laboratory for evaluation.

8.34   Method to prepare urine sediment for dry mounting and routine cytological examination.

Squamous epithelial cells: These line the distal third of the urethra, the vagina and the prepuce. They are large, flat or rolled cells that have angular sides and usually a single small, condensed nucleus, or they may be anucleate (Figure 8.35). A variable number of squamous epithelial cells is most commonly observed with lower urinary tract contamination of voided or catheterized samples. Squamous epithelial cells should not be present in samples collected by cystocentesis. A significant number of squamous epithelial cells are very rarely seen in cystocentesis samples due to squamous cell carcinoma of the bladder or due to squamous metaplasia of the bladder, which can occur with transitional cell carcinoma or chronic bladder irritation. Squamous epithelial cells may also be found if the uterine body of an intact female was unintentionally penetrated during urine sample collection.

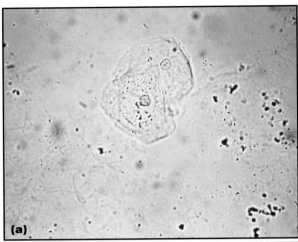
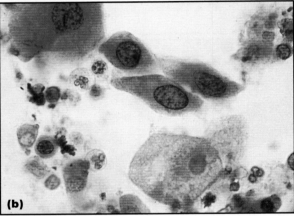

8.35   **(a)** Squamous epithelial cells in canine urine sediment. Note their angular borders, abundant translucent cytoplasm and single condensed nucleus. (Unstained; original magnification X400) **(b)** Mixed population of epithelial cells and leucocytes in canine urine sediment. Three transitional epithelial cells are found (top left). Note their pleomorphism and relatively large nuclei. An angular squamous epithelial cell is present (bottom). Some leucocytes with segmented nuclei and fewer small round cells are scattered throughout the field. (SediStain™; original magnification X400)

Transitional epithelial cells: These line the renal pelves, ureters, bladder and proximal two thirds of the urethra. They are highly pleomorphic, variably sized cells that are smaller than squamous epithelial cells and two to four times larger than leucocytes (see Figures 8.35b and 8.36a). They may be round, oval, pear-shaped, polygonal or caudate, and often have granular cytoplasm with a single nucleus that is larger than that of squamous epithelial cells. There should be fewer than five transitional epithelial cells per low power field in normal urine sediment. A greater number of transitional epithelial cells are seen in urine samples collected by catheterization or in patients with inflamed, hyperplastic or neoplastic mucosa. Transitional epithelial cells with caudate morphology specifically line the renal pelves (Figure 8.36b). These cells are rarely observed in urine sediments and are an abnormal finding that can sometimes be seen in patients with pyelonephritis, renal pelvic calculi or other pathology involving the renal pelves.

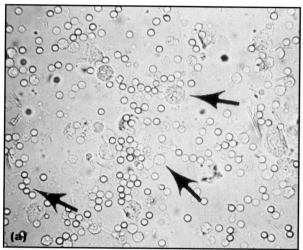

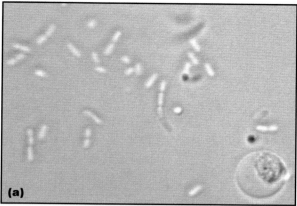

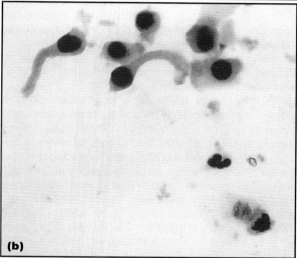

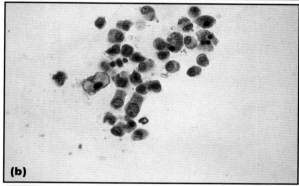

8.36 **(a)** Size comparison of cells in an active canine urine sediment. Erythrocytes are the smallest cells (left arrow), leucocytes are larger than erythrocytes (middle arrow) and transitional epithelial cells are larger than leucocytes (right arrow). Squamous epithelial cells are the largest cells (not pictured). (Unstained; original magnification X400) **(b)** Caudate transitional epithelial cells (top) exfoliated from the renal pelvis of a cat with pyelonephritis. Beneath the epithelial cells, two smaller neutrophils are found. (New methylene blue stain; original magnification X400)

8.37 **(a)** Rounded renal tubular epithelial cell and bacteria in canine urine sediment. A small round cell is present (lower right) that can be presumptively identified as a renal tubular epithelial cell based upon the eccentric placement of its round nucleus. There are several bacilli in the background. (Unstained; original magnification X500) **(b)** A large number of cuboidal to low columnar renal tubular epithelial cells in feline urine sediment. Most cells are cuboidal or low columnar with eccentric nuclei. Fewer cells are rounded. Though not identified within a cast, this large number of renal tubular epithelial cells is abnormal and suggests an active tubular lesion. (New methylene blue stain; original magnification X400)

Renal tubular epithelial cells: Cuboidal to low columnar renal tubular epithelial cells often become small round cells once they have exfoliated into urine (Figure 8.37a) and are not always easily distinguished from leucocytes or small transitional epithelial cells. Unless they are found within a tubular cast, the presence of renal tubular epithelial cells is not considered a dependable indicator of renal disease, since a low number of tubular cells are sloughed normally and since other similarly sized cells (e.g. small transitional epithelial cells, leucocytes) may be mistakenly identified as renal tubular epithelial cells in wet-mount preparations. Observation of a large number of these cells with their cuboidal to low columnar morphology intact is a rare abnormal finding, however, that would indicate active renal tubular disease (Figure 8.37b).

Neoplastic epithelial cells: These are occasionally identified in urine sediment (Figure 8.38). In a patient that has a bladder or urethral mass, the urine sediment finding of atypical transitional epithelial cells in the absence of inflammation is suggestive of transitional cell carcinoma. Neoplastic transitional epithelial cells may exfoliate in cohesive sheets or individually. They are identified by their malignant features, such as high nuclear:cytoplasmic ratio, variable cell and nuclear size, clumped chromatin with prominent nucleoli, and mitotic activity. However, when inflammation is present, it is not possible to distinguish hyperplastic epithelial cells, which develop similar cytological features, from neoplastic epithelial cells. Since it is quite common for bladder tumours to become secondarily inflamed, definitive diagnosis using urine cytology alone is often not possible. In these instances, additional diagnostic information (e.g. imprint cytology or histology of catheter biopsy material) may be helpful in making a definitive diagnosis. Other less commonly observed tumours include rhabdomyosarcoma, urothelial papilloma and squamous cell carcinoma.

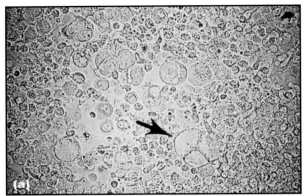

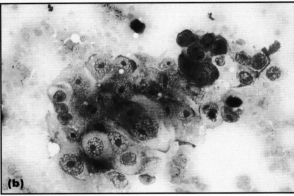

8.38 **(a)** A large number of neoplastic epithelial cells in canine urine sediment. It is apparent that the nuclear:cytoplasmic ratio is markedly increased, although a stained preparation would improve visualization of nuclear details. The arrow is pointing to a cohesive cell cluster. (Unstained; original magnification X400)
(b) Neoplastic epithelial cells in a dry-mounted canine urine sediment prepared for routine cytology as described in Figure 8.34. There is a cohesive sheet of neoplastic transitional epithelial cells. Note the absence of inflammation and the presence of morphological changes consistent with malignancy (i.e. variation in cell and nuclear sizes, very high nuclear:cytoplasmic ratio, open chromatin pattern and prominent, large nucleoli). Compare the morphology of these cells to the non-neoplastic transitional epithelial cell in Figure 8.42b. Several erythrocytes are also present in the background. (Diff Quik®; original magnification X500)

The veterinary bladder tumour antigen (v-BTA) test is a rapid latex agglutination assay that is designed to be used as a screening test for early diagnosis of transitional cell carcinoma by detecting an antigen that is produced by the tumour and released into the urine. This test is associated with a high rate of false-positive results, which may occur due to haematuria, pyuria, 4+ glucosuria or 4+ proteinuria. Therefore, this test would not be useful in patients that have an advanced transitional cell carcinoma associated with haematuria and pyuria, which often occur secondarily to bladder neoplasia. To decrease the possibility of false-positive reactions, the test should be performed upon the supernatant of centrifuged urine. However, some investigators feel that the test has an unacceptable number of false-positive reactions, even in dogs with normal urine sediment. Using the supernatant of centrifuged urine, the specificity of the test has been reported as 46% in unhealthy patients with urinary tract

disease other than transitional cell carcinoma. The specificity increased to approximately 86% in clinically normal animals or in animals with non-urinary tract disease (Henry *et al.*, 2003).

In its current form, this assay is unlikely to be useful as a screening test for use in the general canine population. Because of the low incidence of bladder tumours in dogs (<2% of canine cancers) and the high frequency of false-positive test reactions, an unacceptable number of animals may be subjected to invasive and costly diagnostic procedures in order to prove a false reaction. However, this test may have some utility in selected at-risk canine populations, such as obese, geriatric dogs from urban areas with lower urinary tract signs and breed predisposition for transitional cell carcinoma (e.g. Scottish Terriers, Shetland Sheepdogs, Beagles, Wire-Haired Fox Terriers, West Highland White Terriers) (Mutsaers *et al.*, 2003), when a negative result can be used to help exclude the possibility of transitional cell carcinoma in a high-risk individual.

Blood cells, infectious agents and other sediment findings

Highly alkaline or dilute urine or improper sample storage may significantly reduce the number of cells in the urine sediment (see Figures 8.7 and 8.26). During microscopic examination care should be taken to distinguish erythrocytes from lipid droplets. Lipid droplets are quite variably sized, refractile, greenish discs that are usually smaller than erythrocytes, often float above the plane of focus and never exhibit the biconcave appearance of erythrocytes (Figure 8.39). They are frequently observed in feline urine. Beyond their potential to be misidentified as erythrocytes, they are of little significance.

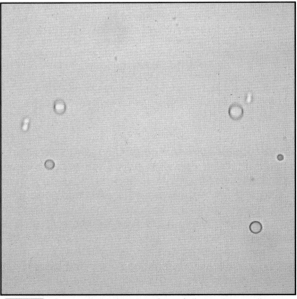

8.39 Seven lipid droplets from feline urine sediment, floating in different focal planes. Note their variable size, refractile, jewel-like appearance and greenish hue, all of which are features that distinguish them from erythrocytes (not pictured). (Unstained; original magnification X400)

Erythrocytes: Erythrocytes are quite translucent and may be pale orange due to their haemoglobin content. Erythrocyte shape varies with the tonicity of the urine. They may:

- Maintain their biconcave disc morphology
- Shrivel, becoming crenated in concentrated urine
- Swell, becoming rounded in dilute urine (Figure 8.40).

There should be fewer than five erythrocytes per high power field. However, the number observed can be influenced by collection method (see Figure 8.4). Haematuria can be a component of pathology seen with haemorrhagic diathesis (e.g. thrombocytopenia), infection, inflammation, necrosis, neoplasia, toxicity (e.g. cyclophosphamide) or trauma (see Chapter 1).

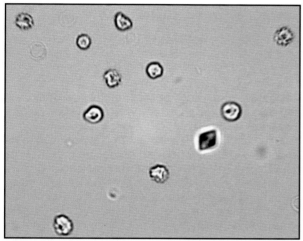

8.40 Variable erythrocyte morphology in canine urine sediment. Ten pale orange, crenated erythrocytes are present along with three colourless erythrocyte ghosts. Compare with Figures 8.17a and 8.36a. A single diamond-shaped calcium oxalate dihydrate crystal is in the middle of the field. (Unstained; original magnification X500)

Leucocytes: In a sample collected by cystocentesis, there should be fewer than three leucocytes per high power field. In a sample collected by catheterization or midstream voiding, there should be fewer than eight leucocytes per high power field. Being larger than erythrocytes and smaller than epithelial cells, leucocytes are intermediate in size compared with other cells that may be present in the sediment (see Figure 8.36a). They are usually round with a stippled appearance and greyish internal structure that transmits less light than erythrocytes; segmented nuclei are frequently visualized (see Figures 8.35b and 8.41). Some leucocytes contain granules that are occasionally visible as refractile structures within the leucocyte. These cells may be referred to as *glitter cells*.

Observation of pyuria with concurrent bacteriuria indicates active urinary tract inflammation with either primary or secondary bacterial infection (Figure 8.41). Urine culture is useful to identify microorganisms de-

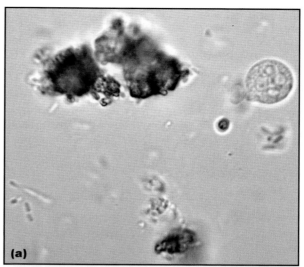

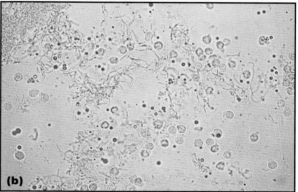

8.41 **(a)** Pyuria, bacteriuria and amorphous urate crystalluria in Dalmatian urine sediment. A leucocyte that has a segmented nucleus is present (right). Note that it is stippled grey and transmits less light than erythrocytes (not pictured). There are several bacilli in the background and two aggregates of brownish-black amorphous urate crystals (middle top and bottom). Compare these with amorphous phosphate crystals in Figure 8.29f. (Unstained; original magnification X500) **(b)** Pyuria and bacteriuria in canine urine sediment. Several leucocytes and bacilli are surrounding a bacterial microcolony (upper left corner) in urine sediment from a dog with bacterial cystitis. (Unstained; original magnification X400)

finitively and to determine their antimicrobial sensitivities. Pyuria is also seen with other causes of genitourinary tract inflammation, such as urolithiasis, neoplasms, prostatitis, pyometra and less common infections by viruses, mycoplasmas or ureaplasmas. Cystocentesis may avoid contamination of the urine sample by leucocytes from the genital tract and aid in localizing the source of pyuria.

Bacteria: The absence of pyuria does not exclude the possibility of a urinary tract infection; therefore *urine sediment evaluation alone cannot be used to exclude definitively the possibility of infectious urinary tract disease.* Silent urinary tract infections (i.e. those lacking a detectable inflammatory response) can be seen with hyperadrenocorticism/hypercortisolaemia, diabetes mellitus and other immunosuppressed states

(Figure 8.42). Also, leucocytes and bacteria may be diluted below the detection limit of light microscopy in polyuric conditions when large volumes of dilute urine are produced (e.g. pyelonephritis). At least 10,000 bacilli/ml or 100,000 cocci/ml are required for detection by light microscopy.

Bacteria may be observed in urine sediment for reasons other than urinary tract infection (e.g. overgrowth after collection) (Figure 8.43). When microorganisms are observed in stained wet mounts, it is necessary to distinguish them from contaminants (see Figure 8.17b) by confirming their presence in

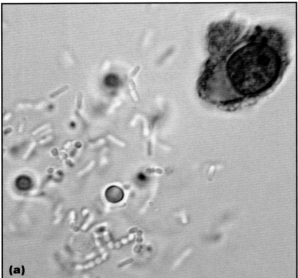

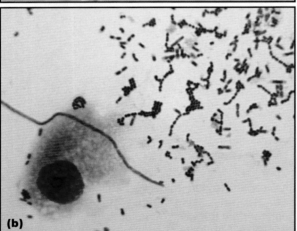

8.42 Bacteriuria in urine sediment from a glucosuric Miniature Schnauzer. The dog was isosthenuric (specific gravity 1.008) and mildly glucosuric (5.6 mmol/l). **(a)** A mixed population of bacteria (bacilli and cocci) is present near a transitional epithelial cell (right). Note the absence of pyuria. (New methylene blue stain; original magnification X500) **(b)** Bacteriuria in dry-mounted urine sediment from a glucosuric Miniature Schnauzer. This slide was prepared using the method described in Figure 8.34. Several cocci, small bacilli and large bacilli are present with a single transitional epithelial cell. This method of slide preparation improves visualization of bacterial morphology and increases the sensitivity and specificity for the detection of bacteriuria. (Wright-Giemsa stain; original magnification X500)

Urinary tract infection

Sample contamination during micturition or catheterization

Sample contamination during processing (e.g. by staining)

In vitro bacterial overgrowth

8.43 Causes of bacteriuria.

Observed bacteria represent contaminants of the urine sample incurred during collection or processing

Observed bacteria may actually be non-bacterial structures in the sediment that were mistakenly identified as bacteria during urinalysis

Observed bacteria may not be viable due to:
    Prior antimicrobial administration
    Prolonged urine storage
    Fastidious nutritional and culture requirements (e.g. *Mycoplasma, Ureaplasma*)

Observed bacteria may not grow due to improper culture technique

8.44 Potential causes of a negative urine culture despite identification of bacteria in the urine sediment.

unstained wet mounts or by cytological examination of the dry-mounted sediment pellet (see Figure 8.42b). The latter is a more sensitive and specific method to detect bacteria than wet mounting and permits more accurate identification of bacterial morphology (Swenson *et al.*, 2004). Urine cultures can occasionally be negative, even though bacteria were detected during urinalysis (Figure 8.44). Also, uncommon infections by viruses or highly fastidious microorganisms (e.g. *Mycoplasma, Ureaplasma*) may result in negative urine culture although a urinary tract infection is present.

Urine culture: Cystocentesis is the ideal collection method for urine culture. The likelihood of representative culture results may be enhanced by collection of a randomly timed urine sample (which will probably consist of freshly formed urine that has not stagnated within the bladder) along with inoculation of a culture tube immediately after collection. Afterwards, the culture tube should be refrigerated to prevent overgrowth of robust bacteria.

With routine urine culture, results are reported that simply identify the bacteria present and their respective antimicrobial sensitivities. Quantitative urine culture is an alternative that may be helpful to determine if the bacteria cultured from a urine sample are likely to represent a true infection or if they are likely to be contaminants of the sample. In addition to bacterial identification and elucidation of their antimicrobial sensitivities, quantitative culture enumerates the bacteria as colony-forming units (CFU)/ml, which is determined by serial dilution and plating. Quantitative urine culture can be most beneficial when the urine sample has been collected by transurethral catheterization or by collection of midstream voided urine (Figure 8.45).

Collection method	Significant (cfu/ml)		Questionable (cfu/ml)		Contamination (cfu/ml)	
	Dog	Cat	Dog	Cat	Dog	Cat
Cystocentesis	>1000	>1000	100–1000	100–1000	<100	<100
Catheterization	>10,000	>1000	1000–10,000	100–1000	<1000	<100
Voided	>100,000	>10,000	10,000–100,000	1000–10,000	<10,000	<1000

8.45 Guidelines for interpretation of quantitative urine cultures (see Chapter 23).

Other sediment findings

Dependent on geography, other infectious agents are occasionally identified in urine sediment (Figure 8.46), such as fungi (e.g. *Candida* spp., *Aspergillus* spp., *Blastomyces dermatitidis*, *Cryptococcus* spp.), algae (e.g. *Prototheca* spp.) and nematode ova, larvae or adults (e.g. *Capillaria* spp., *Dirofilaria immitis* and *Dioctophyma renale*). *Trichuris* spp. (whipworm) parasite eggs appear very similar to *Capillaria* spp. parasite eggs. These two types of egg can be distinguished by the positioning of their bipolar caps and the texture of their outer shells. The bipolar caps of *Capillaria* spp. ova are slightly askew, rather than being perfectly

bipolar as they are in *Trichuris* ova. Also, the shells of *Capillaria* ova have a granular appearance, rather than being perfectly smooth as they are in *Trichuris* ova. *Capillaria* are usually an incidental finding in the urine of asymptomatic cats. However, *Capillaria* eggs are rarely identified in cats that present with haematuria, which resolves after fenbendazole administration.

Common contaminants of urine samples include sperm, talc, glass chips, plant pollen, hair and fibres (Figure 8.47; see also Figures 8.29i and 8.33). Aside from sperm, these contaminants can be mistaken for urine crystals (e.g. talc, glass chips), transitional epithelial cells (e.g. plant pollen) or casts (e.g. hair, fibres).

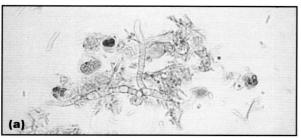

(a)

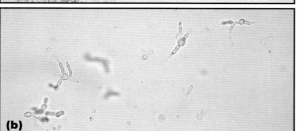

(b)

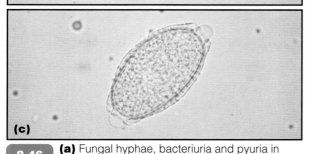

(c)

8.46 **(a)** Fungal hyphae, bacteriuria and pyuria in canine urine sediment. Septate branching fungal hyphae are present surrounded by leucocytes and numerous bacteria. (SediStain™; original magnification X400) **(b)** Budding pseudohyphae of *Candida* in canine urine sediment. **(c)** *Capillaria* ovum in canine urine sediment. A single amber ovum is present surrounded by a few lipid droplets. Note the placement of the bipolar caps which are slightly askew and the granular texture of the outer shell, distinguishing this ovum from that of *Trichuris*. ((b) and (c) Unstained; original magnification X400)

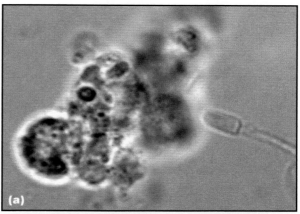

(a)

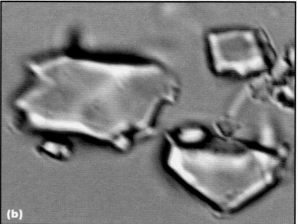

(b)

8.47 **(a)** Pyuria and sperm in a Persian cat with bilateral renomegaly. An aggregate of leucocytes (left) and a single sperm (right) are present. Sperm are a potential contaminant of voided samples. (Unstained; original magnification X1000) **(b)** Glass chip contaminants in canine urine sediment. Glass chips are common contaminants of urine sediments that may be mistaken for crystalluria. (Unstained; original magnification X500)

References and further reading

Albasan H, Lulich JP, Osborne CA *et al.* (2003) Effects of storage time and temperature on pH, specific gravity, and crystal formation in urine samples from dogs and cats. *Journal of the American Veterinary Medical Association* **222**, 176–179

Gary AT, Cohn LA, Kerl ME and Jensen WA (2004) The effects of exercise on urinary albumin excretion in dogs. *Journal of Veterinary Internal Medicine* **18**, 52–55

George JW (2001) The usefulness and limitations of hand-held refractometers in veterinary laboratory medicine: a historical and technical review. *Veterinary Clinical Pathology* **30**, 201–210

Grauer GF, Moore LE, Smith AR and Jensen WA (2004) Comparison of conventional urine protein test strip method and quantitative ELISA for the detection of canine and feline albuminuria. *Journal of Veterinary Internal Medicine* **18**, 418–419 [abstract 127]

Grauer GF, Oberhauser EB and Basaraba RJ (2002) Development of microalbuminuria in dogs with heartworm disease. *Journal of Veterinary Internal Medicine* **16**, 352 [abstract 103]

Henry CJ, Tyler JW, McEntee MC *et al.* (2003) Evaluation of a bladder tumor antigen test as a screening test for transitional cell carcinoma of the lower urinary tract in dogs. *American Journal of Veterinary Research* **64**, 1017–1020

Heuter KJ, Buffington CA and Chew DJ (1998) Agreement between two methods for measuring urine pH in cats and dogs. *Journal of the American Veterinary Medical Association* **213**, 996–998

Holan KM, Kruger JM, Gibbons SN and Swenson CL (1997) Clinical evaluation of a leukocyte esterase test-strip for detection of feline pyuria. *Veterinary Clinical Pathology* **26**, 126–131

Jacob F, Polzin DJ, Osborne CA *et al.* (2005) Evaluation of the association between initial proteinuria and morbidity rate or death in dogs with naturally occurring chronic renal failure. *Journal of the American Veterinary Medical Association* **226**, 393–400

Jensen WA, Grauer GF and Andrews J (2001) Prevalence of microalbuminuria in dogs. *Journal of Veterinary Internal Medicine* **15**, 300 [abstract 113]

Lees GE, Brown SA, Elliot J, Grauer GF and Vaden SL (2005) Assessment and management of proteinuria in dogs and cats: 2004 ACVIM forum consensus statement (small animal). *Journal of Veterinary Internal Medicine* **19**, 377–385

Lees GE, Jensen WA and Simpson DF (2002) Persistent albuminuria precedes onset of overt proteinuria in male dogs with X-linked hereditary nephropathy. *Journal of Veterinary Internal Medicine* **16**, 353 [abstract 108]

Mutsaers AJ, Widmer WR and Knapp DW (2003) Canine transitional cell carcinoma. *Journal of Veterinary Internal Medicine* **17**, 136–144

Osborne CA and Stevens JB (1999) *Urinalysis: A Clinical Guide to Compassionate Patient Care, 1st edn*, pp. 1–214. Veterinary Learning Systems, Bayer Corporation, Shawnee Mission, Kansas

Plier ML, Grindem CB, MacWilliams PS and Stevens JB (1998) Serum fructosamine concentration in nondiabetic and diabetic cats. *Veterinary Clinical Pathology* **27**, 34–39

Raskin RE, Murray KA and Levy JK (2002) Comparison of home monitoring methods for feline urine pH measurement. *Veterinary Clinical Pathology* **31**, 51–55

Rees CA and Boothe DM (2004) Evaluation of the effect of cephalexin and enrofloxacin on clinical laboratory measurements of urine glucose in dogs. *Journal of the American Veterinary Medical Association* **224**, 1455–1458

Stockham SL and Scott MA (2002) Urinary system. In: *Fundamentals of Veterinary Clinical Pathology*. Iowa State Press, Ames

Swenson CL, Boisvert AM, Kruger JM and Gibbons-Burgener SN (2004) Evaluation of modified Wright-staining of urine sediment as a method for accurate detection of bacteriuria in dogs. *Journal of the American Veterinary Medical Association* **224**, 1282–1289

Syme HM and Elliot J (2003) Relation of survival time and urinary protein excretion in cats with renal failure and/or hypertension. *Journal of Veterinary Internal Medicine* **17**, 405 [abstract 106]

Vail DM, Allen TA and Weiser G (1986) Applicability of leukocyte esterase test strip in detection of canine pyuria. *Journal of the American Veterinary Medical Association* **189**, 1451–1453

Walker D, Syme HM, Markwell P and Elliot J (2004) Predictors of survival in healthy, non-azotaemic cats. *Journal of Veterinary Internal Medicine* **18**, 417 [abstract 123]

9

Assessment of renal function

Reidun Heiene and Hervé P. Lefebvre

Introduction

The major role of the kidneys is to maintain the volume and balanced composition of the extracellular fluid. This is achieved by filtering the blood through the glomerulus, and adjusting the composition of the filtrate, as it passes along the tubules, according to the body's requirements. These functions are vital, tightly regulated and closely integrated with the other major regulatory systems in the body.

Assessment of renal function in small animals has been carried out for several decades and often involves a combination of diagnostic tools and functional tests. The interpretation of individual tests or single samples may be hampered by a lack of sensitivity, large biological variability, high cost and/or poor practicability. Knowledge of the relative strengths and weaknesses of each tool is essential to detect the early stages of chronic kidney disease, and to distinguish chronic from acute renal failure. Whereas functional tests may be important in chronic kidney disease, ultrasonography and renal biopsy are often more use-

ful in acute renal failure. A renal function assessment may also be useful for other purposes, such as serial monitoring of renal function or adjustment of a drug dosage regimen. This chapter focuses on the methods available for assessing renal function in dogs and cats, especially in the diagnosis of early stages of chronic kidney disease.

Basic principles

There are several basic principles that need to be taken into consideration.

The different renal functions cannot be assessed simultaneously

The kidney has multiple functions (Figure 9.1) and no single test is able to assess all of them simultaneously. There is, however, a consensus in human and veterinary nephrology that the most relevant and sensitive means of assessing overall renal function is to estimate the glomerular filtration rate (GFR).

9.1 Major renal functions.

Glomerular filtration
- Filters blood at a rate of 60 l/day in a 30 kg dog
- Essential for kidney function
- Clinical relevance: GFR is the best indicator of the overall renal function

Tubular reabsorption and secretion
- Reabsorbs most of the fluid and maintains homeostatic balance in the composition of extracellular fluid
- Clinical relevance: concentrating ability of the kidney, capacity for reabsorption of filtered substances, acid–base disturbances

Renin–angiotensin–aldosterone system
- Controls local glomerular haemodynamics, sodium reabsorption and systemic blood pressure
- Clinical relevance: angiotensin II plays a role in development of systemic hypertension in chronic kidney disease

Erythropoietin
- Stimulates erythrocyte production by the bone marrow
- Clinical relevance: anaemia in chronic kidney disease

Calcitriol
- Stimulates intestinal calcium absorption and bone remodelling, limits parathyroid hormone synthesis
- Clinical relevance: development of renal secondary hyperparathyroidism in chronic kidney disease

Kidney lesions may exist in the absence of renal dysfunction and *vice versa*

A damaged kidney may function normally, and visible lesions may be absent from a functionally impaired kidney. This is apparent:

- After uninephrectomy, when the remaining kidney usually compensates and the GFR returns to normal a few weeks later
- In prerenal causes of acute renal failure (e.g. severe dehydration, when the GFR may drop significantly, even though no lesions can be detected in the renal parenchyma).

Urine composition exhibits considerable fluctuations

Urinalysis remains a cornerstone in the diagnosis of renal failure and is easy to perform (see Chapter 8). Most dogs with chronic kidney disease display polyuria and polydipsia (PU/PD), whereas a large proportion of cats with chronic kidney disease do not. Urine specific gravity, however, fluctuates from day to day and from hour to hour, and shows large inter-individual variability (van Vonderen *et al.*, 1997). Urine sediment may provide information about the processes active in the kidney. Also of importance is the urine protein:creatinine ratio, as proteinuria is known to contribute to the deterioration of renal function (see Chapter 6).

Plasma urea and creatinine levels only increase when renal damage is severe

Due to their wide availability, plasma urea and creatinine analyses are often used in conjunction with urinalysis, in the first step of patient evaluation. These tests are not very sensitive, however, as changes in plasma urea and creatinine are only detectable once most of the renal functional mass has been lost. For this reason, early renal dysfunction can be better identified from measurements of GFR or renal concentrating ability.

Repeated measurements are required

A single blood sample may be sufficient for the diagnosis of renal failure in cases of severe renal dysfunction.

However, the importance of repeated measurements in the early or subclinical stages of chronic kidney disease should be emphasized. Reasons for this include:

- Although an animal may show a trend for its plasma creatinine concentration to increase over time, the values may still remain within the reference ranges
- The reference ranges obtained from books may be too broad for the laboratory or animal in question
- Differences may result simply from analytical and biological variability, and be independent of the pathological process. If, for example, the variability of the assay is about 10%, a difference of 10% between two consecutive measurements cannot be attributed to a change in renal function (Figure 9.2). Such variability needs to be reduced by taking repeated samples under standardized conditions (e.g. fasted animal, same time of day, same laboratory, same assay) (Braun *et al.*, 2003).

Specific tests can be used to distinguish acute from chronic renal failure

Although the history and clinicopathological data associated with acute renal failure and chronic renal failure may be similar, the subsequent treatment and prognosis can be very different (see also Chapter 5).

Ultrasonography is useful for evaluating kidney size, structural changes in renal tissue and circulatory disturbances or for providing evidence of ethylene glycol toxicity.

Renal biopsy (see Chapter 12) is usually only indicated in situations where a histological diagnosis can affect treatment and outcome, as in the case of suspected acute renal failure or glomerulonephritis (see Chapter 6). Biopsy is also the only way to distinguish between amyloidosis and glomerulonephritis in severe proteinuric disease.

Urinary enzymes have been used to detect early renal damage (Grauer *et al.*, 1995), but are not in routine use because of their variable sensitivity and specificity.

The most accurate way of distinguishing between acute and chronic renal failure is to use carbamylated

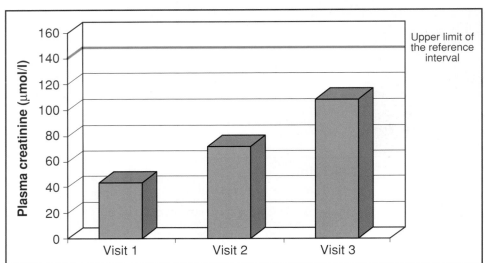

9.2 Renal dysfunction may be detected by repeated measurements in standardized conditions while plasma creatinine is still within the reference ranges. A consecutive increase in plasma creatinine concentration reflects a corresponding decrease in renal function. The critical difference is 35 µmol/l (0.40 mg/dl) for creatinine. The difference observed between visits 3 and 1 can be clinically interpreted as resulting from a decrease in renal function (i.e. a potential reduction in GFR of 50%).

haemoglobin. Isocyanate derived from the urea produced during uraemic states reacts with haemoglobin to form carbamylated haemoglobin, and thus reflects the urea levels of previous weeks. Although this test is not currently performed by commercial laboratories, it can readily be carried out by using capillary electrophoresis and a commercially available test kit (Vaden *et al.*, 1997; Heiene *et al.*, 2001).

Assessment of glomerular function

The ideal markers of GFR are freely filtered, not reabsorbed nor secreted and no extrarenal excretion takes place.

Indirect markers of glomerular function

Azotaemia refers to increased levels of non-protein nitrogen wastes (such as urea and creatinine) in the blood, and may be prerenal, renal or postrenal. Urea and creatinine are indirect markers of renal function. The plasma concentration will depend on the production rate of the marker and on its distribution and elimination (Figure 9.3). A difference between two

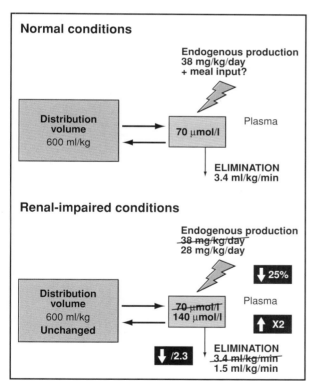

9.3 Plasma concentration is a hybrid parameter which depends on the production, distribution and elimination of the marker. The figure represents the disposition of plasma creatinine concentration in healthy and renal-impaired dogs, according to a classic bicompartmental model (Watson *et al.*, 2002). In healthy conditions, the plasma creatinine concentration is 70 μmol/l (0.79 mg/dl). When GFR is decreased by 2.3, it just reaches the upper limit of the reference interval (140 μmol/l; 1.58 mg/dl). Concomitantly, the production of creatinine has decreased by 25% in the renal-impaired dog due to impaired muscle mass. This decrease in creatinine production has mitigated the effect of the GFR decrease on plasma creatinine.

concentrations measured at two different times in the same subject can only be interpreted if there have been no changes in the production and distribution of the marker.

Creatinine is produced and released at a stable rate by skeletal muscle. It is completely filtered, not reabsorbed and not secreted. Thus, it can serve as an endogenous marker of GFR.

Plasma/serum urea

Urea is synthesized in the liver from ammonia and distributed throughout the body fluids. Urea is mainly eliminated by the kidneys and is freely filtered by the glomeruli, but reabsorbed by the tubules. The rate of reabsorption depends on the tubular urine flow rate and increases as this flow rate decreases (as in dehydration). Urea reabsorption therefore increases in dehydrated animals. Moreover, urea permeability of the collecting duct is influenced by antidiuretic hormone (ADH).

Plasma urea may also increase when protein catabolism is induced by pathological conditions, or when protein intake increases. Significant increases have been observed after food intake, so measurements should only be obtained in fasted animals (after a 10–12-hour fast). An increase in plasma urea may also be caused by fever or infection or by gastrointestinal bleeding (due to protein metabolism).

A decrease in plasma urea may be observed in dogs on a low-protein diet, with severe hepatic failure or portosystemic shunt, or when treated with anabolic steroids. In contrast, an increase may occur in dogs treated with glucocorticoids, antineoplastic agents or tetracyclines.

Thus, for all these reasons, plasma urea is not a good indirect indicator of GFR, but it may provide a useful adjunct to plasma creatinine. A trend towards a relatively higher urea than creatinine value, due to tubular reabsorption, may be observed in prerenal azotaemia. Conversely, a relatively low plasma urea compared to creatinine concentration may indicate severe protein malnutrition in cases of severe chronic kidney disease. The urea:creatinine ratio may thus indicate whether or not a prerenal component is present, but cannot be used reliably to predict the reversibility of azotaemia.

Plasma/serum creatinine

Assays for creatinine are readily available and creatinine concentration is considered the most useful indirect marker for GFR in human and veterinary clinical chemistry. Creatinine is the degradation product of creatine phosphate and creatine which are present in muscle and in food. The volume of distribution of creatinine corresponds to the total body water volume (about 600 ml/kg of body weight). Creatinine is eliminated by glomerular filtration with negligible renal secretion and extrarenal metabolism, and its clearance value provides a good estimate of GFR (see GFR assessment). It is not directly affected by dehydration unless this is severe enough to reduce GFR.

The primary pre-analytical and analytical factors of variation in plasma creatinine are presented in Figure

9.4. The major inter-individual factors of such variation in dogs are age and the ratio of body weight:muscle mass. Plasma creatinine is lower in puppies than in adult dogs and increases progressively to reach the adult basal level at about 1 year. This could potentially be explained by the higher GFR value in very young puppies (Laroute *et al.*, 2005) and later by the increase in muscle mass until adult body size is reached. Creatinine is generally stable in healthy adult dogs up to 8–10 years old, but then decreases. Plasma creatinine increases with body weight and is lower in cachectic dogs and higher in dogs with large muscle mass. It may be increased by dehydration but is not usually altered by physical exercise. Less information is available about the inter-individual factors of variation in cats (Braun *et al.*, 2003).

Creatinine is used to define the clinical stages of chronic kidney disease (IRIS classification www.iris-kidney.com) (see Chapter 11). The IRIS classification scheme enables accurate information about patients to be communicated in texts, case discussions or research. GFR is severely reduced when there is a large increase in plasma creatinine (Figure 9.5). Screening sensitivity, as mentioned previously, can be increased by taking consecutive measurements from the patient over time. To follow the time course of a plasma/serum constituent, the critical difference (determined from the intra-individual and analytical variabilities) has been proposed to judge whether the difference between two consecutive measurements may be safely ascribed to natural variation or not. It has been estimated to be 35 μmol/l (0.40 mg/dl) for plasma creatinine assayed by an enzymatic method in healthy dogs (Jensen and Aaes, 1993). In other words, a change from 40 to 90 μmol/l (0.45–1.02 mg/dl) (i.e. within the reference range) between two consecutive blood samples in the same subject can be interpreted as a significant increase (see Figure 9.2).

Although a reduction in urea, rather than creatinine, is more commonly observed in liver failure, a decrease in plasma creatinine has also been shown in dogs with a portosystemic shunt.

Angiotensin-converting enzyme (ACE) inhibitors are sometimes used in the management of chronic kidney disease in dogs and cats, as clinical studies in human nephrology have shown that ACE inhibitors can reduce progression to end-stage renal diseases. ACE inhibitors may increase plasma creatinine by decreasing glomerular hyperfiltration. In humans, a slight to moderate increase in creatinine over the first weeks of ACE inhibitor treatment seems to be indicative of a long-term positive effect on renal function. Similar increases were not observed in cats when treated with ACE inhibitors.

Factors	Comment
Blood specimen	Creatinine concentration is slightly higher in serum than in plasma. Use the same type of tube for collecting blood when repeating measurements in the same patient
Stability	Creatinine is stable up to 4 days at 4°C in blood, up to 4 days at room temperature in plasma and for at least 3 months at −20°C in plasma.
Food intake	Creatinine may increase following food ingestion up to 12 hours after a meal. The patient should be fasted overnight
Analytical techniques	Specific enzymatic techniques are preferred to the Jaffé reaction. Whereas many analytical interferences can occur with the latter, interferences with the enzymatic reactions are limited to bilirubin

9.4   Pre-analytical and analytical factors contributing to variation in plasma creatinine.

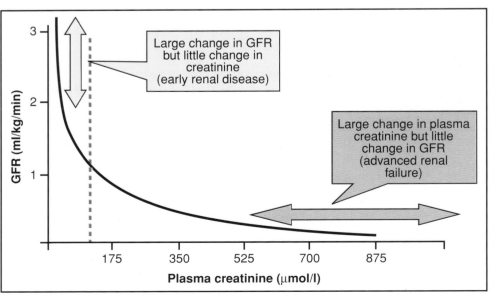

9.5

Relationship between glomerular filtration rate and plasma creatinine concentration. The poor sensitivity of plasma creatinine for the detection of early renal dysfunction is illustrated. The red dashed line corresponds to the upper limit of the reference range in the dog (about 140 μmol/l; 1.58 mg/dl).

Cystatin C

Cystatin C is a small non-glycosylated cysteine proteinase inhibitor (molecular weight 13,350 Daltons), produced by all nucleated cells. Plasma cystatin C concentrations are measured by immunoturbidimetric assay. Cystatin C is a better marker of GFR than serum creatinine in humans, especially in patients exhibiting a small to moderate decrease in GFR. In dogs, a decrease in plasma cystatin C is observed for up to 9 hours after a meal (Braun *et al.*, 2002). The superiority of cystatin C over creatinine as an indirect marker of GFR is highly questionable. They are relatively well correlated with each other (Braun *et al.*, 2002) and with GFR (Almy *et al.*, 2002). The respective sensitivities and specificities (0.78 and 0.98 for cystatin C, and 0.66 and 0.94 for creatinine) are also very similar (Braun *et al.*, 2002). If a more accurate evaluation of GFR is required, it is more useful to measure the clearance of a filtration marker rather than to add cystatin C to the diagnostic panel.

Proteinuria

Proteinuria has received much attention in small animal nephrology over the past few years. It has been shown that proteinuria can be reduced by treatment with ACE inhibitors in humans and dogs (Grauer *et al.*, 2000). It has also been known for more than a decade in human medicine that ACE inhibitors and angiotensin II receptor blockers retard the progression of chronic kidney disease. Although these effects have not yet been reproduced in a general clinical setting in small animals, an increasing body of data supports the notion that these drugs offer 'renoprotection' by reducing proteinuria: the greater the degree of proteinuria, the greater the effect of therapeutic intervention upon life expectancy (Lees *et al.*, 2005).

Proteinuria is quantified by measuring the urine protein:creatinine ratio (UPC) and this should be done when the dipstick protein level of samples exceeds 1+. By relating the protein loss to the creatinine, which is excreted at a constant level, the variation in urine concentration in the 'spot' sample is corrected for. The UPC should be measured for no fewer than 2–3 days to avoid misinterpretation due to day-to-day variation. The results need to be interpreted in conjunction with the urine sediment analysis, as the protein may be due to pyuria if a severe urinary tract infection is present.

Severe proteinuria is the hallmark of glomerular diseases, such as glomerulonephritis or amyloidosis, whereas only a modest increase in UPC is usually observed in animals with chronic kidney disease. Mild proteinuria may be induced by high-protein diets. Corticosteroid treatment, while probably indicated in a small subgroup of glomerulonephritic patients, may sometimes induce severe and life-threatening proteinuria. Proteinuric renal diseases are less common in cats than in dogs.

Microalbuminuria (i.e. urine albumin concentration between 10 and 300 mg/l in dogs) has been proposed as an indicator for the early detection of renal disease in dogs, but is apparently non-specific as microalbuminuria may also increase in non-renal systemic diseases, such as cardiovascular and urogenital diseases and neoplasia (Pressler *et al.*, 2001).

Proteinuria is covered in detail in Chapter 6.

Glomerular filtration rate assessment

There is a consensus in human and veterinary nephrology that GFR is the best indicator of overall renal function. The GFR estimation is simply a particular case of measuring the clearance of a substance from the body. The principles behind the measurement of clearance are explained in Figure 9.6.

Clearance – An estimate of GFR can be obtained by measuring the clearance (CL) of a 'GFR marker substance'. Clearance is a proportionality constant describing the relationship between the rate of transfer of a substance, in amount per unit of time, and its concentration in the urine and/or plasma. Clearance can be thought of as the hypothetical volume of plasma which is completely cleared of the substance during a period of time. Clearance is measured in units of flow and is commonly expressed in ml/min/kg.

The GFR marker – A GFR marker must fulfil the following requirements: it should be freely filtered, not reabsorbed or secreted by the tubule, not metabolized, not toxic and it should only be cleared by the kidneys. If the extrarenal routes of elimination of the marker are negligible, the plasma clearance will be equal to the renal clearance.

Renal clearance – The renal clearance of the GFR marker is equal to the amount of marker excreted in urine (the product of the urine concentration (U) of the marker and the flow (V) of urine collected over a given period of time) divided by its average plasma concentration (P).

$$Renal\ CL = (U \times V)/P$$

Alternatively, after a single injection, the commonly used formula is:

$$Renal\ CL = Ae/AUC$$

(Ae = total amount eliminated in urine, AUC = area under the plasma disappearance curve)

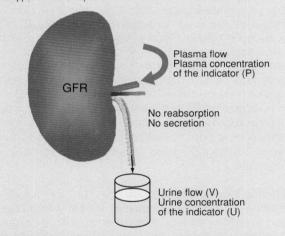

Plasma clearance – The plasma clearance of the marker is calculated by dividing the intravenous dose by the area under the curve (AUC) of the plasma concentration of the marker *versus* time. The exact dose is known and the AUC is calculated manually or by computer. Blood sampling must continue until most of the marker is eliminated to avoid errors in AUC (see Figure 9.7). The time for this varies with the distribution volume of the marker and its clearance, and is thus influenced by renal function such that a lower clearance will necessitate a longer period of sampling.

$$Plasma\ CL = \frac{Dose}{AUC}$$

9.6 Principles of urine and plasma clearance for estimation of glomerular filtration rate (Heiene and Moe, 1998).

An estimation of GFR is particularly useful in the following situations:

- Polyuria/polydipsia without azotaemia
- Borderline increased creatinine values
- Evaluation of drug dosage adjustments for a drug with a low therapeutic index which is eliminated by the kidney
- Suspicion of renal damage after specific events, such as toxic or circulatory collapse
- When renal functional capacity needs to be tested, for example when a nephrectomy is required
- When renal function needs to be monitored over time, such as in clinical trials.

Further population studies are still needed to define valid cut-off values for GFR. The cut-off value may depend on the clearance method and the laboratory. Most published reference values in dogs and cats are between 2 and 5 ml/min/kg. Whatever the method, values lower than 1.5 ml/min/kg can be considered abnormal.

Urinary clearance methods

The urinary clearance of inulin has, for decades, been regarded as the reference ('gold standard') method to which all other methods have been compared. The classic method consists of a 1-hour protocol involving constant infusion and three 20-minute sampling periods. Due to the large body of data published over the years, this method still provides a point of reference. The urinary clearances of endogenous or exogenous creatinine have also been validated in dogs (Bovee and Joyce, 1979; Finco et al., 1991) and used as reference methods. The urinary clearance of exogenous creatinine is currently the method which is the best documented in the veterinary literature. The procedure is described in detail by Finco et al. (1991).

Catheterization of the bladder is required for timed urine collection, however, and this is cumbersome and introduces a risk of infection, so these methods have never been widely used in veterinary practice or in research.

Plasma clearance methods

Plasma clearance methods may lead to errors in certain situations where the marker exhibits extrarenal clearance, or where the pharmacokinetic method used for the calculations is inappropriate in relation to the underlying physiological situation. These methods are nevertheless attractive because they can be performed without urine collection, and the number of plasma samples can be reduced if correction formulae are applied. Such methods are likely to become routinely available for clinical practice as well as research.

Several other plasma clearance and limited sample methods have been published since the last review of renal and plasma clearance methods was published by Heiene and Moe (1998). Although only a few have been thoroughly validated against the reference methods, they provide practical guidelines and reference values from small groups of healthy animals. Several of the methods may be used with reasonable accuracy in a clinical setting, although the elucidation of certain methodological pitfalls still requires further research. Of particular importance is when to terminate sampling. If sampling is stopped too early, the proportion of the area under the curve (AUC) which will need to be estimated by extrapolation will be too large to provide reliable clearance values. Care should be taken when interpreting results in extreme situations, such as in very high or very low renal function, or in very large or very small dogs. At present, the markers with the most practical advantages seem to be creatinine and iohexol.

Methods have been published for testing the plasma clearance of inulin in dogs and cats (Miyamoto, 1998; 2001a). One study provides plasma clearance values for the inulin analogue sinistrin (Haller et al., 1998). However, the method cannot be properly evaluated because sampling was stopped after 2 hours and no estimates of error are included. Inulin is unstable in plasma samples and has to be transported to the laboratory in a frozen state. The laboratory methods are usually cumbersome or expensive and are not widely available. It was also shown in a recent study (Watson et al., 2002), that plasma inulin clearance was significantly higher than urinary clearance of inulin measured simultaneously, suggesting that there are other routes of removal of inulin from plasma.

Plasma clearance methods using the radiocontrast agent iohexol have been described in both dogs and cats (Figure 9.7) (Brown et al., 1996; Heiene and Moe, 1999; Finco et al., 2001; Miyamoto 2001b). Access to routine laboratory analysis is not widely available, but simple laboratory methods are described. Iohexol is stable, so plasma samples can be sent by mail to a central unit. Although toxic reactions have been a concern (allergy, skin reactions, reversible nephropathy), they seem exceedingly rare in view of the widespread clinical use of radiocontrast agents in patients. Toxic reactions are also sometimes observed after inulin injections, and it is difficult to judge whether iohexol truly represents a higher risk of toxicity than other GFR markers. Most toxic reactions occurring after the injection of contrast media are reversible, and the risk is lower at the low dosages recommended for GFR measurement when compared with dosages used for cardiac procedures, computed tomography (CT) or urography.

Recently, the plasma clearance of exogenous creatinine has been described (Le Garreres et al., 2001; Watson et al., 2002) with very encouraging results (Figure 9.8). Laboratory analyses for creatinine are widely available. Although two earlier studies in dogs and cats had indicated the poor performance of plasma creatinine methods (Labato and Ross, 1991; Miyamoto, 1998), the inaccurate plasma creatinine clearance values were most likely to be due to the early termination of sampling in those studies. Creatinine is unusual among the GFR markers in that its volume of distribution and half-life in plasma are approximately three times greater than the corresponding parameters for the other markers. The required sampling times are therefore longer, but this practical constraint is acceptable in cases where renal function has not been se-

Equipment and material required for the test

Iohexol solution 300 mg iodine/ml
Sterile saline (NaCl 0.9%)
Intravenous catheter with stopper, needles, syringes and tubes for blood sampling
Timer

Procedure

1. Ensure that the patient is fasted overnight.
2. Hospitalize the patient for the day. Do not provide food. Water should be available *ad libitum*.
3. Weigh the patient.
4. Take a blood sample for measurement of the basal value (zero sample).
5. Administer the iohexol solution as an intravenous bolus via an intravenous catheter with stopper. Dose: 1 ml/kg for dogs without azotaemia; 0.5 ml/kg for azotaemic dogs.
6. Flush the dead space of the catheter with 2 ml saline after injection. Start the timer immediately. Remove the catheter after rinsing.
7. Sample 1 ml blood at 2 and 3 hours after administration, from a different site to where the injection was made. In azotaemic dogs, samples should be taken at 2, 3 and 4 hours. Use heparinized tubes.
8. Centrifuge the samples and send the plasma to a laboratory.
9. At the time of writing an analysis is commercially available from the Central Laboratory in Oslo, Norway where the clearance value given is corrected by applying a formula to adjust for the reduced number of samples (Renalyzer method; minimum 3 ml of plasma, from 6 ml of blood).
10. Laboratory analysis is likely to be available at Cambridge University Veterinary School, UK, in the near future (Oxford instrument method; minimum 1 ml plasma, 2 ml blood).
11. If laboratory analysis is performed elsewhere (in laboratories with high-performance liquid chromatography (HPLC) or capillary electrophoresis) the clearance value can be calculated manually. Clearance is the actual dose given divided by the area under the plasma disappearance curve (AUC). AUC may be calculated using computer programmes, or manually by drawing the disappearance curve on semilogarithmic paper. The intercept with the X-axis (B) and half life (t $^1/_2$) can be read from the graph:

   $AUC = B/b$

   B = intercept with the X-axis; b = t $^1/_2$/0.693.
12. A correction must be made for the use of a straight line, because a portion of the initial AUC is 'lost'. The correction formulae for the simplified method are:

   $CL_{corrected} = 0.01 + 1.03CL_{2+3h} - 0.06400 (CL_{2+3h})^2$
   for the 2 and 3 hour result

   $CL_{corrected} = -0.03 + 1.06CL_{2+3+4h} - 0.07012 (CL_{2+3+4h})^2$
   for the 2, 3 and 4 hour result.

Advantages

No urine collection
Iohexol is very stable in the sample and may be sent by ordinary mail to the laboratory, without freezing or special precautions
The time for performing the test is only 3–4 hours and the practical procedure is simple

Disadvantages

The expense of iohexol may be an issue for a large dog
Although very rare (1/3,000–1/50,000), adverse reactions have been described (see text)

9.7 Assessment of glomerular filtration rate in dogs by plasma clearance of iohexol (Heiene and Moe, 1998 and 1999).

verely reduced. At present, creatinine is not freely obtainable on the market, but can be prepared in pharmacies and may become commercially available in the near future.

Plasma clearance of the radionuclide 99mTc diethylenetriaminepentaacetic acid (DTPA) or the renal uptake of 99mTc DTPA provide accurate estimates of GFR (Barthez *et al.*, 1998; Kampa *et al.*, 2002), although not necessarily identical to urinary clearance of inulin (Finco, 2005). The most obvious problems associated with these methods are the need for licensed premises and isolation of the animals. However, as more veterinary schools are getting nuclear medicine departments, these methods are becoming increasingly available in academic centres and are thus indirectly accessible to the referring veterinary surgeon.

Equipment and materials required for the test

Creatinine (Sigma Aldrich)
Sterile saline (NaCl 0.9%)
Intravenous catheter with stopper, needles, syringes and tubes for blood sampling
Timer

Procedure

1. Ensure that the patient is fasted overnight.
2. Hospitalize the patient for the day. Do not provide food. Water should be available *ad libitum*.
3. Weigh the patient.
4. Take a blood sample for measurement of the basal value (zero sample).
5. Prepare the creatinine solution (80 mg/ml) by dissolving anhydrous creatinine (Sigma Aldrich) with distilled water or saline, and sterilize by filtration through a 0.2 μm filter.
6. Administer the creatinine solution as an intravenous bolus via an intravenous catheter with stopper. Flush the dead space of the catheter with 2 ml saline after injecting the creatinine solution. Start the timer immediately. Remove the catheter after rinsing.
7. Sample 1 ml blood at 10 minutes, 1, 2, 6 and 10 hours after administration. Other blood sampling strategies have been published.
8. Perform all the creatinine assays in the same batch with the analyser.
9. Determine plasma clearance from the actual dose given and the area under the plasma creatinine *versus* time profile (AUC). The basal value should be subtracted from the observed values following administration.

Advantages

No urine collection
Assays for plasma/serum creatinine are available in most veterinary practices
The overall time for performing the test is short
A blood sample volume of less than 1 ml may be sufficient to perform the test

Disadvantages

Sterile creatinine solution is not commercially available
Repeated blood sampling may be a limit but is generally well tolerated
Hospitalization for 1 day is required

9.8 Assessment of glomerular filtration rate in dogs by plasma clearance of exogenous creatinine (Watson *et al.*, 2002).

Limited sample methods

Correction formulae for use in limited sample methods have been published for iohexol, DTPA and creatinine (Gleadhill and Michell, 1996; Heiene and Moe, 1999; Barthez *et al.*, 2000; Watson *et al.*, 2002).

Another limited sample approach is to make use of a method of standardization to body size that relates GFR to extracellular fluid volume rather than to body weight (Gleadhill and Michell, 1996). Sampling should be done at time zero and at least three other time points and the appropriate correction formula applied. This approach has theoretical advantages that are related to the underlying physiology during clearance measurements.

Assessment of tubular function

One important role of the kidney is to retain or eliminate water according to body requirements. This function requires a sufficient number of nephrons and an intact renal–pituitary axis with respect to vasopressin (antidiuretic hormone), its receptor and the tubular response. Urine-concentrating ability is altered in chronic kidney disease and also in other conditions, such as treatment with glucocorticoids or diuretics, glucosuria, diabetes insipidus and liver failure (see Chapter 2).

Urine specific gravity

Urine specific gravity (SG) shows large inter- and intra-individual variability in healthy conditions (van Vonderen *et al.*, 1997). In veterinary practice, urine SG is measured with a refractometer, as the dipstick test for urine SG is completely unreliable (see Chapter 8).

Abnormal amounts of organic solutes, such as proteins, glucose and amino acids, may lead to an increased urine SG value, but their effects are relatively small, and they rarely produce clinically significant changes in this value in practice. Drugs, such as diuretics and glucocorticoids, indirectly alter urine SG by modifying the concentrating ability. Radiographic contrast media produce substantial direct increases in urine SG.

Urine SG may range from 1.001–1.080 in healthy adult dogs and cats, and tends to be higher in cats than in dogs. Because of the great variability, urine SG should be evaluated in consecutive samples and interpreted in relation to the hydration status of the patient. Persistently low values indicate a need for further diagnostic investigation.

The urine SG value is compared to the value in the blood, which is the same as in the primary glomerular filtrate. Hypersthenuria, hyposthenuria and isosthenuria (urine SG between 1.008 and 1.012) imply that the urine SG is higher than, lower than or similar to that of the glomerular filtrate. Practically, urine SG between 1.013–1.029 for dogs and 1.013–1.034 for cats is considered as minimally concentrated urine.

PU/PD commonly precede uraemia by weeks or months in dogs with chronic kidney disease, whereas approximately half of the cats with chronic kidney disease do not display PU/PD, because they retain some ability to concentrate urine. The relationship between PU/PD and renal function is highly unpredictable in early renal disease.

If renal function is normal then effectively concentrated urine will be present in a dehydrated animal. If urine SG <1.035 (cat) or <1.030 (dog) is observed in a dehydrated animal, it suggests inadequate concentrating ability.

Water deprivation test

The water deprivation test may be indicated for the final evaluation of polyuria/polydipsia, although the advantages do not always outweigh the specific problems related to performing and interpreting this test (DiBartola, 2005). Its only indication is to distinguish between nephrogenic diabetes insipidus (NDI), psychogenic polydipsia and central diabetes insipidus (CDI) (which are all rare). It is contraindicated in azotaemic and/or dehydrated patients and in patients with known renal disease. Patients that are dehydrated have, by definition, already failed the test. The test is difficult to perform, unpleasant for the animal and depends on repeated emptying of the bladder. Details are given in Chapter 2.

Fractional excretion tests

Tests involving the fractional excretion (FE) of electrolytes provide an assessment of tubular function. Fractional excretion is defined as the fraction of filtered electrolytes which escapes reabsorption and consequently is excreted in the urine. It can be calculated by the following equation:

$$FE = \frac{Ue \times V}{Pe \times GFR} \quad \text{(equation 1)}$$

with Ue and Pe the urine and plasma concentrations of the electrolyte, respectively, and V, the volume of urine.

GFR may be estimated by determining urinary endogenous creatinine clearance. Consequently, FE may be calculated using the following equation:

$$FE = \frac{Ue \times Pcreat}{Pe \times Ucreat} \quad \text{(equation 2)}$$

Only 'spot' samples of urine and plasma are required when using equation 2. Reference values have been published for the fractional clearance of electrolytes in healthy cats and dogs, and FE of sodium has been proposed to distinguish prerenal azotaemia from renal parenchymal disease (DiBartola, 2005). Unfortunately, results from spot samples do not correlate well with values measured on 24-hour urine collections over time; there is also considerable intra- and interindividual variation and the results are highly dependent on dietary intake of the electrolyte. The clinical usefulness of these tests is therefore very limited.

Editors' note

With the exception of Chapters 5 and 9, the term chronic renal failure has been discarded in favour of the term chronic kidney disease. Where the severity of the chronic kidney disease needs quantification, this has been provided using the IRIS system (see Chapter 11).

References and further reading

Almy FS, Christopher MM, King DP and Brown SA (2002) Evaluation of cystatin C as an endogenous marker of glomerular filtration rate in dogs. *Journal of Veterinary Internal Medicine* **16**, 45–51

Barthez PY, Chew DJ and DiBartola SP (2000) Effect of sample number and time on determination of plasma clearance of technetium Tc 99m pentetate and orthoiodohippurate sodium I 131 in dogs and cats. *American Journal of Veterinary Research* **61**, 280–285

Barthez PY, Hornof WJ, Cowgill LD, Neal LA and Mickel P (1998) Comparison between the scintigraphic uptake and plasma clearance of 99mTc-diethylenetriaminepentacetic acid (DTPA) for the evaluation of the glomerular filtration rate in dogs. *Veterinary Radiology and Ultrasound* **39**, 470–474

Bovee KC and Joyce T (1979) Clinical evaluation of glomerular function: 24-hour creatinine clearance in dogs. *Journal of the American Veterinary Medical Association* **174**, 488–491

Braun JP, Lefebvre HP and Watson ADJ (2003) Creatinine in the dog: a review. *Veterinary Clinical Pathology* **32**, 162–179

Braun JP, Perxachs A, Péchereau D and De la Farge F (2002) Plasma cystatin C in the dog: reference values and variations with renal failure. *Comparative Clinical Pathology* **11**, 44–49

Brown SA, Finco DR, Boudinot FD *et al.* (1996) Evaluation of a single injection method, using iohexol, for estimating glomerular filtration rate in cats and dogs. *American Journal of Veterinary Research* **57**, 105–110

DiBartola SP (2005) Renal disease: clinical approach and laboratory evaluation. In: *Textbook of Veterinary Internal Medicine, 6th edn*, ed. SJ Ettinger and EC Feldman, pp. 1716–1730. Elsevier Saunders, St. Louis

Finco DR (2005) Measurement of glomerular filtration rate via urinary clearance of inulin and plasma clearance of technetium Tc 99m pentetate and exogenous creatinine in dogs. *American Journal of Veterinary Research* **66**, 1046–1055

Finco DR, Braselton WE and Cooper TA (2001) Relationship between plasma iohexol clearance and urinary exogenous creatinine clearance in dogs. *Journal of Veterinary Internal Medicine* **15**, 368–373

Finco DR, Brown SA, Brown CA *et al.* (1999) Progression of chronic renal disease in the dog. *Journal of Veterinary Internal Medicine* **13**, 516–528

Finco DR, Brown SA, Crowell WA and Barsanti JA (1991) Exogenous creatinine clearance as a measure of glomerular filtration rate in dogs with reduced renal mass. *American Journal of Veterinary Research* **52**, 1029–1032

Gleadhill A and Michell AR (1996) Evaluation of iohexol as a marker for the clinical measurement of glomerular filtration rate in dogs. *Research in Veterinary Science* **60**, 117–121

Grauer GF, Greco DS, Behrend EN *et al.* (1995) Estimation of quantitative enzymuria in dogs with gentamicin-induced nephrotoxicosis using urine enzyme/creatinine ratios from spot urine samples. *Journal of Veterinary Internal Medicine* **9**, 324–327

Grauer GF, Greco DS, Getzy DM *et al.* (2000) Effects of enalapril versus placebo as a treatment for canine idiopathic glomerulonephritis. *Journal of Veterinary Internal Medicine* **14**, 526–533

Haller M, Muller W, Binder H, Estelberger W and Arnold P (1998) Single-injection inulin clearance – a simple method for measuring glomerular filtration rate in dogs. *Research in Veterinary Science* **64**, 151–156

Heiene R and Moe L (1998) Pharmacokinetic aspects of measurement of glomerular filtration rate in the dog: a review. *Journal of Veterinary Internal Medicine* **12**, 401–414

Heiene R and Moe L (1999) The relationship between some plasma clearance methods for estimation of glomerular filtration rate in dogs with pyometra. *Journal of Veterinary Internal Medicine* **13**, 587–593

Heiene R, Vulliet PR, Williams RL and Cowgill LD (2001) Use of capillary electrophoresis to quantitate carbamylated hemoglobin concentrations in dogs with renal failure. *American Journal of Veterinary Research* **62**, 1302–1306

Jacob F, Polzin DJ, Osborne CA *et al.* (2005) Evaluation of the association between initial proteinuria and morbidity rate or death in dogs with naturally occurring chronic renal failure. *Journal of the American Veterinary Medical Association* **226**, 393–400

Jensen AL and Aaes H (1993) Critical differences of clinical chemical parameters in blood from dogs. *Research in Veterinary Science* **54**, 10–14

Kampa N, Wennstrom U, Lord P *et al.* (2002) Effect of region of interest selection and uptake measurement on glomerular filtration rate measured by 99mTc-DTPA scintigraphy in dogs. *Veterinary Radiology and Ultrasound* **43**, 383–391

Labato MA and Ross LA (1991) Plasma disappearance of creatinine as a renal function test in the dog. *Research in Veterinary Science* **50**, 253–258

Laroute V, Chetboul V, Roche L *et al.* (2005) Quantitative evaluation of renal function in healthy Beagle puppies and mature dogs. *Research in Veterinary Science* **79(2)**, 161–167

Le Garreres A, Laroute V, De la Farge F and Lefebvre HP (2001) Comparison of plasma clearances of creatinine and iohexol for glomerular filtration rate assessment in cats. *Journal of Veterinary Internal Medicine* **15**, 317 [abstract]

Lees GE, Brown SA, Elliott J, Grauer GF and Vaden SL (2005) Assessment and management of proteinuria in dogs and cats; 2004 ACVIM Forum Consensus Statement (Small Animal). *Journal of Veterinary Internal Medicine* **19(3)**, 377–385

Miyamoto K (1998) Evaluation of single-injection method of inulin and creatinine as a renal function test in normal cats. *Journal of Veterinary Medical Sciences* **60**, 327–332

Miyamoto K (2001a) Evaluation of plasma clearance of inulin in clinically normal and partially nephrectomized cats. *American Journal of Veterinary Research* **62**, 1332–1335

Miyamoto K (2001b) Use of plasma clearance of iohexol for estimating glomerular filtration rate in cats. *American Journal of Veterinary Research* **62**, 572–575

Pressler BM, Vaden SL, Jensen WA and Simpson D (2001) Prevalence of microalbuminuria in dogs evaluated at a referral veterinary hospital. *Journal of Veterinary Internal Medicine* **15**, 300 [abstract]

Vaden SL (2005) Glomerular diseases. In: *Textbook of Veterinary Internal Medicine, 6th edn*, ed. SJ Ettinger and EC Feldman, pp. 1786–1799. Elsevier Saunders, St. Louis

Vaden SL, Gookin J, Trogdon M *et al.* (1997) Use of carbamylated hemoglobin concentration to differentiate acute from chronic renal failure in dogs. *American Journal of Veterinary Research* **58**, 1193–1196

van Vonderen IK, Kooistra HS and Rijnberk A (1997) Intra- and interindividual variation in urine osmolality and urine specific gravity in healthy pet dogs of various ages. *Journal of Veterinary Internal Medicine* **11**, 30–35

Watson ADJ, Lefebvre HP, Concordet D *et al.* (2002) Plasma exogenous creatinine clearance test in dogs: comparison with other methods and proposed limited sampling strategy. *Journal of Veterinary Internal Medicine* **16**, 22–33

10

Diagnostic imaging of the urinary tract

Ruth Dennis and Fraser McConnell

Introduction

The urinary tract lends itself well to radiographic investigation and no special equipment is required that would not normally be found in a small animal practice. Ultrasonography is also extremely helpful in imaging most areas of the urinary tract, and is complementary to radiography. Advanced imaging techniques (scintigraphy, computed tomography (CT) and magnetic resonance imaging (MRI)) have potential value in selected cases but are not widely used in urinary tract investigations. Cystoscopy can be used to image the lower urinary tract and bladder (see Chapter 14).

Kidneys and ureters

Radiography

Plain (survey) radiographs

Lateral and ventrodorsal (VD) projections are normally used, with the exposure being made during the expiratory pause when there is least superimposition of abdominal structures. In lateral recumbency the kidneys can usually be seen clearly although partly superimposed on each other; this can be minimized by positioning the patient in right lateral recumbency rather than left, allowing the right kidney to slide more cranially and the left kidney caudally. However, since the uppermost kidney rotates slightly around its hilus it may be advantageous in some cases to obtain both right and left lateral recumbent radiographs, thus highlighting different areas of the renal outlines. The VD projection demonstrates the kidneys individually but with greater superimposition of other abdominal structures. The presence of large amounts of ingesta and faeces may hinder interpretation, and the radiographs may need to be repeated following fasting and administration of an enema.

Contrast studies

Contrast techniques can be used to confirm the size, shape and position of the kidneys when these are unclear on plain radiographs. Some information about the internal architecture of the kidneys is given and serial radiographs provide a crude test of kidney function. Contrast studies are essential for demonstrating the ureters, which are rarely seen on plain films. The most commonly used contrast technique is intravenous urography (IVU, excretion urography) using an ionic, water-soluble, iodinated contrast medium such as iothalamate or diatrizoate. If the patient has cardiovascular compromise, a non-ionic, iodinated contrast medium, such as iohexol or iopamidol, is recommended as their lower osmolarity causes less osmotic diuresis than the ionic agents.

All patients should be well hydrated prior to an IVU. Excretion of iodinated media following intravenous administration is largely via the urinary tract, allowing assessment of the kidneys, ureters and, to some extent, the bladder. As with all contrast studies, the patient should be appropriately prepared and plain radiographs obtained first to check exposure factors and to allow comparison with subsequent contrast radiographs.

IVU should be performed with the patient under general anaesthesia or heavy sedation since injection of contrast medium in the conscious patient may cause retching, vomiting and struggling (unpleasant subjective side effects are experienced by human patients). The contrast medium should be given via an intravenous catheter as perivascular leakage causes tissue irritation. If the study is to demonstrate the location of the ureter endings in incontinent patients, a pneumocystogram should be performed first to outline the bladder neck.

High-concentration, low-volume (bolus) IVU:

1. Concentration of contrast medium: 300–400 mg iodine/ml (concentration in mg iodine/ml is given as a number after the trade name), warmed to reduce viscosity.
2. Dose rate: 850 mg iodine/kg body weight (i.e. about 2 ml/kg).
3. Position the patient in dorsal recumbency, as the VD projection is more helpful.
4. Inject warmed contrast medium rapidly into a peripheral vein via a catheter.
5. Obtain the first radiograph immediately.
6. Take further VD radiographs at regular intervals (e.g. 2 minutes, 5 minutes, 10 minutes, 15 minutes) until a clear nephrogram and pyelogram are seen, and then take a lateral projection ± oblique views for ureters.
7. Continue until a diagnosis is made or a normal appearance is confirmed.

8. Use of an abdominal compression band has been recommended to increase opacification of the renal pelvis, but also results in artefactual distension of the pelvis and ureters mimicking mild hydronephrosis.

Low-concentration, high-volume (infusion) IVU:

1. Concentration of contrast medium: 150 mg iodine/ml (more concentrated media can be diluted with 0.9% saline).
2. Dose rate: 1200 mg iodine/kg body weight (i.e. 8 ml/kg).
3. Administer over 5–15 minutes via a giving set and intravenous catheter.
4. Obtain radiographs as above until a diagnosis is made, starting several minutes into the infusion.
5. This technique may produce inferior renal opacification but improved visibility of the ureters due to increased osmotic diuresis.

Renal angiography: This is a more invasive technique which can be used if the kidneys are failing and an IVU is unsuccessful. Concentrated contrast medium (2–5 ml) is deposited in the aorta near the origin of the renal arteries via a femoral arterial catheter. This demonstrates the kidneys by virtue of their blood supply, even when they are not producing urine. Rapid, serial radiographs are required. Renal angiography has largely been replaced by ultrasonography but could potentially be helpful in cases of idiopathic renal haemorrhage.

Normal radiographic appearance

The kidneys lie retroperitoneally in the dorsal abdomen and are most clearly seen when abundant perirenal fat is present. In emaciated animals or those with peritoneal or retroperitoneal fluid they are less clear and their location and size may have to be inferred from the position of adjacent structures such as the small intestine. They appear as smooth-bordered soft tissue opacities and are bean-shaped on the VD view and bean-shaped or elliptical on the lateral view (the uppermost kidney usually rotates about the hilus so that it appears bean-shaped whereas the dependent kidney remains elliptical). Cat's kidneys are more rounded than those of the dog.

The position of the kidneys is slightly variable due to their mobility, especially in the cat, but in the dog the right kidney is cranial and dorsal to the left, allowing differentiation of the two on lateral radiographs. If the descending colon contains faeces it can often be seen to curve around the ventral border of the left kidney. The right kidney is usually approximately level with vertebrae T12–L1. Its cranial pole lies in the renal fossa of the liver's caudate lobe and is often unclear in dogs. Its caudal pole may be seen protruding caudal to the ribcage. The left kidney lies more caudally and is ventral to L2–4; it is usually entirely outside the ribcage and both its cranial and caudal poles can be seen. In the cat, abundant perirenal fat means that both kidneys are usually clearly visible.

The kidneys should be of a similar size, which is usually related to the length of the second lumbar vertebra on the VD radiograph: normal size ranges quoted are 2.75–3.25 times L2 in the dog, 2.1–3.2 times L2 in entire cats and 1.9–2.6 times L2 in neutered cats (Feeney *et al.*, 1979; Shiroma *et al.*, 1999). These figures are a rough guide and a kidney may be enlarged or reduced in size yet still lie within the limits of supposed normality.

The ureters lie in the retroperitoneal space proximally, and enter the peritoneal space distally before terminating in the trigone of the bladder. They are not visible on plain radiographs except in larger, obese dogs in which they are sometimes seen as fine, linear opacities highlighted by retroperitoneal fat.

Following a bolus contrast medium injection the phases of the IVU which can be recognized are:

- A transient *angiogram* (opacification of the renal arteries and veins) may be seen for a few seconds in some individuals, although in most cases the first exposure is made too late or the contrast medium is too diluted by blood for this to be evident. An angiogram phase is not seen following an infusion IVU
- A prolonged *nephrogram* (opacification of the kidney parenchyma) is seen within a minute or so of the injection and can continue for an hour or more (Figure 10.1). Initially, the cortex may opacify more than the medulla
- A *pyelogram* is visible within a few minutes of the injection, with denser opacification of the pelvis and diverticula (recesses) due to concentration of contrast medium in urine. The renal pelvis appears as a curved, T-shaped structure with radiating, paired diverticula, although there is individual variation in its appearance (Figure 10.1). During the pyelogram phase the ureters

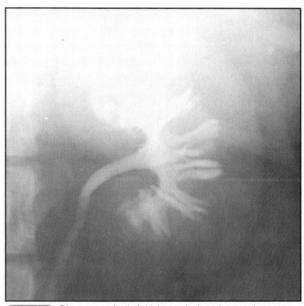

10.1 Close-up of a left kidney during the nephrogram and pyelogram phases of an IVU. The renal pelvis is slightly dilated because abdominal compression had been applied. Although this is no longer performed routinely, this radiograph shows the renal pelvic anatomy well.

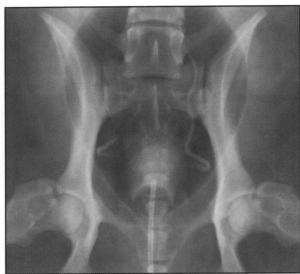

10.2   Normal ureters seen during an IVU in an English Bull Terrier bitch. A pneumocystogram has been performed first to allow the exact location of the ureter terminations with respect to the trigone to be seen.

appear as fine, opaque lines, 1–3 mm diameter, running caudally and following a slightly undulant course; peristalsis creates interruptions in the continuity of these lines. As they enter the trigone of the bladder, the ureters turn back on themselves forming a terminal 'hook', the right ureter end lying more cranially than the left (Figure 10.2). The ureters can also be examined using fluoroscopy with image intensification.

Radiological interpretation

The *kidneys* should be assessed radiographically for the following features:

- Visibility
- Number
- Position and relationship to other organs
- Size
- Shape
- Clarity of outline
- Radiopacity
- Internal architecture (contrast studies)
- Similarity to each other.

The *ureters* should be assessed (on an IVU) for:

- Visibility
- Course
- Diameter
- Margination
- Filling defects
- Termination relative to the trigone.

If an abnormality is detected (e.g. increased size) then a list of possible causes should be compiled, in order of likelihood. If more than one abnormality is present (e.g. increased size and irregular shape) then diseases appearing on each list of possible causes must be regarded as the most likely.

Figure 10.3 lists some conditions which may cause radiographic changes in kidney size, shape or radiopacity. It is important to remember, however, that a kidney may be diseased yet retain its normal radiographic appearance, even with an IVU.

Condition	Enlarged	Reduced size	Irregular	Mineralization
Juvenile nephropathy/ renal dysplasia		✓	✓	
Chronic nephritis/ end-stage kidney disease		✓	✓	✓ Calculi may also be present
Pyelonephritis	✓	✓	✓	Calculi may also be present
Feline infectious peritionitis	✓		✓	
Renal trauma	✓ if subcapsular blood/ urine present			
Renal neoplasm	✓		✓	✓
Renal cyst, abscess, granuloma, haematoma	✓		✓ if large or multiple	✓
Polycystic kidney disease (PKD) (cats)	✓		✓ if large or multiple	✓
Perinephric pseudocysts	✓			
Hydronephrosis	✓	✓ if chronic, mild obstruction		
Hypercalcaemic nephropathy				✓
Chronic renal infarct			✓	
Amyloidosis	✓	✓	✓	

10.3   Summary of causes of radiographic changes in kidney size, shape and opacity. (NB. These changes are not always seen and a normal appearance to the kidney on plain radiographs does not rule out disease.) In some cases renal size may be increased or reduced depending on the stage or chronicity of the disease.

Ultrasonography

Ultrasound examination of the patient with renal disease is not limited to the urinary system, and depending on the presenting problem, examination of other parts of the body may be indicated (e.g. examination of the parathyroid glands may help differentiate chronic kidney disease from acute renal failure). Pathology affecting other organs secondary to urinary tract disease (e.g. gastric mineralization) or an underlying cause of urinary tract disease may also be seen (e.g. portosystemic shunts). For these reasons it is advisable to examine the whole abdomen in a systematic manner. Ultrasonography allows assessment of the internal architecture of the kidneys, prostate and bladder without the need for a contrast study, and usually without requiring general anaesthesia. The indications for renal ultrasonography are similar to those for radiography but ultrasonography has the advantage that it allows guided biopsy (see Chapter 12). If contrast radiographic studies are going to be performed, e.g. pneumocystography, it is preferable to perform ultrasonography first. In severely azotaemic animals ultrasonography is preferred to IVU, as reduced glomerular filtration rate (GFR), renal blood flow and tubular concentrating ability reduce the quality of the IVU.

For all parts of the urinary system a high-frequency transducer (7.5–12 MHz) is ideal, except for very large or obese dogs where a lower-frequency transducer (5 MHz) may be required. Sector or linear transducers can be used; linear transducers suffer less from near-field artefacts but sector scanners require a smaller contact area with the patient. If available, tissue harmonics will give better quality images of the bladder than conventional ultrasonography.

Patient preparation is important and ideally the animal should not have urinated for several hours prior to the study to allow examination with a distended bladder. Rehydration of a dehydrated animal will improve image quality. The examination should take place in a quiet, darkened room and most patients can be imaged without the need for sedation or anaesthesia. If Doppler examination of the kidneys is being performed the animal should preferably be unsedated.

Kidneys

Normally the hair should be clipped at the appropriate site and the skin cleaned with spirit before applying the acoustic gel. In long-haired animals it may be possible just to part the hair and wet the skin and hair with spirit, although it is then impossible to examine the rest of the abdomen adequately. It is often easiest to position the animal in lateral recumbency and image the non-dependent kidney through the uppermost flank. The animal can then be turned over and the contralateral kidney imaged. A flank approach is less likely to suffer from interference caused by bowel gas. Alternatively, the animal can be positioned in dorsal recumbency and the transducer placed on the flank or ventral abdomen, especially in smaller animals.

To locate the kidneys, the transducer is placed just caudal to the costal arch, ventral to the epaxial muscles, and a sweep is made dorsoventrally. The left kidney is located caudal to the head of the spleen and lateral to the aorta. The right kidney lies more cranially and is often under the ribcage in dogs, in which case an intercostal approach may be required with the transducer placed over one of the last two intercostal spaces. If a sector transducer is being used a stand-off pad may be helpful to image the superficial structures in the near-field in cats and small dogs. The kidneys should be evaluated in at least two planes (transverse and sagittal) and also in the dorsal plane if possible.

In some animals the kidneys, particularly the left, are mobile and may be located in the mid or, rarely, caudal abdomen. If the kidney cannot be found despite searching it may be possible to locate it or confirm aplasia by identifying the renal arteries, which arise laterally from the aorta in the mid abdomen, via a dorsal window through the flank. The left renal artery lies slightly caudal to the right. The renal arteries are the first visible paired arteries caudal to the coeliac and cranial mesenteric arteries, which are single and arise from the ventral surface of the aorta. Occasionally there may be disease of the renal arteries or veins or evaluation may be required to monitor surgery (e.g. renal transplant) in which case examination of the hilar vessels is indicated. B-mode images may be unreliable for the detection of acute thrombi and Doppler ultrasonographic evaluation may be required.

Normal ultrasonographic appearance: There is considerable variation in the normal appearance of the kidneys. The kidneys should be similar in length and the renal cortices should be smooth and uniform with no focal bulges or depressions. In some animals a thin, hyperechoic capsule may be seen. Three distinct regions can normally be identified within the kidney: cortex, medulla and pelvis (Figure 10.4). The normal renal cortex has a fine uniform echotexture, and is always hyperechoic to the medulla. The cortical echogenicity can be compared to the adjacent spleen (left kidney) or liver (right kidney). The renal cortex is normally hypoechoic relative to spleen, and has similar echogenicity to the liver in dogs. The echogenicity of the cortex varies in cats according to reproductive status: pregnant female and neutered male cats often have relatively hyperechoic cortices. In normal cats the renal cortex may be isoechoic to spleen. Increased cortical echogenicity results in increased contrast between the medulla and cortex, which can be marked in some normal cats. Feline kidneys with hyperechoic cortices tend to be larger than less echogenic kidneys. This is due to fat deposition within the cortical tubular epithelium.

The medulla is very hypoechoic but may be slightly more echogenic adjacent to the pelvis. It is divided into pyramids, which may mimic cysts when seen obliquely. In some animals, especially cats, a thin, complete or incomplete hyperechoic band may be seen within the outer medulla, parallel to the corticomedullary boundary – the 'medullary rim sign' (Figure 10.4c). This sign is due to calcium deposits in the lumen of the proximal renal tubules and, in the absence of other ultrasonographic renal changes, is likely to be a normal finding. However, a medullary rim sign has also been reported in association with a number of diseases, including nephrocalcinosis, feline infectious peritonitis (FIP), acute tubular necrosis, ethylene glycol toxicity and chronic interstitial nephritis.

The renal sinus is composed of dense fibroadipose tissue. It appears very hyperechoic and may show faint distal acoustic shadowing. Interlobar arteries and veins lie in grooves within the pelvic diverticula and are seen as linear hypo-/anechoic structures running from the renal pelvis towards the cortex (Figure 10.4b). The arcuate arteries are surrounded by similar connective tissue and appear as small hyperechoic foci with anechoic centres adjacent to the corticomedullary junction. Shadowing or refraction of sound often results in acoustic shadowing from the diverticula and artery walls, which should not be mistaken for areas of mineralization (Figure 10.4d). Anechoic blood vessel lumens should not be mistaken for small renal cysts; differentiation is possible using colour-flow Doppler ultrasonography (Figure 10.5).

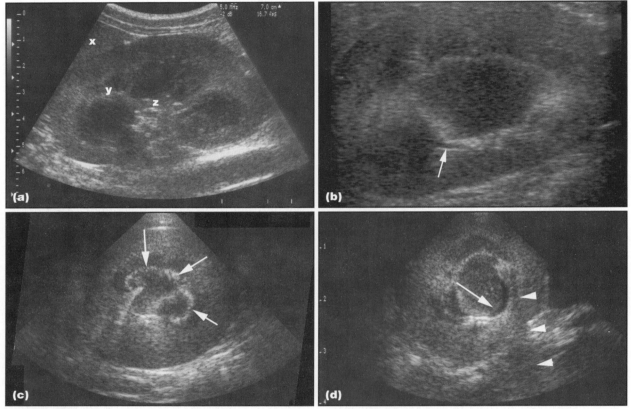

10.4 **(a)** Longitudinal (sagittal) ultrasonographic image of a normal dog's kidney. Note the clear differentiation between the renal cortex (x), medulla (y) and pelvis (z). **(b)** Longitudinal ultrasonographic image of a normal cat's kidney. An interlobar blood vessel can be seen running from the pelvis towards the cortex (arrowed). **(c)** Transverse ultrasonographic image of a normal cat's kidney. The thin echogenic line (arrowed) within the outer medulla parallel to the corticomedullary junction is known as the 'medullary rim sign'. **(d)** Transverse ultrasonographic image of a normal cat's kidney. There is mild dilation of the renal pelvis (arrowed), which is physiological in this case (pyelectasia) secondary to intravenous fluid therapy. There is distal acoustic shadowing (arrowheads) from a renal diverticulum, which should not be mistaken for an area of mineralization.

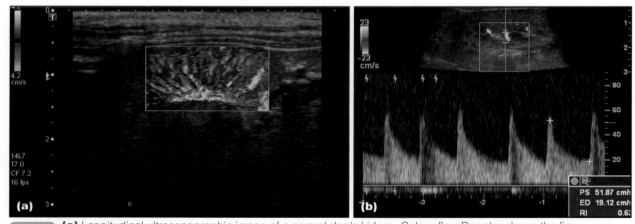

10.5 **(a)** Longitudinal ultrasonographic image of a normal dog's kidney. Colour-flow Doppler shows the fine branching pattern of the vascular supply to the renal cortex. This gives information on the spatial distribution of blood vessels and a global view of renal vascularity. **(b)** Pulsed-wave Doppler ultrasound examination of blood flow within an arcuate artery of a cat's kidney. The renal resistive index is measured from the Doppler waveform.

In the normal animal the lumen of the renal pelvis is either not seen or appears as a thin anechoic structure in the centre of the sinus. The lumen of the renal pelvis is Y- or V-shaped and is best seen on transverse and sagittal plane images. If visible it is recognized as a thin anechoic band adjacent to the renal crest and highlighted by the echogenic fat pad of the renal sinus. The renal pelvis may be mildly dilated up to 2 mm (pyelectasia) following diuresis, intravenous fluid therapy or in polyuric conditions. Physiological pyelectasia may be unilateral or bilateral.

Kidney length should be measured from a dorsal or sagittal plane image with the kidney maximized on the image. Kidney length in cats is reported to be 30–43 mm but may be up to 53 mm. The majority of feline kidneys are 33–43 mm in length and outside this range the kidney should be carefully examined for alteration in structure. There is a wide normal range of renal size in dogs and evaluation is usually subjective. A linear relationship exists between renal length (L) and body weight (Wt), given by the formula L(cm) = 0.07Wt + 4.75; diuresis may result in mild renal enlargement due to increased size of the medulla. Renal volume may be a more accurate method of evaluating renal size although it is rarely measured. It may be estimated using the formula for a prolate ellipsoid (V = L × W × D × 0.523; where V = volume, L = length, W = width and D = diameter). The kidneys should be similar in size, with the smaller kidney not comprising less than 37% of the total renal volume.

Ultrasonography yields more information about the internal architecture of the kidney, but diffuse changes are harder to recognize than focal lesions. Even diffuse alterations in echogenicity or architecture are non-specific findings and, in many cases, ultrasound-guided fine needle aspiration or ultrasound-guided biopsy is required (see Chapter 12). In the case of focal lesions, the minimum size at which they can be detected depends on the equipment used (especially the frequency of the transducer), the size of the patient and the experience of the operator. Fluid-filled structures are more easily seen than solid lesions, and with experience and high-quality equipment, cysts smaller than 2 mm diameter can be detected in cats undergoing ultrasonographic screening for polycystic kidney disease (PKD). Ultrasonography will normally be the first line of investigation for renal disease, where it is available.

Renal resistive index: Renal blood flow can be assessed using Doppler ultrasonography and in some cases can be used to identify renal disease in the absence of structural abnormalities. The most common measurement used is **renal resistive index (RRI)**. This is a unitless index and is obtained from a pulsed-wave Doppler measurement of the interlobar or arcuate arteries (see Figure 10.4b):

$$RRI = \frac{Peak\ systolic\ velocity - End\ diastolic\ velocity}{Peak\ systolic\ velocity}$$

Elevated RRI is reasonably specific (but not very sensitive) in indicating renal disease, although it does not indicate what the underlying disease process is. An elevated RRI is most commonly seen in acute and interstitial diseases and is due to a relative reduction in diastolic flow compared to systolic flow. An elevated RRI may also be seen in extrarenal diseases, such as hypoadrenocorticism, and in processes that alter renal haemodynamics.

Ureters

The proximal ureters and renal pelvis are imaged as for the kidneys. It may be difficult to differentiate ureters from hilar blood vessels and colour-flow Doppler may be beneficial, the renal pelvis and ureter showing no blood flow. The distal ureters may be imaged as for the bladder neck. If the entire ureter is dilated it may be possible to follow it from kidney to bladder, although bowel gas often interferes with the image.

The ureter has an anechoic lumen and a single echogenic wall layer, often showing peristalsis. The terminal ureter may occasionally be seen as a thin anechoic structure adjacent to the bladder neck and terminating at the ureteric papilla. A small blood vessel runs in the same region and should not be mistaken for a ureter. In many animals the ureteric papillae can be seen as small semicircular projections in the mucosa. Ureteric jets (episodic echogenic jets of urine arising from the papillae) may often be seen with modern equipment due to differences in specific gravity between urine in the bladder and ureter. A low dose of furosemide 15–20 minutes prior to the ultrasound examination may increase visibility of jets. Furosemide will, however, result in a poor IVU and is best avoided if an IVU is going to be performed soon after the ultrasound examination or if urinalysis is required. The jets may also be seen with colour-flow Doppler, although reduction of the pulse-repetition frequency and wall filter may be required. Other techniques suggested for visualizing ureteric jets include withholding water from the animal for a few hours then allowing it to drink just before examination, or emptying the bladder and infusing saline.

Renal masses – general radiographic principles

The origin of abdominal masses seen radiographically can often be deduced by evaluating the resultant displacement of other organs. The kidneys lie in the retroperitoneal space and so remain dorsal in the abdomen, displacing other organs ventrally and contralaterally. Right renal masses produce ventral displacement of the ascending colon and small intestines on the lateral radiograph and medial displacement of these structures on the VD view. Left renal masses result in ventral displacement of the descending colon and small intestines on the lateral view and medial displacement on the VD view (Figure 10.6).

Ultrasonography may be helpful to confirm the renal origin of the mass if recognizable kidney tissue remains. If the whole of the normal kidney architecture is destroyed, diagnosis of the origin of the mass is harder and relies on the inability to find a normal kidney and the recognition of other normal organs.

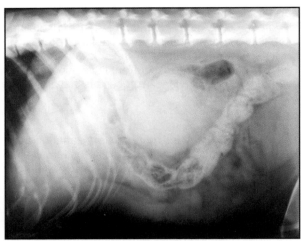

10.6 Abdominal mass due to a tumour of the left kidney in an 11-year-old Bearded Collie. The mass has caused ventral displacement of the descending colon and small intestines.

Congenital absence of a kidney

Bilateral absence is rapidly fatal and such cases are unlikely to require imaging. Unilateral absence is an occasional finding, the right kidney being more often aplastic. It is important to confirm the presence of a second kidney if a nephrectomy is to be performed.

Radiography

- Absence of one kidney with compensatory hypertrophy of the other; confirmed with IVU.
- Remaining kidney enlarged but shows normal architecture.
- Differential diagnosis – kidney present but small and non-functional.

Ultrasonography

- Changes as for radiography.
- Absence may be proved by showing that the renal artery and veins are not present.

Juvenile nephropathies and hypoplasia (familial in certain breeds)

Radiography

- Kidneys small and either smooth or irregular in outline.
- IVU confirms the size and shape but with delayed and poor opacification.
- Renal secondary hyperparathyroidism may result in demineralization of the skull and dystrophic calcification of soft tissue structures, such as gastric rugae and major blood vessels.

Ultrasonography

- Cannot be differentiated ultrasonographically from other chronic or end-stage renal diseases but young age and breed may be suggestive.
- Changes include reduced kidney size, irregular

cortical margins, reduced corticomedullary differentiation, dilated and distorted renal pelvis, parenchymal mineralization (hyperechoic with or without distal acoustic shadowing) and the formation of small cysts.
- Glomerulocystic kidney disease may cause increased renal size with normal shape and increased cortical echogenicity.

Acute nephritis

Radiography

- Usually normal.
- IVU may show poor or absent opacification depending on renal function.

Ultrasonography

- Non-specific changes; may be normal.
- Doppler changes may be suggestive (increased RRI) but are also non-specific.
- Increase in size and cortical echogenicity, mild pelvic dilation and perinephric effusion may all occur.
- Specific changes suggesting underlying cause may be seen in some cases:
  - Ureteric obstruction
  - Ethylene glycol poisoning initially causes an increase in echogenicity of the cortex (within 3.5 hours), closely followed by an increase in echogenicity of the medulla, resulting in reduced corticomedullary differentiation. The renal cortex becomes iso- to hyperechoic to the spleen by 5–8 hours and in some cases the medulla may become as echogenic as the cortex. Relatively less increase in echogenicity of the corticomedullary junction and central medulla may result in a hypoechoic band ('halo sign') at the corticomedullary junction. The presence of a halo sign is a poor prognostic indicator and associated with anuria
  - Leptospirosis – increased renal size with increased renal cortical echogenicity and often mildly dilated pelves and perinephric effusion. A broad, distinct, well marginated band of increased echogenicity in the medulla may be specific for leptospirosis.

Chronic nephritis (progressing to end-stage renal disease)

Radiography

- Small, irregular kidneys which may show patchy mineralization or calculi (Figure 10.7).
- IVU confirms size and shape but with poor opacification.
- Renal secondary hyperparathyroidism (see above) may be present but the radiographic manifestations are most marked when renal disease occurs in young animals as the skeleton is maturing.

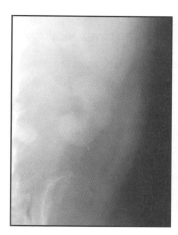

10.7 Close-up of the shrunken and irregular left kidney of a 2-year-old English Bull Terrier with chronic kidney disease due to renal dysplasia. An IVU has been performed and has increased the opacity of the kidney slightly, showing that there is still some residual renal function. The opacity medial to the kidney is an enlarged nipple.

Ultrasonography

- Non-specific changes and may be normal.
- Most commonly reduced (uncommonly increased) corticomedullary differentiation (Figure 10.8a).
- Reduced cortical thickness occasionally visible.
- Diffuse increase in cortical echogenicity, which may be uniform or patchy (Figure 10.8b).
- In later stages there is reduced renal size with irregularity of cortical margins.
- The renal pelvis is often mildly dilated due to polyuria.
- End-stage kidneys may be unrecognizable as kidneys but location aids correct identification (Figure 10.8c).

- Small areas of mineralization (hyperechoic foci with or without distal acoustic shadowing) often seen in advanced stages.

Pyelonephritis

Radiography

- The kidney may be normal, mildly enlarged or small and irregular, depending on the severity and chronicity of the condition.
- Renal calculi may be present concurrently (see below).
- IVU shows mild dilation of the renal pelvis and ureter and debris shows as filling defects.
- May be secondary to an ectopic ureter.
- Differential diagnosis – mild obstructive hydronephrosis.

Ultrasonography

- In the acute stages the kidneys may be normal or show only mild pelvic dilation and mild increase in kidney size.
- Chronic pyelonephritis usually results in dilation of the pelvis and proximal ureter (usually mild to moderate); a hyperechoic mucosal margin may be seen.
- Reduced corticomedullary differentiation, increased cortical echogenicity (which may be patchy) or hypoechoic foci.

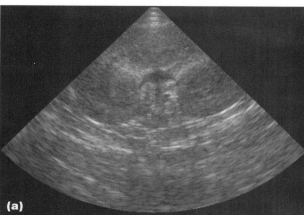
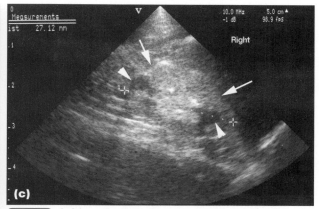
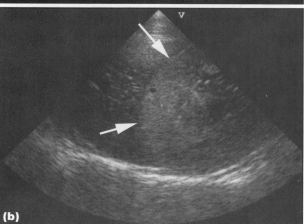

10.8 **(a)** Longitudinal ultrasonographic image of the kidney of a Shetland Sheepdog with chronic kidney disease of unknown aetiology. There is reduced corticomedullary differentiation and mild dilation of the renal pelvis. These are non-specific changes and are seen in many renal diseases. **(b)** There is increased echogenicity of the renal cortex (arrowed) in this Basset Hound. The echogenicity of the right kidney can be compared to the adjacent liver and in this case the renal cortex is of much greater echogenicity than the liver. This is a non-specific finding seen in many diseases, and can also be seen in some normal animals. **(c)** End-stage renal disease in a cat. The ultrasonographic findings of reduced size, irregular cortices (arrowed) and loss of normal architecture are typical findings of chronic, end-stage renal disease, irrespective of the cause. In this case there is also cyst formation within the poles of the kidney (arrowheads).

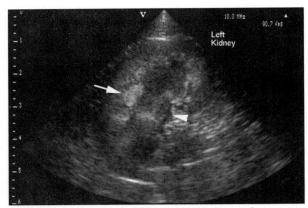

10.9 Longitudinal ultrasonographic image from a dog with pyelonephritis. There are patchy areas of increased echogenicity within the renal parenchyma (arrowed) and mild dilation of the renal pelvis (arrowhead). Diagnosis was based upon urinalysis and culture.

- Focal hyperechoic regions may be seen within the renal crest and medulla (Figure 10.9).
- The renal pelvis may have irregular margins and the contents may be echogenic or contain gas (resulting in reverberation artefact or 'dirty' shadowing) or calculi.

Renal calculi

Most renal calculi are struvite (associated with urinary tract infection) and are radiopaque. Calcium oxalate uroliths are also radiopaque; the opacity of xanthine, urate and cystine calculi is variable (often radiolucent) and depends on their size and exact composition.

Radiography

- Mineralized opacities seen in the renal pelvis on both lateral and VD views (must be differentiated from end-on nipples on the VD view) (Figure 10.10).
- Large calculi may extend into the diverticula or down the proximal ureter ('stag-horn calculi').
- Calculi may also be seen elsewhere in the urinary tract.
- IVU may obscure radiopaque calculi but show radiolucent calculi as filling defects in the pyelogram.

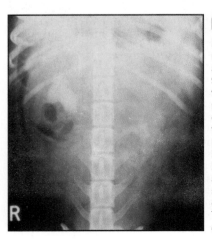

10.10

Plain ventrodorsal radiograph of the abdomen of a 9-year-old Beagle with large, radiopaque calculi present in the pelvis and proximal ureter of both kidneys. The left kidney is small and irregular, suggesting chronic nephritis. The right kidney outline is unclear.

- Pyelonephritis may be present too (see above).
- IVU will differentiate calculi from nephrocalcinosis (see below).
- IVU may flush calculi into the ureter or bladder via osmotic diuresis.

Ultrasonography

- Uroliths have a similar ultrasonographic appearance irrespective of composition.
- Uroliths are hyperechoic and show distinct, clean, distal acoustic shadowing. The presence and nature of the shadowing depends upon the frequency and focal zones of the transducer and the shape, size and surface characteristics of the calculus.
- It may be difficult to differentiate calculi from parenchymal mineralization. However, they are often associated with pelvic dilation. Calculi may be confidently diagnosed if they are surrounded by fluid or are clearly within the renal pelvis.
- Concurrent changes due to chronic kidney disease are often present.

Feline infectious peritonitis

Radiography

- The kidneys may be enlarged and irregular on plain radiographs.
- Uneven nephrogram on IVU.

Ultrasonography

- May result in enlarged and irregular kidneys.
- Focal, hyperechoic nodules or a diffuse increase in cortical echogenicity (Figure 10.11)
- There may be a thin rim of perinephric fluid/infiltrate.
- Changes in other organs may also be seen, e.g. nodules in enlarged liver or lymph nodes, the presence of ascites.
- Similar changes may be seen with multicentric neoplasia.

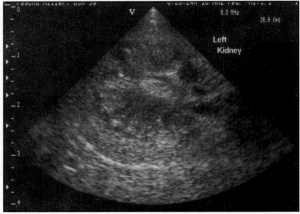

10.11 Transverse ultrasonographic image of the kidney of a Persian kitten with FIP. There is increased cortical and medullary echogenicity. The renal medulla is abnormal with a striated appearance.

Renal trauma

Renal trauma usually follows blunt abdominal injury, such as a road traffic accident (RTA).

Radiography

- Loss of serosal detail in the retroperitoneal or peritoneal spaces due to haemorrhage or urine leakage.
- Change in shape of the kidney (rupture) or smooth increase in size (subcapsular urine or blood accumulation).
- IVU may show absent nephrogram (renal artery transected), uneven nephrogram or contrast extravasation.

Ultrasonography

- Loss of normal architecture if the kidney is ruptured.
- Haematomas are variable in appearance – anechoic/hypoechoic lesions or complex masses.
- Complex appearance of retroperitoneal space or free fluid if retroperitoneal haemorrhage or renal/ureteric rupture has occurred.
- Subcapsular fluid (anechoic or echogenic) if perinephric haemorrhage has resulted.
- IVU is more sensitive than ultrasonography for detecting ureteric rupture.

Renal neoplasia

Malignant renal tumours occur more commonly than benign tumours, and a wide variety of histological types is seen. They may be primary or metastatic, and may occur unilaterally or bilaterally. The kidneys are often involved alone or with more widespread lymphoma, and in cats renal and nasal lymphoma may occur concurrently; renal lymphoma in cats must be differentiated from FIP. A syndrome of renal cystadenomas, dermatofibrosis and uterine leiomyomas occurs in the German Shepherd Dog, usually recognized clinically in middle age.

Radiography

- Plain films may show increased kidney size and irregular shape, although a normal appearance does not rule out neoplasia.
- Often only one pole is affected.
- Dystrophic mineralization may be present.
- An IVU will confirm the renal origin of the mass (Figure 10.12).
- Nephrogram appears patchy, with areas of poor opacification and contrast pooling.
- Pelvis distorted and may contain filling defects due to tumour tissue or haemorrhage.
- Proximal ureter often mildly dilated.
- IVU findings are non-specific and cannot differentiate benign from malignant disease.
- A search for metastases should be made, looking especially for lung nodules.

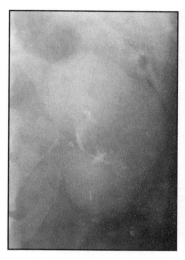

10.12 Close-up IVU of the left kidney of an 11-year-old crossbred dog with haematuria. Although the cranial and caudal poles of the kidney appear normal, the central part is swollen and fails to opacify normally with contrast medium. The renal pelvis is compressed and distorted. The appearance indicates a renal mass, most likely to be neoplastic. Following nephrectomy the histological diagnosis was adenocarcinoma.

Ultrasonography

- Usually expansile and cause enlargement of the kidney and loss of normal shape (lymphoma may cause diffuse enlargement with normal shape). In advanced stages the entire kidney may be obliterated.
- Primary renal tumours are usually complex or solid and cause focal disruption of the normal architecture (Figure 10.13). Histological type cannot be determined ultrasonographically and other masses, e.g. organizing abscess, granuloma, haematoma, may appear similar.
- Metastatic and multicentric tumours often appear as multifocal, hypoechoic nodules.
- Lymphoma – multiple hypoechoic nodules are most commonly seen but diffuse increase in cortical echogenicity also occurs, usually in combination with increased size and alterations in shape (Figure 10.14).
- Renal cystadenomas are usually bilateral with variable anechoic/hypoechoic cysts and nodules with or without a heterogenous solid component.

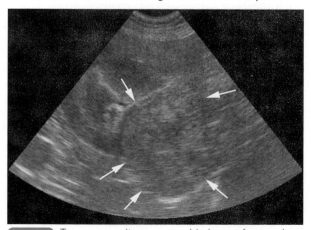

10.13 Transverse ultrasonographic image from a dog with a primary renal tumour confirmed by biopsy. There is a large parenchymal mass replacing renal tissue and extending into the perirenal tissues (arrowed). Primary renal tumours often occur within the poles of the kidneys and disrupt the normal parenchyma. (Metastatic tumours may be solitary or multiple.)

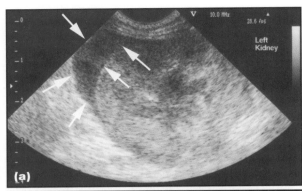

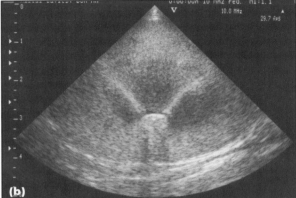

10.14 **(a)** Transverse ultrasonographic image of the kidney of a cat with renal lymphoma. The perirenal tissue is abnormal with a hypoechoic mass (arrowed) of tissue adjacent to the renal cortex. This may be perirenal or subcapsular and is not uncommon in cats with renal lymphoma. Similar subcapsular fluid/tissue accumulations may be seen with FIP, acute renal failure, trauma and some cases of perinephric effusions/infections. **(b)** Longitudinal ultrasonographic image of the kidney of a cat with renal lymphoma. The kidney is enlarged and shows increased cortical echogenicity and thickness. These are non-specific findings and diagnosis was based upon renal cytology.

Renal cysts, abscesses, granulomas and haematomas

Solitary renal cysts are an occasional incidental finding in dogs and cats. PKD is common in Persian cats and related breeds, such as the exotic shorthair, and ultrasonographic screening programmes exist. A genetic test is also now available for feline PKD (see Chapter 7). Renal abscesses and granulomas are unusual.

Radiography

- With small lesions the kidney appears normal on plain radiographs.
- With numerous or large lesions an increase in size and/or irregular shape occurs.
- Cysts may occasionally calcify.
- IVU shows spherical filling defects in the parenchyma, which may distort the pelvis.
- A radiograph taken 24 hours after an IVU may show contrast medium uptake into cysts and haematomas but not into abscesses or granulomas.

Ultrasonography

- Irrespective of aetiology, the appearance of cysts is similar; cysts are usually round, thin-walled, with anechoic contents and distal acoustic enhancement.
- It may be difficult to differentiate cysts from hypoechoic nodules; lack of distal enhancement, the presence of internal echoes, thick irregular walls or irregular shape warrant monitoring or further investigation.
- Cysts may be seen in association with other renal diseases, e.g. renal cystadenoma (see above).
- PKD usually affects both kidneys. One or more cysts ranging in size from 1–2 mm up to several centimetres become apparent from a few weeks or months of age but become more conspicuous with time as they enlarge. The cysts are usually spherical but may distort and become irregular in shape (Figure 10.15). They are thin-walled, anechoic and show distal acoustic enhancement; some may mineralize in which case hyperechoic regions with or without shadowing may be seen. Cysts are usually cortical or at the corticomedullary junction but if medullary are harder to see. In severely affected animals the kidneys are enlarged and irregular. PKD may be associated with cysts elsewhere in the abdomen, predominantly liver and pancreas.
- Renal abscesses have a variable appearance and may be seen in association with pyelonephritis or present as focal renal hypoechoic or complex masses (Figure 10.16) or as subcapsular fluid. Abscesses usually have a thick wall and contain moderately echogenic fluid. Solid, heterogenous nodules may be seen in some cases. As the appearance of focal renal lesions is non-specific, cytology is required for diagnosis.

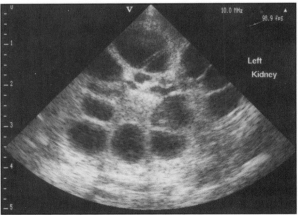

10.15 Longitudinal ultrasonographic image from a Persian cat with PKD. This cat is severely affected with numerous large, anechoic cysts and virtually no recognizable renal tissue. Some affected cats may have only one small cyst (<2 mm diameter), which may be easily overlooked. In some cases the cysts may appear hyperechoic with reverberation artefact due to mineralization of the cyst.

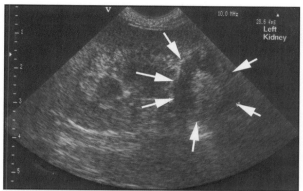

10.16 Longitudinal ultrasonographic image from a cat with a renal abscess due to mycobacterial infection. There is an irregular, thick-walled lesion within the caudal pole (arrowed) which was confirmed by aspiration. Differential diagnoses include neoplasia, granuloma and haematoma.

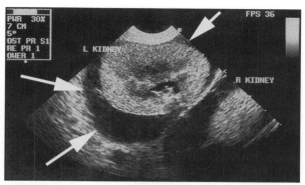

10.17 Longitudinal ultrasonographic image of bilateral perinephric pseudocysts in a cat. The kidneys are surrounded by anechoic fluid contained by a thin wall (arrowed). The kidneys are abnormal with mild pelvic dilation and loss of corticomedullary differentiation. (Courtesy of Cambridge University Veterinary School.)

- Renal haematoma – hypoechoic or complex mass possibly associated with perinephric haemorrhage.
- Differential diagnoses for thick-walled, cavitary lesions include abscess, granuloma, haematoma and neoplasia.

Perinephric (perirenal) pseudocysts

Accumulation of modified transudate associated with renal impairment (possibly secondary to effects on lymphatic drainage) is seen most often in older, male cats and is usually bilateral. Uriniferous pseudocysts or urinomas occur when urine leaks from a kidney or ureter and becomes encapsulated in fibrous tissue. The leak is usually due to trauma, iatrogenic damage or rupture secondary to urolithiasis. This condition is more likely to be unilateral, and can resolve after appropriate treatment.

Radiography

- Plain radiographs show smooth enlargement of the 'kidney' shadow, which may be massive.
- IVU is required to show the kidneys themselves and can therefore help to suggest the cause.

Ultrasonography

- Circumscribed fluid collection (often very large) surrounding the affected kidney (Figure 10.17).
- The fluid is usually anechoic but may be hypoechoic.
- Pseudocysts are usually unichambered with a thin hyperechoic capsule surrounding the fluid and attaching to the renal hilus. Less commonly the pseudocyst is septated with attachments to the kidney surface.
- Rarely the pseudocyst may arise from one pole of the kidney rather than surrounding the whole kidney.
- The kidney is usually abnormal in appearance reflecting concurrent chronic kidney disease.
- Differential diagnoses include perinephric

abscess and haematoma, though these often produce more echogenic perinephric fluid. Exudation/infiltrate seen with FIP, lymphoma (see Figure 10.14a) and acute renal failure may result in very small volumes of subcapsular/perinephric fluid and should not be mistaken for the large fluid collections seen with perinephric pseudocyst or urinoma.

Hydronephrosis

Hydronephrosis is the dilation of the renal pelvis and diverticula, and often the ureter too, due to chronic obstruction or infection. It is commonly seen with ectopic ureters. The radiographic and ultrasonographic appearance depends on the severity of the condition.

Radiography

- Kidney size may be normal, reduced (in cases of chronic, mild obstruction) or show varying degrees of enlargement.
- The outline may be rounded, with loss of the hilar notch.
- Mild or moderate hydronephrosis is seen as rounding and increase in size of the pelvis and diverticula on IVU; the diverticula may be lost.
- In severe cases, most of the kidney fails to opacify on IVU and only a thin rim of functioning tissue is seen (Figure 10.18a).
- A 24-hour radiograph may show contrast medium uptake within the mass due to slow excretion.

Ultrasonography

- Dilation of the renal pelvis results in an anechoic band within the centre of the renal sinus and often concurrent dilation of the proximal ureter (Figure 10.18b) (easiest to see in transverse plane images).
- As the hydronephrosis becomes more severe there is widening of the diverticula and cortical atrophy, ultimately ending in a septated, cystic appearance to the kidney.

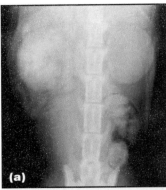

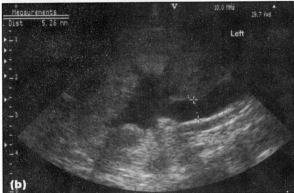

10.18 **(a)** IVU in a 4-year-old domestic shorthaired cat with a previous history of RTA, showing severe hydronephrosis of the left kidney. Only a thin rim of functioning tissue around the periphery of the kidney has opacified, suggesting that this surrounds a large collection of fluid. **(b)** Longitudinal ultrasonographic image from a Jack Russell Terrier with hydronephrosis and hydroureter secondary to an ectopic ureter. The renal pelvis and proximal ureter and renal diverticula are dilated.

- A careful examination for evidence of any underlying obstruction should be made.
- The dilated ureter should be followed if possible from kidney to trigone. Most cases of obstruction occur at the bladder neck.
- Masses or other lesions involving the ureters may be seen in the retroperitoneal tissues.

Nephrocalcinosis

Nephrocalcinosis has various causes, including chronic kidney disease, ethylene glycol poisoning, hyperadreno-corticism, hypercalcaemia (various aetiologies) and hypervitaminosis D. Ultrasonography is more sensitive for detection of calcification than radiography.

Radiography

- Patches and lines of parenchymal mineralization.
- If very advanced, a radiopaque line may seen along or near to the corticomedullary junction.
- Depending on the cause, the kidney may also be small and irregular.
- Differential diagnosis – calculi or mineralization of a tumour; superimposed ingesta or end-on nipple.

Ultrasonography

- Diffuse increase in cortical echogenicity and a hyperechoic band at corticomedullary junction; shadowing variably present.
- Should not be confused with the medullary rim sign seen in some normal animals.
- Parenchymal mineralization (hyperechoic with distal acoustic shadowing) is seen in many chronic or end-stage renal diseases and is not specific for hypercalcaemia.

Renal infarcts

Renal infarcts may be single or multiple. Imaging is also helpful in a search for a source for the infarcts, such as endocarditis.

Radiography

- Usually nothing on plain radiographs, although large, chronic infarcts may result in an indented area to the outline.
- Wedge-shaped areas of non-opacification of the nephrogram on IVU.

Ultrasonography

- May be an incidental finding in older animals, more common in dogs.
- Infarcts are wedge-shaped with apex towards the medulla and are most obvious in the cortex (Figure 10.19).
- Acute infarcts may be hypoechoic and may be seen within 24 hours.
- Subacute or chronic infarcts are usually hyperechoic.
- Chronic infarcts result in a depression in the surface of the kidney.

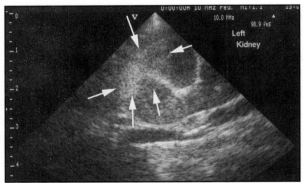

10.19 Longitudinal ultrasonographic image of the cranial pole of a cat's kidney, showing an acute renal infarct (arrowed), secondary to hypertrophic cardiomyopathy. Small chronic renal infarcts are commonly seen in older animals.

Idiopathic renal haemorrhage

A rare condition, often with no findings on radiography or ultrasonography other than filling defects in the pyelogram due to blood clots, although this may be helpful to identify the affected side (see Chapter 1). The main role of imaging is to rule out structural disease.

Amyloidosis

Radiography

- Unpredictable change in size or shape of the kidney.

Ultrasonography

- In cats usually reduced renal size and increased medullary echogenicity.
- In dogs affected kidneys may be small, normal or increased in size with increased cortical echogenicity and often irregularity of the renal cortical margins.
- Other signs associated with amyloidosis may be seen, e.g. ascites, hepatic changes, thrombus formation. Abdominal ultrasonography is useful in identifying the cause of ascites.

Ureteric ectopia

Ectopic ureters are usually congenital, and may be unilateral or bilateral. Ectopia may also be acquired due to accidental surgical ligation of a ureter at ovariohysterectomy. Female animals are more likely to show clinical signs than males. Certain dog breeds show an increased incidence (e.g. Golden Retriever); ectopic ureters are unusual in cats. Ectopic ureters usually terminate in the urethra or vagina.

Radiography

- Plain radiographs are usually normal (bladder may be small if both ureters are ectopic) although a severely dilated ureter may be visible.
- IVU with pneumocystogram shows abnormal terminations of one or both ureters (Figure 10.20a).
- Due to peristalsis, several radiographs may be required to confirm where the ureters terminate; in dogs they may appear to end with the normal terminal hook but then turn again to extend further caudally along the wall of the bladder; in cats the bladder is usually bypassed.
- Ectopic ureters are usually dilated due to strictures at their openings or to ascending infection from stagnant urine.
- Absence of contrast medium accumulation in the bladder suggests bilateral ectopia, but presence of contrast medium does not preclude a bilateral condition as urine can leak forwards into the bladder.
- Retrograde (vagino)urethrography can also be used to show the ureter endings in some cases, and is preferred to IVU by some people.
- Secondary changes due to hydronephrosis, hydroureter or pyelonephritis may be seen in severe cases, and are circumstantial evidence for ectopia even if the ureter endings are not clearly seen.

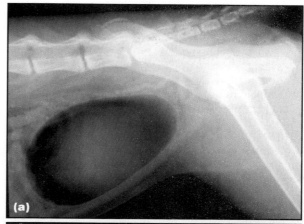
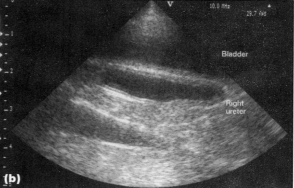

10.20 **(a)** Pneumocystogram and IVU in a 10-month-old male domestic shorthaired cat with urinary incontinence. The ureters can be seen extending caudal to the bladder neck and terminating in the region of the urethra. One of the ureters is markedly dilated. The diagnosis is bilateral ectopia. **(b)** Longitudinal ultrasonographic image of the bladder and right ureter. There is dilation of the ureter due to ectopia. Dilated ureters can be differentiated from fluid-filled small intestines by the thinner walls and lack of distinct layering of the ureter when compared with small intestine. In many cases ureters show slow peristalsis, which differentiates them from blood vessels. If the dilated ureter can be followed to the kidney or bladder this allows correct identification.

Ultrasonography

- Ectopic ureters can often be identified ultrasonographically.
- The terminal ureters are most easily visualized from a transverse image at the level of the bladder neck.
- Concurrent hydroureter and hydronephrosis are often present (see Figure 10.18b).
- It may be possible to follow the dilated ureter from the kidney to its termination. If the ureter can be seen to terminate in an abnormal location (e.g. urethra or vagina) a definitive diagnosis of ectopia can be made. In some cases the ureter can be seen to extend caudal to the trigone but the termination may not be visible (Figure 10.20b).
- Visualization of a ureteric jet arising from a normally-positioned papilla effectively rules out

an ectopic ureter although theoretically a double opening ureter is possible. However, turbulence at the bladder neck may be seen with ectopic ureters and should not be mistaken for a normal ureteric jet.
- If the bladder neck is intrapelvic it may not be possible to visualize the ureteric openings or jets, making the diagnosis of ectopia impossible.

Ureterocele

Ureterocele is a congenital, localized ureteric dilation, usually within the bladder wall. It may be associated with an ectopic ureter.

Radiography

- Plain radiographs are unremarkable.
- Cystography may show a filling defect arising from the bladder wall in the trigone area.
- IVU shows focal ureteric dilation.
- Secondary hydronephrosis may occur if the ureter becomes obstructed.

Ultrasonography

- Focal, cystic dilation of the ureter is present, which may be within the bladder or adjacent to the bladder neck.
- Other signs of ureteric ectopia, if present.

Hydroureter

Ureteric dilation due to obstruction (e.g. calculus, bladder neck tumour) or ascending infection.

Radiography

- If the dilation is severe, a tubular, soft-tissue-opacity viscus may be seen on plain radiographs.
- Usually an IVU is required, and shows the ureter to be dilated, tortuous and lacking in peristaltic breaks.
- Distension of the renal pelvis is also seen (hydronephrosis) with or without an enlarged or shrunken kidney.
- Depending on the cause, other radiographic features may also be seen.

Ultrasonography

- If possible the ureter should be followed from the kidney to the bladder to determine whether an obstructive lesion is present.
- Dilated ureters are thin-walled, tubular structures usually with anechoic luminal contents (see Figure 10.20b).
- It may be possible to follow a dilated ureter from the kidney to the bladder, which allows correct identification.
- Doppler examination of the kidneys may be helpful in some cases in differentiating obstructed from unobstructed ureters, but has low sensitivity and specificity (increased RRI).
- May be mistaken for other tubular structures, but

can be differentiated from small intestines by lack of layering of the ureteric wall, and from the uterus and blood vessels by the presence of peristalsis in the ureter.
- Obstruction occurs most commonly at the trigone, e.g. bladder neck neoplasia.

Ureteric calculi

Calculi may also be present in the kidneys (where ureteric calculi originate) and bladder.

Radiography

- Small, mineralized opacities are seen in the region of a ureter, although they cannot be distinguished from ingesta on plain radiographs (except if present on more than one occasion).
- IVU confirms their ureteric location and may show hydroureter and hydronephrosis proximally.
- Radiolucent calculi are only seen on IVU.
- The osmotic effect of the IVU may flush calculi into the bladder.
- Following calculus impaction, stricture may develop (see below).

Ultrasonography

- Ureteric calculi are often associated with dilation of the ureter and the intraluminal location is usually obvious, although bowel gas may interfere with assessment.
- Calculi are seen as hyperechoic structures within the lumen of the ureter causing acoustic shadowing or reverberation artefacts (Figure 10.21).

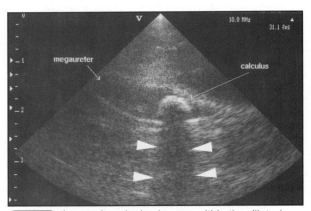

10.21 A ureteric calculus is seen within the dilated ureter on ultrasonography. Most calculi are hyperechoic and show distal acoustic shadowing (arrowheads) as in this case. Calculus type cannot be determined ultrasonographically.

Ureteric rupture

Ureteric rupture can occur following trauma, e.g. RTA, or be iatrogenic at laparotomy.

Radiography

- There is increased opacity in the retroperitoneal and possibly peritoneal spaces, obscuring the kidneys; this may not be apparent until several days after trauma (differential diagnosis – retroperitoneal haemorrhage).

- IVU shows leakage of contrast medium into the retroperitoneal space, although the site of leakage may be unclear.
- Distal ureter may fail to opacify.
- Ureter is dilated proximal to the rupture; subsequently may form a stricture.
- Para-ureteral urinoma may arise, producing a retroperitoneal mass.

Ultrasonography

- Ultrasonography is less sensitive than contrast radiography for demonstrating ureteric rupture.
- Accumulations of fluid (urine) within the retroperitoneal space.
- Urinomas appear as cystic masses, being anechoic/very hypoechoic, usually sharply demarcated, with or without a thin septa.
- Related changes in the kidneys or retroperitoneal space may be seen, e.g. hydronephrosis.

Ureteric stricture (post trauma, post calculus, neoplasia, iatrogenic)

Radiography

- Severe or chronic stricture may produce hydronephrosis or an end-stage kidney recognizable on plain radiographs.
- A dilated, fluid-opacity ureter may also be seen proximal to the stricture if the secondary ureteric dilation is marked.
- IVU will confirm these findings, but serial radiographs or fluoroscopy with image intensification may be needed to differentiate a stricture from a peristaltic contraction.
- The site of the stricture may be smooth or irregular, the latter suggesting primary ureteric pathology.
- Depending on the cause, other radiographic findings may also be present.

Ultrasonography

- Dilation of ureter proximal to the stricture is usually seen.
- Identification of the cause of stricture is often difficult; a mass or calculus at the site of the stricture may be seen in some cases.

Bladder

Radiography

Plain radiographs
The most helpful projection for demonstrating the bladder is the lateral view, with the hindlegs pulled as far caudally as possible to prevent superimposition of the limb musculature. The VD view may give extra information about the position of the bladder but the bladder

neck is obscured by the spine and sacrum. The presence of large amounts of faeces may impair interpretation and an enema may be required, especially if contrast studies are planned.

Contrast studies
Contrast studies of the bladder (cystograms) are used to demonstrate its integrity and position when these are not clear from the plain radiographs. Indications for cystography include haematuria, dysuria, stranguria and pollakiuria, as well as investigation of abdominal masses, hernia contents and suspected bladder trauma. More importantly, they are used to show the thickness of the bladder wall, changes to the mucosal surface and the presence of intraluminal masses, calculi or other debris. Although catheterization of the bladder is possible in the conscious animal, sedation or anaesthesia is recommended for cystography in order to allow non-manual restraint during the exposure.

Pneumocystography:

1. Catheterize and completely drain the bladder (measure the amount of urine removed, as an indication of the minimum amount of air that can be safely injected).
2. Inject air slowly using a syringe and three-way tap.
3. Palpate the abdomen periodically: stop when the bladder becomes slightly turgid or if back-pressure to injection is felt (check for rebound on the syringe).
4. Amount of air required varies: about 20 ml for a cat and 250 ml for a large dog. It varies greatly depending on body size and the presence of any pathology.

Rupture of the bladder due to over-inflation is possible, especially in male animals, and it is safer to have to repeat an exposure, following addition of further air, than to over-inflate. Both under- and over-inflation can result in false diagnoses.

In animals with severe haematuria or recent trauma, air embolus is a theoretical risk and the use of carbon dioxide or nitrous oxide, rather than room air, has been recommended by some authorities.

Pneumocystography is valuable for identifying the bladder and showing its position and wall thickness but it gives little information about the mucosal surface. In addition, small tears may be overlooked since escaping air mimics intestinal gas, and small calculi and other luminal contents may be over-exposed.

Positive-contrast cystography: This is performed as above but using water-soluble, iodine-containing contrast medium (150–200 mg iodine/ml); more concentrated solutions can be diluted with normal saline. Undiluted solutions should be avoided since their high osmolarity may irritate the mucosa.

Positive-contrast cystography is more expensive than pneumocystography and is usually reserved for suspected cases of bladder rupture; otherwise it offers little advantage over pneumocystography.

Double-contrast cystography:

1. After draining the bladder instil a small amount of dilute (150–200 mg/ml iodine) water-soluble contrast medium, 0.5–10 ml, depending on the size of the animal.
2. Roll the patient and massage the bladder area to ensure even distribution of contrast medium over the mucosa.
3. Inject air slowly using a syringe and a three-way tap as for a pneumocystogram.
4. Obtain lateral, VD and oblique radiographs.

A double-contrast study produces optimal mucosal detail. Positive contrast medium adheres to inflamed or ulcerated areas and residual contrast medium forms a useful central 'puddle' in the dependent part of the bladder, within which calculi and debris are visible as radiolucent filling defects.

If the bladder cannot be catheterized, a positive-contrast cystogram can be produced by performing an IVU, since excreted contrast medium will mix with urine already present in the bladder. However, it is not possible to control the degree of bladder distension using this method and it should be used only as a last resort.

Pitfalls in cystography:

- Failure to perform an enema may result in masking of lesions by superimposed faeces.
- With incomplete urine drainage, air superimposed over the residual urine puddle may mimic bladder wall thickening.
- Rapid injection of air into residual urine or positive contrast medium creates air bubbles (Figure 10.22).
- Insufficient bladder distension creates a false appearance of bladder wall thickening, or allows indentation of its outline by adjacent organs.
- Overdistension may mask subtle wall thickening.
- Too much positive contrast medium may 'drown' small luminal structures, such as calculi; they may be over-exposed on pneumocystography.

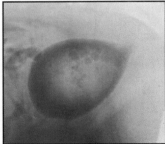

10.22 Double-contrast cystogram in a Labrador with haematuria. Within the central contrast medium puddle are several irregular filling defects, caused by blood clots. Caudodorsally, at the edge of the contrast medium puddle, is a number of discrete, round, coalescing radiolucencies, which represent air bubbles. Their location at the edge of the contrast medium puddle helps to differentiate them from true filling defects such as calculi.

- Insufficient number of projections may fail to skyline lesions.
- Overlying bowel gas may be mistaken for a luminal filling defect.

Normal radiographic appearance

The bladder is seen on most plain radiographs as a pear-shaped, homogenous, soft tissue structure in the caudal abdomen, ventral to the colon, although its position varies with its size. It is outlined by fat in the mesentery and bladder ligaments. The bladder neck can be seen tapering caudally towards the pelvic inlet. In the cat, the bladder lies more cranially than in the dog and the bladder neck is often very long and narrow or even not visible. If the bladder is completely empty, it may be intrapelvic and hard to detect, particularly if the hindlegs have been insufficiently retracted. On the VD radiograph, the bladder is sometimes seen lying obliquely with its apex to one side of the abdomen, especially if the animal has previously been lying on its side.

Following pneumocystography or double-contrast cystography, the bladder wall can be seen as a thin, uniform, soft tissue structure, 1–2 mm wide. Under-inflation of the bladder may give rise to the erroneous appearance of bladder wall thickening but this can be recognized by a flaccid appearance to its outline, which is indented by adjacent organs. Bladder wall thickness is harder to assess on positive-contrast cystography. Using double-contrast cystography, the mucosal surface is highlighted by a faint covering of contrast medium while the rest pools under gravity in the centre of the bladder shadow. Some vesicoureteral reflux is occasionally seen.

Radiological interpretation

The bladder should be assessed radiographically for the following features:

- Presence of a bladder shadow
- Integrity
- Position and relationship with other organs
- Size
- Shape
- Radiopacity
- Internal architecture and luminal contents (contrast studies).

Ultrasonography

A linear transducer is preferred for the bladder as near-field artefacts seen with sector transducers often interfere with visualization of the near wall, although a sector transducer can be used with a stand-off pad to overcome this problem (Figure 10.23). A sector transducer may be required to evaluate the prostate and bladder neck in animals with an intrapelvic bladder.

Careful adjustment of the machine settings is required for bladder examination to avoid artefacts, which are common. The power and gain should not be too high and the time-gain compensation set to minimize side-lobe artefacts and spurious low-level echoes within the urine (Figure 10.24).

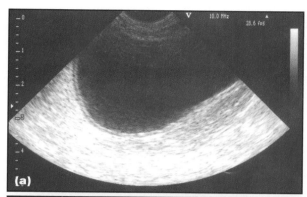

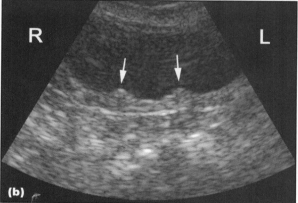

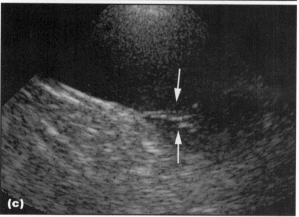

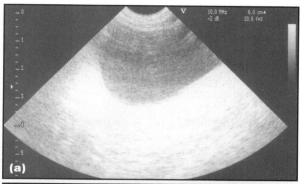

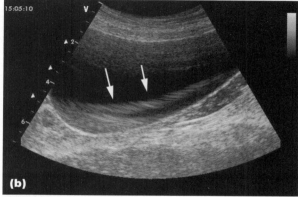

10.24 **(a)** Ultrasound image of the bladder with inappropriate machine settings. To obtain diagnostic images of the urinary tract it is important to pay attention to the ultrasound controls. Artefacts within the bladder are commonly seen due to poor technique. In this case the gain is too high, resulting in spurious echoes within the bladder and the urine appearing echogenic. This should not be mistaken for an abnormality. This is the same dog as Figure 10.23(a). **(b)** Ultrasound image of the bladder with a grating-lobe artefact (arrowed). Grating and side-lobe artefacts are common in the bladder and may be mistaken for sediment. They can be differentiated from sediment by the curved appearance of the artefact and by repositioning the animal (sediment should move). Altering the gain may also reduce the artefact.

10.23 **(a)** Longitudinal ultrasonographic image of the normal canine bladder. The image was obtained with a sector transducer, which results in poor near-field definition and prevents clear evaluation of the bladder wall nearest to the transducer (top of image). To assess this area a stand-off pad or linear transducer should be used. The normal bladder wall is uniform in thickness with a three-layered appearance. Wall thickness is dependent upon the degree of distension of the bladder. **(b)** Transverse ultrasonographic image of the normal canine bladder at the level of the trigone. The two focal wall thickenings (arrowed) are normal ureteric papillae and represent the vesiculoureteric junctions. In many animals the left ureteric papilla is slightly caudal to the right. If the bladder neck is intrapelvic, the ureteric papillae may not be visible. **(c)** Ureteric jets of urine (arrowed) may be seen in many normal animals on ultrasonography. Visualization of the jet is thought to be due to differences in specific gravity of the urine within the bladder and ureter. Visibility and frequency of ureteric jets may be increased by administering a low dose of diuretic to the animal. Echogenic urine can be seen entering from the bladder at level of the ureteric papillae.

In most animals the bladder can be examined without clipping the ventral body wall. It can be imaged from a ventral or lateral approach and is easiest to evaluate if it is reasonably full. If the bladder is completely empty it can be located by angling the transducer caudally into the pelvic canal. Normally it lies immediately cranial to the pubis and ventral to the colon in the caudoventral abdomen. It may be helpful to examine the bladder both with the animal standing and in recumbency to differentiate movable bladder calculi from gas or mineralization within the wall. The bladder should be evaluated in both sagittal and transverse planes. Careful attention should paid to the cranioventral bladder wall, a common site of disease, which may be overlooked in the near-field.

The bladder must be differentiated from other cystic structures in the caudal abdomen, e.g. paraprostatic cysts. In some cases this may be difficult and it may be helpful to catheterize the bladder and possibly to inject agitated saline. In cases of bladder retroflexion and intrapelvic displacement it may be possible to image the malpositioned bladder through a caudal pelvic window with the transducer placed lateral to the anus and directed cranially into the pelvic canal.

In animals with cystitis the bladder is often empty due to frequent urination. In these cases distension of the bladder with saline may be required for full examination. Care should be taken not to introduce air bubbles, which may mimic calculi.

Normal ultrasonographic appearance

The bladder wall has a three-layered appearance with hyperechoic serosa and mucosa sandwiching a hypoechoic muscularis. The layering is less distinct than in the small intestine and is not usually seen if the bladder is empty or in regions of the bladder wall not perpendicular to the ultrasound beam. When the bladder is almost empty the mucosa has a wrinkled appearance and the wall has a uniform hypoechoic appearance, which should not be over-interpreted as pathology. The bladder wall should be fairly even in thickness but is slightly thinner caudoventrally. Its thickness is variable and dependent upon body weight and degree of bladder distension:

- In dogs the bladder wall measures 1–1.5 mm when moderately distended and 2–3 mm when nearly empty
- In cats the bladder wall normally measures 1.3–1.7 mm.

The ureteric papillae are seen with high-frequency transducers in most animals, and appear as two small, convex projections protruding from the mucosa of the dorsal bladder wall (see Figure 10.23b). Jets of echogenic urine ('ureteric jets') may be seen originating from the ureteric papillae in some normal animals (see Figure 10.23c).

The urine should be anechoic, although in normal cats with concentrated urine it is not uncommon to see small, mobile, non-shadowing, hyperechoic foci floating within the urine. These should not be mistaken for sediment, which settles in the dependent portion of the bladder. Artefacts are commonly seen in the bladder and careful technique is needed. Side-lobe and grating-lobe artefacts result in spurious echoes within the lumen that mimic sediment (see Figure 10.24b). They can be differentiated from true sediment as side-lobe artefacts have a curved interface and do not re-suspend with agitation of the bladder. Reverberations and near-field artefact result in loss of visibility of the near bladder wall.

The colon lies dorsal to the bladder. It has a curved hyperechoic interface with reverberation or shadowing due to gas, and should not be mistaken for a bladder calculus. Repositioning the animal, e.g. so that it is standing, will cause calculi to move to the dependent portion of the lumen which differentiates them from colonic gas or bladder wall mineralization.

Bladder volume may be estimated ultrasonographically and has a reasonable correlation with measurement of urine volume after bladder catheterization (Atalan *et al.*, 1999). Bladder volume measurement is most accurate with the animal in dorsal recumbency and using the formula:

Bladder volume (ml) = $0.625 \times L \times W \times (DL + DT)/2$

where L is length in sagittal plane, W is width in transverse plane, and DL and DT are depth measurements from sagittal and transverse images, respectively. This may be used to measure residual urine volume, which may be increased in neurogenic or dysuric conditions, and may also be used to monitor response to treatment. Mean normal residual urine volume has been reported as 0.2–0.4 ml/kg in dogs.

Bladder diverticula

Radiography

- Congenital urachal diverticula are visible on cystography as outpouchings of the lumen into the cranioventral bladder wall.
- Chronic cystitis is often a sequel (see below).
- Traumatic diverticula are due to bulging of mucosa through torn bladder wall muscle, seen as change in bladder shape on plain radiographs. Blood clots may be present.

Ultrasonography

- Small outpouching, most commonly at the apex.
- Often mild thickening of bladder wall adjacent to the diverticulum.
- Acquired diverticula may occur at any location.

Patent pervious urachus

This is rare in small animals; it is more common in large animals.

Radiography

- Plain radiographs show an elongated bladder shadow extending towards the umbilicus.
- Cystography confirms communication between bladder and umbilicus.

Ultrasonography

- Urachal cyst (thin-walled cyst attached to the serosa) or a visible communication between umbilicus and bladder is seen.

Cystitis

Radiography

- Acute cystitis produces no radiographic changes, unless blood clots are present and seen on cystography.
- Chronic cystitis rarely produces changes on plain radiographs, although the bladder may be small due to pollakiuria or poor distensibility.
- Double-contrast cystography is the technique of choice and shows diffuse bladder wall thickening, especially cranioventrally (where irritant material collects when the animal is upright) (Figure 10.25a). This is unlike tumours, which occur most

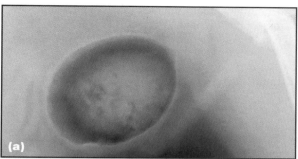

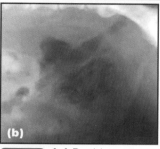

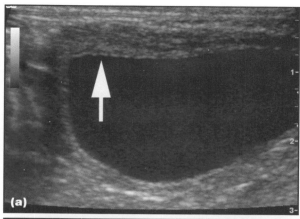

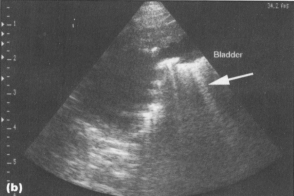

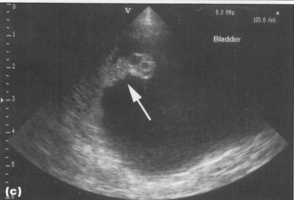

10.25 **(a)** Double-contrast cystogram in a 7-year-old domestic shorthaired cat with haematuria, pollakiuria and urinary tenesmus. The bladder wall is thickened and irregular, especially along its cranioventral margin, with adherence of positive contrast medium indicating mucosal inflammation. Filling defects in the central contrast medium puddle are likely to be due to blood clots and other luminal debris. **(b)** Caudal abdominal radiograph of a 15-year-old diabetic collie bitch who was showing signs of cystitis. Numerous streaks of gas are visible in the region of the bladder, and a normal bladder outline is not evident. Subsequent pneumocystography showed that the gas was largely trapped in the bladder wall.

frequently in the region of the bladder neck.
- Contrast medium adheres to inflamed and ulcerated areas, especially at the apex; urachal diverticula are occasionally seen and may be primary or secondary.
- Debris may be visible as filling defects within the contrast medium puddle.
- Mucosal lifting may be seen in cats with cystitis as air or positive contrast medium dissects into the bladder wall.
- Polypoid cystitis produces severe, diffuse changes which can only be differentiated from diffuse neoplasia by biopsy.
- Differential diagnosis includes bladder wall hypertrophy secondary to chronic outflow obstruction, although this is more diffuse.
- Emphysematous cystitis (usually associated with diabetes mellitus) produces streaks and patches of gas which, on cystography, are shown to be within the bladder wall rather than luminal (Figure 10.25b).

Ultrasonography

- May be normal in acute cases.
- Radiography is more sensitive than ultrasonography for identifying mild wall thickening.
- Most commonly seen abnormality is thickening of cranioventral wall gradually merging with normal wall (Figure 10.26a).

10.26 **(a)** Longitudinal ultrasonographic image of the bladder of a dog with chronic cystitis. The cranioventral aspect of the bladder wall is thickened (arrowed) but gradually resumes a normal thickness caudally (on the right of the image). In some cases the mucosa may be irregular and there may be alteration in echogenicity of the wall. If the bladder is poorly distended the wall will appear thicker and this can mimic the changes seen with cystitis. **(b)** Emphysematous cystitis in a dog. Gas within the bladder wall is seen ultrasonographically as hyperechoic areas with reverberation artefact (arrowed). Radiographs confirmed the presence of gas within the bladder wall. Differential diagnosis would include a mineralized bladder wall or mass (but not usually with reverberation artefact). Gas within the wall will not move with position of the animal, which helps differentiate it from calculi or gas within the bladder lumen. **(c)** Longitudinal ultrasonographic image of the bladder of a dog with polypoid cystitis. Polyps (arrowed) most commonly arise from the cranial aspect of the bladder as in this case. They usually have a thin base but some have a larger base, resembling a bladder tumour. Biopsy is required to rule out neoplasia.

- Increased echogenicity of mucosal layer and blurring of layering are seen.
- Wall may appear hypoechoic if oedematous.
- In severe cases may see fibrosis or mineralization of wall which appears hyperechoic with or without shadowing.
- Sediment in lumen; blood clots are seen in severe cases.
- Emphysematous cystitis results in hyperechoic foci with reverberation artefacts; these may be difficult to differentiate from mineralization in some cases. There may be concurrent gas within the lumen which rises to the non-dependent portion (whilst sediment settles dependently) (Figure 10.26b).
- Polypoid cystitis is usually seen as thin-necked masses protruding on a stalk into the lumen; less commonly it appears as broad-based masses resembling neoplasia. Biopsy is required to confirm polypoid cystitis and exclude neoplasia (Figure 10.26c).

Bladder calculi

Radiography

- Struvite, oxalate and carbonate calculi are radiopaque and visible on plain radiographs unless very small.
- On a recumbent radiograph they will appear in the centre of the bladder shadow, since this area is lowest.
- Double-contrast cystography is the technique of choice – all types of calculi appear as well defined filling defects in the centre of the contrast medium puddle, whereas air bubbles collect around the periphery of the contrast medium puddle and usually coalesce (Figure 10.27).

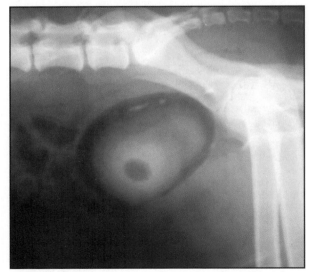

10.27 Double-contrast cystogram performed in a 3-year-old male Cocker Spaniel. A rounded filling defect is seen in the centre of the contrast medium puddle and is due to a large calculus. The calculus was of similar radiopacity to urine and was hard to see on plain radiographs. Compare with the air bubbles shown in Figure 10.22.

- Pneumocystography may result in small calculi being over-exposed and hard to see.
- Signs of chronic cystitis and/or blood clots may also be present.

Ultrasonography

- Cannot differentiate calculi type ultrasonographically.
- Radiography is more accurate in determining number of calculi.
- Calculi are hyperechoic, rounded and show distal acoustic shadowing in almost all cases (Figure 10.28).
- Twinkling artefact may be seen within calculus with colour-flow Doppler.
- Usually mobile and move to dependent portion of the bladder; occasionally small calculi are adherent to bladder wall.
- May be concurrent signs of cystitis.
- Differential diagnoses – normal colon, gas or soft tissue mineralization.

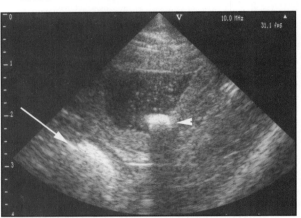

10.28 Transverse ultrasonographic image of the bladder of a cat with cystitis and bladder calculus (arrowhead). Urinary calculi are hyperechoic and usually, although not always, show clean distal acoustic shadowing as in this case (the acoustic shadowing is the black band extending distal to the calculus). Calculi move to the dependent portion of the bladder, which helps differentiate them from gas bubbles (which rise to the non-dependent part) and the colon (which does not move with positioning). Gas within the descending colon (arrowed) should not be mistaken for a bladder calculus.

Bladder haemorrhage

Radiography

- Plain radiographs are unremarkable.
- Pneumocystography shows irregular soft tissue mass(es) within the bladder lumen; if attached to the wall they may mimic tumours.
- With double-contrast cystography, blood clots are seen as irregular filling defects in the contrast medium puddle.
- Blood clots may be broken up or flushed out using saline, whereas true masses will remain constant in appearance.

Ultrasonography

- Blood clots are usually hyperechoic, irregular, lacy masses often located in the dependent part of the lumen. Larger or adherent clots may be hypoechoic and mimic mural masses (Figure 10.29a).
- Diffuse bladder wall thickening with or without irregular mucosal surface (Figure 10.29b).
- Rapid return of bladder wall thickness to normal following successful treatment (approximately 1 mm reduction per day).
- Doppler examination may help to differentiate a blood clot from a mass in some cases (no blood flow is seen in clots) but lack of visualization of a Doppler signal does not rule out a mass.
- Localized haematoma may appear as a focal hypoechoic mass within the wall.
- If associated with generalized coagulopathy, may see evidence of haemorrhage elsewhere.

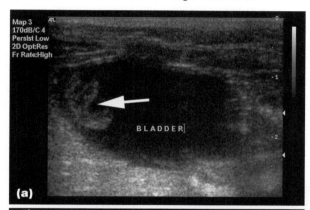

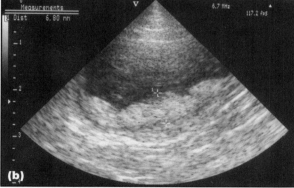

10.29 **(a)** Ultrasonographic image of the bladder of a dog following abdominal trauma. There is a large blood clot adherent to the bladder wall (arrowed). Adherent clots may mimic bladder masses but they are often lacy in appearance and may be mobile. If in doubt flushing the bladder with sterile saline may help move the clot. Colour-flow Doppler may show blood flow within a mass but absence of Doppler signal does not exclude a mass. (Courtesy of Cambridge University Veterinary School.) **(b)** Longitudinal ultrasonographic image of the bladder of a dog with warfarin toxicity. Haemorrhage results in diffuse thickening of the wall, which is most marked dorsally in this view (bottom of image). The bladder wall changes resolved over several days following treatment for the coagulopathy. The ultrasonographic findings are non-specific and diagnosis was based upon history and response to treatment.

Bladder trauma

Rupture is more common in males than in females, because of the much longer, less distensible urethra. The possibility of bladder or urethral rupture should always be considered in cases of pelvic or hindlimb fracture. Rupture may occur spontaneously in the presence of severe bladder wall disease or outflow obstruction.

Radiography

- Bladder contusion without rupture may result in a change of bladder shape, poor distensibility, focal wall thickening and intraluminal blood clots.
- Recent, small tears may be overlooked on plain radiographs, since a bladder shadow may still be visible.
- With larger or older tears the bladder outline is lost, free abdominal fluid collects and obscures normal serosal detail.
- Urine peritonitis produces ileus, with static, dilated intestinal loops.
- Confirmed by positive-contrast retrograde urethrocystography; one is more likely to demonstrate small tears with positive contrast medium than with air (small amounts of air leaking out mimic gastrointestinal gas) (Figure 10.30).

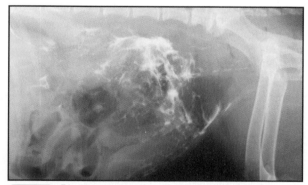

10.30 Bladder rupture in a Springer Spaniel. A double-contrast cystogram has been performed and, although leaking air is hard to differentiate from gastrointestinal gas, there is clearly extravasation of positive contrast medium from the bladder lumen.

Ultrasonography

- Usually bladder is small and may be difficult to identify if collapsed; defect in bladder wall not usually seen.
- Free anechoic abdominal fluid is present, which is most easily seen in the caudal abdomen between small intestines and serosa of bladder.
- Effusion may be cellular in more chronic cases.
- Injection of agitated saline into the bladder via a urinary catheter is confirmatory of bladder rupture if bubbles appear in fluid outside the bladder.
- Differential diagnoses – an artefactual, focal area of reduced echogenicity within the bladder wall with a hypoechoic band extending distally may be seen with ascites ('pseudolesion'). This is due to refraction of sound and should not be mistaken for a genuine defect.

Bladder neoplasia

Most bladder tumours arise in the trigone or bladder neck area, and may involve the urethra. Obstruction of the ureter endings can give rise to hydroureter and hydronephrosis. The histological type of tumour cannot be assessed with imaging, although most are transitional cell carcinomas.

Radiography

- Plain radiographs are usually normal, unless a very large mesenchymal tumour has distorted the bladder outline or has calcified.
- The bladder may be small (if poorly distensible) or large (if obstruction has occurred).
- Cystography shows bladder wall masses or thickening, which is more severe yet more focal than with cystitis, and is less commonly at the apex (c.f. cystitis) (Figure 10.31a).
- Precancerous bladder polyps are seen as pedunculated masses.
- Contrast medium adheres to ulcerated and inflamed surfaces of epithelial tumours and blood clots may be present.
- There may be hydroureter/hydronephrosis on IVU.
- There may be sublumbar lymphadenopathy and pulmonary metastases.
- Bladder rhabdomyosarcoma in young dogs has been associated with hypertrophic osteopathy (Marie's disease).

Ultrasonography

- Usually broad-based masses are seen (Figure 10.31b), but occasionally they are diffuse and mimic cystitis.
- Epithelial tumours usually result in focal wall thickening with irregular mucosal surface and loss of layering (Figure 10.31c).
- The masses are often heterogenous in appearance and may be partly mineralized.
- In severe cases the entire bladder lumen may be obliterated and the bladder may appear solid.
- Smooth muscle tumours are less common and appear as hypoechoic submucosal masses.
- Hydroureter/hydronephrosis may be seen if there is ureteric obstruction by the mass.
- There may be lymphadenopathy in the sublumbar area, usually medial iliac lymph nodes.
- Differential diagnosis – polypoid cystitis, granulomatous cystitis and adherent blood clots may all mimic bladder tumours.
- Ultrasound-guided catheter biopsy reduces the risk of seeding tumour cells along a needle tract that exists with percutaneous biopsy.

Bladder displacement

The bladder may be displaced by pressure from other organs or by passage through a hernia or rupture. In some instances, plain radiographs will show the displaced bladder shadow, but urethrocystography may be

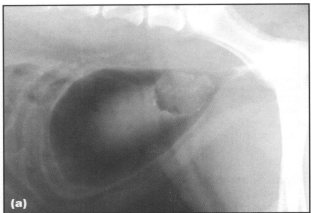

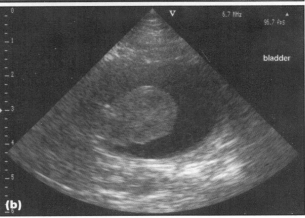

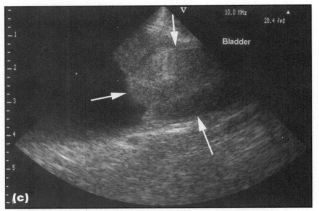

10.31 **(a)** Bladder neck mass due to transitional cell carcinoma in a 6-year-old crossbred dog with haematuria and pollakiuria. The tumour is seen as an irregular mass at the bladder neck, outlined by contrast medium from a double-contrast cystogram. The rest of the bladder appears normal. **(b)** Transverse ultrasonographic image of the bladder of a Labrador with transitional cell carcinoma. A broad-based mass is present extending into the lumen of the bladder. Differential diagnosis would be polypoid cystitis, although polyps are not usually as large, broad-based or infiltrative as in this case. **(c)** Longitudinal ultrasonographic image of the bladder neck of a Scottish Terrier with a tumour in the trigone. Cranial is to the left of the image. The bladder neck is replaced by homogenous soft tissue (arrowed). Biopsy confirmed transitional cell carcinoma.

necessary for confirmation. Ultrasonography provides a quick and easy method for bladder identification.

The bladder position may change as follows:

- Ventral displacement by:
  - Enlarged colon, uterus or uterine stump
  - Sublumbar swelling
  - Paraprostatic cyst ·
  - Ventral or inguinal hernia.
- Dorsal or lateral displacement by:
  - Paraprostatic cyst.
- Cranial displacement by:
  - Prostatomegaly
  - Paraprostatic cyst
  - Enlarged uterus or uterine stump.
- Caudal displacement by:
  - Mid-abdominal mass
  - Perineal hernia
  - Short urethra.

Urethra

Radiography

Plain radiographs

The normal urethra is not visible as a discrete structure. In the female, much of the urethral area is obscured by the pelvis on both lateral and VD radiographs and pathology can only be recognized if gross swelling displaces or compresses the rectum. Even then, the urethral origin of the mass cannot be confirmed with certainty.

In the male the urethra is much longer, consisting of prostatic, ischial and penile segments. Although the urethra is not visible on plain radiographs, lateral views may be useful in the diagnosis of urolithiasis. In larger dogs radiography of the complete length of the urethra requires more than one film, using a higher exposure for the intrapelvic portion and a lower exposure for the urethra beyond the ischial arch. Pulling the hindlegs forwards assists in demonstration of the distal urethra.

Contrast studies

Indications for contrast studies of the urethra include haematuria, dysuria, stranguria, urinary incontinence, urethral discharge and trauma. Urethrography is best performed under general anaesthesia, especially in females.

Retrograde urethrography (males): Some authorities recommend performing a pneumocystogram first to produce back pressure against which to distend the urethra, but it may be better to perform the study before a catheter has been passed along the whole length of the urethra, in order to assess its 'native' state. The technique is as follows:

1. Catheterize the urethra with the widest catheter possible, pre-filled with saline to avoid producing air bubbles.
2. Position the tip of the catheter distal to the area under investigation.

3. Hold the sheath tightly around the catheter.
4. Inject 1 ml/kg, dilute, water-soluble contrast medium fairly rapidly (possibly preceding with 2% lidocaine to reduce muscle spasm).
5. Expose immediately after the end of the injection, taking appropriate safety precautions. Lateral views are usually most helpful. VD views can give extra information about the prostatic urethra: the slight obliquity from the VD position will prevent superimposition of the urethra over itself or over bony structures.

Dilute, iodinated contrast media (150–200 mg iodine/ml) as described for positive-contrast cystography can be used, but mixing with an equal volume of sterile KY jelly produces a more viscous medium and better urethral distension. The mixture should be made up well in advance, since small air bubbles introduced at mixing can mimic genuine filling defects due to calculi. It should be stored in a dark place as iodinated media degrade in light.

Retrograde vaginourethrography (females):

1. A pneumocystogram may be performed first, especially if the bladder is not full.
2. Remove the Foley catheter and cut the tip off beyond the inflatable bulb to prevent it passing too far into the vagina; in cats a non-cuffed catheter is used.
3. Pre-fill the catheter with saline and place the catheter tip just inside the vulval lips, holding the vulva closed around the catheter using gentle bowel clamps.
4. Inflate the bulb of the catheter.
5. Inject a little 2% lidocaine then dilute (150–200 mg iodine/ml) water-soluble contrast medium up to 1 ml/kg over 5–10 seconds (CARE – vaginal rupture has been reported).
6. Expose immediately. Lateral views are standard but an oblique VD (to prevent superimposition of the vagina and urethra) may also be helpful.

Normal radiographic appearance

The male urethra is seen on urethrography to be a smooth-walled tube of fairly uniform diameter, although reactive peristalsis may cause slight variations in its width (Figure 10.32a). The prostatic portion is often slightly wider. The female urethra is short and appears narrow radiographically; it is hard to distend since contrast medium is able to escape into the bladder and vagina at either end. The vestibule and vagina are also seen (Figure 10.32b).

Radiological interpretation

The urethral area should be assessed on plain radiographs for evidence of soft tissue swelling or the presence of radiopaque calculi. Following urethrography, it can be examined for stricture, mucosal irregularity, filling defects or contrast medium leakage.

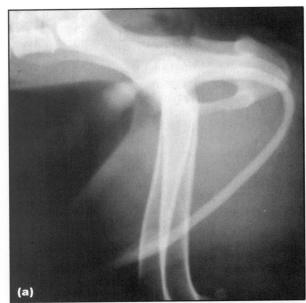

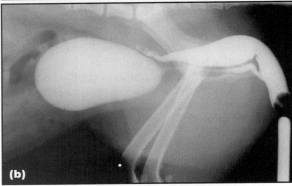

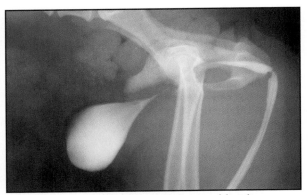

10.33 Uterus masculinus in a 4-year-old male neutered Cocker Spaniel with haematuria and urinary tenesmus. During retrograde urethrography contrast medium fills a cavitary structure arising from the pelvic urethra and outlines internal mucosal folds. Penile structures are reduced in size. The diagnosis was confirmed following surgical removal of the structure.

10.32 **(a)** Normal retrograde urethrogram in a male dog, following pneumocystography. **(b)** Normal retrograde vaginourethrocystogram in a bitch, outlining the vestibule, vagina, cervix, urethra and bladder. The inflated bulb of the Foley catheter is seen as a filling defect in the vestibule.

Ultrasonography

Ultrasonography has limited applications for imaging intrapelvic structures, although proximal urethral disease may be seen ultrasonographically. In the dog, the proximal urethra may be imaged by following the urethra caudally from the bladder neck through the prostate, which is easiest in a transverse plane. It is seen as a uniform hypoechoic tract in the centre of the prostate and an anechoic lumen may be seen if it is dilated. The intrapelvic urethra is not visible unless small transrectal transducers are available, and use of these requires sedation or general anaesthesia. The ischial urethra may be seen by placing the transducer on the perineum. A linear transducer with stand-off pad is preferred for evaluating the penile urethra, although the os penis may prevent full evaluation. The urethra is hard to examine in the cat.

Intersex/hermaphrodite

In cases of intersex, retrograde (vagino)urethrography is invaluable in understanding the anatomy of the lower urogenital tract (Figure 10.33).

Sphincter mechanism incompetence ('short urethra') – females

A retrograde vaginourethrogram may show caudal displacement of the bladder and an unusually short urethra (see Chapter 3). However, this is a functional disease and radiography is mainly indicated to rule out ectopic ureters as a cause for the clinical signs.

Urethritis

- Plain radiographs are unremarkable.
- Retrograde urethrography shows irregular urethral filling if severe.
- Differential diagnosis – urethral neoplasia.

Urethral calculi

Radiography

- In dogs, most urethral calculi are radiopaque (Figure 10.34).

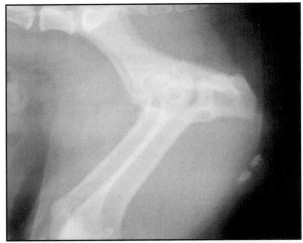

10.34 Two large, irregular, radiopaque urethral calculi in a 6-year-old male Bichon Frise with urethral obstruction. Following surgical removal, analysis showed them to be a mixture of calcium oxalate and ammonium phosphate crystals.

- In male dogs, they usually lodge at the ischial arch or at the base of the os penis.
- In cats, obstructing material is a radiolucent plug.
- In females, calculi must be large to cause obstruction since small calculi are easily voided.
- Retrograde urethrography shows all types of calculus as consistent radiolucent filling defects (air bubbles appear similar but will not distend the urethra).
- Retrograde urethrography is also helpful for demonstrating strictures secondary to urethral calculi.

Ultrasonography

- Appearance of urethral calculi is as for ureteric and bladder calculi.

Urethral rupture
Urethral rupture may occur due to trauma, e.g. RTA, or may be iatrogenic due to repeated catheterization, especially in obstructed cats.

Radiography

- Plain radiographs are usually unremarkable unless there are skeletal injuries or escape of urine into the peritoneal cavity.
- Retrograde urethrography shows contrast medium extravasation into periurethral soft tissues (Figure 10.35).
- If the rupture is near the bladder neck, contrast medium may pass into the peritoneal cavity.
- It may not be possible to identify the exact site of rupture.

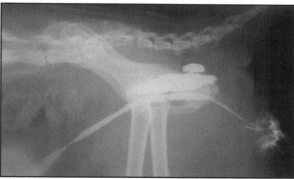

10.35 Retrograde urethrogram of a 7-year-old neutered male domestic shorthaired cat with urethral rupture following repeated catheterization for urethral obstruction. A large volume of contrast medium has extravasated into the pelvic soft tissues, although the exact site of rupture is not clear.

Urethral neoplasia
Urethral neoplasia occurs more frequently in females than in males.

Radiography

- Plain radiographs may show urinary retention and/or an intrapelvic soft tissue mass compressing the rectum.

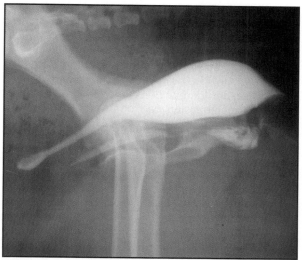

10.36 Urethral tumour in an 8-year-old collie bitch with dysuria, shown by retrograde vaginourethrography. The contrast medium demonstrates a stricture in the mid part of the urethra; distal to this the urethra is dilated due to the pressure of injection, and the urethral walls are irregular. The radiological differential diagnosis is severe urethritis, although stricture formation would be less likely than with neoplasia.

- Retrograde (vagino)urethrography shows narrowing and irregular filling of the urethra with roughened mucosa and filling defects of variable size (Figure 10.36).
- The vagina or bladder neck may also be involved and the exact origin of the tumour may not be clear.
- Sublumbar swelling may be seen if there is metastasis to local lymph nodes; check for lung metastases.
- Differential diagnosis – severe urethritis.

Ultrasonography

- Urethral tumours have a similar appearance to prostatic tumours and it may not be possible to identify the origin of a mass in male dogs.

Urethral stricture
Urethral stricture may occur due to trauma, neoplasia, prostatic disease or previous surgery or urolithiasis.

Radiography

- Plain radiographs are usually unremarkable; urine retention may be evident.
- Retrograde urethrography with the catheter tip distal to the stricture shows a consistent narrowing of the contrast medium column, which may be distended on the distal (catheter) side of the obstruction due to back pressure of the contrast medium.
- The stricture must be consistent on all radiographs to be considered genuine, since peristaltic waves will produce a similar appearance.

Prostate

Radiography

Plain radiographs
The lateral view is taken with the hindlegs extended caudally, as for the bladder. Although large amounts of faeces in the colon can be a problem, a small amount of faecal material is actually helpful since it delineates the descending colon and highlights any colonic displacement or compression due to prostatic enlargement.

Contrast studies
If there is doubt following study of plain films, cystography confirms which, of two or more soft tissue masses, is the bladder and which is the prostate. Delineation of the bladder by cystography shows the prostatic size more clearly, since the prostate is pulled cranially by a full bladder. Air in the catheter highlights the position of the prostatic urethra within the gland, and allows assessment of symmetry. Retrograde positive-contrast urethrography will allow a more complete evaluation of the prostatic urethra. If the colon is empty, instillation of air or barium into the rectum may help to show secondary large bowel displacement.

Normal radiographic appearance
The prostate surrounds the proximal urethra and lies in a variable position in the caudal abdomen and/or the pelvic canal, depending on its size and the degree of bladder distension. It is small and intrapelvic in young and castrated male animals and is not usually visible in entire male cats. In the dog, the prostate is seen as a smooth, rounded soft tissue mass just behind the bladder neck on lateral radiographs and it may be discernible between the shafts of the ilia on the VD view. Its bilobed conformation is sometimes evident radiographically. The size of the prostate varies greatly between individual dogs, tending to enlarge gradually during middle age before atrophying in old age. The variability in size and the presence of subclinical benign prostatic hypertrophy has meant that attempts to define a normal size range have so far proved fruitless.

Retrograde urethrography shows that the urethra lies more or less centrally in the prostate, being slightly above the midline on the lateral view. The prostatic part of the urethra is usually slightly wider than the rest of the urethra. A small amount of leakage of contrast medium into parenchymal cysts is not necessarily a pathological finding.

Radiological interpretation
The prostate should be examined radiographically for the following features:

* Position and relationship with other organs
* Size
* Shape
* Margination (clarity of borders)
* Radiopacity
* Width, margination and integrity of urethra (contrast studies).

Whilst imaging techniques can be used to demonstrate changes in prostatic size, shape, opacity and internal architecture, the findings tend to be non-specific and a definitive diagnosis usually rests on laboratory tests or biopsy (see Chapter 20). This is particularly true of prostatic ultrasonography, since cystic hyperplasia, prostatitis, neoplasia and abscessation may produce similar echo patterns, and may co-exist in any given patient. Prostatic disease is rare in cats.

Radiological findings in prostatic disease can be summarized as follows:

* Enlarged size is most likely to be due to benign prostatic hyperplasia, squamous metaplasia under hormonal influence, cyst formation, abscessation and neoplasia
* Asymmetry is most likely to be due cyst formation, abscessation and neoplasia
* Calcification is most likely to be due to chronic prostatitis or neoplasia
* Irregularity or loss of clarity of prostatic outline is due to prostatitis or neoplasia
* Stricture of the urethra on retrograde urethrography is likely to be due to neoplasia or chronic prostatitis
* Sublumbar soft tissue swelling and lumbosacral or pelvic new bone is due to neoplasia.

Ultrasonography
A high-frequency sector transducer should be used for imaging the prostate. In entire male dogs the prostate is imaged as for the bladder neck, using a prepubic approach. To locate the prostate, first identify the bladder, then angle or move the transducer caudally to visualize the cranial urethra and prostate. In some dogs the prostate cannot be seen clearly due to its intrapelvic location and a better view may be obtained if an assistant pushes the prostate cranially per rectum with a gloved finger. The prostate in cats is not normally visible, and in neutered male dogs is only seen as a small, fusiform-shaped area of hypoechoic tissue surrounding the proximal urethra (Figure 10.37a).

The normal prostate in an entire dog should be relatively hyperechoic and symmetrically bilobed with fine echotexture (Figure 10.37b). A thin, hyperechoic capsule may be seen when the ultrasound beam is perpendicular to the capsule. On transverse images the prostate is peach-shaped, reflecting its bilobed nature. The centrally located urethra is hypoechoic and is seen as a linear band on sagittal images and a circular spot in the transverse plane. On transverse images it occasionally may be surrounded by a subtle, butterfly-shaped hyperechoic region of collagenous tissue; dorsally and ventrally are slightly hypoechoic regions corresponding with glandular tissue. However, this detailed structural appearance is rarely seen and in most dogs the prostate appears uniform. On sagittal images the prostate is round or pear-shaped with the urethra joining the bladder neck cranially.

The prostate increases in size with age and with body weight and there is some breed variation (Scottish Terriers have relatively larger prostates than other breeds). In older dogs it is not uncommon to see small

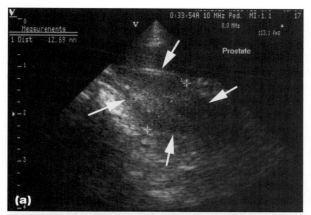

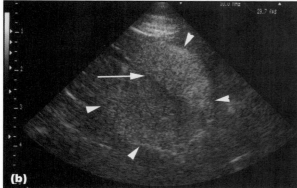

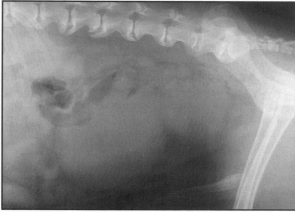

10.38 Caudal abdominal radiograph of an 11-year-old entire male German Shepherd Dog with prostatomegaly. Two rounded soft tissue masses are visible, the cranial of which was shown to be the bladder on ultrasonography. The enlarged prostate displaces the bladder cranially and colon dorsally; it retains a bilobed shape and smooth outline which suggests benign rather than malignant disease.

10.37 **(a)** Longitudinal ultrasonographic image of the prostate (arrowed) in a neutered dog. In neutered dogs the prostate is small and reduced in echogenicity compared with intact dogs. The prostate should be symmetrical with smooth margination. **(b)** Longitudinal ultrasonographic image of the normal canine prostate in an entire dog. The prostate has smooth margins (arrowheads) and is symmetrical in shape with a fine even echotexture. The hypoechoic line (arrowed) running through the middle of the prostate is the prostatic urethra. The apparent area of increased echogenicity within the prostate at the top of the image is artefactual.

cysts as incidental findings, which probably reflect benign prostatic hyperplasia. Formulae exist for measuring prostate volume but are rarely used and size is usually assessed subjectively or by clinical examination.

Benign prostatic hyperplasia

Radiography

- Plain films show an increase in prostatic size, which may compress the colon and rectum and displace the bladder cranially (Figure 10.38).
- The prostate remains symmetrical, round and smoothly marginated.
- Cystography is helpful to confirm the bladder position and to delineate the cranial aspect of the prostate.
- Retrograde urethrography confirms symmetry about the urethra.
- Small amounts of contrast medium may extravasate into the prostatic parenchyma, especially if cystic changes are present.
- If the condition is clinically significant, the urethra may be narrowed.

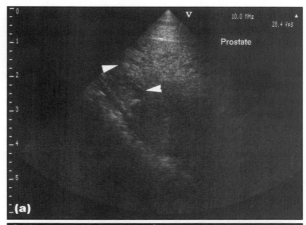

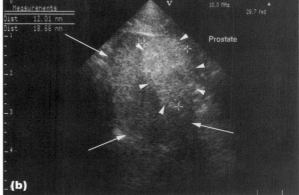

10.39 **(a)** Benign prostatic hyperplasia in a Bearded Collie seen with ultrasonography. The entire prostate has an abnormal mottled appearance with several small parenchymal cysts (arrowheads). The prostate is still normal in shape and size. The changes are non-specific and may also be seen with prostatitis. **(b)** Ultrasound image of the prostate of a Boxer with nodular prostatic hyperplasia (confirmed by biopsy). A focal, well circumscribed hyperechoic nodule (arrowheads) is present within the ventral aspect (top of image) of the prostate (arrowed). Differential diagnosis would include neoplasia.

Ultrasonography

- The prostate may be of normal size and shape or may be enlarged.
- Enlargement is normally symmetrical with the urethra remaining centrally located; asymmetrical enlargement is seen less commonly.
- The prostate remains clearly marginated and there is no extension into adjacent soft tissues or regional lymphadenopathy.
- Small parenchymal cysts are not uncommon (Figure 10.39a).
- There may be diffuse increase in parenchymal echogenicity, a subtle mottled echotexture or focal hyperechoic nodules (Figure 10.39b).

Prostatic and paraprostatic cysts

These may occur due to neoplasia, retention of secretions or Müllerian duct vestiges. They may be multiple.

Radiography

- Plain films show enlarged, asymmetrical prostate (intraprostatic cysts) or multiple soft tissue masses in the caudal abdomen or pelvic canal (paraprostatic cysts) (Figure 10.40a).
- Paraprostatic cysts may calcify.
- Cystography is usually necessary to identify the bladder, which may be displaced in any direction by paraprostatic cysts.
- Contrast medium does not usually enter the cysts during urethrography.

Ultrasonography

- Paraprostatic cysts may be very large and may be confused with the bladder but often lie dorsal to the bladder and craniodorsal to the prostate (Figure 10.40b).
- Caudal location occurs, particularly in conjunction with perineal hernia.
- Often pedunculated, in which case confirming direct communication with the prostate may be difficult.
- Cyst walls are usually thin and may be mineralized; they are occasionally thick-walled and irregular.
- Cyst contents may vary from anechoic to echogenic and sedimentation may be seen.
- Septation is variable and occasionally the cysts have a complex appearance.
- Concurrent prostatic disease is often visible.

Prostatitis

Radiography

- Acute prostatitis may produce a mild increase in size (unlikely to be dramatic and therefore cannot be differentiated from benign hypertrophy).
- If severe, inflammation or rupture of the prostatic capsule causes loss of clarity of the prostatic outline, progressing to peritonitis.

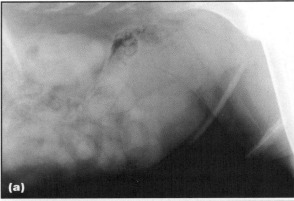

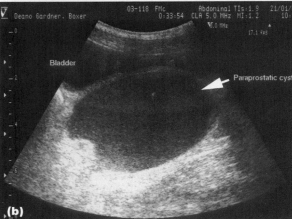

10.40 **(a)** Caudal abdominal radiograph of an 11-year-old entire male Red Setter with dysuria and a palpable caudal abdominal mass. A large, soft tissue mass is seen between the colon dorsally and the bladder ventrally, and extends beyond the bladder neck to the area of the prostate. Ultrasonography showed complex, septated soft tissue containing floccular fluid. The final diagnosis was paraprostatic cyst. **(b)** Longitudinal ultrasonographic image of the caudal abdomen of a Labrador with dysuria. A large, thin-walled, egg-shaped cystic structure (arrowed) is present dorsal to the bladder, which is the smaller fluid-filled structure at the top of the image. The cyst was filled with echogenic fluid, and the walls were mineralized on radiographs. If there are multiple cystic structures it may be difficult to determine ultrasonographically which one is the bladder unless it can be followed caudally to the urethra. Catheterizing the bladder will allow correct identification. In this case the large cyst was seen to be arising from the prostate by a thin stalk, consistent with it being a paraprostatic cyst (confirmed at surgery).

- Chronic prostatitis produces an irregular outline and dystrophic calcification may be recognized.
- Retrograde urethrography may show urethral narrowing, especially in chronic cases.

Ultrasonography

- May be normal and any changes are non-specific.
- Acute prostatitis may result in diffuse or focal decrease or increase in echogenicity.
- Focal mineralization may be present in chronic cases but is less common than with neoplasia.

- Localized peritonitis is seen as a fluid accumulation adjacent to the prostate and an increased echogenicity of peritoneal fat.

Prostatic abscessation

Radiography

- Plain films show enlarged, asymmetrical prostate (cystography may be required to confirm position of bladder).
- Rupture of abscess produces peritonitis.
- Retrograde urethrography confirms asymmetry of the prostate, but radiography cannot differentiate solid from liquid material within the gland.

Ultrasonography

- Often asymmetry and enlargement of the prostate.
- Irregular cavities within the parenchyma.
- Contents may be anechoic or echogenic with or without sedimentation within fluid.
- Gas within abscesses causes reverberation artefact.
- Ultrasound-guided drainage of abscesses may be therapeutic as well as diagnostic.

Prostatic neoplasia

Radiography

- Prostate may be enlarged (sometimes grossly), although a normal size does not preclude neoplasia.
- Urinary retention may be present.
- Neoplasia is the commonest cause of prostatic parenchymal calcification.
- Metastasis to sublumbar lymph nodes provokes reactive periosteal new bone on caudal lumbar vertebrae, sacrum and pelvis (diagnostic for neoplasia).
- Retrograde urethrography may show urethral stricture or contrast extravasation (Figure 10.41a).
- Prostate is usually asymmetrical about the urethra.

Ultrasonography

- There is usually enlargement of the prostate, which is often asymmetrical.
- There is a diffuse decrease in echogenicity with focal areas of increased echogenicity, resulting in a complex or heterogenous appearance.
- Areas of mineralization, irregular margination and extension into the periprostatic tissues are suggestive of neoplasia but may also be seen with prostatitis (Figure 10.41b).
- Irregular anechoic/hypoechoic cavities are common and may represent cyst formation or central necrosis.
- Loss of the capsule is often seen.

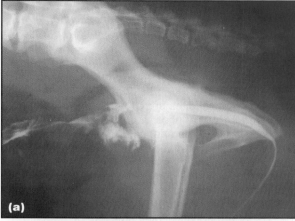

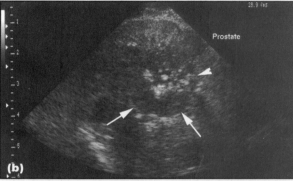

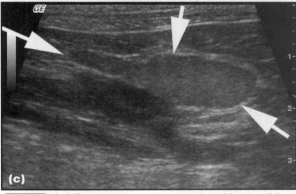

10.41 **(a)** Retrograde urethrogram in a 10-year-old neutered male German Shepherd Dog with dysuria due to prostatic neoplasia. Contrast medium extravasates into the region of the prostate gland, which is ill defined. Caudal to this is a urethral stricture. No significant sublumbar changes are seen in this case, the new bone ventral to the lumbosacral junction being attributable to spondylosis. The final diagnosis was transitional cell carcinoma. **(b)** Ultrasound image of the prostate of a dog with prostatic carcinoma. The margins of the prostate are irregular (arrowed) and the parenchyma is heterogenous with areas of calcification, which appear as hyperechoic foci (arrowhead). Ultrasound-guided fine needle aspiration confirmed the diagnosis.
(c) Longitudinal ultrasonographic image of an enlarged medial iliac lymph node (arrowed). The lymph node lies adjacent to the distal aorta, which is seen as an a hypoechoic structure below the lymph node on this image, at the level of the aortic trifurcation. Enlargement of the medial iliac lymph nodes may be seen with any pathology in the pelvis, caudal abdomen or hindlimbs and is non-specific. Cytological examination is required to differentiate reactive or inflammatory changes from neoplastic infiltration.

- Enlargement often asymmetrical.
- May be local spread to bladder, peritoneum or sublumbar lymph node (Figure 10.41c).

Nuclear medicine (scintigraphy)

Nuclear medicine is the use of radioactive elements or radionuclides for diagnostic purposes. The radionuclide is usually bound to another compound to form a radiopharmaceutical (radiolabelling). The properties of the label used determine the distribution of the radiopharmaceutical within the body, which is detected using a 'gamma camera', a technique known as scintigraphy. If a dynamic study is performed the change in uptake of the radiopharmaceutical over time can be measured.

The use of scintigraphy is limited to practices with gamma cameras and the facilities for administering radiopharmaceuticals and for subsequent patient isolation (this is for 24 hours, following administration of the most commonly used radionuclide technetium). Monitoring equipment must also be available for detecting environmental contamination and radiation emitted by the patient.

As it is essentially a functional tool, the use of nuclear imaging for small animal urology is usually confined to the assessment of renal function, although crude structural information may also be obtained and evaluation of ureteric obstruction is also possible. Scintigraphy has also been used in small animals to document communication of the urinary system with the thorax, and for the localization of ectopic kidneys. The changes in uptake seen with different renal diseases are, however, non-specific and other imaging techniques are preferable to assess renal structure.

The most common indication for renal scintigraphy is measurement of glomerular filtration rate (GFR). GFR can be measured using the plasma clearance of radionuclides, typically technetium 99m-diethylenetriaminepentaacetic acid (Tc 99m DTPA). In addition to allowing measurement of total GFR, by using a gamma camera it is possible to measure individual GFR for each kidney, which is indicated when the relative contribution of each kidney to total renal function is important, e.g. prior to unilateral nephrectomy (Figure 10.42). Scintigraphy is less accurate than plasma clearance methods for GFR measurement (see Chapter 9).

Tc 99m may be bound to a variety of compounds for renal imaging and the choice of radionuclide depends upon the type of scan being performed (Figure 10.43).

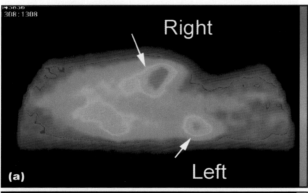

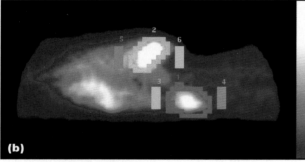

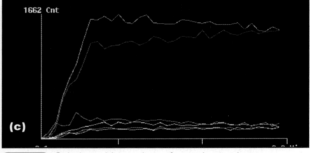

10.42 Scintigraphic study performed on a dog to assess individual kidney GFR. **(a)** Dorsal plane image of activity over 3 minutes. Tc-DTPA is eliminated via the kidneys, which can be identified as areas of increased uptake (arrowed). There is greater activity within the right kidney (uppermost kidney) compared with the left. **(b)** Dorsal plane image during a Tc-DTPA study. Regions of interest (ROI) have been drawn around each kidney and adjacent tissue at the poles. Using this image and ROIs, time activity curves of the kidneys and background can be generated. **(c)** Time activity curves to assess GFR. The activity in the left (red line) and right (yellow line) kidneys can be measured individually. Using the individual uptake curves the GFR for each kidney can be calculated. Although there is a difference between the two kidneys in this case, measurement of GFR was within normal limits for each kidney.

Radiopharmaceutical	Main method of localization	Use
Tc-mercaptoacetyltriglycine (MAG3)	Tubular excretion	Measurement of effective renal plasma flow. Gives better images than Tc-DTPA at low GFRs
Tc-dimercaptosuccinic acid (DMSA)	Binds to renal cortex via tubular uptake	Renal morphology and qualitative measurement of individual renal function
Tc-diethylenetriaminepentaacetic acid (DTPA)	Glomerular filtration	Measurement of GFR (individual and global)

10.43 Technetium radiopharmaceuticals used for renal imaging.

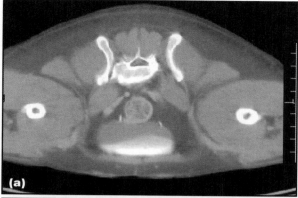

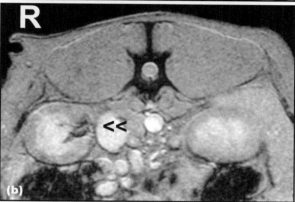

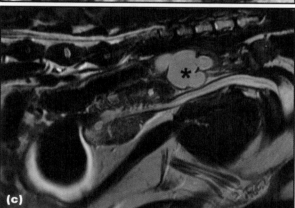

Computed tomography and magnetic resonance imaging

CT and MRI are advanced imaging techniques that are becoming increasingly available in small animal medicine.

CT is based on differential absorption of X-ray photons by tissues, and effectively produces a cross-sectional radiograph. The resultant images not only give three-dimensional information about the tissues under investigation but also give greatly increased contrast. Scanning times are fairly short and respiratory motion is not usually a problem, although the patient needs to be sedated or anaesthetized for the procedure. Most scanners produce primary images in the transverse plane, and reformatting of data into other planes results in some loss of detail.

MRI uses a combination of a powerful magnetic field and radio energy to produce cross-sectional images that demonstrate the distribution of hydrogen nuclei within the body's tissues. Soft tissue detail is much greater than with CT, and images can be acquired in any plane. However, scan times are much longer than for CT and so movement blur may be a problem for thoracic and abdominal studies. Nevertheless, useful images can often be obtained.

Indications for CT or MRI of the urinary tract in small animals are few, as a combination of radiography and ultrasonography will usually provide the information required about the extent of a lesion. However, the three-dimensional anatomical information produced by CT and MRI may be helpful if surgery of an extensive lesion is planned, especially to detect invasion of tumours into adjacent tissues. As with other techniques, the images are usually non-specific for the histological nature of tissue. CT intravenous urography has been described as being superior to other established diagnostic imaging techniques for diagnosing canine ureteral ectopia (Samii *et al.*, 2004). Figure 10.44 shows examples of the use of CT and MRI in imaging the urinary tract.

10.44 **(a)** CT scan of the abdomen of a male Golden Retriever following intravenous injection of iodinated contrast medium, in order to perform an intravenous urogram. The ureters are normal and seen in cross-section as two small, radiopaque dots dorsal to the bladder. (Picture courtesy of the Royal Veterinary College Queen Mother Hospital.) **(b)** Transverse MR image of the abdomen of a 5-year-old Staffordshire Bull Terrier with haematuria, at the level of the kidneys. The image has been obtained using a gradient echo technique; this is highly sensitive for haemorrhage which is seen as a signal void (black area). In this dog, ultrasonography and an IVU were unremarkable but the MRI scan showed an area of haemorrhage in the right kidney (arrowheads). The final diagnosis was idiopathic renal haemorrhage. **(c)** Intrapelvic paraprostatic cyst in a 7-year-old entire male Bernese Mountain Dog (*). This midline sagittal T2-weighted fast spin echo image shows an irregular but well defined, fluid-filled structure in the pelvic canal dorsal to the urethra and caudodorsal to an enlarged prostate gland. The dog had been showing signs of dyschezia and rectal examination revealed a soft, intrapelvic mass. Confirmation of prostatic cyst was made at surgery.

References and further reading

Atalan G, Barr FJ and Holt PE (1999) Assessment of urinary bladder volume in dogs by use of linear ultrasonographic measurements. *American Journal of Veterinary Research* **59**, 10–15

Biller DS, Schenkman DI and Bortnowski H (1991) Ultrasonographic appearance of renal infarcts in a dog. *Journal of the American Animal Hospital Association* **27**, 370–372

Costello M (2001) Ultrasonography of the urinary bladder. *UK Vet* **6**, 60–63

Cuypers MD, Grooters AM, Williams J and Partington BP (1997) Renomegaly in dogs and cats. Part 1: Differential diagnosis. *Compendium of Continuing Education for the Practicing Veterinarian* **19**, 1019–1032

Daniel GB, Mitchell SK, Mawby D, Sackman JE and Schmidt D (1999) Renal nuclear medicine: a review. *Veterinary Radiology & Ultrasound* **40**, 572–587

Dennis R, Kirberger RM, Wrigley RH and Barr FJ (2001) Urogenital tract. In: *Handbook of Small Animal Radiological Differential Diagnosis*, pp. 185–208. WB Saunders, London

Feeney DA, Thrall DE, Barber DL, Culver DH and Lewis RE (1979) Normal canine excretory urogram; effects of dose, time, and individual dog variation. *American Journal of Veterinary Research* **40**, 1596–1604

Geisse AL, Lowry JE, Schaeffer DJ and Smith CW (1997) Sonographic evaluation of urinary bladder wall thickness in normal dogs. *Veterinary Radiology and Ultrasound* **38**, 132–137

Grooters AM, Cuypers MD, Partington BP, Williams J and Pechman RD (1997) Renomegaly in dogs and cats. Part 2: Diagnostic approach. *Compendium of Continuing Education for the Practicing Veterinarian* **19**, 1213–1229

Gunn-Moore D (2000) Feline lower urinary tract disease: an update. *In Practice* **22**, 534–542

Hotston-Moore A (2001) Urinary incontinence in adult bitches 1. Investigation. *In Practice* **23**, 534–540

Hotston-Moore A (2001) Urinary incontinence in adult bitches 2. Differential diagnosis and treatment. *In Practice* **23**, 588–595

Lamb CR and Gregory SP (1994) Ultrasonography of the ureterovesicular junction in the dog: a preliminary report. *Veterinary Record* **134**, 36–38

Lamb CR, Trower ND and Gregory SP (1996) Ultrasound-guided catheter biopsy of the lower urinary tract: technique and results in 12 dogs. *Journal of Small Animal Practice* **37**, 413–416

Lamb CR and Gregory SP (1998) Ultrasonographic findings in 14 dogs with ectopic ureter. *Veterinary Radiology and Ultrasound* **39**, 218–223

Morrow KL, Salman MD, Lappin MR and Wrigley R (1996) Comparison of resistive index to clinical parameters in dogs with renal disease. *Veterinary Radiology and Ultrasound* **37**, 193–199

Nyland TG, Fisher PE, Doverspike M, Hornof WJ and Olander HJ (1993) Diagnosis of urinary tract obstruction in dogs using duplex Doppler ultrasonography. *Veterinary Radiology and Ultrasound* **43**, 348–352

Ruel Y, Barthez PY, Mailles A and Begon D (1998) Ultrasonographic evaluation of the prostate in healthy intact dogs. *Veterinary Radiology and Ultrasound* **39**, 212–216

Samii VF, McLoughlin MA, Mattoon JS *et al.* (2004) Digital fluoroscopic excretory urography, digital fluoroscopic urethrography, helical computed tomography, and cystoscopy in 24 dogs with suspected ureteral ectopia. *Journal of Veterinary Internal Medicine* **18**, 271–281

Shiroma JT, Gabriel JK, Carter RL, Scruggs SL and Stubbs PW (1999) Effect of reproductive status on feline renal size. *Veterinary Radiology and Ultrasound* **40**, 242–245

Stonehewer J (1997) Differential diagnosis of urinary tenesmus in the dog. *In Practice* **19**, 134–143

White RAS, Herrtage ME and Dennis R (1987) The diagnosis and management of paraprostatic and prostatic retention cysts in the dog. *Journal of Small Animal Practice* **28**, 551–574

Williams J and Niles J (1999) Prostatic disease in the dog. *In Practice* **21**, 558–575

11

Staging chronic kidney disease

Jonathan Elliott

Introduction

The terminology in current use to describe the different stages of chronic kidney disease (CKD) is confusing and is applied in different ways by different authorities. In 1998, the International Renal Interest Society (IRIS) was formed and one of its main purposes was to devise, through consensus and debate, a staging system for CKD. The system would allow better communication of the concepts underlying the diagnosis and management of this complex disease syndrome to general veterinary practitioners and veterinary students throughout the world. This group now has representation from 10 different countries. The staging system first proposed has been utilized by members of the IRIS Board and refined on the basis of this use. In addition, feedback has been obtained from the American and European Societies of Veterinary Nephrology and Urology and modifications made according to this feedback.

In veterinary medicine staging systems have been used for defining heart failure, where a modification of a system used in human medicine is routinely applied. Similarly, the IRIS system for staging CKD is based on systems used in human medicine. It should be viewed as a work in progress. As more information is published in the form of original studies involving the diagnosis, prognosis and management of CKD in dogs and cats, modifications to this staging system and the treatment recommendations that go with it (see Chapter 18) will be made. The concepts upon which staging is based are presented in Chapter 5 and the application of the IRIS staging system to the management of CKD is presented in Chapter 18. The purpose of this chapter is to define the staging system precisely, explain the reasoning that underlies it and describe its appropriate application.

Selecting dogs and cats to be staged

The IRIS staging system only applies to dogs and cats with stable CKD. In other forms of disease affecting kidney function, the plasma creatinine concentration (upon which the staging system is based) can change dramatically over a short period of time. Hence, staging is not appropriate under these circumstances. The approach to the azotaemic animal is outlined in Chapter 5. In summary, it is important to:

- Determine the cause of the azotaemia:
  - Prerenal
  - Primary intrinsic renal
  - Postrenal
- If the cause is primary intrinsic kidney disease, then the clinician needs to determine whether the kidney disease is:
  - Acute
  - Decompensated chronic (sometimes termed 'acute on chronic')
  - Chronic.

The important point for the purposes of staging is that only stable CKD can be staged accurately by the proposed method. It is possible that cases of acute kidney disease (or decompensated chronic kidney disease) will stabilize into a chronic form after 4–8 weeks of management, at which point staging might be appropriate.

Staging system

Plasma creatinine is utilized as the major factor for staging as this is the most readily available test of kidney function for veterinary practitioners (Figure 11.1). The limitations of plasma creatinine are well recognized and are outlined in Chapter 9. The staging system would undoubtedly be improved should a practical method be devised of adjusting plasma creatinine concentration to take account of body condition score in general, and muscle mass in particular, since these govern the rate of production of creatinine. Such correction factors are available in human medicine but the complexity of devising appropriate systems for veterinary practice should not be underestimated. In addition, the IRIS group expects that measurement of glomerular filtration rate (GFR) by a plasma clearance method may replace plasma creatinine concentration as the major criterion for staging. Validation of practical methods of measuring GFR, which can be applied to general practice, is ongoing and will represent a significant advance in veterinary nephrology once careful research has been published.

The staging system based on plasma creatinine recognizes that a large proportion of kidney tissue has to be damaged before a rise in plasma creatinine concentration is detectable. Hence stage I and early stage II encompass plasma creatinine concentrations

Stage	Creatinine	Comments

I	<125 μmol/l (<1.4 mg/dl) (dogs)
	<140 μmol/l (<1.6 mg/dl) (cats)
		Non-azotaemic
		Some other renal abnormality present:
		    Inadequate urine-concentrating ability without identifiable non-renal cause
		    Abnormal renal palpation and/or abnormal renal imaging findings
		    Proteinuria of renal origin
		    Abnormal renal biopsy results
		    Increasing plasma creatinine concentrations noted on serial samples

II	125–179 μmol/l (1.4–1.9 mg/dl) (dogs) 140–249 μmol/l (1.6–2.7 mg/dl) (cats)	Mild renal azotaemia (lower end of the range lies within the reference range for many laboratories but the insensitivity of creatinine as a screening test means that animals with creatinine values close to the upper reference limit often have excretory failure) Clinical signs usually mild or absent
III	180–439 μmol/l (2.0–4.9 mg/dl) (dogs) 250–439 μmol/l (2.8–4.9 mg/dl) (cats)	Moderate renal azotaemia Many extrarenal clinical signs may be present
IV	>440 μmol/l (>5.0 mg/dl) (dogs and cats)	Severe renal azotaemia Many extrarenal clinical signs are usually present

11.1 The IRIS staging system based on plasma creatinine.

which are well within or in the upper end of the reference ranges for most laboratories. For an animal to be classified in stage I, therefore, some other abnormality has to have been detected which makes the clinician suspect a disease process is ongoing within the kidney. This could include:

- Inadequate urine-concentrating ability in the absence of an extrarenal cause
- The detection of renal proteinuria (see Chapter 6)
- Abnormal size or shape of the kidneys detected on palpation and confirmed by diagnostic imaging

- Abnormal findings on kidney biopsy
- Increasing plasma creatinine concentrations (even though they remain within the laboratory reference range) noted on serial plasma samples.

The precise plasma creatinine concentrations used to divide the different stages outlined in Figure 11.1 were reached by consensus and debate. They were based on clinical experience of the Board members and from data derived from longitudinal studies. For example, Figure 11.2 shows survival curves for cats presenting to first

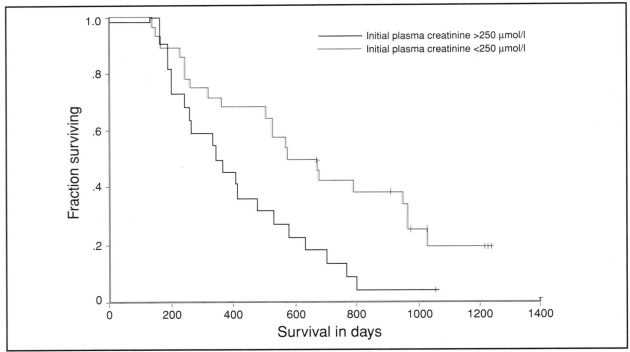

11.2 Effect of presenting plasma creatinine concentration on long-term survival of cats with chronic kidney disease. Kaplan–Meier survival curves from 50 cats entered into a prospective study (Elliott *et al.*, 2000). Cats have been divided into two groups based on their initial plasma creatinine concentration at entry to the study as either stage II (creatinine <250 μmol/l (<2.8 mg/dl); all cats in this group had plasma creatinine concentrations >177 μmol/l (>2.0 mg/dl)) or stage III (creatinine >250 μmol/l (>2.8 mg/dl); all cats in this group had plasma creatinine concentrations <440 μmol/l (<5.0 mg/dl)).

opinion veterinary practice in stage II or stage III. As can be seen, there is a significant difference between the survival times of these two groups of cats.

It is likely that some animals with CKD pass through all these stages if their kidney disease progresses. Some animals, however, will remain stable within one stage and die of some other disease before their kidney disease has had chance to progress. Cases may be presented to the veterinary surgeon at any stage depending on how observant their owner is and how open they are to routine health screening being practised. Figure 11.3 depicts progression of kidney dis-

ease through these four stages and overlies the IRIS staging system with some of the terminology that has been used previously to describe these different stages of kidney disease. This is an adaptation of Figure 5.5. The IRIS staging system defines these stages more precisely than terms that were commonly used in the past. For example:

- Stage I is equivalent to 'early renal disease – non-azotaemic'
- Late stage I to early stage II is equivalent to 'renal insufficiency'

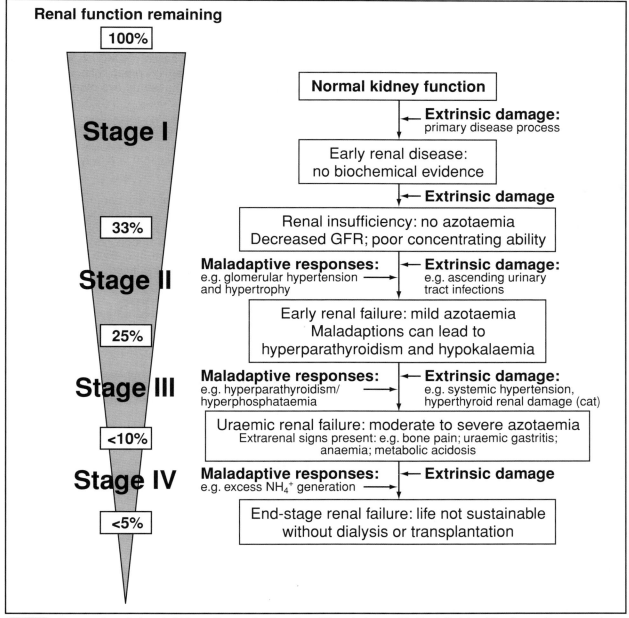

11.3 Progression of chronic kidney disease to show the different stages. On the left side of the figure, the percentage of remaining functioning tissue GFR/number of nephrons) is shown and overlaid by the stages defined by the IRIS group. On the right of the figure, the flow diagram describes the stages using older terminology which has been employed less precisely in the past. In addition, potential factors influencing progression from one stage to the next are shown. Initially extrinsic factors (the primary disease processes) are responsible for causing loss of functioning nephrons. Once the animal has reached late stage II/stage III, then maladaptive responses to loss of functioning nephrons and consequences of the uraemic syndrome may contribute to further kidney damage (so-called 'intrinsic progression').

- Late stage II to early stage III is equivalent to 'early renal failure – mild azotaemia'
- Late stage III to early stage IV is equivalent to 'uraemic renal failure'
- Late stage IV is equivalent to 'end-stage renal failure'.

The staging system will be useful to provide practitioners with prognostic information and to determine the likely consequences of the kidney disease, which will need to be addressed by management protocols at different stages. For example, Figures 11.4 and 11.5 show the prevalence and severity of hyperparathyroidism and metabolic acidosis across stages II to IV of CKD. This has implications for management recommendations at the different stages. Chapter 18 uses the IRIS staging system to make recommendations for the management of CKD in dogs and cats.

Substaging of chronic kidney disease

In addition to staging cases of CKD on the basis of plasma creatinine, the IRIS group recommends that cases are substaged based on two other diagnostic factors, namely:

- The quantity of protein excreted in urine (see Chapter 6)
- The systemic arterial blood pressure (see Chapter 13).

Assessment of both of these parameters is important because proteinuria and systemic hypertension can occur at any of the four stages of CKD. Also, in human medicine, each is an independent risk factor for progressive renal injury and, as such, warrants specific treatment protocols to be instituted.

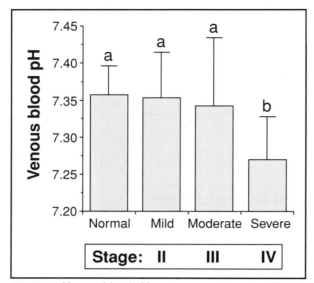

11.4 Venous blood pH measurements in cats with naturally occurring CKD. Blood pH measurements were made using a patient-side monitor. The reference range devised from 28 aged normal cats was 7.27–7.44. None of the cats in stage II, 3 of 20 (15%) in stage III and 10 of 19 (52.4%) in stage IV had venous blood pH below 7.27 and so were considered to be acidaemic. Columns that bear a different letter are significantly different from each other (one way ANOVA followed by Fishers test; P<0.05) (Elliott *et al.*, 2003).

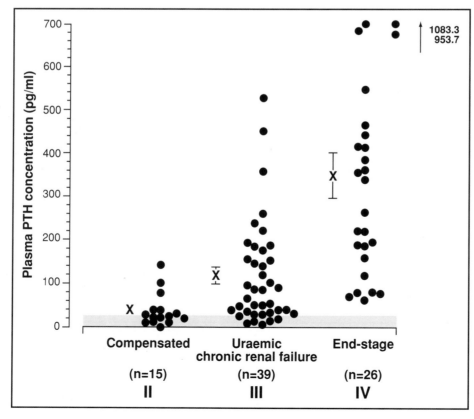

11.5 A scattergram showing the distribution of plasma parathyroid hormone (PTH) concentrations in cats at different stages of CKD. This represents a cross-sectional study of 80 cats presenting to first opinion practices at initial diagnosis of CKD. Plasma PTH concentrations were measured using an intact immunoradiometric assay. The classification system used was based on clinical presentation rather than plasma creatinine concentration. Nevertheless, plasma creatinine concentrations in the three groups were for the majority of cases equivalent to IRIS stages II, III and IV. PTH concentrations outside the laboratory reference range were found in 47% of cats in stage II, 87% of cats in stage III and 100% of cats in stage IV. (Reproduced with permission from Barber and Elliott, 1998.)

Substaging based on protein in the urine

Chapter 6 discusses in detail the diagnostic approach to identifying protein in the urine and classifying proteinuria as:

- Prerenal
- Renal
- Postrenal.

The substaging of cases based on proteinuria refers only to renal proteinuria. Prerenal and postrenal causes should be ruled out if the substaging system recommended below is to be utilized. Figure 11.6 presents the substaging system to be adopted.

UPC value (calculated using mass units)	Interpretation
<0.2 (dogs and cats)	Non-proteinuric (NP)
0.2–0.4 (cats) 0.2–0.5 (dogs)	Borderline proteinuric (BP)
>0.4 (cats) >0.5 (dogs)	Proteinuric (P)

11.6 Substaging on urine protein:creatinine ratio (UPC).

The above recommendations have been modified in light of the most recent ACVIM Consensus Statement on Proteinuria (Lees *et al.*, 2005). It is important to recognize that persistent proteinuria is more likely to be pathological than transient proteinuria. As discussed in Chapter 6, therefore, substaging based on urine protein:creatinine ratio (UPC) should demonstrate persistence of proteinuria, ideally by collection of at least three urine samples over at least a 2-week period.

The action required, having identified an animal as being either proteinuric or borderline proteinuric, depends on the stage of CKD according to the plasma creatinine concentration. A UPC >0.5 in a dog with a plasma creatinine concentration of 350 μmol/l (3.96 mg/dl) (stage III) is far more significant than such a UPC in a dog with a plasma creatinine concentration of 100 μmol/l (1.13 mg/dl) (stage I). The reason for this is

that as the mass of functioning nephrons declines, so the filtered load of protein presented to the tubules is reduced. Hence, the appearance of relatively low amounts of protein in the urine attains higher significance.

Current recommendations for interventions according to the stage of CKD are as follows:

- Stage I
  - UPC >2.0 and persistent – investigate for underlying cause and introduce antiproteinuric therapy (see Chapter 19)
  - UPC <2.0 – continue to monitor to determine whether proteinuria is worsening
- Stages II–IV (see Chapter 18 for further details)
  - UPC in the proteinuric range (>0.5 (dog) or >0.4 (cat)) – investigate for underlying cause and introduce antiproteinuric therapy (see Chapter 18)
  - UPC in the borderline proteinuric range (0.2–0.4 (cat) or 0.2–0.5 (dog)) – monitor closely to determine whether proteinuria is worsening.

A further reason proteinuria is singled out for special attention in animals with CKD is that there is good evidence that it is a prognostic indicator in dogs and cats with CKD. A longitudinal study in dogs with naturally occurring CKD has demonstrated that animals with UPCs >1.0 have a threefold higher risk of suffering a uraemic crisis when compared with dogs presented with UPCs <1.0 (Jacob *et al.*, 2005). In cats with CKD, proteinuria is an independent risk factor for all-cause mortality (Syme *et al.*, 2006).

Substaging based on systemic arterial blood pressure

The application of indirect blood pressure measurement techniques to clinical practice (see Chapter 13) means that this important physiological parameter can and should be assessed in dogs and cats with CKD. High blood pressure can be damaging to the kidneys (Figure 11.7), and kidney disease can give rise to problems with blood pressure regulation, leading to inappropriately high blood pressure. In addition, high blood pressure can cause damage to other target

Risk	Systolic (mmHg)	Diastolic (mmHg)	Classification according to evidence of extrarenal complications
Minimal or no (N)	<150	<95	Minimal or no risk of end-organ damage Highly unlikely to see evidence of extrarenal damage at this level
Low (L)	150–159	95–99	Low risk of end-organ damage If no extrarenal complication seen (Lnc) If evidence of extrarenal complications seen (Lc)
Moderate (M)	160–179	100–119	Moderate risk of end-organ damage If no extrarenal complications seen (Mnc) If evidence of extrarenal complications seen (Mc)
High (H)	≥180	≥120	High risk of end-organ damage If no extrarenal complications seen (Hnc) If evidence of extrarenal complications seen (Hc)

11.7 Substaging on blood pressure. c = Extrarenal complications detected; nc = No extrarenal complications present.

organs, such as the heart (left ventricular hypertrophy), the eye (hypertensive retinopathy) and the brain, leading to extrarenal signs and morbidity in the CKD patient. For these reasons the IRIS group recommends that all patients with CKD have their blood pressure measured regardless of the stage of their kidney disease. Antihypertensive treatment may be appropriate, depending on the level of risk and/or the presence of end-organ damage. Hence, blood pressure is used to substage dogs and cats according to the risk of end-organ damage and whether there is evidence of extrarenal end-organ damage.

Extrarenal complications of hypertension might include:

- Left ventricular concentric hypertrophy in the absence of structural/valvular heart problems identified
- Ocular abnormalities compatible with damage by high blood pressure, such as hyphaema or hypertensive retinopathy
- Neurological signs – dullness and lethargy, seizures.

The IRIS group recognizes there are a number of different methods available for measuring blood pressure and the veterinary profession has not agreed a standardized approach. These blood pressure recommendations are therefore to be used as a guide; they will be useful provided practitioners standardize their approach within their own practice and ensure the technique used remains the same for a given animal from one visit to the next. Details concerning the measurement technique, which is important to standardize, are discussed in Chapter 13. It is also recognized that within dog breeds there are some differences with regards to blood pressure reference ranges. If dealing with a breed known to have higher blood pressure than average (e.g. sight hounds), the following adaptation of the staging system can be adopted:

- Minimal-risk category <10 mmHg above the breed reference range
- Low to moderate-risk category 10–40 mmHg above the breed reference range
- High-risk category >40 mmHg above the breed reference range.

In the same way that proteinuria was categorized based on persistence, blood pressure risk should also be based on multiple sequential measurements to document persistence of risk. This recommendation applies when there is no evidence of extrarenal end-organ damage. If extrarenal end-organ damage (e.g. hypertensive retinopathy) is identified then treatment should begin immediately these signs are recognized (see Chapters 13 and 18). If no evidence of extrarenal end-organ damage is recognized, the following actions are recommended:

- For patients found persistently to be in the low-risk category – re-evaluate every 2 months to determine whether blood pressure is increasing
- For patients found persistently to be in the moderate-risk category – re-evaluate and if blood pressure persistently remains in this category based on multiple measurements made over 2 months, institute treatment
- For patients in the high-risk category – re-evaluate over 7 days and if blood pressure persistently remains in this category based on multiple measurements made over this time, institute treatment.

Conclusions

The IRIS scheme thus allows CKD in dogs and cats to be staged on the basis of the fasting blood creatinine concentration and further characterized according to urine protein content and systemic blood pressure. Figure 11.8 presents an algorithm for the complete staging system applied to a cat. A similar algorithm can be produced for the dog. The following examples serve to illustrate the entire staging system:

- A proteinuric (UPC 1.2) dog with systolic blood pressure of 154 mmHg (but no evidence of extrarenal damage) and blood creatinine concentration 260 μmol/l (2.94 mg/dl) would be classified as stage III-P-Lnc
- A dog with borderline proteinuria (UPC 0.4), blood creatinine concentration 550 μmol/l (6.22 mg/dl) and blood pressure of 130 mmHg (with no evidence of extrarenal damage) would be classified as stage IV-BP-N
- A non-proteinuric (UPC 0.12) cat with systolic blood pressure of 210 mmHg, bilateral retinal detachment and blood creatinine concentration of 180 μmol/l (2.03 mg/dl) would be classified as stage II-NP-Hc.

The IRIS staging system reflects current knowledge and opinion about CKD in dogs and cats and will continue to develop as the results of new research are published. Consistent and widespread use of such staging should aid practitioners with prognosis in CKD, providing a framework for logical treatment plans (see Chapter 18) and facilitating communication between veterinary surgeons about this complex disease syndrome.

Acknowledgement

The author wishes to acknowledge all the IRIS Board members who contributed to the generation of this staging system. They are: S Brown (USA), C Brovida (Italy), J-P Cotard (France), L Cowgill (USA), J Elliott (UK), M-J Fernandez del Palacio (Spain), S Gnass (Germany), G Grauer (USA), R Heiene (Norway), A Huttig (Germany), A Kosztolich (Austria), H Lefebvre (France), AR Michell (UK), R Mitten (Australia), D Polzin (USA), J-L Pouchelon (France), R Santilli (Italy), T Watanabe (Japan) and D Watson (Australia).

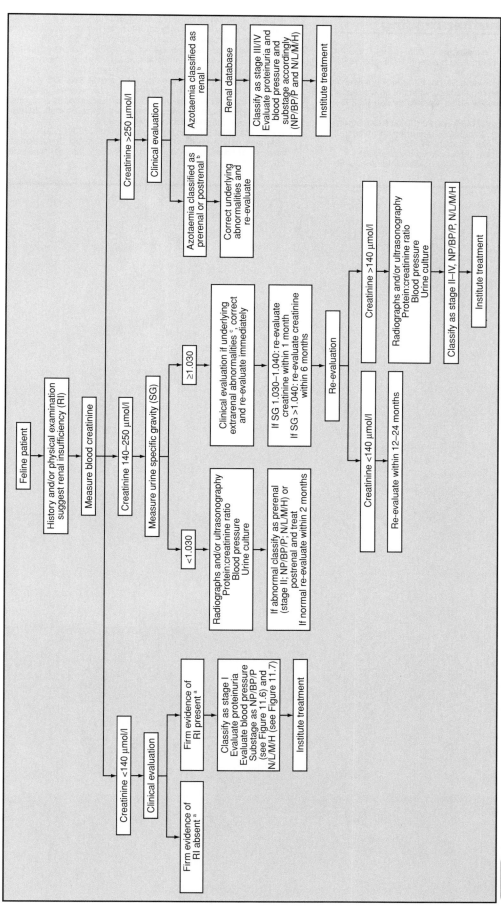

11.8 An algorithm applying the IRIS staging system to a cat suspected of having chronic kidney disease. [a] In the setting of a low value for serum creatinine (<125 µmol/l (<1.4 mg/dl) in dogs or <140 µmol/l (<1.6 mg/dl) in cats) firm evidence of renal disease would usually be morphological, such as abnormal renal architecture on survey radiographs, abnormal renal ultrasonography findings or biopsy diagnosis of renal disease. [b] The classification of prerenal azotaemia (generally due to dehydration or renal ischaemia) or postrenal azotaemia (generally due to ureteral or urethral obstruction, or rupture of part of the urinary tract) will depend on careful evaluation of history, physical examination and other clinical findings. This determination may require additional tests, based on clinical judgement. For example, radiographic studies and/or abdominal paracentesis (with analysis of ascitic fluid creatinine concentration) may be required to establish a diagnosis of ruptured urinary bladder in an azotaemic cat with a history of blunt abdominal trauma. The classification of azotaemia as renal is based on the presence of azotaemia with no identifiable prerenal or postrenal causes. As a general guide, dogs and cats with renal azotaemia usually have a urine specific gravity <1.030. [c] These abnormalities may include any prerenal factor that leads to dehydration or systemic arterial hypotension or postrenal factors such as ureteral or urethral obstruction, or urinary tract rupture. BP = Borderline proteinuric; H = High; L= Low; M = Moderate; N = No or minimal; NP = Non-proteinuric; P = Proteinuric; RI = Renal insufficiency; SG = Specific gravity. (For further information on proteinuria substaging and blood pressure substaging on risk of extrarenal damage, see Figures 11.6 and 11.7, respectively.)

References and further reading

Barber PJ and Elliott J (1998) Feline chronic renal failure: calcium homeostasis in 80 cases diagnosed between 1992 and 1995. *Journal of Small Animal Practice* **39**, 108–116

Elliott J, Rawlings JM, Markwell PJ and Barber PJ (2000) Survival of cats with naturally occurring renal failure: effect of conventional dietary management. *Journal of Small Animal Practice* **41**, 235–242

Elliott J, Syme HM, Reubens E and Markwell PJ (2003) Assessment of acid–base status of cats with naturally occurring chronic renal failure. *Journal of Small Animal Practice* **44**, 65–70

International Renal Interest Society: www.iris-kidney.com

Jacob F, Polzin DJ, Osborne CA *et al.* (2003) Association between initial systolic blood pressure and risk of developing a uremic crisis or of dying in dogs with chronic renal failure. *Journal of the American Veterinary Medical Association* **222**, 322–329

Jacob F, Polzin DJ, Osborne CA *et al.* (2005) Evaluation of the association between initial proteinuria and morbidity rate or death in dogs with naturally occurring chronic renal failure. *Journal of the American Veterinary Medical Association* **226**, 393–400

Lees GE, Brown SA, Elliott J, Grauer GF and Vaden SL (2005) Assessment and management of proteinuria in dogs and cats: 2004 ACVIM Forum Consensus Statement (small animal). *Journal of Veterinary Internal Medicine* **19**, 377–385

Syme HM, Markwell PJ, Pfeiffer DU and Elliott J (2006) Survival of cats with naturally occurring chronic renal failure is related to severity of proteinuria. *Journal of Veterinary Internal Medicine* **20**, 528–535

12

Renal biopsy

Shelly L. Vaden and Cathy A. Brown

Introduction

Dogs and cats with renal diseases can often be described as having acute renal failure, chronic kidney disease (CKD) or a glomerulopathy based on the patient history and results of physical examination and clinical laboratory tests. However, renal biopsy may be required in order to establish a definitive diagnosis, determine the severity of the lesion and formulate an optimal treatment plan. Despite the need for renal biopsy, practitioners may be reluctant to perform one on their patients because of concern over expense and potential complications, as well as the belief that the rendered diagnoses may lack consistency. The expense and complication rate can be minimized by correct patient selection and use of proper technique for one of several methods. Consistent and accurate diagnoses are more likely to be obtained when renal biopsy specimens are appropriately processed and evaluated. This chapter summarizes the indications, contraindications, techniques and complications of renal biopsy, as well as the appropriate processing and evaluation of the renal biopsy specimen.

Indications

Renal biopsy is indicated only when having an accurate histological diagnosis is likely to alter patient management. Patients whose management is most likely to be altered by results of a renal biopsy include those with protein-losing nephropathy (i.e. glomerular disease) or acute renal failure (Figure 12.1). Client factors that need to be considered include the ability to incur the expense of the procedure and proper evaluation of the specimen, as well as the desire to pursue additional treatment of their dog or cat, as may be indicated by the histological diagnosis.

Renal biopsy is generally not indicated in patients with chronic kidney disease (stage IV and possibly stage III). Results are unlikely to alter the prognosis, therapy or outcome in these patients. Furthermore, there is an increased risk of complications from renal biopsy in people with chronic kidney disease (Parrish, 1992). Renal biopsy results may also aid in the formulation of an accurate prognosis (e.g. whether or not there is evidence of tubular cell regeneration in acute renal failure).

Protein-losing nephropathy
May be one of the more important factors in successful management of specific glomerular diseases
Identify and treat potential underlying diseases before biopsy. Biopsy may not be needed if proteinuria resolves after effective treatment of an underlying disease
Low yield in patients with CKD stage IV
Appropriate evaluation may require light, electron and immunofluorescent microscopy

Acute renal failure
May be indicated in patients with persistently severe uraemia or oliguria, or those that deteriorate during appropriate medical management
May help determine aetiological diagnosis that may lead to specific therapeutic measures
May facilitate prognostication
Light microscopic evaluation may be sufficient. However, samples should be collected for electron and immunofluorescent microscopy in the event that the primary disease is glomerular

Mass lesions
May be needed if mass aspiration cytology is non-diagnostic

12.1 Indications for renal biopsy.

Contraindications and other considerations

A thorough patient evaluation prior to renal biopsy should identify any existing contraindications to the procedure (Figure 12.2). This evaluation process should include obtaining a current history, performing a complete physical examination, measuring systemic blood pressure, analysing results of a biochemical profile, complete blood count, urinalysis and coagulation profile, and assessing size, shape, contour and internal architecture of the kidney via abdominal ultrasonography.

Dogs and cats with moderate to severe thrombocytopenia (platelet counts $<80 \times 10^9/\mu l$), dogs with prolonged one-stage prothrombin time (OSPT >1.5 x normal) and cats with prolonged activated partial thromboplastin time (APTT >1.5 x normal) had a greater risk of haemorrhage from ultrasound-guided biopsy procedures in one study (Bigge *et al.*, 2001). Severe azotaemia (serum creatinine >442 µmol/l (4.99 mg/dl)), uncontrolled systemic hypertension, administration of

Chronic kidney disease late stage III and stage IV
Severe azotaemia (serum creatinine >442 µmol/l (4.99 mg/dl))
Severe anaemia
Uncorrectable coagulopathy
Administration of NSAID within previous 5 days
Uncontrolled hypertension
Severe hydronephrosis
Large or multiple renal cysts
Perirenal abscess
Extensive pyelonephritis
Inexperienced operator
Incomplete patient immobilization

12.2 Contraindications for renal biopsy.

Percutaneous

Ultrasound guidance
Preferred method for dogs >5 kg and all cats
Blind or palpation technique
Better suited for cats; rarely performed in dogs
Keyhole technique
Used in dogs when ultrasound guidance not available
Laparoscopy
Requires specialized equipment and expertise; preferred method of some clinicians

Surgical

Wedge biopsy
Preferred method for dogs <5 kg; animals with isolated areas of kidney that need to be avoided; or animals undergoing laparotomy for another reason

12.3 Methods used to obtain renal biopsy specimens.

a non-steroidal anti-inflammatory drug (NSAID) within the previous 5 days and operator inexperience also may increase the risk of patient haemorrhage. These patient abnormalities may not be absolute contraindications to renal biopsy; however, the clinician should be prepared to monitor such patients for severe haemorrhage following the biopsy and have suitable blood products from a compatible donor available to administer to the patient if needed.

Severe hydronephrosis is a contraindication to renal biopsy because of the possibility that the needle might penetrate a distended renal pelvis that is under increased pressure, and the increased risk of transecting the larger arteries located in the corticomedullary junction and the medulla. Kidney biopsy is generally not recommended when there are large or multiple renal cysts because biopsy might induce renal pain or renal cyst infection, and a specimen that contains large cysts may have limited diagnostic value. Renal pain develops after rupture of the cyst because of release of cystic fluid into the perirenal tissues. While the risk of inducing cyst infections through renal biopsy is low, poor antibiotic penetration into the cyst fluid makes these infections particularly difficult to treat.

Perirenal abscessation and extensive pyelonephritis are contraindications to renal biopsy because of the possibility of seeding the abdomen with bacteria or other infectious agents. Ideally, urinary tract infections should be eliminated prior to renal biopsy. Some authors have included a solitary kidney as a contraindication to biopsy; however, this may be performed if proper technique is used and other contraindications are not present.

Procurement of the specimen

Renal biopsy samples can be obtained using one of several techniques (Figure 12.3). Regardless of the method selected, only cortical tissue should be obtained. In most cases, evaluation of cortical tissue alone is diagnostic. When the kidney is penetrated more deeply, the risk of serious haemorrhage increases if the corticomedullary junction, medulla or

pelvis is penetrated because renal vessels progressively increase in size from the surface of the kidney towards the renal pelvis. Furthermore, biopsy of the medulla has been reported to cause large areas of infarction and fibrosis (Osborne *et al.*, 1972; Nash *et al.*, 1983).

If possible, the biopsy specimen should be taken from either the cranial or caudal pole of the kidney because it is easier to stay in a larger portion of cortex in these locations. In the dog with generalized renal disease, the right kidney is often preferred over the left kidney for renal biopsy because it is more stable, as the caudate lobe of the liver provides resistance to movement during the biopsy procedure. Conversely, the left kidney is more movable during the procedure but can be found in a more caudal position, providing easier access in some deep-chested dogs. Feline kidneys are located more caudally in the abdomen compared with canine kidneys. Both feline kidneys can be easily localized and immobilized making both equally suitable for renal biopsy.

Once collected, renal biopsy specimens should be divided into three pieces, each of which contains glomeruli. The largest piece should be placed in formalin, a smaller piece should go into a fixative suitable for electron microscopy (e.g. 4% formalin plus 1% glutaraldehyde in sodium phosphate buffer) and another small piece should either be frozen or placed in a fixative suitable for immunofluorescent microscopy (e.g. ammonium sulphate-N-ethylmaleimide fixative, also known as Michel's solution). While light microscopy may be highly suggestive of a particular glomerular disease, particularly with more advanced disease, electron microscopy is required to verify the presence of deposits, to detect small deposits not evident by light microscopy, to identify the location of the deposits in the glomerulus (subendothelial, subepithelial, intramembranous, mesangial) and to detect basement membrane or podocyte abnormalities. Immunofluorescent microscopy is used to determine the specific nature of the immune deposits (IgG, IgA, IgM, complement) and further defines the disease process.

Patient sedation or anaesthesia

The patient must be immobilized if proper renal biopsy technique is to be used. The likelihood that serious complications will develop may increase if the patient is not properly immobilized. Providing general anaesthesia to the patient also allows for the procurement of a higher quality biopsy specimen (Vaden *et al.*, 2005). General anaesthesia is most likely to produce complete immobilization of the patient. Although some very ill patients may be immobilized by sedatives alone, incomplete anaesthesia of the peritoneum may result in sudden abdominal movement during the biopsy procedure.

Percutaneous renal biopsy

Percutaneous renal biopsy can be performed using one of several techniques, all of which use a needle to obtain the biopsy specimens. Many needles are available in various gauges and lengths that theoretically could be used for renal biopsy. The authors prefer either a 16 or 18-gauge needle that is 9 cm in length for renal biopsy. Use of a 14-gauge biopsy needle was associated with a greater likelihood that biopsy specimens contained medulla in one study (Vaden *et al.*, 2005). The selected needle should be one in which the cannula does not move deeper into the tissue during activation. Needles that have throw mechanisms that go beyond where the tip of the needle is placed at the beginning of the procedure allow for limited control of the depth of the biopsy and may be associated with an increased risk of penetration of the needle into the medulla.

While the Tru-cut biopsy needle was once the needle of choice for renal biopsy, it is no longer recommended because it can be difficult to use and improper technique can yield poor-quality specimens and result in unnecessary trauma to the kidney. Likewise, the Vim-Silverman needle is no longer routinely used for renal biopsy. The authors prefer disposable spring-loaded biopsy needles. These needles can easily be operated using only one hand. The spring-loaded stylet of the needle, which is visible by ultrasonography, is advanced first. The cutting cannula is activated when the operator fully depresses the plunger. The specimen is retrieved from the specimen notch when the needle is removed from the animal. Alternatively, automatic spring-loaded biopsy guns can be used. These guns are loaded with disposable needles of appropriate gauges and lengths that are available from a variety of manufacturers. The weight and size of the gun can make its use more difficult when compared with the spring-loaded biopsy needle. The operator needs to have large, strong hands and experience with the needle to use the gun single-handedly with ease.

Obtaining a good quality biopsy specimen with limited damage to the kidney requires the use of a sharp biopsy needle. A small stab incision through the skin at the entry site for the biopsy needle keeps the needle sharp as it passes through the skin. Because needles become dull after several biopsies are performed, and the needles are relatively inexpensive, re-use of these disposable needles is generally not recommended. Prior to activation of the cutting mecha-nism, the tip of the needle should be placed through the renal capsule to prevent sliding of the needle along the capsule and to avoid tearing the capsule. However, care should be taken not to penetrate too deeply beyond the renal capsule prior to activation as this may limit the amount of cortex in the sample. In most cases, at least two quality cortical samples should be obtained when a percutaneous method is used. After biopsy, digital pressure should be applied to the kidney trans-abdominally for approximately 5 minutes to minimize haemorrhage.

Percutaneous biopsy using ultrasound guidance

Percutaneous renal biopsy using ultrasound guidance (Figure 12.4) is the renal biopsy method of choice for dogs that are larger than 5 kg and for all cats that do not have other contraindications for renal biopsy. Ultrasonography is used to identify and examine the kidneys, establish that many of the contraindications for renal biopsy are not present, and guide correct placement of the biopsy needle through the cortex. While the relative hyperechogenicity of the normal renal cortex allows for easy differentiation from the medulla, differentiation may be more difficult in diseased kidneys.

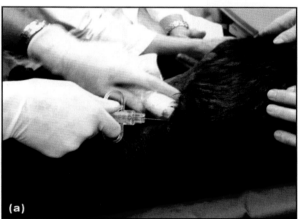

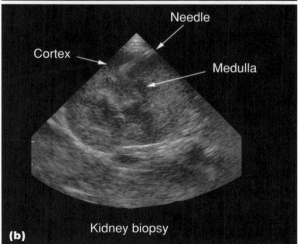

12.4 **(a)** Ultrasound-guided renal biopsy in a dog. Note that the probe is held in one hand while the needle is held in the other hand. **(b)** The ultrasonographic image of the dog in (a). This image is used to guide the needle to the kidney and through the cortex. (Reprinted from Vaden SL (2004) with permission from Elsevier.)

The patient is placed in left lateral recumbency for biopsy of the right kidney or in right lateral recumbency for biopsy of the left kidney. The hair over the biopsy site is removed, the skin is aseptically prepared and sterile coupling gel is applied. A sterile sleeve is placed over the ultrasound probe. The kidneys are scanned for general examination of the renal architecture and for selection of the biopsy site. The tip of the needle is guided through the stab incision in the skin and to and through the renal capsule with one hand while the probe is held with the other (see Figure 12.4). The biopsy specimen is taken using the method that is appropriate for the selected needle, making sure that the needle remains in the renal cortex (Figure 12.5). Although some clinicians prefer to use the needle guides that are available for the ultrasound probe, the authors do not use these. The guides are probe-specific and not available for all probes. Some ultrasonographers find the guides to be confining. The requirement of specific computer software for operation of the guides can make their usage rather expensive.

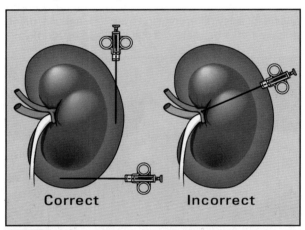

12.5 Schematic demonstrating the correct and incorrect method of directing the renal biopsy needle. Note that the needle should remain in the renal cortex, preferably in either the cranial or caudal pole. The needle should not cross the corticomedullary junction nor enter either the renal medulla or pelvis. (Reprinted from Vaden SL (2004) with permission from Elsevier.)

Blind or palpation technique

Performing renal biopsy with guidance by palpation is rarely done in dogs because their kidneys are more cranially located and can be difficult to immobilize by palpation. Blind biopsy is more frequently performed in feline kidneys, which are relatively more caudal in position and more easily immobilized. With the cat in lateral recumbency, the uppermost kidney is localized by palpation. The hair is clipped from the area over the kidney and the skin is aseptically prepared. A small stab incision is made through the skin. While one hand immobilizes the kidney, the other hand advances the needle through the stab incision and directs it towards the cranial or caudal pole of the kidney. The tip of the needle is stabbed just through the capsule, making sure the angle is such that the needle will pass only through renal cortex. The cutting mechanism of the needle is then activated.

Keyhole technique

The keyhole technique can be used in dogs if ultrasound guidance is not available. The dog is placed in left lateral recumbency for biopsy of the right kidney. The dog's back should be facing the surgeon. The hair in the lumbar fossa is clipped and the skin is aseptically prepared. An oblique, paralumbar 7.5–10 cm skin incision is made on a line that bisects the angle between the last rib and the edge of the lumbar musculature. If the incision is made too far caudal or ventral, it may be impossible to palpate the kidney. If the incision is made too far dorsal, a large, vascular muscle mass will need to be dissected. An incision that is too cranial may lead to puncture of the intercostal artery. The muscle fibres are separated along muscle planes and the peritoneum is incised. The peritoneal incision must be large enough to allow for easy insertion of the surgeon's index finger over the caudal pole of the kidney. The index finger holds the kidney against the edge of the lumbar musculature. The other hand inserts the biopsy needle through a separate small stab incision in the lateral body wall. The biopsy needle is guided into the peritoneal cavity and the tip of the needle is stabbed just through the capsule making sure the angle is such that the needle will pass only through renal cortex. The needle cutting mechanism is activated as appropriate for the selected needle.

The need to displace the kidney a considerable distance prior to biopsy when the keyhole technique is used may be the cause of artefacts that are sometimes reported in samples obtained with this method (e.g. peritubular and glomerular capillary congestion and extravasation of erythrocytes into the tubular lumina and Bowman's space).

Laparoscopic biopsy

Laparoscopy is a rigid endoscopic procedure performed under sterile conditions that is used to examine the peritoneal cavity after establishment of a pneumoperitoneum. Laparoscopy offers an advantage over the other percutaneous biopsy techniques in that direct visualization and inspection of the kidneys through insertion of the laparoscope allows for visual control of the biopsy. Visualization of the kidneys increases the chance that biopsy will yield diagnostic tissue, particularly if focal lesions are present. When compared with surgery, laparoscopy is less invasive and can be performed more quickly, allowing for comparatively less patient morbidity. Like surgery, other abdominal organs can be inspected and biopsy specimens collected, if necessary, although complete abdominal exploration is not possible. Haemorrhage following biopsy can be monitored during laparoscopy and direct pressure can be applied with the laparoscope or laparoscopic tools if needed. Laparoscopy requires appropriate equipment and operator expertise.

Contraindications specific to laparoscopy include peritonitis, extensive abdominal adhesions, hernias, obesity, coagulopathies and operator inexperience. Creation of air emboli, pneumothorax or subcutaneous emphysema, the introduction of gas into a hollow viscus, damage to internal organs with the Verres needle or trocar and cardiac arrest are reported complications of laparoscopy. Evacuation of the urinary bladder and colon prior to penetration into the abdomen will reduce the chance that these organs are punctured. Operator experience and attention to detail, as well as the use of a surgically placed port instead of the Verres needle, may reduce the risk of these complications. None of these complications were reported in either of two studies of laparoscopic renal biopsy performed in dogs and cats (Grauer *et al.*, 1983; Vaden *et al.*, 2005).

Laparoscopy can be performed through a right lateral, left lateral or midline incision. The right kidney is readily visible in dogs in left lateral recumbency. To separate the abdominal wall from the organs, a pneumoperitoneum is created via injection of carbon dioxide through the Verres needle or a surgically placed trocar and cannula unit. If the Verres needle technique is used, the trocar and cannula unit for the laparoscope are then inserted through a small (1 cm) skin incision. Once the assembly is in the abdomen, the trocar is removed from the cannula and replaced by the laparoscope. The abdominal organs can be systematically inspected. A biopsy needle can then be introduced into the abdomen through a separate site. The renal biopsy is performed while observing the procedure through the laparoscope.

Surgical biopsy

Surgical biopsy may be the preferred method in dogs that are small (<5 kg) or in animals that either have isolated areas in the kidney (e.g. large cysts) that need to be avoided during the biopsy procedure or are undergoing laparotomy for another reason. Likewise, surgical biopsy may be safer in some animals that have other listed contraindications to biopsy. A surgical wedge biopsy is preferred over a surgical needle biopsy because of better control over the depth of biopsy and the volume of tissue collected with a wedge biopsy. Surgical wedge biopsy specimens were five times more likely to be of good quality than were surgical needle biopsy specimens in one study (Vaden *et al.*, 2005).

The surgical biopsy can be obtained through a paracostal incision, if only one kidney is to be examined and a biopsy performed, or a cranial midline abdominal incision if other intra-abdominal procedures are to be performed or both kidneys need to be examined prior to biopsy. The paracostal incision is made with the patient in lateral recumbency. The incision is parallel and 2 cm caudal to the last rib. The oblique muscles are divided between fibres and retracted. The kidney is located after separating the transverse abdominal muscle.

The kidney can be elevated through the incision by placing umbilical tape around both poles. Exposure of the kidney may be difficult through the paracostal incision if the animal is obese. Following exposure, the kidney is immobilized with thumb and forefinger prior to biopsy. A wedge-shaped incision is made through the capsule and into the cortex. Tissue forceps are used gently to lift the biopsy wedge while the scalpel blade is used to sever any remaining attachments. Monofilament, absorbable suture material (e.g. 1.5 metric (4/0

USP)) in a simple continuous pattern is used to close the renal capsule. Pressure is applied with thumb and forefinger to appose the edges during suturing.

Care of the patient following renal biopsy

During the first several hours after renal biopsy, isotonic fluids should be given intravenously in amounts needed to produce diuresis. Theoretically, this will decrease the chance that blood clots will form in the renal pelvis or ureter and cause obstruction to urine flow. The patient should be kept relatively quiet and in the hospital for 24 hours after biopsy to reduce the risk of serious haemorrhage that may occur if the blood clot becomes dislodged from the biopsy site. The patient's packed cell volume should be evaluated 24 hours after biopsy in all animals or sooner if a concern arises that major bleeding is occurring. Dogs should be walked only on a leash for 72 hours after biopsy. The colour of urine should be monitored for several days after renal biopsy. Gross haematuria is common after renal biopsy and usually resolves within 24 hours. Persistent gross haematuria warrants re-evaluation of the kidneys and biopsy site.

Complications

Renal biopsy minimally affects renal function and the frequency of severe complications is relatively low when proper technique is employed (Osborne, 1971; Jeraj *et al.*, 1982; Grauer *et al.*, 1983; Hager *et al.*, 1985; Wise *et al.*, 1989; Leveille *et al.*, 1993; Minkus *et al.*, 1994; Groman *et al.*, 2004; Vaden *et al.*, 2005). While complications following renal biopsy are limited, reported frequency has varied between 1% and 18% (Figure 12.6). Differences in biopsy technique and patient status at the time of biopsy undoubtedly contribute to this wide range of reported complication rates. Patient factors that are reported in association with the development of complications in dogs include age

Arteriovenous fistula formation

Biopsy of non-renal tissue (e.g. liver, adrenal gland, fat, muscle, connective tissue, spleen)

Cyst formation

Death

Haemorrhage:
    Microscopic haematuria
    Macroscopic haematuria
    Perirenal haematoma
    Intrarenal haematoma
    Intra-abdominal haemorrhage due to laceration of vessel or other organ or vessel

Hydronephrosis

Infarction and thrombosis

Infection

Scar formation and fibrosis

12.6 Reported complications of renal biopsy.

(>4 years), body weight (<5 kg) and presence of severe azotaemia (serum creatinine >442 μmol/l (4.99 mg/dl)) (Vaden *et al.*, 2005). In one study, having a radiologist or internist perform the biopsy appeared to be associated with the development of complications (Vaden *et al.*, 2005). The use of percutaneous methods to collect the renal biopsy samples or sedation or injectable anaesthesia instead of general anaesthesia may have led to this association.

Between 20% and 70% of dogs and cats are reported to develop microscopic haematuria after renal biopsy (Minkus *et al.*, 1994; Vaden *et al.*, 2005). Microscopic haematuria is self-limiting, generally resolving within 48–72 hours. Macroscopic haematuria is less common, developing in approximately 1–4% of dogs and cats after renal biopsy. If the kidneys are examined carefully by ultrasonography after biopsy, small perirenal haematomas are identified commonly. Severe haemorrhage, often severe enough to require blood transfusion, was the most common reported complication in one study, occurring in 9.9% of dogs and 16.9% of cats (Vaden *et al.*, 2005). Hydronephrosis developing secondary to obstruction of the renal pelvis or ureter by a blood clot is an uncommon complication of renal biopsy. Death from renal biopsy is also uncommon, occurring in 3% or fewer dogs and cats.

Histological changes following renal biopsy have been well documented. Linear infarcts representing needle tracts associated with varying amounts of atrophy and fibrosis appear to be common after renal biopsy. Retention cysts can also be found in association with the needle tract and probably form secondary to tubular obstruction (Sweet *et al.*, 1969). Severe renal parenchymal changes of haemorrhage, thrombosis, infarction and fibrosis correlate with the presence of major renal vessels or medulla in the biopsy specimen (Osborne *et al.*, 1972; Nash *et al.*, 1983). Performing multiple kidney biopsies does not appear to produce more damage than a single biopsy, providing the biopsy needle remains in cortical tissue (Nash *et al.*, 1986).

Despite renal histological changes, renal biopsy had minimal effect on renal function in one study (Drost *et al.*, 2000). However, the effect of renal biopsy on the kidney should not be taken lightly. It is possible that renal biopsy in an animal with pre-existing renal disease could contribute to progressive loss of renal function in association with some of these major histological changes.

Morphological classification of renal disease

The normal renal cortex contains scattered glomeruli and numerous tubules within a scant interstitium (Figure 12.7). Most of the tubules in the cortex are proximal as the proximal tubule is much longer than the distal tubule. Proximal tubules have microvilli, have a larger diameter, contain fewer cells and are more numerous in cross-section due to their longer length. Distal tubules have more closely packed cells, the cells are cuboidal and they have a sharper luminal border.

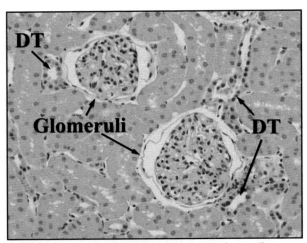

12.7 Normal renal cortex containing glomeruli, tubular cross-sections and scant interstitium. Most tubular profiles are proximal in origin, with fewer distal tubules (DT) present. (H&E stain; original magnification X100)

Tubules are normally in close apposition, as the normal cortical interstitium contains only peritubular capillaries, scant matrix and scattered interstitial cells. All of these renal components are initially evaluated in slides stained with haematoxylin and eosin (H&E) in order to determine lesion distribution, severity and the primary site of renal disease (interstitial or glomerular).

Non-glomerular causes of acute renal failure such as acute tubular necrosis (ATN) and acute tubulointerstitial nephritis may be diagnosed using routine H&E stains (Figure 12.8). ATN may be caused by ischaemic or toxic insults. Ischaemic ATN is difficult to detect histologically, as the morphological lesions are focal and mild. The injury usually results in sublethal cell injury, seen as cell swelling, brush border loss and tubular dilation. This type of injury is due to decreased renal blood flow associated with hypotension/ shock, blood loss, hypovolaemia or sepsis. While

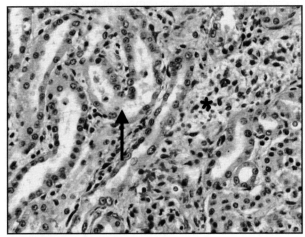

12.8 Acute tubular necrosis in a dog with acute leptospirosis. Proximal tubules are dilated with attenuation of the epithelium, brush border loss and occasional sloughing of necrotic epithelial cells into the lumen (arrowed). The tubules are no longer touching due to expansion of the interstitium with oedema and erythrocytes (*). (H&E stain; original magnification X200)

ischaemic ATN is a common cause of acute renal failure in people, it is rarely documented in animals. Dogs with acute septicaemic leptospirosis, prior to the development of serum antibody titres and interstitial nephritis, may develop icterus and severe acute renal failure with only mild acute tubular degeneration histologically (see Figure 12.8); this ATN is attributed to both ischaemia and toxic factors released by the spirochaetes (Davila de Arriaga *et al.*, 1982).

Nephrotoxic ATN is more commonly recognized in dogs and cats. Tubular epithelial necrosis primarily affects the proximal tubule with the severity of the necrosis dependent on the offending toxin/toxicant (Figure 12.9). The susceptibility of the proximal tubule cells to toxic injury is a reflection of their large microvillus surface area, their high oxygen requirements and their normal absorptive and excretory function, which may actually lead to excretion of toxins/toxicants into this segment.

The cortical interstitium is inconspicuous in the normal kidney and tubules are in close apposition. The cortical interstitial compartment may be expanded by oedema, blood (see Figure 12.8), inflammatory (Figure 12.10a) or neoplastic cells, or fibrous connective

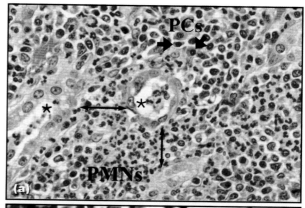

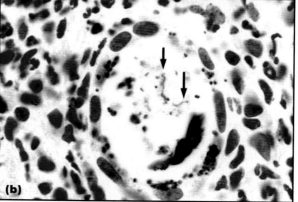

12.10 **(a)** Subacute puruloplasmacytic tubulointerstitial nephritis in a dog with leptospirosis. Tubules are separated (double arrows) by large numbers of neutrophils (PMNs), plasma cells (PCs, arrowed) and fewer macrophages. Neutrophils are also present within tubules (⋆). (H&E stain; original magnification X200) **(b)** Typical positive leptospiral immunohistochemistry, showing clumps of positive staining material in interstitial macrophages, tubular epithelial cells and the tubular lumen. Intact spirochaetes (arrowed) are also present within the tubular lumen. (Avidin-biotin-peroxidase method, haematoxylin counterstain; original magnification X400)

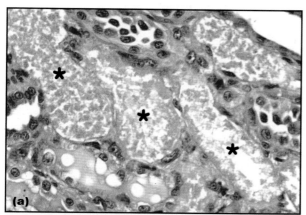

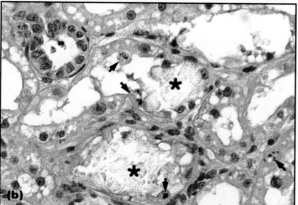

12.9 **(a)** Toxic acute tubular necrosis in a cat with Easter lily toxicosis. Segments of the proximal tubule are devoid of viable epithelium, and are lined or filled with necrotic cellular debris (⋆). **(b)** Toxic acute tubular necrosis in a cat with ethylene glycol toxicosis. Tubules are mildly dilated and the epithelium is attenuated with individual cell necrosis and karyorrhexis (arrowed). Histological diagnosis is dependent on the finding of large numbers of oxalate crystals (⋆) within tubules. (H&E stain; original magnification X400)

tissue, resulting in separation of the tubules. Tubulointerstitial diseases in cats and dogs are often infectious in aetiology, and some of these infectious diseases, such as feline infectious peritonitis and subacute leptospirosis, may be confirmed with immunohistochemical staining (Figure 12.10b). Interstitial fibrosis, recognizable with H&E stains, is better appreciated with a Masson's trichrome stain. Fibrosis is indicative of chronic disease, and the severity of fibrosis is positively correlated with the degree of renal dysfunction. Interstitial fibrosis is a poor prognostic indicator, as it is associated with irreversible renal injury and nephron loss.

The glomerulus is a tuft of highly branched capillaries that invaginate into an extension of the proximal tubule. The afferent arteriole enters and arborizes to form the glomerular capillary tuft and exits as the efferent arteriole; these arterioles enter and exit at the vascular pole (Figure 12.11). The capillary loops are supported by scaffolding made up of mesangial cells and their surrounding extracellular mesangial matrix. The capillary tuft is draped by glomerular basement membrane (GBM), and is covered by a layer of inter-

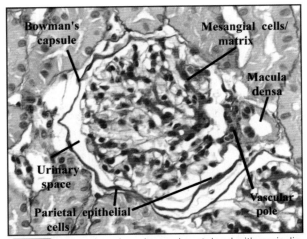

12.11 Normal canine glomerulus stained with periodic acid–Schiff haematoxylin (PASH). The basement membranes of Bowman's capsule, tubules and the glomerular capillaries, and the mesangial matrix stain dark pink. (PASH stain; original magnification X400)

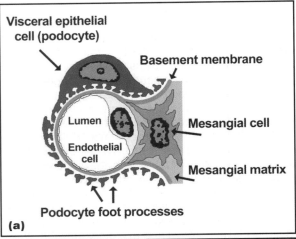

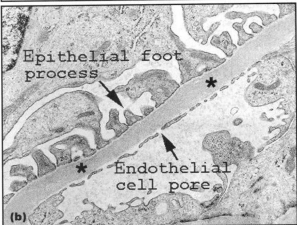

12.12 **(a)** Diagram of normal glomerular capillary. **(b)** Electron micrograph of the normal glomerular capillary wall. Note the fenestrated capillary endothelium that results in endothelial cell pores, the glomerular basement membrane (∗) and the podocyte foot processes. (Reprinted from Vaden SL (2005) with permission from Elsevier. Original images courtesy of JC Jennette, Chapel Hill, NC, School of Medicine, University of North Carolina.)

digitating visceral epithelial cells (podocytes). The glomerular filtration barrier consists of endothelium, GBM and podocytes (Figure 12.12). Proteinuria results when there is disruption of the filtration barrier, which may be caused by the deposition of immune complexes, complement or amyloid, by a change (either acquired or congenital) in the composition of the GBM, or by injury to the endothelial cells or podocytes. Glomerular injury may also affect mesangial cells, resulting in mesangial cell proliferation and/or increased production of mesangial matrix. Injury primarily affecting mesangial cells is not typically associated with significant proteinuria.

Glomerular involvement seen by light microscopy may be focal (less than 50% of glomeruli involved) or generalized (all or almost all glomeruli involved). Within an affected glomerulus, the lesion may be segmental (only part of the capillary tuft affected) or global (the entire tuft involved). While most glomerular diseases in dogs and cats are generalized and global, focal segmental disease may also occur.

The goal of renal biopsy in glomerular diseases is to identify accurately the specific changes occurring in the glomerulus in order to determine the prognosis and potential treatment options for the identified glomerular disease. The number of glomeruli present in the biopsy specimens should be recorded as a measure of the adequacy of the biopsy; a minimum of five glomeruli should be present. Glomeruli should be evaluated for cellularity, matrix increase, amyloid deposition, hyalinization, necrosis, fibrin thrombosis, crescents, protein deposits, adhesions and glomerular basement membrane changes. As thicker sections will appear more cellular, have more mesangial matrix and have thicker capillary loops, renal biopsy specimens should be routinely sectioned and evaluated at 2–3 μm. Biopsy samples with glomerular deposits suggestive of amyloid (Figure 12.13) should be cut at 7 μm, stained with Congo red or standard toluidine blue, and viewed with polarized light to confirm this diagnosis.

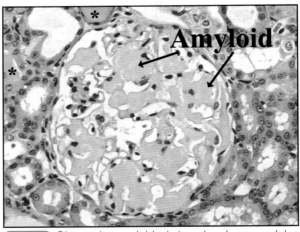

12.13 Glomerular amyloidosis in a dog. Large nodular accumulations of eosinophilic homogenous material (amyloid, arrowed) displace nuclei to the periphery. Glassy eosinophilic casts (∗), indicative of proteinuria, are present in distal tubules. (H&E stain; original magnification X400)

Periodic acid–Schiff haematoxylin (PASH) and Masson's trichrome stains, in addition to H&E, should be used when evaluating glomerular morphology in diseases other than amyloidosis. Basement membrane, mesangial matrix and cell cytoplasm (including podocytes and endothelium) stain pink with PASH, and trichrome stains basement membrane blue, immune deposits within the capillary walls magenta and mesangial matrix (type IV collagen) blue–grey. In the normal glomerulus stained with PASH (see Figure 12.11), the thickness of the capillary walls should be assessed in peripheral capillary loops, and when cut at a right angle the normal loops will be thin, uniform and crisp. The mesangial matrix can be seen as disconnected branches containing mesangial cells. Matrix typically surrounds one or two mesangial cell nuclei; mesangial matrix expansion is present if matrix extends to encircle more cells. More than three mesangial cell nuclei in close proximity are indicative of mesangial hyperplasia.

Membranous glomerulonephritis (MGN) (Figure 12.14) and membranoproliferative glomerulonephritis (MPGN) (Figure 12.15) are immune-mediated diseases associated with the deposition of immune complexes and/or complement in the glomerulus. Immune complexes may be observed on either side of the glomerular basement membrane, in the mesangium or in a combination of these sites (see Figure 12.12). Immune complexes are thought to occur in these areas primarily via *in situ* formation – the antigen is filtered across the endothelium, but then 'sticks' or implants within the glomerulus due to characteristics of the antigen (i.e. size, charge). The implanted antigen then combines with antibody, forming antigen–antibody complexes. Alternatively, there may be trapping of preformed circulating immune complexes. Changes in the filtration barrier and consequent proteinuria are the result of the response to these immune complexes.

In MGN, complexes are present on the subepithelial side of the basement membrane and induce the

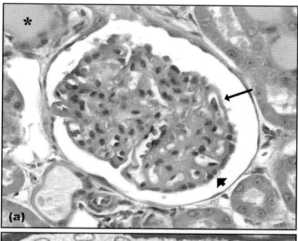

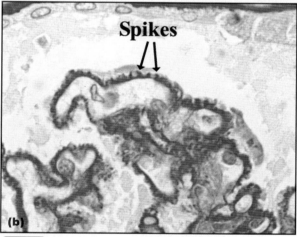

12.14 Membranous glomerulonephritis (MGN) in a cat. **(a)** MGN is characterized by normal glomerular cellularity with thickening of the capillary loops (long arrow). In this cat, podocytes (short arrow) are hypertrophied, which is a non-specific change that may be associated with protein leakage. (H&E stain; original magnification X400) **(b)** PASH stain demonstrating well developed subepithelial spikes that form around unstained immune deposits. (PASH stain; original magnification X600)

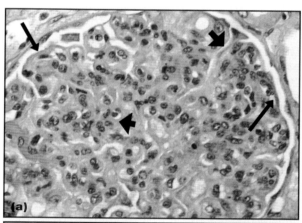

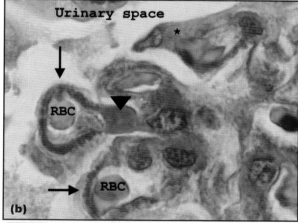

12.15 Membranoproliferative glomerulonephritis (MPGN) in a dog. **(a)** MPGN is characterized by glomerular hypercellularity (short arrows) and thickening of the capillary loops (long arrows). (H&E stain; original magnification X400) **(b)** Trichrome stain demonstrating large magenta deposits within capillary walls (arrowed), with fine deposits also present in mesangial areas (arrowhead). Podocyte hypertrophy (*) is also present. Erythrocytes (RBCs) are present in the capillary lumen. Mesangial matrix and basement membrane stain blue with this stain. (Masson's Trichrome stain; original magnification X600)

production of more basement membrane material, which may eventually incorporate the immune deposits. The cellularity of the tuft remains normal. With light microscopy, the capillary loops are prominent, and spikes may be evident with PASH as the basement membrane extends between the unstained immune deposits (see Figure 12.14).

In MPGN, the immune complexes are present on the subendothelial aspect of the glomerular basement membrane (and may also be present in subepithelial and/or mesangial areas), and in this location they are associated with proliferation of resident glomerular cells (see Figure 12.15a). With trichrome stain, magenta immune deposits may be observed (see Figure 12.15b). Glomerular crescents occur in some cases of MPGN, and are indicative of severe injury to the capillary wall. Breaks or gaps in the GBM allow the passage of fibrinogen, and later macrophages, into the urinary space. Fibrin and macrophages induce parietal epithelial cell proliferation, and glomerular crescents form. Glomerular diseases with significant crescent formation are typically more severe and have a rapidly progressive clinical course.

While light microscopy may be highly suggestive of MPN or MPGN, particularly with more advanced disease, electron microscopy is required to verify the presence of deposits, to detect small deposits not evident by light microscopy, and to identify the location (subendothelial, subepithelial, intramembranous and/or mesangial) of the deposits in the glomerulus. Immunofluorescence further defines the disease process, by determining the specific nature of the immune deposits (IgG, IgA, IgM and/or complement).

Focal segmental glomerulosclerosis (FSGS) is the most common cause of the nephrotic syndrome in adult people, but this lesion is seldom recognized in nephrotic dogs and cats. It differs from amyloidosis and glomerulonephritis in that only some glomeruli are affected (i.e. it is focal) and the lesion affects only a portion of the capillary tuft (i.e. it is segmental). Glomerulosclerosis, which may be focal in nature, also occurs in dogs and cats as a consequence of decreased functioning renal mass in animals with chronic kidney disease, but these animals are not severely proteinuric. On light microscopy, FSGS is characterized by hypercellularity and mesangial expansion of portions of the glomerulus (Figure 12.16). Secondary changes, such as hyalinosis and adhesions of the sclerotic portion of the tuft to Bowman's capsule, are common. With a PASH stain, hyalinosis appears as glassy eosinophilic material in the capillary wall; this material is serum lipoproteins, which have leaked across the damaged portion of the glomerular basement membrane.

Some glomerular diseases are associated with no or non-specific changes on light microscopy, further underscoring the importance of electron microscopy in the diagnosis of glomerular disease. Inherited defects in the structure of the glomerular basement membrane, involving mutations in type IV (basement membrane) collagen, have been described in several breeds of dog. The light microscopic lesions are variable, depending on the stage of the disease, and are non-

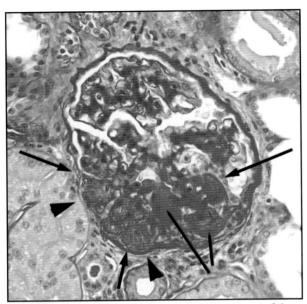

12.16 Glomerulosclerosis in a dog. A segment of the capillary tuft is hypercellular with loss of the capillary spaces (arrowed). The sclerotic segment is adhered to Bowman's capsule (arrowheads) and there are areas of hyalinosis (lines). (PASH stain; original magnification X400)

specific, so diagnosis of this disease is absolutely dependent on electron microscopy. Affected dogs have diffuse irregular splitting of the GBM and foot process effacement (Figure 12.17). Minimal change disease is a disease of podocytes characterized by essentially normal glomeruli on light microscopy with diffuse podocyte foot process effacement on electron microscopy. Minimal change disease is the most common cause of the nephrotic syndrome in children, and accounts for 15–20% of cases in adults. This is an important lesion to detect, as it is steroid-responsive in people and, without treatment, may progress and become non-steroid-responsive.

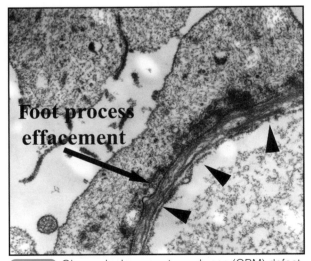

Foot process effacement

12.17 Glomerular basement membrane (GBM) defect in a young dog. Ultrastructurally, the GBM shows diffuse splitting with a multilayered appearance (arrowheads) and spreading (effacement) of the podocyte foot processes.

References and further reading

Bigge LA, Brown DJ and Pennick DG (2001) Correlation between coagulation profile findings and bleeding complications after ultrasound-guided biopsies: 434 cases (1993–1996). *Journal of the American Animal Hospital Association* **37(3)**, 228–233

Davila de Arriaga AJ, Rocha AS, Yasuda PH and De Brito T (1982) Morpho-functional patterns of kidney injury in the experimental leptospirosis of the guinea-pig (*L. icterohaemorrhagiae*). *Journal of Pathology* **138(2)**,145–161

Drost WT, Henry GA, Meinkoth JH *et al.* (2000) The effects of a unilateral ultrasound-guided renal biopsy on renal function in healthy sedated cats. *Veterinary Radiology and Ultrasound* **41**, 57–62

Grauer GF, Twedt DC and Mero KN (1983) Evaluation of laparoscopy for obtaining renal biopsy specimens from dogs and cats. *Journal of the American Veterinary Medical Association* **183(6)**, 677–679

Groman RP, Bahr A, Berridge BR and Lees GE (2004) Effects of serial ultrasound-guided renal biopsies on kidneys of healthy adolescent dogs. *Veterinary Radiology and Ultrasound* **45(1)**, 62–69

Hager DA, Nyland TG and Fisher P (1985) Ultrasound-guided biopsy of the canine liver, kidney and prostate. *Veterinary Radiology* **26**, 82–88

Jeraj K, Osborne CA and Stevens JB (1982) Evaluation of renal biopsy in 197 dogs and cats. *Journal of the American Veterinary Medical Association* **181(4)**, 367–369

Leveille R, Partington BP, Biller DS and Miyabayashi T (1993) Complications after ultrasound-guided biopsy of abdominal structures in dogs and cats: 246 cases (1984–1991). *Journal of the American Veterinary Medical Association* **203(3)**, 413–415

Minkus G, Reusch C, Horauf A *et al.* (1994) Evaluation of renal biopsies in cats and dogs – histopathology in comparison with clinical data. *Journal of Small Animal Practice* **35**, 465–472

Nash AS, Boyd JS, Minto AW and Wright NG (1983) Renal biopsy in the normal cat: an examination of the effects of a single needle biopsy. *Research in Veterinary Science* **34(3)**, 347–356

Nash AS, Boyd JS, Minto AW and Wright NG (1986) Renal biopsy in the normal cat: examination of the effects of repeated needle biopsy. *Research in Veterinary Science* **40(1)**, 112–117

Osborne CA (1971) Clinical evaluation of needle biopsy of the kidney and its complications in the dog and cat. *Journal of the American Veterinary Medical Association* **158(7)**, 1213–1228

Osborne CA, Low DG and Jessen CR (1972) Renal parenchymal response to needle biopsy. *Investigative Urology* **9**, 463–469

Parrish AE (1992) Complications of percutaneous renal biopsy: a review of 37 years' experience. *Clinical Nephrology* **38(3)**, 135–141

Sweet EI, Davidson AJ and Hayslett JP (1969) Complications of needle biopsy of the kidney in the dog. A radiological and pathological correlation. *Radiology* **92(4)**, 849–854

Vaden SL (2004) Renal biopsy: methods and interpretation. *Veterinary Clinics of North America: Small Animal Practice* **34**, 887–908

Vaden SL (2005) Glomerular diseases. In: *Textbook of Veterinary Internal Medicine, 2nd edn*, ed. SJ Ettinger and EC Feldman, pp. 1787–1789. Elsevier

Vaden SL, Levine JF, Lees GE *et al.* (2005) Renal biopsy: a retrospective study of 283 dogs and 65 cats. *Journal of Veterinary Internal Medicine* **19(6)**, 794–801

Wise LA, Allen TA and Cartwright M (1989) Comparison of renal biopsy techniques in dogs. *Journal of the American Veterinary Medical Association* **195(7)**, 935–939

13

Measurement of blood pressure

Rebecca L. Stepien and Jonathan Elliott

Introduction

'Systemic hypertension' (HT) refers to the persistent elevation of systemic arterial blood pressure (BP) and is typically classified as primary ('essential') or secondary HT. In veterinary medicine, secondary HT (hypertension that occurs as a complication of another disease) is by far the most common type. Acute or chronic renal disease is the most common predisposing cause of HT in dogs and cats.

Hypertension in renal disease

Prevalence

Renal disease is a well recognized cause of HT in both dogs and cats. Approximately 60% of dogs with chronic kidney disease and 80–90% of dogs with proteinuria are reported to have systemic HT (Cowgill and Kallet, 1983), although some have reported a lower prevalence (Michell *et al.*, 1997). In cats with renal disease, HT is similarly common and has been documented in approximately 20% (Syme *et al.*, 2002) to 60% (Kobayashi *et al.*, 1990) of cats with naturally occurring chronic kidney disease.

Pathophysiology

Despite the prevalence of kidney disease in many species, the pathophysiology of renal disease-related HT remains unclear. Contributory abnormalities at the level of the kidney include both anatomical and functional changes:

- Inappropriate dilation of the afferent glomerular arteriole is a recognized abnormality in both dogs and cats with renal disease and diminishes the ability of the afferent arteriole to protect the glomerulus from variations in systemic BP
- Diseased nephrons exhibit decreased filtration, impaired sodium excretion and excessive renin secretion that is resistant to feedback mechanisms
- The increased renin secretion stimulates production of angiotensin II and, subsequently, aldosterone. Angiotensin II also has a direct stimulatory effect on the sympathetic nervous system (SNS), increasing vascular tone, and, in the diseased kidney, preferential vasoconstriction of the efferent arteriole

- The combination of renin–angiotensin–aldosterone system (RAAS) activation with SNS stimulation and the kidneys' inability to compensate by increasing sodium excretion leads to increased systemic BP.

Although many individual events in this complicated pathophysiological pathway are not yet well understood in dogs and cats, consideration of the RAAS and SNS contributions to HT in animals with renal disease provides possible mechanistic targets for therapy of HT beyond direct arterial wall relaxation. More research is required to understand the pathophysiology of HT as a complication of kidney disease.

Clinical effects of systemic hypertension

The effects of HT are often insidious, and animals with substantial elevations in BP may not be perceived as having any clinical signs of HT. Although rare, large vessel complications (e.g. dissecting aortic aneurysm) of HT may occur, elevations in BP appear to be most damaging at the capillary level and lead to 'end-organ' damage. End-organ damage may be noted as either:

- Functional change (e.g. ventricular hypertrophy in response to increased afterload, epistaxis due to capillary damage)
- Chronic progressive deterioration of organ function (e.g. progression of glomerular lesions and proteinuria in renal patients with HT)
- Acute catastrophic abnormalities associated with haemorrhage (e.g. hyphaema) or oedema formation (e.g. retinal detachment, cerebral oedema).

The organ systems most at risk for HT-related damage in veterinary patients include those systems which are normally protected from variations in perfusion pressure by local control of vascular tone and include the eyes, brain and kidneys. In these systems, loss of local vasoconstrictive mechanisms paired with increased systemic BP may lead to damage at the capillary level. Although left ventricular hypertrophy has been documented in both people and pet species with HT and regresses with successful antihypertensive therapy, the congestive heart failure and cardiovascular morbidity related to chronic HT in people have not been frequently reported in cats and dogs.

Studies in dogs have established that a sustained systolic BP of >160 mmHg is associated with progressive renal damage and retinal damage, and the degree of BP elevation is related to the degree of damage (Brown *et al.*, 2000). Acute increases in BP most typically result in ocular or neurological signs, but chronic HT may lead to less obvious clinical signs (e.g. gallop rhythm) or clinical signs that may be masked by manifestations of concurrent diseases (e.g. worsening of pre-existing proteinuria) (Figure 13.1). In the kidneys, the magnitude of the increase above 160 mmHg is correlated to the amount of damage that occurs (Finco, 2004). Clinical signs of HT in dogs and cats may be dramatic on occasion (Figure 13.2). Many animals with systemic HT, however, may not exhibit outward clinical abnormalities, or have subtle changes in de-

meanour, appetite or activity that may be attributed by the owner to aging or concurrent systemic illnesses.

Recognition and therapy of HT in renal disease patients may prevent development of catastrophic ocular lesions (Mathur *et al.*, 2002) or may limit or slow progression of end-organ damage (Brown *et al.*, 2001; Snyder *et al.*, 2001; Brown *et al.*, 2003). In the same way that controlling hyperglycaemia in diabetic patients limits clinical signs and progression of disease, therapy of HT in renal patients should be viewed as a method of improving quality of life, avoiding life-threatening crises and slowing progressive renal damage.

Body system	Typical abnormalities
Eyes	Retinal haemorrhage Retinal effusion Retinal detachment Hyphaema Vitreal haemorrhage Vascular tortuosity
Nervous system	Changes in attitude or appetite Evidence of intracranial lesions: • Changes in mentation, usually decreased • Seizures (focal facial or generalized)
Renal system	Decreased urine-concentrating ability Worsening of proteinuria
Cardiovascular system	New murmur, typically mitral insufficiency Arrhythmia Gallop rhythm Left ventricular hypertrophy on echocardiographic examination
Other	Epistaxis

13.1 Typical clinical signs associated with systemic HT, listed by body system. This list is not exhaustive. Animals with renal disease should have BP measurement performed regardless of outward clinical signs.

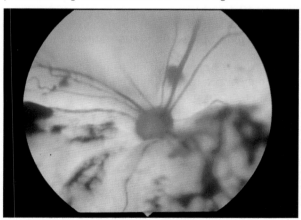

13.2 Hypertensive retinopathy and choroidopathy in a cat. The cat was presented for acute onset of blindness and had a systolic BP of 200 mmHg. The lack of crisp detail in some areas is a result of complete detachment and forward displacement of the retina. Dark areas represent previous, resolving areas of haemorrhage. The red areas on the left side of the image represent more recent haemorrhage. The black spot with the blood vessel crossing it (upper right) represents choroidal haemorrhage.

Measurement of blood pressure

Identification of patient population
Dogs or cats with acute renal failure or chronic kidney disease have a high prevalence of HT and should have their BP evaluated at first identification of the renal abnormalities. Patients with evidence of ocular or intracranial neurological abnormalities (see Figure 13.1) should have their BP evaluated immediately. Diagnosis of systemic HT in patients with acute malignant signs (e.g. retinal detachment, neurological signs) warrants immediate and aggressive antihypertensive therapy with close monitoring until the BP is decreased and clinical signs abate (Figure 13.3). For patients without outward clinical signs of HT, elevated BP values should be confirmed by one or more recheck measurements before commencing antihypertensive therapy.

Hypertensive patients on therapy require periodic re-evaluation of BP. If no outward signs of HT are present, weekly rechecks are recommended until a satisfactory response to therapy is documented. When a satisfactory result is confirmed, BP should be re-evaluated at least every 3 months unless problems develop sooner. Chronic kidney disease patients without HT at the time of diagnosis should have their BP monitored over time for development of HT.

Documentation of measurements
BP is discussed in terms of systolic and diastolic values. In people, combined HT (systolic and diastolic values elevated), isolated systolic and isolated diastolic HT have differing morbidity and mortality rates, but systolic BP elevations are stronger measures for predicting renal, cerebrovascular and cardiovascular risk than diastolic BP elevations. Little information about the prevalence and importance of diastolic HT in dogs and cats is available and some commonly used measurement systems (i.e. Doppler sphygmomanometry) do not provide reliable diastolic BP readings, rendering *systolic BP* the most frequently discussed BP value in veterinary clinical use.

Regardless of the technique used, the value reported as representative of a BP recording event should be the average of multiple serial measurements. If a representative value needs to be recorded from a continuous arterial BP monitoring system, a paper recording of at least five cardiac cycles should be printed and measured with the final value calculated as

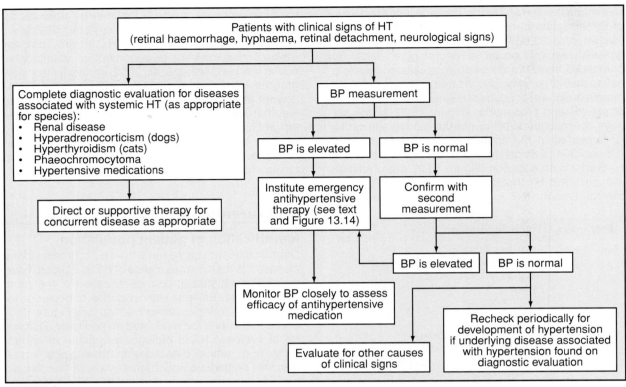

13.3 Suggested BP evaluation sequence for dogs or cats with clinical signs of systemic HT.

the average of five systolic and diastolic values. If required, the mean arterial pressure (MAP) values can be estimated using the following formula:

$$MAP = DBP + (0.3 \times [SBP-DBP])$$

where DBP is diastolic blood pressure and SBP is systolic blood pressure.

When non-invasive methods are used, the first reading is typically discarded, and the mean of three to five measurements, with 30 seconds to 1 minute between readings, is recorded as the representative BP. In all cases, the technique used and the cuff size and position (if applicable) should be recorded with the results. Recording the heart rate during measurement may assist in interpretation of results.

Standardizing measurement techniques

Consistency and attention to the technique of BP measurement is more important than which method is used. Most important is standardization of the procedure in the clinic; BP should be measured the same way in similar patients (e.g. anaesthetized *versus* conscious *versus* critically ill). Ideally, one or two operators are responsible for this diagnostic procedure in a clinic and should be trained to perform the test and record the results uniformly. For each BP measurement session, the following information should be recorded:

- Date and time of measurement
- Technique used (if more than one technique is available)

- Cuff size (if non-invasive technique)
- Measurement site (specify which leg *versus* tail)
- Present medications, last date/time of administration
- Previous BP measurement date and results
- Heart rate matched to each BP reading (see techniques).

Overview of measurement techniques

For an overview of measurement techniques see Figures 13.4 and 13.5.

Invasive blood pressure measurement

- Invasive BP measurement, using either acute arterial puncture or an indwelling arterial catheter, provides the most accurate measurement of actual intra-arterial pressure.
- The invasiveness of acute arterial puncture combined with the increased level of technical capability necessary for this technique make it impractical for use on typical clinical outpatients. For occasional patients in which precise knowledge of arterial pressure is needed, acute arterial puncture is feasible by an experienced practitioner.

Non-invasive blood pressure measurement

- Oscillometric methods employ a cuff positioned on a limb or at the tailhead. The cuff is automatically inflated and deflated according to machine settings and displays a numerical result

Factor	Direct (arterial puncture)	Doppler	Oscillometric
Measurement principle	Direct measurement of intra-arterial pressure	Detects movement of blood cells (blood flow)	Detects vibrations (oscillations in the blood vessel wall)
Output	Pressure trace with machine-read numerical systolic, diastolic and mean pressure with heart rate	Systolic BP only (estimates of diastolic pressure are unreliable)	Systolic, diastolic and mean BP with heart rate
Cuff and detection system	No cuff required, detection system is a pressure transducer	A cuff and a flow detection device are applied separately	The detection system is incorporated into the cuff
Influence of heart rate	Accurate at all heart rates	Affects precision of measurement if cuff not deflated slowly	Machines will not work accurately at very high heart rates unless specifically adapted to do so
Time taken to obtain consistent results	1–2 minutes after local anaesthetic is injected	Usually takes 5–10 minutes to obtain consistent readings – operator determines whether results are acceptable	May take 15–30 minutes to obtain consistent readings – machine determines whether results are acceptable and provides no output if they are not

13.4 Comparison of various aspects of BP measurement techniques.

Technique	Indications	Contraindications	Advantages	Disadvantages	Comments
Acute arterial puncture (invasive)	Acute, accurate single measurement. Confirm BP in patient with conflicting results or unmeasurable BP by non-invasive methods	Bleeding disorders. Cats	Accurate reflection of instantaneous BP. Maintains accuracy at higher heart rates or during arrhythmias	Technically challenging. May be more stressful for patient. Risk of haemorrhage. Displayed instantaneous numerical data may not match true BP during arrhythmias	Seldom used for clinical BP measurement
Indwelling arterial catheter (invasive)	Continuous BP monitoring in hospitalized patients. During or following anaesthesia. During acute therapy of life-threatening hypertension	More difficult in cats	Continuous reporting. Accurate at any BP. Maintains accuracy at higher heart rates or during arrhythmias. Can be compared with simultaneous ECG. Many monitors may also have oscillometric capabilities	Technical skill required to place and maintain patent catheter. Risk of haemorrhage	Continuous flushing systems prevent catheter clotting
Doppler ultrasonography (non-invasive)	Clinical BP measurement in dogs and cats. Single measurement or intermittent monitoring	None	Most inexpensive of non-invasive methods. Familiar technology to client and clinician. Can be used in dogs and cats	Variable, underestimates systolic BP by 5–20 mmHg. Less accurate at subnormal pressures. Requires prolonged manipulation of paws, resented by some pets. Reliant on subjective skill of person making measurement	Preferred method for cats. Especially useful in nervous and trembling dogs
Oscillometry (non-invasive)	Clinical BP measurement in dogs and cats. Single measurement or monitoring. Dogs, anaesthetized and some conscious cats	More expensive of non-invasive methods. May not read at high heart rates or during arrhythmias	Automated so less reliant on subjective judgement of person making measurement. Automated repeat measurements useful during anaesthetic monitoring. Less 'hands-on' manipulation once cuff is placed. Little technical skill required. Returns immediate numerical results. Can be used in dogs and cats	May not successfully measure values at high heart rates or during arrhythmias. Variable, underestimates systolic BP by 5–20 mmHg. Inaccurate at low BP. Incorrect cuff size or position markedly decrease accuracy	Tailhead most commonly used cuff site for cats

13.5 Indications and contraindications for use and advantages and disadvantages of different BP measurement techniques. Detailed descriptions of measurement techniques are outlined in the text. ECG = Electrocardiogram.

for systolic, mean and diastolic BP, as well as heart rate for each reading. The readings are based on oscillations detected in the arterial wall. Oscillometric methods are most accurate when used in dogs, although accurate measurements can be obtained from cats using tailhead or proximal forelimb cuff sites.

- Doppler sphygmomanometric methods use a cuff placed on a limb or tailhead, with manual or fixed positioning of a piezoelectric crystal over a superficial artery distal to the cuff. The cuff is manually inflated until the audible sound of blood flow in the limb ceases, and then deflated until the sound is heard once again. The BP at the time of recurrence of the sound of blood flow is noted as systolic pressure. Doppler sphygmomanometry can be used in cats or dogs, and is the method of choice in cats.

Technical aspects of measurement

Further details on the technical aspects of BP measurement may be found in Stepien and Rapoport (1999).

Acute arterial puncture

Equipment:

- 1–2 ml of lidocaine hydrochloride in small syringe with a 25–27 gauge needle for local anaesthetic infiltration.
- 20–23 gauge needle attached to a pressure transducer.
- Invasive BP monitor with data screen and printer.
- Hair clippers, if needed.
- Heparinized saline flush (approximately 10 ml) (Figure 13.6).

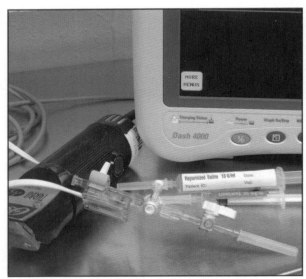

13.6 Equipment required for acute arterial puncture (direct BP measurement). From left: hair clippers, sterile disposable pressure transducer attached to 23-gauge needle, 10 ml heparinized saline, 1–2 ml lidocaine hydrochloride to provide local anaesthesia. Background: haemodynamic monitor with electrocardiogram and invasive and oscillometric BP measurement capabilities.

Technique:

1. Restrain the patient in comfortable lateral recumbency and allow to acclimatize to position.
2. Palpate the femoral arterial pulse in the femoral triangle on the medial proximal thigh and clip hair over site, if necessary.
3. Infiltrate the skin and subcutaneous tissue over the palpable femoral pulse with 1–2 ml of lidocaine hydrochloride, using a small gauge needle to decrease discomfort. Allow the local anaesthetic to take effect (approximately 5 minutes).
4. Attach a 20, 21 or 23-gauge needle (smaller gauge needle for smaller patients) to a pressure transducer attached to a commercial BP monitoring system. Flush the transducer and needle with heparinized saline to be sure no bubbles are present.
5. Zero the transducer at the level of the patient's sternum (right atrial level).
6. Palpate the femoral arterial pulse again, and slowly advance the needle into the artery while watching the pressure tracing on the monitor screen (Figure 13.7). When a waveform is obtained, print a sample of at least five to ten cardiac cycles.
7. Once a tracing has been obtained, withdraw the needle and immediately apply firm manual pressure to the area over the needle puncture for at least 5 minutes to ensure haemostasis.
8. Measure systolic and diastolic BP off the tracing (Figure 13.8). MAP can be calculated as noted above, if desired. Typically, the results of three to five cardiac cycles are averaged to obtain representative pressures for the session.

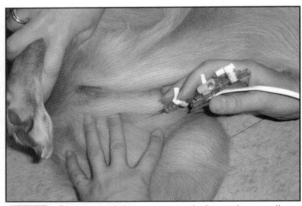

13.7 Direct arterial puncture technique: the needle attached to a pressure transducer is slowly advanced into the palpable femoral artery at the level of previous dermal and subcutaneous anaesthetic block.

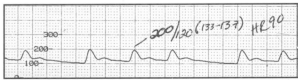

13.8 Sample of a BP tracing obtained via direct arterial puncture. Systolic (200 mmHg), diastolic (120 mmHg) and mean (133–137 mmHg) values are indicated. The heart rate is 90 bpm.

9. Recording of the heart rate during pressure measurement assists in assessment of the stress level of the patient during the procedure.

Oscillometric blood pressure measurement

Equipment:

- Commercial automated oscillometric BP monitor, with either print or data storage capability.
- A variety of cuff sizes based on patient limb circumference.
- Pliable measuring tape to measure patient limb circumference (Figure 13.9).

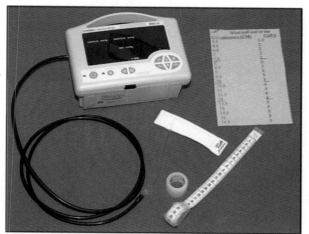

13.9 Equipment required for oscillometric BP measurement. A flexible measuring tape (lower right) is used to measure the circumference of the cuff site. A previously devised 'cuff size chart' (upper right) may be useful for rapid choice of cuff size. An automated oscillometric monitor is attached to the appropriately sized cuff, and light tape may be used to secure the cuff in position once it is wrapped around the extremity to be used for measurement.

Technique:

1. Restrain the patient in comfortable position and allow time and reassurance for acclimatization. The position of the patient is dependent on patient temperament and mobility and on the planned position of the cuff (limb cuffs should not be used in standing animals):
   - Cuff on forelimb at level of radius: sternal or lateral recumbency or sitting (Figure 13.10a)
   - Cuff on proximal forelimb at level of humerus (cats): sternal recumbency
   - Cuff on distal hindlimb at level of metatarsus (median artery): lateral recumbency preferred, sternal recumbency may be used if leg is in gentle extension (Figure 13.10b)
   - Cuff on proximal tailhead: sternal or lateral recumbency, or standing if immobile.
2. Measure the circumference of the limb or tail at the intended cuff site. The *width* of the cuff selected should be approximately 40% of the circumference of the cuff site. A chart can be prepared in advance to aid rapid cuff selection.

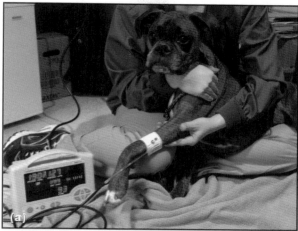

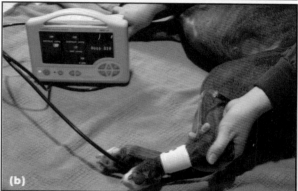

13.10 Oscillometric BP measurement. **(a)** A forelimb cuff is used to measure BP with an automated oscillometric device. Note that during measurement, the limb is supported comfortably such that the cuff is at the level of the right atrium (thoracic inlet). The monitor displays systolic/diastolic pressure (e.g. 190/127 mmHg) with mean pressure (144 mmHg) beneath. Heart rate is displayed at the bottom (93 bpm). **(b)** A hindlimb cuff is positioned distal to the hock, with the dog in lateral recumbency. The limb is gently supported during readings so that the cuff is at the level of the right atrium (sternum in lateral recumbency). A reading has not yet been obtained in this dog.

3. Wrap the cuff snugly around the limb with the centre of the inflatable bladder of the cuff positioned over the artery and attach to the BP monitor.
4. Gently position limb so that the cuff is at the level of the right atrium during readings (no repositioning required if tail cuff is used):
   - Sternum if patient is in lateral position
   - Thoracic inlet level if patient is sternal or sitting.
5. Record at least six measurements in succession, allowing approximately 30 seconds to 1 minute between measurements to allow for limb reperfusion.
6. Discard the first reading and any readings with clearly spurious results, and average the results of the remaining readings to obtain a representative figure for systolic, diastolic and mean pressures, respectively.
7. Note the heart rate associated with the BP

readings. If the heart rate is clearly incorrect, BP measurement may be spurious. In addition, high heart rate during recording may indicate high patient stress levels and possible elevated BP due to stress of procedure.

Doppler blood pressure measurement

Equipment:

- Commercial Doppler amplifier with attached piezoelectric crystal for detection of blood flow.
- Sphygmomanometer previously calibrated for accuracy.
- A variety of cuff sizes based on patient limb circumference.
- Pliable measuring tape to measure patient limb circumference.
- Ultrasound coupling gel.
- Hair clippers and isopropyl alcohol, if desired, for preparation of site prior to crystal application (Figure 13.11).

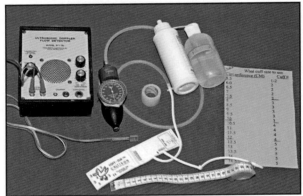

13.11 Equipment required for Doppler sphygmomanometric measurement of BP in dogs and cats. The signal amplifier (upper left) is attached to a piezoelectric crystal (lower centre). An inflatable bulb syringe attached to a manometer (upper centre) is used to inflate an appropriately sized cuff. Coupling gel and isopropyl alcohol (upper centre-right) are used to dampen fur.

Technique:

1. Restrain the patient in comfortable position and allow time and reassurance for acclimatization. The position of the patient is dependent on patient temperament and mobility and on the planned position of the cuff:
   - Cuff on forelimb at level of radius: sternal or lateral recumbency or sitting position
   - Cuff on hindlimb proximal to hock (tibial level): lateral recumbency preferred, sternal recumbency may be used if leg is in gentle extension during measurement.
2. Measure the circumference of the limb or tail at the intended cuff site. The *width* of the cuff selected should be approximately 40% of the circumference of the cuff site (Figure 13.12a). A chart can be prepared in advance to aid rapid cuff selection.

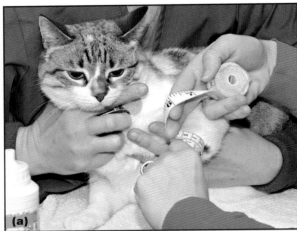

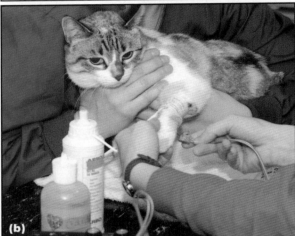

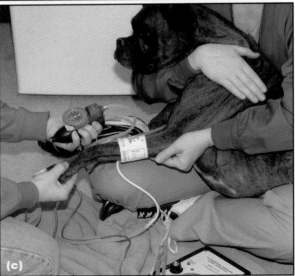

13.12 Doppler BP measurement. **(a)** The cat is held gently in position and a flexible measuring tape is used to measure the circumference of the limb at the level of cuff placement. The cuff size used is noted in the patient's record. **(b)** Coupling gel is applied to the Doppler crystal just before application on to the ventral portion of the metacarpal arch in a cat. The patient is held comfortably with the cuff at the level of the right atrium. **(c)** A bulb syringe attached to a manometer is used to inflate the BP cuff positioned on the distal forelimb of a dog. During measurements, the leg is held gently, so that the cuff is at the level of the right atrium.

3. Wrap the cuff snugly around the limb and attach to sphygmomanometer.
4. Clip or dampen hair as needed at site of Doppler crystal application (palmar or plantar arterial arch), apply coupling gel and hold or tape crystal in position (Figure 13.12b). Verify correct position by listening for clear pulsatile sounds of flow in the artery beneath the crystal. Adjust the crystal position or angle as necessary to improve signal strength if sounds are soft, distant or muffled.
5. Gently position limb so that the cuff is at the level of the right atrium during readings:
   - Sternum if patient is in lateral position
   - Thoracic inlet level if patient is sternal or sitting.
6. While listening to sound of flow, inflate the cuff using the bulb manometer to approximately 20 mmHg greater than the pressure needed to cut off flow sounds (Figure 13.12c).
7. Slowly deflate the cuff (1–3 mmHg per second) and note the pressure at which pulsatile sounds of flow recur. This pressure is recorded as the systolic pressure.
8. Completely deflate the cuff and count the heart rate in the approximately 30 seconds between pressure readings. A heart rate can be recorded with each BP reading.
9. Record at least six measurements in succession, allowing approximately 30 seconds to 1 minute between measurements to allow for limb reperfusion.
10. Discard the first reading and average the results of the remaining readings to obtain a representative figure for systolic pressure and heart rate. High heart rate may indicate increased levels of patient stress, which may have affected readings.

Interpretation of blood pressure results

Interpretation of BP results involves consideration of the numerical results of reliable BP measurement in conjunction with knowledge of the patient's diagnosis, clinical condition and temperament. Elevated BP values are not invariably an indication for antihypertensive therapy, especially in situations in which disease or procedure-related stress may have lead to spuriously increased values. Conversely, mild to moderate elevations in patients with overt clinical signs of hypertensive damage (e.g. retinal detachment) are an indication for immediate therapy.

Normal values generated using direct and indirect methods in cats (Bodey and Sansom, 1998; Belew et al., 1999; Sparkes et al., 1999) and dogs (Cowgill and Kallet, 1983; Bodey and Michell, 1996; Stepien and Rapoport, 1999) are available, but there is no single number in any species that represents a value necessitating therapeutic intervention. BP elevations form a continuum of values with increasing potential for causing acute or chronic end-organ damage; establishment of a single value that is considered to be 'treatable' is clinically unfeasible, and subclinical end-organ damage has been documented with even mild or moderate BP elevations.

Studies of the sensitivity and specificity of Doppler and oscillometric measurement techniques suggest that BP >160 mmHg, measured with a non-invasive technique, is a reasonable diagnostic cut-off value for diagnosis of HT in dogs (Stepien et al., 2003). Current recommendations for both species suggest that systolic BP >160 mmHg or diastolic BP >95 mmHg, measured by any method, are reasonable values at which concern is warranted (Cowgill, 2001; Hypertension Consensus Panel, 2002) but the decision to begin antihypertensive therapy is considered as a second question after elevated BP has been documented. General guidelines for interpretation of systolic BP in both cats and dogs are expressed in terms of risk of end-organ damage and are associated with recommendations for further action. A suggested algorithm for BP evaluation in patients with renal disease is outlined in Figure 13.13.

Blood pressure <150/95 mmHg: minimal risk for end-organ damage

BP in this range is considered to impose minimal risk of end-organ damage. No immediate therapy is indicated. In animals with documented renal disease, especially those with proteinuria, intermittent re-evaluation of BP is indicated. If proteinuria is present, therapy with angiotensin converting enzyme (ACE) inhibitors may be warranted (Grauer et al., 2000).

Blood pressure 150/95 to 160/100 mmHg: low risk for end-organ damage

Animals with BP in this range rarely have clinical signs solely attributable to HT. If renal disease is present, BP should be monitored over time to ensure that systolic BP remains <160 mmHg and renal disease should be treated appropriately. Some animals with stress-related elevations may have BP in this range. For these animals, home measurement of BP may be helpful to reduce the effect of patient stress.

Blood pressure 160/100 to 180/120 mmHg: moderate risk of end-organ damage

BPs in this range may be associated with clinical signs of HT. If clinical signs are present, antihypertensive therapy is indicated. If no renal disease is apparent after careful diagnostic evaluation of these patients, effective antihypertensive medication should be continued and the animal should be evaluated for other causes of HT (e.g. hyperadrenocorticism) and monitored for clinical evidence of causative disease over time (e.g. chronic kidney disease may not be identifiable in early stages but may become more obvious over time). If BP is documented to be in this range in a patient with known renal disease, concurrent therapy with antihypertensive medications and therapy for renal disease is warranted even if no clinical signs of HT are present.

Blood pressure >180/120 mmHg: high risk for end-organ damage

Patients with BP in this range are at high risk for end-organ damage. If ocular or neurological signs are present in renal patients with BP values in this range,

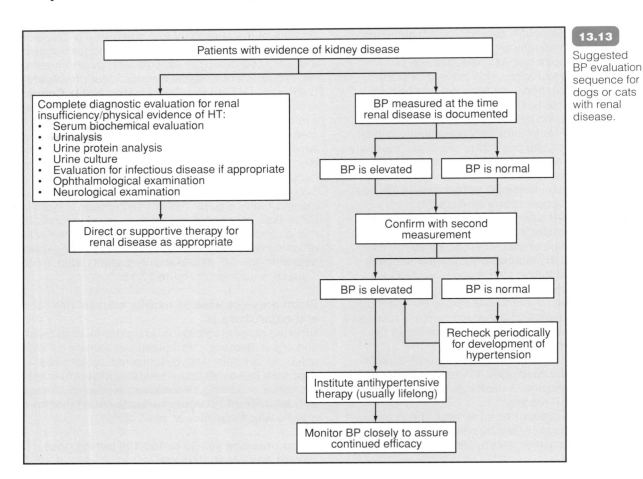

13.13

Suggested BP evaluation sequence for dogs or cats with renal disease.

Flowchart:

Patients with evidence of kidney disease

→ Complete diagnostic evaluation for renal insufficiency/physical evidence of HT:
• Serum biochemical evaluation
• Urinalysis
• Urine protein analysis
• Urine culture
• Evaluation for infectious disease if appropriate
• Ophthalmological examination
• Neurological examination

→ Direct or supportive therapy for renal disease as appropriate

→ BP measured at the time renal disease is documented

→ BP is elevated / BP is normal

→ Confirm with second measurement

→ BP is elevated / BP is normal

→ Recheck periodically for development of hypertension

→ Institute antihypertensive therapy (usually lifelong)

→ Monitor BP closely to assure continued efficacy

aggressive emergency antihypertensive therapy should be initiated, but antihypertensive therapy is indicated even if no overt signs of HT are noted but known renal disease is present. Occasionally, apparently healthy animals have BP measurements in this range. These animals should be retested several times, screened for underlying disease as appropriate and carefully observed over time for evidence of clinical HT.

Therapy of systemic hypertension in renal patients

The goals of antihypertensive therapy include:

• Prevention or limitation of immediate catastrophic damage to eyes and nervous system
• Prevention of chronic damage to microvasculature in target organs (e.g. kidney, brain)
• Limitation of harmful adaptive processes (i.e. cardiac hypertrophy).

In human hypertensive patients, the current recommendation for a numerical goal of antihypertensive therapy is a BP <130/80 mmHg (Chobanian et al., 2003) in renal patients, although the precise BP target following treatment is likely to depend on the severity of proteinuria. Similar information regarding appropriate clinical goals in veterinary patients is not available. One study suggested that a reduction in BP to approximately 165 mmHg in severely hypertensive cats with signs of ocular damage prevented further ocular damage (Elliott et al., 2001). In dogs, sustained systolic BP of >160 mmHg was associated with progressive renal failure and uraemic crises in dogs with renal disease (Brown et al., 2000; Jacob et al., 2003). This implies that BP reductions to <160 mmHg may be at least partially protective against further renal damage. A reasonable numerical goal for antihypertensive therapy in dogs and cats appears to be to decrease systolic BP to <160 mmHg chronically.

Despite the large number of drugs available to treat hypertension in people, therapy of systemic hypertension in dogs and cats is still under-researched in the clinical population. Recommendations are frequently based on anecdotal information and theoretical concerns, especially in dogs. As controlled clinical trials accumulate, better information regarding rational choices of antihypertensive medications will guide clinical decision-making.

Other management considerations include:

• *Diet*. Although normal cats do not have increases in BP related to salt loading (Luckschander et al., 2004), it is not clear that the same is true in cats or dogs with renal failure. A diet moderately restricted in sodium content is a reasonable recommendation for patients with HT and may assist in the control of BP by decreasing circulating blood volume

• *BP-elevating medications.* Some hypertensive patients may respond to discontinuation of other medications that tend to raise BP (e.g. phenylpropanolamine, corticosteroids). In patients receiving fluid therapy, reductions in the amount of fluid administered may allow for easier management of HT with vasodilating medications, but renal function should be monitored closely.

Emergency therapy

Emergency therapy of HT in dogs and cats (Figure 13.14) is primarily guided by the level of concern generated by clinical signs in the patient. The presence of ocular or neurological signs in conjunction with BP >160 mmHg is an indication for aggressive intervention. Rapid oral (e.g. hydralazine) or intravenous therapy (e.g. nitroprusside) with vasodilating agents is warranted. Nitroprusside or acepromazine can be used intravenously for rapid reduction of BP; the short half-life of nitroprusside makes it easy to titrate to effect (i.e. hypotension can be quickly rectified by decreasing the infusion rate). Reduction of systolic BP to <180 mmHg acutely may provide relief from clinical signs and prevent further damage in the short term. Acepromazine is available in most clinics and can be used in an emergency situation, but the longer-lasting effects of the drug make it harder to titrate to effect. Higher doses of acepromazine may result in over-sedation, hypotension and compromise of renal function, especially in geriatric patients; it should, therefore, be used with caution. Animals receiving emergency therapy for HT with overt clinical signs should be hospitalized and their BP monitored closely during the first 12–24 hours of therapy.

Long-term therapy

The success of long-term antihypertensive therapy depends on:

• The severity of the HT
• The type of medication used
• Owner factors, such as medication administration and recheck compliance
• The temperament of the patient.

The natural volatility of pet animals in the unusual situation of the hospital makes artefactual BP measurements a daily occurrence. In order to minimize artefact, all abnormal measurements should be confirmed and all measurements should be performed under optimal conditions. In addition, the importance of medication compliance and adherence to a rational recheck schedule should be emphasized to the pet's owner. Lastly, a partial but inadequately decreased BP in response to the initial medication should not be viewed as a therapeutic failure but as a reflection of the pet's individual drug response.

Given the complex pathophysiology of HT in renal patients, it is perhaps unsurprising that many approaches can be attempted to control HT. The clinical observation that multiple medications may be needed to control BP reflects our present understanding of compensatory mechanisms in the cardiovascular sys-

Medication	Indication	Mechanism	Dose	Comments
Acepromazine maleate	Acute HT	Blocks SNS-mediated vasoconstriction	D/C: 0.02–0.05 mg/kg i.v., start at lowest dose and monitor carefully	Extreme caution in renal and aged patients
Amlodipine besylate	Chronic HT	Direct vasodilation (sustained release)	D/C: 0.05–0.2 mg/kg orally q24h	Alone or with other medications
Angiotensin converting enzyme inhibitors: • Benazepril • Enalapril maleate	Chronic HT Proteinuric renal disease	↓ AT-II formation: • ↓ AT-II-mediated vasoconstriction • ↓ SNS stimulation • ↓ aldosterone formation (↓ sodium and water retention)	Benazepril: D/C: 0.25–0.5 mg/kg orally q12–24h Enalapril maleate: D: 0.5 mg/kg orally q12–24h C: 0.25–0.5 mg/kg orally q24h	May only lead to small reductions in BP in cats
β-antagonists: • Atenolol • Propranolol	Chronic HT	Blocks SNS-mediated renin secretion ↓ HR and stroke volue Effects on central nervous system to lower BP	Atenolol: D: 0.25–1.0 mg/kg orally q12h (start low and work up) C: 6.25–12.5 mg orally q24h Propranolol: D: 0.2–1.0 mg/kg orally q8h C: 2.5–5.0 mg orally q8–12h	Most helpful added to other medications
Hydralazine hydrochloride	Acute HT Chronic HT	Direct vasodilation	D/C: 0.5–2 mg/kg orally q12h, start at low end of dose, titrate to effect	Monitor closely when used with other medications
Nitroprusside sodium	Acute HT	Direct vasodilation	D/C: 0.5–5 µg/kg/min as continuous infusion, start low and titrate to effect with continuous BP monitoring	Invasive BP monitoring recommended during use

13.14 Medications commonly used to treat hypertension in dogs and cats. Note: doses given are approximate and should be used based on the discretion of the attending clinician. AT-II = Angiotensin II; BP = Blood pressure; C = Cats; D = Dogs; HR = Heart rate; HT = Hypertension; SNS = Sympathetic nervous system.

tem. Direct-acting vasodilator drugs are the most successful in causing acute reduction of BP, but SNS-mediated increases in HR and aldosterone-mediated sodium and water retention may moderate the effects of the vasodilation (Figure 13.15). As a result, a multiple blockade theory of BP management may have better results than monotherapy in some animals. In this system, additional medications may be used to block the compensatory effects caused by one medication (Figure 13.16). In this regard, some types of medications (e.g. diuretics, aldosterone antagonists and β-antagonists) that have little apparent antihypertensive effect alone may have additive effects when given with other medications. Lastly, some medications with vasoactive effects have additional indications in patients with renal disease. ACE inhibitors have beneficial effects on proteinuria and intraglomerular pressure in renal patients beyond their often modest antihypertensive effects (Grauer *et al.*, 2000; Brown *et al.*, 2001, 2003), and thus may be added to other more efficacious antihypertensive medications to take advantage of the non-systemic BP effects of these medications.

Cats

Amlodipine besylate (a long-acting dihydropyridine calcium antagonist) is the current antihypertensive medication of choice for cats and has proven to control BP in both induced and naturally occurring renal disease in cats (Snyder, 1998; Elliott *et al.*, 2001; Mathur *et al.*, 2002). Recent information has raised the concern that amlodipine as a single medication in animals with renal disease may expose the glomerulus to higher pressures, due to efferent arteriolar constriction caused by local increases in RAAS activity. If so, cats with renal disease may benefit from therapy with both ACE inhibitors and amlodipine.

Beta-blocking agents, such as atenolol or propranolol, may be useful adjunctive therapy, especially in hyperthyroid cats, but beta-blocking agents are less successful when administered alone for management of HT. The additive effects of amlodipine and beta blockers have not been studied in cats.

ACE inhibitors (e.g. enalapril or benazepril) have proven to be variable in their efficacy in controlling hypertension in cats (Steele *et al.*, 2002) but may have other beneficial effects (e.g. aldosterone antagonism)

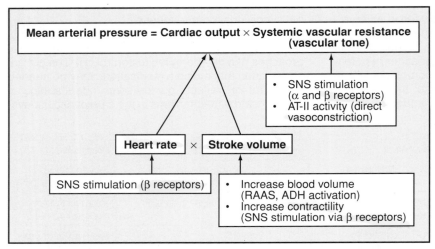

13.15 Cardiovascular compensatory mechanisms that support BP. Activity of the sympathetic nervous system, renin–angiotensin–aldosterone system and antidiuretic hormone act to support heart rate, stroke volume and vascular tone to maintain mean arterial pressure. ADH = Antidiuretic hormone; AT-II = Angiotensin II; RAAS = Renin–angiotensin–aldosterone system; SNS = Sympathetic nervous system.

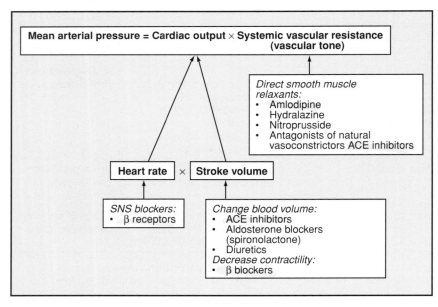

13.16 Effect of various classes of antihypertensive medications on the compensatory mechanisms of the cardiovascular system.

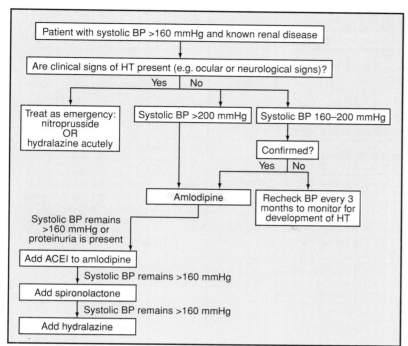

13.17 Approach to therapy of HT in cats with renal disease. Cats with known renal disease and systolic BP repeatedly >160 mmHg are considered candidates for antihypertensive therapy. Animals with systolic BP >160 mmHg without clinical signs should have the BP confirmed at rechecks. Cats with systolic BP ≥200 mmHg or clinical signs of HT should be treated immediately. Target systolic BP is <160 mmHg. ACEI = Angiotensin converting enzyme inhibitor

in these patients. Other oral agents such as hydralazine may be useful in some situations but have not undergone wide clinical study.

A typical sequence of medications for long-term control of HT in cats with renal disease is presented in Figure 13.17. In most cases, approximately 1–2 weeks should elapse before a medication is considered to be inadequate to control BP.

Dogs

Little clinical information regarding the comparative success of different antihypertensive medications in dogs with renal disease has been published. In general, dogs with renal disease and HT may be more resistant to antihypertensive medications than cats (see Figure 13.14).

ACE inhibitors are useful for therapy of HT related to protein-losing renal diseases in dogs, decreasing both BP and renal protein loss (Grauer *et al.*, 2000). ACE inhibitors alone may be expected to decrease systolic BP by about 10% in responsive dogs, and may be effective as monotherapy in dogs with mild HT. In dogs not adequately responsive to ACE inhibitors alone, other drugs may be added or substituted (Figure 13.18).

Amlodipine besylate is commonly added for control of HT in dogs if ACE inhibitors alone are inadequate, but higher doses may be needed to obtain clinical effects compared to cats (see Figure 13.14). Adverse effects may be seen at higher doses and caution is advised when increasing amlodipine doses for BP control in dogs. Hydralazine can be added to ACE inhibitor and amlodipine therapy with caution and close monitoring.

Lastly, when standard doses of these initial medications are tolerated but not adequate to control BP, addition of an ACE inhibitor, a beta-blocking agent in tachycardic animals or a diuretic/aldosterone antago-

nist (spironolactone) may be helpful. If more than two medications are required to control HT, careful review of the medications with the patient's owner is helpful to ensure compliance, and lack of response should be confirmed with recheck measurements.

Monitoring the hypertensive renal patient

At the time antihypertensive therapy is initiated, a review of the patient's renal care should be performed and optimal management (including ACE inhibitors for proteinuric patients) ensured. Initial antihypertensive therapy in non-emergency patients should be administered for 7–14 days before BP is rechecked. If BP is controlled adequately, it can be evaluated every 1–3 months as needed, based on the patient's clinical condition. Frequent rechecks of the patient's renal and electrolyte status are recommended, beginning at the first BP recheck. Progression of the renal disease over time as well as therapy of HT may affect these parameters adversely (Elliott *et al.*, 2001). Although cats with renal disease treated with amlodipine tend to have a consistent BP response that is stable over time (Figure 13.19) (Elliott *et al.*, 2001), dogs may need periodic adjustment in their medications, with the number of medications needed to control HT increasing over time. In some cases, decreasing renal function or a change in clinical condition may lead to adverse drug effects (e.g. hyperkalaemia in dehydrated patients receiving ACE inhibitors). Patients with renal disease tend to lose weight over time; doses of antihypertensive medications that were necessary initially may lead to hypotension if patients sustain significant weight loss. In general, antihypertensive medications in hypotensive patients should be adjusted to render a systolic BP >110 mmHg. Carefully monitored fluid therapy with short-term discontinuation of antihypertensive medications may be necessary to 'rebalance' dehydrated, hypotensive renal patients.

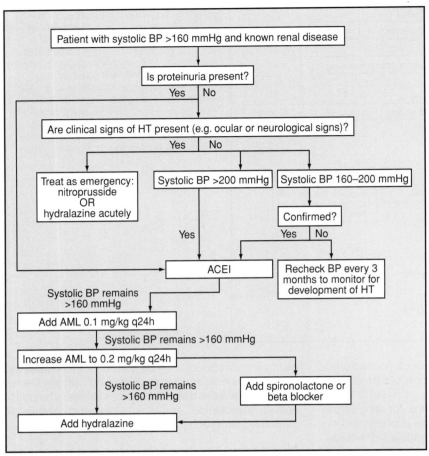

13.18 Approach to therapy of HT in dogs with renal disease. Dogs with known renal disease and systolic BP repeatedly >160 mmHg are considered candidates for antihypertensive therapy. Animals with systolic BP >160 mmHg without clinical signs should have the BP confirmed at rechecks. Dogs with systolic BP ≥200 mmHg or clinical signs of HT should be treated immediately. Target systolic BP is <160 mmHg. Before adding medications, owner compliance should be checked and lack of BP response confirmed by rechecking. ACEI = Angiotensin converting enzyme inhibitor; AML = Amlodipine.

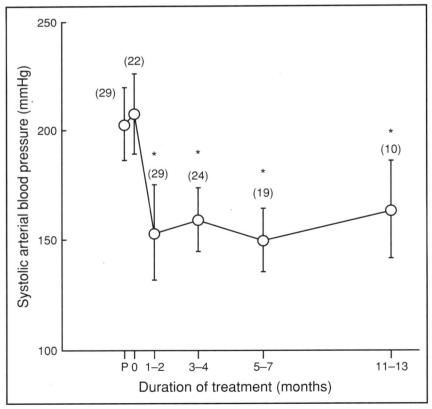

13.19 Response of 29 hypertensive cats to amlodipine treatment. Two pre-treatment BP measurements were made in 22 cats (P and 0). The time in months following introduction of treatment is shown and represents a range at each point. The readings taken during treatment (∗) show significant difference from the pre-treatment value (paired Student's t-test with Bonferroni's correction). Note the stable BP achieved in response to chronic amlodipine administration. (Reproduced with permission from Elliott *et al.*, 2001.)

References and further reading

Belew AM, Barlett T and Brown SA (1999) Evaluation of the white-coat effect in cats. *Journal of Veterinary Internal Medicine* **13**, 134–142

Bodey AR and Michell AR (1996) Epidemiological study of blood pressure in domestic dogs. *Journal of Small Animal Practice* **37**, 116–125

Bodey AR and Sansom J (1998) Epidemiological study of blood pressure in domestic cats. *Journal of Small Animal Practice* **39**, 567–573

Brown SA, Brown CA and Hendi R (2000) Does systemic hypertension damage the canine kidney? *Journal of Veterinary Internal Medicine* **14**, 351 [abstract]

Brown SA, Brown CA, Jacobs G *et al.* (2001) Effects of the angiotensin converting enzyme inhibitor benazepril in cats with induced renal insufficiency. *American Journal of Veterinary Research* **62(3)**, 375–383

Brown SA, Finco DR, Brown CA *et al.* (2003) Evaluation of the effects of inhibition of angiotensin converting enzyme with enalapril in dogs with induced chronic renal insufficiency. *American Journal of Veterinary Research* **64(3)**, 321–327

Chobanian AV, Bakris GL, Black HR *et al.* (2003) Seventh report of the Joint National Committee on prevention, detection, evaluation, and treatment of high blood pressure. *Hypertension* **42**, 1206–1252

Cowgill LD (2001) Systemic hypertension: overview and importance. *Proceedings, 19th Annual Veterinary Medical Forum*, Denver, CO, American College of Veterinary Internal Medicine

Cowgill LG and Kallett AJ (1983) Recognition and management of hypertension in the dog. In: *Current Veterinary Therapy VIII: Small Animal Practice*, ed. RW Kirk and JD Bonagura, pp. 1025–1028. WB Saunders, Philadelphia

Elliott J, Barber PJ, Syme HM and Rawlings JM (2001) Feline hypertension: clinical findings and response to antihypertensive treatment in 30 cases. *Journal of Small Animal Practice* **42**, 122–129

Finco DR (2004) Association of systemic hypertension with renal injury in dogs with induced renal failure. *Journal of Veterinary Internal Medicine* **18**, 289–294

Grauer GF, Greco DS, Getzy DM *et al.* (2000) Effects of enalapril vs. placebo as a treatment for canine idiopathic glomerulonephritis. *Journal of Veterinary Internal Medicine* **14**, 526–533

Hypertension Consensus Panel (2002) Current recommendations for diagnosis and management of hypertension in cats and dogs [report]. *Dallas, 20th Annual Veterinary Medical Forum*

Jacob F, Polzin DJ, Osborne CA *et al.* (2003) Association between initial systolic blood pressure and risk of developing a uremic crisis or of dying in dogs with chronic renal failure. *Journal of the American Veterinary Medical Association* **222(3)**, 322–329

Kobayashi DL, Peterson ME, Graves TK *et al.* (1990) Hypertension in cats with chronic renal failure or hyperthyroidism. *Journal of Veterinary Internal Medicine* **4**, 58–62

Luckschander N, Iben C, Hosgood G, Gabler C and Biourge V (2004) Dietary salt does not affect blood pressure in healthy cats. *Journal of Veterinary Internal Medicine* **18**, 463–467

Mathur S, Syme H, Brown CA *et al.* (2002) Effects of the calcium channel antagonist amlodipine in cats with surgically induced hypertensive renal insufficiency. *American Journal of Veterinary Research* **63(6)**, 833–839

Michell AR, Bodey AR and Gleadhill A (1997) Absence of hypertension in dogs with renal insufficiency. *Renal Failure* **19(1)**, 61–68

Snyder P (1998) Amlodipine: A randomized, blinded clinical trial in 9 cats with systemic hypertension. *Journal of Veterinary Internal Medicine* **12**, 157–162

Snyder PS, Deena S and Galin LJ (2001) Effect of amlodipine on echocardiographic variables in cats with systemic hypertension. *Journal of Veterinary Internal Medicine* **15**, 52–56

Sparkes AH, Caney SMA, King MCA and Gruffydd-Jones TJ (1999) Inter- and intraindividual variation in Doppler ultrasonic indirect blood pressure measurements in healthy cats. *Journal of Veterinary Internal Medicine* **13**, 314–318

Steele JS, Henik RA and Stepien RL (2002) Effects of ACE-inhibition on blood pressure and the renin-angiotensin-aldosterone system in cats with hypertension associated with chronic renal disease. *Veterinary Therapy* **3(2)**, 157–166

Stepien RL and Rapoport GS (1999) Clinical comparison of three methods to measure blood pressure in nonsedated dogs. *Journal of the American Veterinary Medical Association* **215(11)**, 1623–1628

Stepien RL, Rapoport GS, Henik RA, Wenholz L and Thomas CA (2003) Comparative diagnostic test characteristics of oscillometric and Doppler ultrasonographic methods in the detection of systolic hypertension in dogs. *Journal of Veterinary Internal Medicine* **17**, 65–72

Syme HM, Barber PJ, Markwell PJ and Elliott J (2001) Prevalence of systemic hypertension in cats with chronic renal failure and evaluation of associated risk factors [abstract]. *British Small Animal Veterinary Association Congress Scientific Proceedings*, 506

Syme HM, Barber PJ, Markwell PJ and Elliott J (2002) Prevalence of systolic hypertension in cats with chronic renal failure at initial evaluation. *Journal of the American Veterinary Medical Association* **220(12)**, 1799–1804

14

Cystoscopy

Larry G. Adams

Introduction

The principal form of endoscopy for the urinary tract in veterinary medicine is transurethral cystoscopy. Although it has been underutilized, transurethral cystoscopy is an integral part of the diagnostic evaluation of dogs and cats with recurrent or persistent lower urinary tract disease (McCarthy, 1996; Cannizzo et al., 2001; McCarthy, 2005). Cystoscopy allows visualization and biopsy of any lesions in the bladder and urethra. The most common indications for cystoscopy are listed in Figure 14.1 and include evaluation of urinary incontinence, haematuria, recurrent urinary tract infection, urinary tract trauma, urolithiasis and neoplasia.

Endourology refers to an area of human medicine involving closed urological surgical procedures (diagnostic and therapeutic) performed through instruments such as cystoscopes, nephroscopes and ureteroscopes. Veterinary surgeons are progressing from use of cystoscopes primarily for diagnostic evaluation of the lower urinary tract to more advanced diagnostic and therapeutic endourological techniques.

Equipment

Several rigid and flexible endoscopes designed for use in humans may be used for transurethral cystoscopy in dogs and cats. Figure 14.2 shows the tips of flexible and rigid cystoscopes used in small animals. The size of the patient's urethra dictates the size of cystoscope. Because male dogs have smaller diameter and longer urethral length, 2.5 mm (7.5 French) diameter, 70–100 cm long flexible ureteroscopes may be utilized for transurethral cystoscopy. Rigid cystoscopes used for diagnostic cystoscopy typically have a 30-degree upward angle view. Forward viewing (0-degree lens) cystoscopes are available for some therapeutic procedures such as laser lithotripsy. For bitches weighing approximately 5–30 kg, 2.7 mm diameter and 18 cm long, rigid paediatric cystoscopes allow transurethral cystoscopy. For bitches smaller than 5 kg body weight and female cats, a 1.9 cm diameter, 18 cm long paediatric cystoscope is small enough to pass through the urethra in most animals. For larger bitches, 4.0 mm diameter, 30 cm long cystoscopes allow for access to the cranial aspect of the urinary bladder.

Problem	Use	Comments
Urinary incontinence	Examine for ectopic ureters or other developmental abnormalities Injection of periurethral bulk-enhancing agents	More sensitive than contrast radiography Treatment of refractory urinary incontinence due to urethral incompetence
Haematuria	Determine source of haematuria	Treatment also possible for some causes
Recurrent urinary tract infection (UTI)	Examine for anatomical abnormalities or uroliths that might contribute to UTI Obtain mucosal biopsy specimen for culture	Abnormalities of the lower urinary tract are readily detected, more difficult to detect kidney involvement in UTI Cultures of mucosal biopsy specimens are more sensitive than urine culture alone
Urinary tract trauma	Examine integrity of the lower urinary tract Assist in placement of indwelling catheter past urethral tears	Cystoscopy is able to detect small perforations or tears of the urinary tract Placement of guidewire past urethral tears facilitates catheter placement without enlarging tears
Urolithiasis	Removal of uroliths via flushing, basket retrieval or voiding urohydropropulsion Obtain uroliths for quantitative analysis or culture via basket retrieval Fragment larger uroliths via laser lithotripsy	Cystoscopy is sensitive for detection of small uroliths before and after voiding urohydropropulsion Basket retreival allows for removal of irregular stones that may be difficult to remove by urohydropropulsion See Chapter 15 regarding laser lithotripsy
Neoplasia	Determine extent and location of neoplasia Obtain biopsy samples for cytology and histopathology	Cystoscopy is sensitive for detecting urethral involvement Use the largest biopsy instrument that will pass through the working channel

14.1 Indications for cystoscopy.

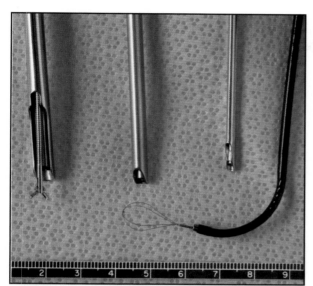

14.2 Photograph of the tip of rigid and flexible cystoscopes used for cystoscopy. From left to right: 4.0 mm rigid cystoscope within 19 French cystoscopy sheath (5 French biopsy instrument in working channel); 2.7 mm diameter rigid cystoscope with 14.5 French sheath; 1.9 mm diameter rigid cystoscope with 9 French sheath; and 2.5 mm diameter flexible ureteroscope with stone basket in the working channel.

The 7.5 French ureteroscope and 9 French paediatric rigid cystoscope sheath each have a 1.2 mm working channel which accepts 3 French working instruments. The larger working channels in the 14.5 and 19 French cystoscope sheaths accept 5 French working instruments. Laser fibres may be passed through the working channel for laser lithotripsy (see Chapter 15). Guidewires may also be passed through the working channel of rigid and flexible cystoscopes for passage proximally in the urinary tract.

Working instruments that are most commonly used during cystoscopy include biopsy forceps, graspers, stone baskets and urological guidewires. These instruments are generally available in 3 French and 5 French sizes, depending on the size of the working channel within the cystoscope sheath. Use of the largest biopsy forceps that the working channel will accommodate provides for larger biopsy specimens.

Flexible tipped urological guidewires are available in a variety of sizes and designs for endourological procedures. Guidewires may be used as working wires, such that scopes or catheters are passed over the guidewire, or as safety wires to maintain a pathway into the portion of the urinary tract being manipulated. Guidewires may be placed past urethral tears or obstructions under visual guidance via cystoscopy, and then an indwelling catheter can be passed over the guidewire to bypass the tear or obstruction. Without visual placement of the guidewire, retrograde placement of a catheter using a blind technique risks enlarging the urethral tear. Flexible tipped guidewires can also be passed through the cystoscope into the ureteral orifice to obtain retrograde ureteral access.

Diagnostic techniques

Routine cystoscopic examination of the lower urinary tract

Prior to cystoscopy the hair around the vulva in bitches and around the prepuce in male dogs is clipped and the skin surrounding the area is cleaned using standard presurgical cleaning. Female dogs and cats may be positioned in dorsal, ventral or lateral recumbency with the vulva positioned at the end of the table. Dorsal recumbency is the most useful position for access to the vulva for passage of the cystoscope. If the animal is positioned in sternal recumbency, a sterile drape should be placed under the animal after the vulvar area is clipped and prepared and the vulva is positioned several centimetres caudal to the edge of the examination table. Male dogs and cats are placed in lateral recumbency and the penis is exteriorized by an assistant.

The cystoscope and all related equipment should be sterile. For all cystoscopic procedures, aseptic principles are observed, including wearing sterile gloves. If the procedure involves use of ancillary equipment, such as biopsy forceps, guidewires or stone baskets, the operator should also wear a sterile surgical gown to avoid contamination of the equipment during repeated passage in and out of the working channel. The sterile, isotonic irrigation solution (i.e. normal saline) should be warmed.

Routine cystoscopy should follow a normal protocol to inspect all aspects of the lower urinary tract before focusing on any obvious abnormalities, to avoid overlooking any less obvious changes. In females, the cystoscope may be passed blindly with the blunt obturator using a technique identical to urethral catheterization, or it may be passed under visual guidance with fluid distension of the urethra. The disadvantages of blind passage include the potential of causing apparent lesions in the urethra or overlooking significant urethral lesions until the cystoscope is withdrawn at the end of the procedure. Therefore, the author prefers to inspect the urethra during initial passage of the cystoscope under visual guidance. The cystoscope should be passed retrograde into the vestibule and into the urethra without entering the body of the vagina, to avoid contamination of the scope tip with normal vaginal flora.

Once the cystoscope is in the urinary bladder, the urine is drained and the bladder is lavaged with sterile warm isotonic solution and then refilled. This process is repeated as necessary to provide clear visualization of the bladder lumen. Overdistension of the urinary bladder should be avoided and the irrigation solution is allowed to flow by gravity with the fluids positioned no higher than 80 cm above the patient. Overdistension may result in bleeding from iatrogenic trauma to the mucosa with resultant impaired visualization of the urinary tract.

Normal bladder mucosa allows for easy visualization of submucosal blood vessels (Figure 14.3). Oedema or inflammation of the bladder wall makes the vessels more difficult to visualize and may completely obscure the smaller vessels. Normal ureteral orifices are

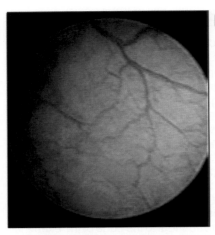

14.3

Normal appearance of bladder mucosa in a bitch. Note the visibility of the large and small blood vessels in the submucosa of the bladder wall.

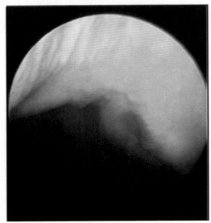

14.4

Normal ureteral openings in a bitch. Urine can be seen flowing into the urinary bladder from the left ureteral orifice. The urine is visible because the urinary bladder is distended with normal saline.

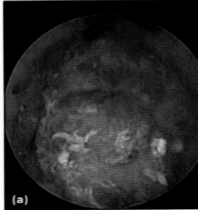

14.6

Variable appearance of transitional cell carcinoma in dogs.
(a) Large haemorrhagic and partially necrotic mass in the urinary bladder.
(b) Papillary nature of transitional cell carcinoma is the most common appearance in dogs.
(c) Papillary structure of transitional cell carcinoma. Note the blood vessel extending to the tip of the papillary structure, which is highly suggestive of transitional cell carcinoma.

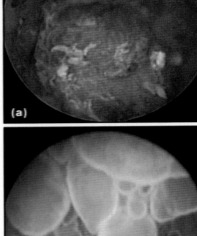

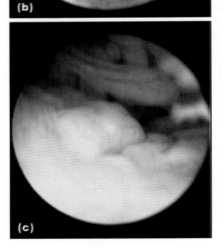

C-shaped with the opening of the C pointing medially (Figure 14.4). In cats, the ureteral orifices are more caudally positioned than in dogs and the ureteral orifices appear to be in the proximal urethra in some cats. The positions of both ureteral orifices are identified within the trigone region and urine should be seen entering the bladder from each orifice.

The bladder mucosa should be visually inspected throughout the entire urinary bladder. If a 30-degree view cystoscope is utilized, the scope should be rotated 180 degrees along the long axis to view the dependent portion of the bladder and inspect for uroliths, masses or other lesions (Figures 14.5 and 14.6).

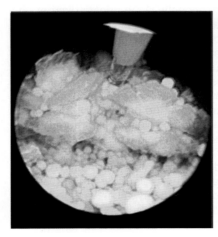

14.5

Calcium oxalate uroliths in the urinary bladder with multiple smaller uroliths. A 550 μm diameter flexible quartz laser fibre is positioned near the surface of the urolith (see Chapter 15).

Masses or polyps

Masses or polyps in the urinary bladder may be visualized and biopsies performed during cystoscopy. Transitional cell carcinoma, the most common neoplasm of the lower urinary tract in dogs and cats, has a variable cystoscopic appearance (see Figure 14.6). Polypoid cystitis in dogs is a benign lesion that often occurs secondary to urolithiasis and/or chronic urinary tract infection (UTI) (Figure 14.7). Definitive differentiation of transitional cell carcinoma from polypoid cystitis requires histopathological evaluation of biopsy specimens obtained during cystoscopy (or surgery). Placement of the biopsy forceps across the base of a pedunculated or papillary lesion often allows removal of a large biopsy sample from the lesion.

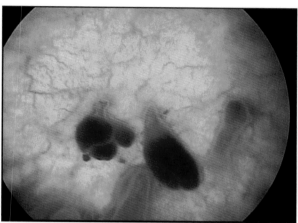

Polypoid cystitis in the apex of the urinary bladder of a dog.

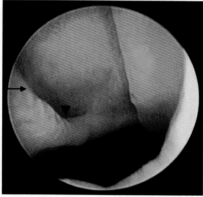

Ectopic left ureteral opening (arrowhead) in the proximal urethra of a spayed Bulldog bitch with urinary incontinence. Note the ridge (arrowed) extending from the lip of the ureteral opening down the urethra. Such malformations of the urethra often contribute to concurrent urethral incompetence. The bladder lumen is visible in the ventral portion of the image.

Diagnostic evaluation of recurrent urinary tract infection

Cystoscopy is useful for diagnostic evaluation of dogs with recurrent UTI to look for anatomical defects and to obtain biopsy specimens for cytology, histopathology and microbiological culture. Figure 14.2 shows biopsy forceps that have been passed through the working channel of a rigid cystoscope; these are used to perform mucosal biopsies. In a study comparing urolith cultures and cultures of mucosal biopsy specimens obtained during cystotomy to routine urine cultures, cultures of mucosal biopsy specimens or uroliths were able to detect infection in 18% of dogs that was not detected by concurrent urine culture (Hamaide *et al.*, 1998). Similarly, the author has observed that cultures of mucosal biopsy specimens obtained via cystoscopy can also detect organisms not isolated by simultaneous urine culture. Biopsies for culture and histopathology should also be performed on any lesions present in the lower urinary tract from dogs with recurrent UTI. Multiple small follicles are often present in the lower urinary tract of dogs with chronic UTI; this has been termed follicular cystitis. Biopsy and culture of one or more follicles confirms the chronic nature of the UTI and may facilitate identification of the infecting organism(s). Follow-up cystoscopy can be used to document regression of follicular cystitis after effective management of the UTI, although this is not essential. Uroliths may be retrieved from the bladder or urethra aseptically for culture using stone baskets.

Ectopic ureters

Recent studies confirm that cystoscopy is more sensitive than excretory urography for identification of ectopic ureters and associated anatomical defects (Cannizzo *et al.*, 2003). The normal ureteral openings should be visualized within the trigone of the urinary bladder (see Figure 14.4) and ectopic ureteral openings are usually detected in the urethra (Figure 14.8) or in the vaginal vestibule (uncommon). If there is doubt about the patency of suspected ectopic ureteral openings, flexible tipped urological guidewires may be passed retrograde into the suspect ureteral opening under visual guidance and imaged by fluoroscopy or radiog-

raphy. The guidewire may be left in place while the cystoscope is withdrawn, then a ureteral catheter may be fed over the guidewire and retrograde contrast studies may be performed to determine the anatomical configuration of the ureters.

Concurrent urethral malformation is common in dogs with ectopic ureters (Cannizzo *et al.*, 2003). Urethral conformation is evaluated during initial visual passage of the cystoscope for shape and for the presence of any ectopic ureteral openings within the urethra. The normal urethra in female dogs and cats has a single prominent dorsal ridge extending most of the length of the urethra. In dogs with ectopic ureters, ureteral troughs are often seen as ridges that extend down the urethra from the edge of the ectopic ureteral openings. Abnormalities of the vaginal vestibule, such as paramesonephric septal remnants, are also common concurrent developmental abnormalities seen in dogs with ectopic ureters (Cannizzo *et al.*, 2003).

Localization of haematuria

During cystoscopy the source of gross haematuria can usually be definitively localized to the genital tract, urethra, bladder or left or right kidney and ureter. This approach is more accurate than predicting the localization of haematuria based on when blood is noted during voiding. Bleeding lesions in the lower urinary tract can be confirmed and sometimes treated depending on the nature of the lesion (e.g. uroliths, neoplasia). Localization of upper urinary tract haematuria can be determined by either direct visualization of gross haematuria from the ureteral orifice (Figure 14.9) (Cannizzo *et al.*, 2001; McCarthy, 2005) or by retrograde catheterization of each ureter (Senior and Newman, 1986). In humans, ureteroscopy may be used further to localize and treat the source of upper urinary tract haematuria rather than performing nephrectomy for treatment of renal haematuria (Tawfiek and Bagley, 1998).

The author has performed ureteroscopy in three dogs with renal haematuria. The source of the haematuria could be visualized within the renal pelvis of the

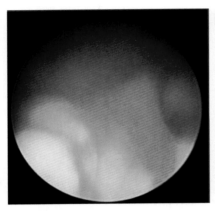

14.9
Grossly haemorrhagic urine from the left ureteral orifice in a 2-year-old spayed bitch Weimaraner with renal haematuria.

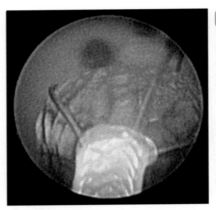

14.10
Urolith trapped in stone basket and positioned near the end of the cystoscope prior to removal.

kidney in two of the three dogs. In one of these dogs, electrocautery of the bleeding vessel resolved the haematuria. In a previously reported dog with renal haematuria, ligation of the branch of the renal artery supplying the renal 'bleed' also resolved the renal haematuria without nephrectomy (Mishina *et al.*, 1997).

Therapeutic techniques

Periurethral injections of bulk-enhancing agents
An alternative therapy for dogs with refractory urinary incontinence due to confirmed urethral incompetence includes cystoscopically guided periurethral injections of bulk-enhancing agents (glutaraldehyde cross-linked collagen) (Arnold *et al.*, 1996; Barth *et al.*, 2005). Periurethral injection of collagen narrows the urethral lumen and allows for more effective closure of the urethra by existing urethral pressure. Periurethral injection of collagen resolved urinary incontinence in 53% of dogs; an additional 22% were improved with concurrent administration of phenylpropanolamine (Arnold *et al.*, 1996). In a second study, 68% of dogs were continent after collagen injection; for an average of 17 months (Barth *et al.*, 2005). Repeat cystoscopic injections of collagen are required in some dogs to maintain continence, however.

Stone baskets
Stone baskets may be used to remove uroliths from the lower urinary tract, provided the uroliths are smaller than the dilated urethra. Stone baskets are usually passed through the working channel of the cystoscope (see Figure 14.2), the basket is opened, and once the urolith is engaged in the basket, the basket is closed around the urolith and positioned at the end of the cystoscope (Figure 14.10). Then the cystoscope and basket containing the urolith are slowly withdrawn through the urethra with direct visualization to ensure there is no bulging of the urothelium around the urolith edges, which may indicate the urolith is becoming wedged in the urethra. This technique may be safely used to remove some uroliths that will not readily pass during voiding urohydropropulsion; however, caution is required to avoid getting the urolith wedged in the urethra.

Ellik evacuator
During cystoscopy with a rigid cystoscope, the telescope is removed leaving the cystoscope sheath in place in the urethra with the tip of the sheath just inside the trigone. An Ellik evacuator is attached to the cystoscope sheath and the bladder is rapidly lavaged to flush sterile saline into and out of the bladder using the bulb attachment. The design of the Ellik evacuator allows the aspirated uroliths to gravitate to the bottom chamber while fluid in the top chamber is flushed into and out of the bladder (Adams and Senior, 1999). This technique can be used to collect uroliths smaller than the diameter of the cystoscope sheath, and thus allows for removal of larger uroliths than a standard urinary catheter. This technique may be used to remove small uroliths completely from the urinary bladder or to obtain smaller uroliths for quantitative analysis and culture. This technique may also be used to remove urolith fragments after intracorporeal lithotripsy (Adams and Senior, 1999). See Chapter 15 for additional details.

Removal of polyps or tumours
Cystoscopy is useful for documenting the extent and location of lower urinary tract neoplasia and for obtaining biopsy samples for cytology and histopathology from lesions within the bladder or urethra. Some polyps or tumours with narrow stalks can be removed using biopsy instruments, electrocautery snares or with the holmium–YAG laser or diode lasers (McCarthy, 2003) (see Chapter 15). This allows for larger sample size for histopathology. The author has removed a solitary transitional cell carcinoma that had a narrow-based stalk using the holmium–YAG laser followed by fulguration of the base. Benign polyps (e.g. polypoid cystitis) may also be removed from the bladder using the holmium–YAG laser.

Urethral stricture dilation
Urethral strictures can be easily detected during cystoscopy. If the stricture is too small to allow passage of a 7.5 French flexible cystoscope, a flexible tipped guidewire may be passed through the strictured area under fluoroscopic guidance. If needed, a ureteral catheter may be passed over the guidewire and retrograde contrast studies may be performed to delineate the extent and severity of the urethral stricture. Alternatively, contrast medium may be injected through the

working channel of flexible cystoscopes to perform retrograde contrast studies. Urethral strictures may be dilated over the guidewire using serially enlarging dilators (e.g. Amplatz renal dilators or ureteral dilation catheters) or appropriately sized balloon dilation catheters (Senior, 1992). Urethral strictures may recur after dilation and may require re-dilation or incision to release fibrous bands. The author has successfully dilated proximal urethral strictures in two male and two female cats. In one female cat, follow-up cystoscopy showed partial narrowing of the previous stricture site, although it was not severe enough to impair urine flow.

Risks and complications

In the author's experience, complications from routine cystoscopy are uncommon; however, potential complications include iatrogenic UTI and trauma to the urinary tract, such as perforation or rupture of the urethra or urinary bladder. Passage of rigid cystoscopes should be done as atraumatically as possible and only under visual guidance to avoid urethral trauma. Insertion of too large a cystoscope for the patient's size is an avoidable error that could lead to urethral trauma. Although some authors previously recommended urethral dilation prior to passage of larger cystoscopes, this approach has been rendered unnecessary by utilization of appropriate-sized small-diameter rigid and flexible cystoscopes.

Iatrogenic UTI can be avoided by use of appropriate aseptic technique and minimizing mucosal trauma. Additionally, irrigation of large volumes of sterile isotonic solutions, normally done to provide clear visualization of the urinary tract, further serves to remove any bacteria introduced by passage of the cystoscope from the non-sterile distal urethra and vaginal vestibule into the urinary bladder. Routine administration of prophylactic antibiotics is not required unless the cystoscope is passed up the urethra several times during the procedure or there are additional predisposing factors to the establishment of UTI, such as mucosal injury, neoplasia or urethral stricture.

References and further reading

Adams LG and Senior DF (1999) Electrohydraulic and extracorporeal shock-wave lithotripsy. *Veterinary Clinics of North America: Small Animal Practice* **29**, 293–302

Arnold S, Hubler M, Lott-Stolz G and Rusch P (1996) Treatment of urinary incontinence in bitches by endoscopic injection of glutaraldehyde cross-linked collagen. *Journal of Small Animal Practice* **37**, 163–168

Barth A, Reichler IM, Hubler M, Hassig M and Arnold S (2005) Evaluation of long-term effects of endoscopic injection of collagen into the urethral submucosa for treatment of urethral sphincter incompetence in female dogs: 40 cases (1993–2000). *Journal of the American Veterinary Medical Association* **226**, 73–76

Cannizzo KL, McLoughlin MA, Chew DJ and DiBartola SP (2001) Uroendoscopy. Evaluation of the lower urinary tract. *Veterinary Clinics of North America: Small Animal Practice* **31**, 789-807

Cannizzo KL, McLoughlin MA, Mattoon JS *et al.* (2003) Evaluation of transurethral cystoscopy and excretory urography for diagnosis of ectopic ureters in female dogs: 25 cases (1992—2000). *Journal of the American Veterinary Medical Association* **223**, 475–481

Hamaide AJ, Martinez SA, Hauptman J and Walker RD (1998) Prospective comparison of four sampling methods (cystocentesis, bladder mucosal swab, bladder mucosal biopsy, and urolith culture) to identify urinary tract infections in dogs with urolithiasis. *Journal of the American Animal Hospital Association* **34**, 423–430

McCarthy TC (1996) Cystoscopy and biopsy of the feline lower urinary tract. *Veterinary Clinics of North America: Small Animal Practice* **26**, 463–482

McCarthy TC (2003) Transitional cell carcinoma. *Veterinary Medicine* **98**, 96

McCarthy TC (2005) Cystoscopy. In: *Veterinary Endoscopy.* ed. TC McCarthy, pp. 49–135. Elsevier Saunders, St. Louis

Mishina M, Watanabe T, Yugeta N *et al.* (1997) Idiopathic renal hematuria in a dog; the usefulness of a method of partial occlusion of the renal artery. *Journal of Veterinary Medical Science* **59**, 293–295

Senior DF (1992) Urethral dilation. In: *Kirk's Current Veterinary Therapy 11: Small Animal Practice*, ed. RW Kirk and JD Bonagura, pp. 880–882. WB Saunders, Philadelphia

Senior DF and Newman RC (1986) Retrograde ureteral catheterization in female dogs. *Journal of the American Animal Hospital Association* **22**, 831–834

Tawfiek ER and Bagley DH (1998) Ureteroscopic evaluation and treatment of chronic unilateral hematuria. *Journal of Urology* **160**, 700–702

15

Lithotripsy

Jody P. Lulich, Larry G. Adams and Carl A. Osborne

Introduction

In the 1970s it was fortuitously recognized that shock waves generated by collision with raindrops produced unusual pitting patterns on the metal surface of supersonic aircraft during high-speed flight. Researchers theorized that the elliptical contour of one part of the plane's fuselage resulted in the convergence of shock waves on to another focal point of the aircraft, accelerating metal fatigue. Based on these observations, scientists at Dornier, a German aerospace firm, embarked on a programme to develop a system for the production of shock waves that could be reproducibly focused at a solitary point, with the goal of fragmenting urinary stones. This technique was called extracorporeal shock wave lithotripsy (ESWL). On 7 February 1980, at the University of Munich, ESWL was successfully used to fragment uroliths in the kidney of a human patient (Chaussy and Fuchs, 1989). Since that time, the development of ESWL has become a smashing success in terms of revolutionizing treatment of uroliths in humans. The term lithotripsy is derived from the Greek words 'lith' meaning stone, and 'tripsis' meaning to crush. A lithotriptor is a device for crushing or disintegrating uroliths.

ESWL was followed by development of intracorporeal techniques whereby instruments used to generate high-energy wavelengths were directly applied to the surface of uroliths viewed through an endoscope. Compared to surgery, lithotripsy is highly effective, minimally invasive and associated with less risk to the patient. Notably, use of ESWL and intracorporeal endoscopic laser lithotripsy to treat human patients with nephroliths resulted in a significant reduction in iatrogenic loss of renal function associated with surgical intervention (Holman *et al.*, 2002).

Widespread success of extracorporeal and intracorporeal techniques of lithotripsy to treat kidney and ureteral stones in humans prompted veterinary surgeons to consider its feasibility for management of uroliths in dogs and cats.

Extracorporeal shock wave lithotripsy

ESWL is fragmentation of uroliths using shock waves generated outside the body. ESWL is effective for fragmentation of uroliths in the upper urinary tract of dogs (Block *et al.*, 1996; Adams and Senior, 1999). Shock wave lithotripsy (SWL) uses repeated shock waves to fragment nephroliths into many small pieces that can pass spontaneously through the excretory system. All common urolith compositions are amenable to fragmentation by SWL, with the exception of cystine (Williams *et al.*, 2003). In humans, cystine uroliths have highly variable susceptibility to SWL with many cystine nephroliths being resistant to fragmentation.

The components of a shock wave lithotriptor include an energy source for generating the shock waves, a focusing device to concentrate the shock wave energy to a focal point (F2), a coupling medium to transmit the shock waves and allow the shock waves to enter the patient's body, and an imaging system for positioning the urolith within F2. Shock wave lithotriptors are referred to as water bath or dry lithotriptors, based on the coupling medium utilized. Water bath lithotriptors have been used successfully to treat upper tract uroliths in dogs (Figure 15.1). Dry lithotriptors (Figure 15.2) have also been successfully used to treat nephroliths and ureteroliths in dogs (Lane, 2004).

Dogs and cats require general anaesthesia for SWL treatment because of the precise positioning required in addition to providing analgesia during the SWL therapy. Compared with voltages used to generate the shock waves in humans, lower voltages are

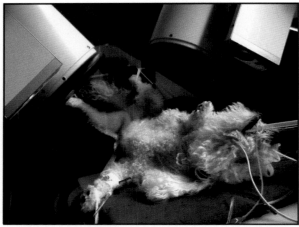

15.1 A 15-year-old spayed Bichon Frise bitch positioned in a water bath lithotriptor during SWL. The flash from the spark discharge which generates the shock wave is visible underneath the dog. Image intensifiers for the biplanar fluoroscopy are also visible.

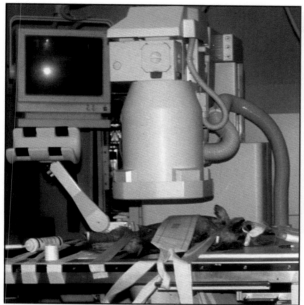

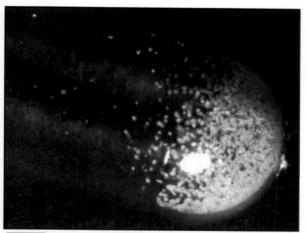

15.3 Voided nephrolith fragments in a 10 ml tube. A dog voided the fragments 48 hours after SWL.

15.2 Dry lithotripsy treatment of nephroliths in a 12-year-old spayed Lhasa Apso bitch. A fluoroscopy imaging system is visible immediately above the dog and the shock wave generator is positioned against the lateral body wall. A 3-litre bag is positioned between the shock wave generator and the dog to facilitate targeting the shock wave at the appropriate depth to position the stone within the focal spot.

recommended to minimize renal injury. Likewise, newer data suggest that slower treatment rates may result in less renal injury and better urolith fragmentation; the authors recommend treatment at approximately 60 shocks/minute.

Efficacy

SWL treatment of canine nephrolithiasis and ureterolithiasis results in fragmentation of the uroliths in approximately 85% of cases with the fragments being small enough to pass through the excretory pathway (Adams and Senior, 1999). Dogs with bilateral nephroliths may receive SWL treatment of both kidneys in one session; however, for dogs with large bilateral nephroliths, SWL treatment of the kidneys may be intentionally staggered with treatments administered 2–4 weeks apart to minimize the risk of bilateral ureteral obstruction during passage of fragments. Ureteroliths appear to be more resistant to fragmentation by SWL than nephroliths and approximately 50% of patients may require more than one treatment for complete fragmentation (Adams and Senior, 1999).

Fragments from SWL may pass rapidly or they may take several months to pass to the urinary bladder then be voided out through the urethra with urine (Figure 15.3). Voiding urohydropropulsion is necessary to remove nephrolith fragments in some dogs if the fragments accumulate in the urinary bladder. In humans, SWL has been considered successful if the patient is stone-free or if the remaining fragments are clinically silent and are smaller than 2 mm in diameter. Recent studies suggest that residual fragments are more likely to cause symptomatic stone episodes in the future.

Thus the optimal outcome in humans following SWL is stone-free rather than having any remaining fragments (Lingeman *et al.*, 2002). Of the dogs the authors have treated using SWL, more than half have retained some <1 mm stone fragments in the recesses of the renal pelvis despite the fact that these fragments were small enough to pass through the ureter. In some of these patients, new nephroliths have formed 1–4 years after SWL, and the remaining fragments may have served as a nidus for stone re-formation. Calcium oxalate stones also tend to recur in dogs that are stone-free; these dogs are frequently documented as recurrent stone formers.

Indications

Not every dog with nephroliths or ureteroliths requires treatment of their uroliths. The term inactive nephroliths refers to small nephroliths that are not causing clinical signs, are not associated with obstruction or infection and do not enlarge over time. Inactive nephroliths may not require treatment but should be monitored for obstruction or enlargement. Indications for treatment of nephroliths in dogs include (Adams and Senior, 1999):

- Large or progressively enlarging nephroliths
- Nephroliths associated with recurrent urinary tract infection
- Uroliths causing partial or complete obstruction of the renal pelvis or ureter
- Dogs with renal failure
- Nephroliths in a solitary functional kidney.

Ureteroliths may pass through the ureter spontaneously and may be monitored for passage unless they are causing moderate to severe obstruction or are associated with infection. Dogs with ureteroliths causing severe obstruction or that do not pass within 1–2 months are candidates for SWL; however, ureteroliths may be more difficult to treat using SWL than nephroliths.

Potential complications

Although SWL is safer than open surgical removal of nephroliths and ureteroliths, complications may occur in some patients. The most common complication is

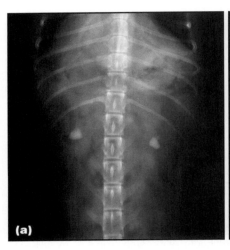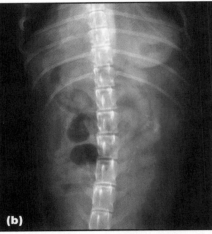

15.4 Abdominal radiographs of a 9-year-old spayed Miniature Poodle bitch with bilateral calcium oxalate nephroliths, **(a)** before SWL and **(b)** 24 hours after SWL, revealing multiple urolith fragments passing through both ureters. The fragments passed spontaneously without any associated clinical signs.

partial to complete obstruction of the ureter during passage of stone fragments. Transient ureteral obstruction has occurred in approximately 10% of canine patients treated with SWL (Figure 15.4). Dogs with large nephroliths are more likely to have ureteral obstruction during passage of the fragments; therefore, SWL may not be ideal for smaller dogs with large stone burdens (nephroliths more than 2–3 cm in diameter).

Other complications are uncommon but may include shock wave-induced pancreatitis, cardiac arrhythmias and urosepsis. Pancreatitis occurs in approximately 2–3% of dogs treated with the HM-3 water bath lithotripter (Daugherty *et al.*, 2004). The focal spot of this lithotripter is larger than the kidney of small dogs; therefore, shock wave energy is partially focused on the pancreas adjacent to the right kidney, which may cause enough pancreatitic trauma to induce pancreatitis. Cardiac arrhythmias are rare and are believed to result from secondary shock waves that are reflected off the gantry or other areas within the water bath. Treatment of infected nephroliths may liberate bacteria into the bloodstream from infected urine in the renal pelvis (so-called urosepsis); therefore, perioperative antibiotics are recommended for any nephroliths that may be complicated by urinary tract infection (Lingeman *et al.*, 2002).

Intracorporeal lithotripsy

The application of SWL has provided new effective treatment options for the management of renal and ureteral stones in dogs (Adams and Senior, 1999). However, the majority of naturally occurring uroliths in dogs are located in the lower urinary tract rather than the kidneys and ureters. For example, uroliths from more than 240,000 dogs have been submitted to the Minnesota Urolith Center for analysis since 1981: in 98% of cases, uroliths were retrieved from the urinary bladder and/or urethra. Unfortunately, SWL is not a reliable form of treatment for bladder stones because of their tendency to move out of the focal point of converging shock waves, resulting in reduced fragmentation. Fortunately, this obstacle has been overcome by fragmenting bladder stones with the aid of cystoscopes to guide various types of newly developed lithotriptors directly to the stones' surface. Several forms of energy (electrohydraulic, ultrasonic and ballistic) can be delivered through the cystoscope and each device has its advantages and disadvantages (Figure 15.5). Because of the versatility of the laser lithotriptor and the authors' familiarity with laser lithotripsy, the remaining discussion applies to holmium–YAG laser lithotripsy in companion animal practice.

Device	Principle	Advantages	Disadvantages
Electrohydraulic	Electric shock produces shock wave	Flexible probe allows use with flexible scopes Minimal cost for equipment	Narrowest margin of safety Failure to fragment hard stones Most likely to cause tissue and equipment damage
Ultrasound	Piezoelectric-generated sound waves mechanically fragment stone	Safe Efficiently fragments large stones Can evacuate stone fragments through probe	Semirigid probes impair use with flexible endoscopes Conversion of vibrational energy to heat requires sufficient irrigation to prevent tissue damage
Pneumatic	Compressed air-driven spike mechanically fragments stone	Safe When combined with ultrasound lithotripsy fragmentation time is reduced	Semirigid probes impair use with flexible endoscopes
Holmium–YAG laser	Excited crystal produces photothermal effect	Flexible, narrow probes permit use with all cystoscopes Fragments all types of stones	Most expensive Safety glasses/training may be required Less efficiently fragments larger stone burdens

15.5 Advantages and disadvantages of several methods of intracorporeal lithotripsy.

The origin of intracorporeal laser lithotripsy

The term 'laser' is an acronym for 'Light Amplification by Stimulated Emission of Radiation'. A laser is a device which transmits light of various frequencies into an extremely intense, small and nearly non-divergent beam of monochromatic radiation in the visible region with all the waves in phase. Lasers are capable of mobilizing immense heat and power when focused in close range.

Use of laser energy for intracorporeal lithotripsy is a relatively new concept. In 1968, investigators first reported *in vitro* fragmentation of uroliths with a ruby laser. However, because fragmentation of stones was associated with generation of heat that would probably be sufficient to damage adjacent tissues, it could not be used to treat patients. Likewise, carbon dioxide laser energy was considered to be unsuitable for clinical use because it could not be delivered through non-toxic fibres. However, in 1986 researchers using a 504 nm, pulsed dye laser successfully and safely treated human patients with ureteroliths. The holmium–YAG laser is the newest device available for clinical lithotripsy.

Holmium (Ho) is a rare-earth element named after Sweden (the Greek word 'holmia' means Sweden) in honour of the Swedish chemist who discovered it. A holmium–YAG (Ho:YAG) laser is a laser whose active medium is a crystal of yttrium, aluminium and garnet (YAG) doped with holmium, and whose beam falls in the near infrared portion of the electromagnetic spectrum (2100 nm).

The mechanism of stone fragmentation with the holmium–YAG laser is mainly photothermal, and involves a thermal drilling process rather than a shock wave effect. Holmium–YAG laser energy is transmitted from the crystal to the urolith via a flexible quartz fibre. To achieve optimum results, the quartz fibre tip must be guided with the aid of a cystoscope so that it is in direct contact with the surface of the urolith.

Efficacy

Laser lithotripsy has been reported to effectively eliminate urinary stones in humans, horses, goats and pigs (Razvi *et al.*, 1996; Howard *et al.*, 1998; Hallard *et al.*, 2002). *In vitro* studies revealed that the holmium–YAG laser consistently shattered canine stones of all types (i.e. calcium oxalate, cystine, struvite, silica and urate) into extractable fragments (<3.5 mm in diameter) in less than 30 seconds (Wynn *et al.*, 2002).

Safety

It is logical to question whether or not lasers capable of shattering stones would also damage tissues comprising the urinary bladder. However, damage to the bladder wall is minimal because the energy of the holmium–YAG laser is delivered in a pulsed fashion and readily absorbed by water. Therefore, continuous irrigation of the urinary bladder during lithotripsy quickly absorbs and disperses stray energy. Under these conditions the thermal effect of the holmium laser is localized to within 1–2 mm of the quartz fibre tip. In a prospective study of 598 human patients with kidney or ureteral stones fragmented by laser lithotripsy, complications were only observed in one patient (ureteral

trauma) (Sofer *et al.*, 2002). These results suggest that when properly used, laser lithotripsy can be safe in dogs and cats. To promote their safe operation, laser use is generally associated with a set of requirements related to national or institutional safety standards (e.g. protective eyewear, safety shut-off devices), as well as operator training requirements.

Lithotripsy in female dogs and cats

Laser lithotripsy is performed via cystoscopy in anaesthetized patients (Figure 15.6). Although patient positioning is often the choice of the operator, the authors position bitches in dorsal recumbency. A rigid cystoscope is passed retrograde into the vestibule and into the urethra to allow visualization of urocystoliths. The bladder is lavaged with a sterile warm isotonic solution (i.e. normal saline, lactated Ringer's) and then refilled. During lithotripsy, continuous irrigation is provided to wash debris from the bladder as stones are fragmented. The laser energy is delivered via a quartz lithotripsy fibre that is passed through the working channel of the cystoscope. The fibre is placed in contact with the stone surface using the aiming beam of the fibre. A foot-operated switch will activate and deactivate the release of energy from the lithotriptor. The energy selected will vary depending on the size and location of the stones; however, initial settings to fragment most stones have been 0.6–0.7 Joules at 8–10 Hertz. The force and frequency of laser pulses can be increased to fragment a larger more stationary urolith, or decreased if excessive stone movement following deployment of higher energies inhibits laser fibre-to-stone contact.

Once uroliths have been shattered such that they are small enough to pass through the urethra, fragments can be removed by a variety of methods. Larger fragments are initially removed with a stone basket to verify that the size is sufficiently small to allow removal by antegrade voiding. If larger fragments are safely retrieved through the urethra, additional fragmentation is not needed. Subsequently, voiding urohydropropulsion is performed to evacuate remaining pieces. Other methods include use of stone evacuators and spontaneous voiding.

In some instances, bladder inflammation and trauma during lithotripsy result in extravasation of blood and subsequent clot formation. If the clot entraps stone fragments and remains adherent to the bladder wall, complete evacuation of stone fragments may not be possible. In the authors' experience, most blood clots resolve in 24 hours. At that time the residual stone burden can be removed by voiding urohydropropulsion or allowed to pass by spontaneous voiding.

Lithotripsy in male dogs

In male dogs, the size of the os penis and flexure of the urethra limits the size and deflectability of cystoscopes that can be introduced into the urinary bladder. However, small diameter (7.5 French), flexible endoscopes used for evaluation of human ureters can easily be inserted into the urethra and bladder of most dogs weighing more than 6–8 kg. When using flexible cystoscopes, the fibreoptic lithotriptor probe can

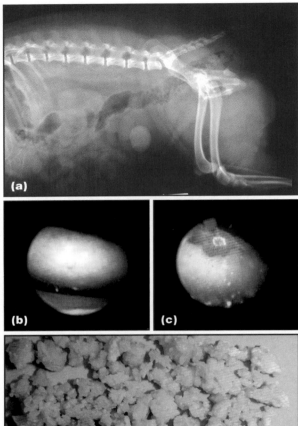

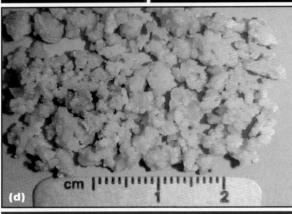

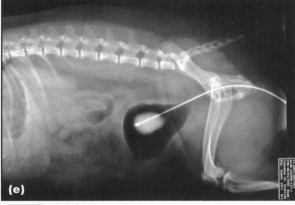

15.6 **(a)** Survey lateral abdominal radiograph of a 4-year-old spayed Pug bitch with a large urocystolith. **(b)** Cystoscopic view of the large stone in the lumen of the bladder before and **(c)** after initiation of laser lithotripsy. A 365 μm diameter flexible quartz laser fibre is positioned near the surface of the urolith. After creating a crater in the stone, further laser application shattered the stone into multiple fragments. **(d)** Multiple stone fragments that were removed with a stone basket and voiding urohydropropulsion. **(e)** Lateral view of a double-contrast cystogram obtained following lithotripsy and retrieval of stone fragments.

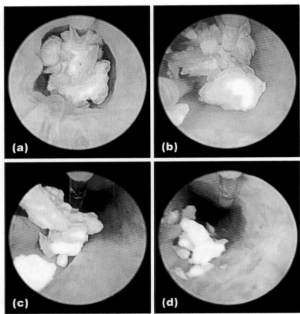

15.7 **(a)** Calcium oxalate urolith in the urethra prior to fragmentation with laser lithotripsy. A 550 μm diameter flexible quartz laser fibre is positioned near the surface of the urolith. **(b)** Initial fragmentation of urolith after 2 seconds of laser lithotripsy. **(c)** Fragmentation of urolith after 35 seconds of laser lithotripsy. **(d)** Complete fragmentation of urolith after approximately 2 minutes of laser lithotripsy.

be inserted through the working channel of the ureteroscope to deliver laser energy to shatter stones. It is usually more efficient and effective to basket bladder stones and place them in the urethra prior to fragmentation (Figure 15.7). Urethroliths are more easily fragmented because their movement out of the laser field is inhibited.

The small diameter of the urethra in male cats currently prohibits application of intracorpreal lithotripsy in this situation without incorporating more invasive procedures.

References and further reading

Adams LG and Senior DF (1999) Electrohydraulic and extracorporeal shock-wave lithotripsy. *Veterinary Clinics of North America: Small Animal Practice* **29**, 293–302

Block G, Adams LG, Widmer WR and Lingeman JE (1996) Use of extracorporeal shock wave lithotripsy for treatment of spontaneous nephrolithiasis and ureterolithiasis in dogs. *Journal of the American Veterinary Medical Association* **208**, 531–536

Chaussy CG and Fuchs GJ (1989) Current state and future developments of noninvasive treatment of human urinary stones with extracorporeal shock wave lithotripsy. *Journal of Urology* **141**, 782–789

Daugherty MA, Adams LG, Baird DK, Siems JJ and Lingeman JE (2004) Acute pancreatitis in two dogs associated with shock wave lithotripsy. *Journal of Veterinary Internal Medicine* **18**, 441 (A)

Davidson EB, Ritchey JW, Higbee RD, Lucroy MD and Bartels KE (2004) Laser lithotripsy for treatment of canine uroliths. *Veterinary Surgery* **33**, 56–61

Grasso M and Chalik Y (1998) Principles and applications of laser lithotripsy: experience with the holmium laser lithorite. *Journal of Clinical Laser Medicine and Surgery* **16**, 3–7

Hallard SK, House JK and Geroge LW (2002) Urethroscopic and laser lithotripsy for the diagnosis and treatment of obstructive urolithiasis in goats and pot-bellied pigs. *Journal of the American Veterinary Medical Association* **220**, 1831–1834

Holman CDJ, Wisniewski ZS, Semmens JB and Bass AJ (2002)

Changing treatment for primary urolithiasis: impact on services and renal preservation in 16679 patients in western Australia. *BJU International* **90**, 7–15

Howard RD, Pleasant RS and May KA (1998) Pulsed dye laser lithotripsy for treatment of urolithiasis in two geldings *Journal of the American Veterinary Medical Association* **212**, 1600–1603

Lane IF (2004) Lithotripsy: an update on urologic applications in small animals. *Veterinary Clinics of North America: Small Animal Practice* **34**, 1011–1025

Lingeman JE (1997) Extracorporeal shock wave lithotripsy: development, instrumentation, and current status. *The Urologic Clinics of North America* **24**, 185–211

Lingeman JE, Lifshitz DA and Evan AP (2002) Surgical management of urinary lithiasis. In: *Campbell's Urology, 8th edn,* ed. PC Walsh, pp. 3361–3451. WB Saunders, Philadelphia

Mulvaney WP and Beck CW (1968) The laser beam in urology. *Journal of Urology* **99**, 112–115

Razvi HA, Denstedt JD, Chun SS and Sales JL (1996) Intracorporeal lithotripsy with the holmium:YAG laser. *Journal of Urology* **156**, 912–914

Sofer M, Watterson JD, Wollin TA *et al.* (2002) Holmium:YAG laser lithotripsy for upper urinary tract calculi in 598 patients. *Journal of Urology* **167**, 31–34

Watson GM and Wickham JE (1986) Initial experience with a pulsed dye laser for ureteric calculi. *Lancet* **1**, 1357–1358

Williams JC, Chee Saw K, Paterson RF *et al.* (2003) Variability of renal stone fragility in shock wave lithotripsy. *Urology* **61**, 1092–1096

Wynn VM, Davidson EB, Higbee RG *et al.* (2002) In vitro assessment of Ho:YAG laser lithotripsy for the treatment of canine urolithiasis. *Proceedings of SPIE (International Society for Optical Engineering), Prog Biomed Opt Imaging* **4609**, 241–246

16

Peritoneal dialysis and haemodialysis

Julie R. Fischer

Introduction

Strictly speaking, *dialysis* refers to the net movement of solutes and water across a semipermeable membrane according to concentration gradients. In medicine, dialysis effects the removal of toxic solutes and excess fluids from the body via indirect exposure of the patient's blood to a sugar and electrolyte solution. This process becomes clinically useful in the following situations:

- When the body cannot eliminate waste solutes and/or fluids due to failure of renal excretory function
- When intractable fluid overload occurs (usually associated with renal or cardiac failure)
- When the presence of a toxin or toxicant requires specifically augmented excretory function.

Dialysis provides metabolic stability to patients who would otherwise die from the polysystemic sequelae of severe renal failure, and dramatically enhances removal of certain endogenous and exogenous toxic substances from the bloodstream.

Two basic forms of dialysis are used in clinical veterinary practice: *peritoneal dialysis* (PD) and *haemodialysis* (HD). This chapter discusses: the basic technical, physical and physiological principles of PD and HD; the identification of patients well suited for dialysis; and the relative advantages, disadvantages and potential risks and complications of these therapies. As the availability of dialytic therapy and awareness of its utility increase among veterinary surgeons and pet owners, dialytic management will probably become the standard of advanced care for animals with severe intractable uraemia.

Principles of dialysis

Physical principles

The basic physical principles are the same for PD and HD: the patient's blood interfaces indirectly with a contrived solution, termed the *dialysate*, across a semipermeable membrane. The dialysate is formulated to favour movement of permeable waste molecules (e.g. urea, creatinine, phosphorus) out of the plasma, to maintain physiological plasma concentrations of permeable substances (e.g. sodium, chloride, glucose, calcium) and to replenish or load permeable molecules that have been depleted from the plasma (e.g. bicarbonate). In the case of PD, the vessel-rich peritoneum serves as the interface, the dialysis membrane (Figure 16.1); in the case of HD, the interface occurs extracorporeally across the many membranes of a

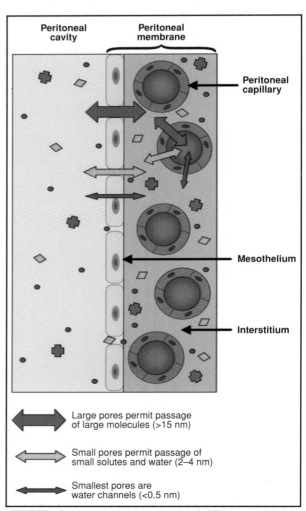

16.1 Schematic representation of diffusion across the peritoneal membrane. Water and solutes diffuse out of peritoneal capillaries and across the peritoneal membrane through pores in the membrane. The largest pores (green arrow) permit passage of large molecules (e.g. small proteins), the mid-size pores (yellow arrow) permit passage of small solutes and water and the smallest pores (red arrow) are water channels only.

Within figure:

Peritoneal cavity

Peritoneal membrane

Peritoneal capillary

Mesothelium

Interstitium

Large pores permit passage of large molecules (>15 nm)

Small pores permit passage of small solutes and water (2–4 nm)

Smallest pores are water channels (<0.5 nm)

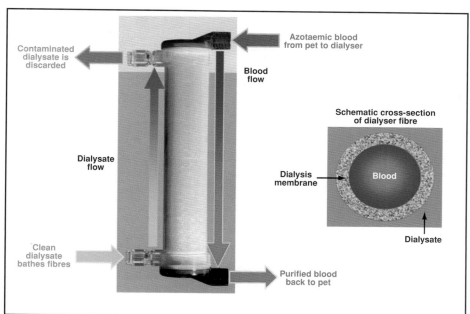

Dialyser flows and schematic cross-section of dialyser fibre. In HD, blood flows through many hollow fibres encased in the plastic shell of the dialyser. Dialysate flows in a counter-current direction in the plastic shell, bathing the blood-filled fibres. The counter-current flow of blood and dialysate maximizes the concentration gradient across the dialyser membranes and thus maximizes diffusion across the membranes.

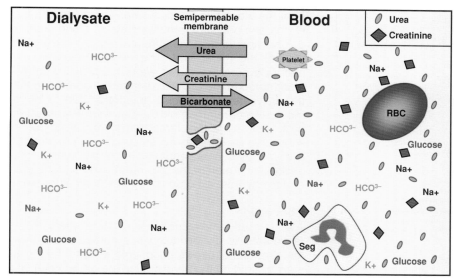

16.3 Schematic representation of diffusion in HD. Dissolved solutes diffuse across the semipermeable dialysis membrane through membrane pores. Molecular movement occurs in both directions, but net transfer occurs according to the concentration gradient of each solute, as indicated by the arrows. Pore size precludes loss of cellular elements from the blood, as well as larger molecules such as proteins. The dialysate is formulated to maintain physiological concentrations of diffusible substances such as glucose and sodium.
HCO_3^- = Bicarbonate; K^+ = Potassium; Na^+ = Sodium; RBC = Red blood cell; Seg = Segmented neutrophil.

hollow-fibre dialyser (Figure 16.2), through which the patient's blood is pumped. In both types of dialysis, removal of dissolved solutes and excess fluid occurs across the dialysis membrane by the processes of diffusion, ultrafiltration and convection.

Diffusion

Diffusive dialysis relies on the random molecular motion of dissolved particles. As these particles arbitrarily encounter the dialyser membrane, they can move from one side of the membrane to the other through membrane channels (see Figures 16.1 and 16.3). Likelihood of contact with a membrane channel is directly proportional to the concentration of a given particle type and its thermodynamic energy. Thermodynamic energy is inversely proportional to molecular mass; thus, at equal concentrations smaller molecules diffuse more readily than larger molecules (e.g. urea diffuses more readily than creatinine). If concentra-

tions of a solute become equal on both sides of the membrane (i.e. filtration equilibrium is achieved), diffusion across the membrane still occurs but net transfer of that solute will be zero. Maintenance of the concentration gradient between blood and dialysate, and therefore maintenance of diffusive dialysis, is accomplished by periodic (in PD) or continuous (in HD) replacement of dialysate, thus preventing filtration equilibrium. The large majority of solute removal during a standard PD or HD session occurs by simple diffusion.

Ultrafiltration

Ultrafiltration is the process by which excess plasma water is removed, and is accomplished differently in PD and HD (Figures 16.14 and 16.15). PD uses hyperosmolal dialysate to draw fluid into the peritoneal cavity. The dialysate osmolality is usually adjusted by varying the dextrose concentration (though some newer dialysate solutions use amino acids as the osmotic

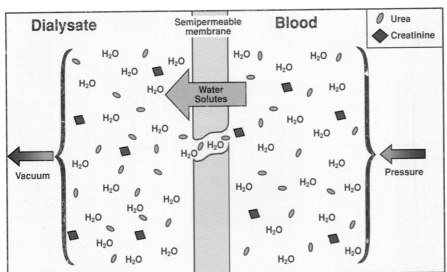

Schematic representation of ultrafiltration and convection in HD. Positive pressure on the blood side and negative pressure on the dialysate side of the dialysis membrane combine to draw water and solute molecules through the membrane pores in processes called ultrafiltration and convection (solvent drag), respectively. Note that the concentration of dissolved solute in the blood remains the same in these processes, since solutes and water are simultaneously moved through the pores. The arrow represents the direction of net movement of solutes and water.

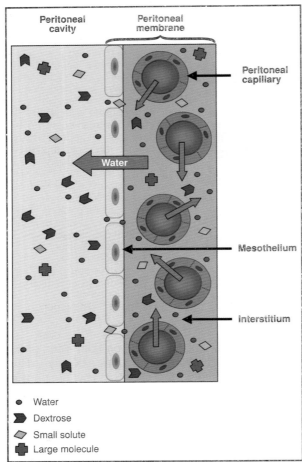

16.5 Schematic representation of ultrafiltration and convection in PD. The peritoneal cavity has been filled with dialysate that is hyperosmolal to the blood due to the dialysate dextrose concentration (blue arrowheads). Water (red ovals) follows the osmotic gradient and diffuses out of the capillaries into the peritoneal membrane interstitium and then into the peritoneal cavity. Though water diffusion occurs in both directions, net water movement is into the peritoneal cavity as indicated by the red arrow. Some dissolved solutes are carried with the water molecules into the peritoneal cavity by convection.

agent), and different dextrose concentrations permit different rates of fluid removal. HD uses a pressure gradient across the dialysis membrane to move water from the blood into the dialysate. The outward transmembrane pressure generated by the blood pump is complemented by a vacuum applied to the dialysate side of the membrane. The resulting outward net hydraulic pressure draws water molecules from the blood through the dialyser membrane pores and into the dialysate. The precise amount of fluid to be removed is programmed into the dialysis delivery system by the operator at the start of treatment. The amount of water that can be moved across the HD membrane during a given time depends on the hydraulic permeability of the membrane, the membrane surface area and the hydrostatic gradient across the membrane.

Convection

Also termed *solvent drag*, convection refers to the movement of dissolved solutes across the dialysis membrane that occurs in conjunction with the movement of fluid during ultrafiltration in both PD and HD. Convection plays a minor role in solute removal during standard PD and HD, and does not occur in the absence of ultrafiltration (see Figures 16.4 and 16.5). Some HD techniques maximize the contribution of convective solute removal by performing simultaneous high-rate ultrafiltration and intravenous fluid replacement. When combined with HD this process is called *haemodiafiltration* and maximizes removal of middle molecular weight solutes (~12,000 kD).

Peritoneal dialysis

PD requires minimal specialized equipment and is not technically difficult to perform. PD is, however, extremely labour-intensive, and demands close attention to issues of sterility during the procedures.

Performance of PD requires insertion of a large-bore catheter into the abdomen, and the degree and durability of that catheter's function are the chief determinants of success or failure of PD in a given patient.

Most catheters are variations of silastic tubing with multiple fenestrations and one or more, commonly two, Dacron velour cuffs along the length of the tubing (Figure 16.6). The fenestrated portion of the tubing is positioned in the peritoneal cavity, and the cuffs are designed for placement in the rectus sheath and in the subcutaneous tunnel created between the point of rectus penetration and skin exit. Fibroblast migration into the cuffs anchors the catheter in place and provides a physical barrier to dialysate leakage and ingress of infectious agents. Catheter placement may be performed percutaneously, laparoscopically or via

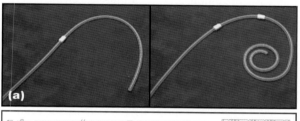

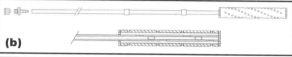

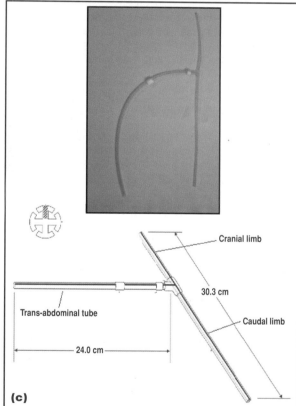

Cranial limb

30.3 cm

Trans-abdominal tube

Caudal limb

24.0 cm

(c)

16.6 Peritoneal dialysis catheters. **(a)** Tenckhoff single-cuffed, straight acute PD catheter (left) and double-cuffed, spiral chronic PD catheter (right). (Courtesy of Cook Inc., Bloomington.) **(b)** Acute peritoneal dialysis catheter with two Dacron cuffs and coaxial intraperitoneal portion (lower drawing is cross-section of coaxial portion). (Courtesy of Smiths Medical PM, Waukesha.) **(c)** Ash Advantage fluted-T catheter (left) with schematic cross-section of fluted portion (upper middle) and labelled catheter schematic (right). (Courtesy of Medigroup Inc., Oswego.)

laparotomy. Laparotomy provides the option of simultaneously performing a partial or complete omentectomy, which substantially increases and prolongs catheter function. If the clinician anticipates that the need for PD will exceed 24 hours, omentectomy is recommended (Labato and Ross, 2005).

PD is accomplished by infusion of dialysate into the abdomen through the catheter, allowing the dialysate to remain in the abdomen for a prescribed *dwell time*, draining the fluid into a waste bag and then repeating the process. Exchanges can be performed with a straight transfer set but, ideally, the dialysate bag, catheter and drain bag should be connected by a closed 'Y' system that permits abdominal drainage followed by dialysate infusion without disconnection of the catheter (Figure 16.7). Prior to draining the abdomen, a small amount of clean dialysate should be flushed through the line into the drain bag. The abdomen is then drained, and subsequently filled with fresh dialysate for the next dwell. This drain-then-infuse sequence flushes any contaminants that may have entered the system during connection into the drain bag instead of into the abdomen, and in humans markedly reduces the incidence of septic peritonitis. Each infuse-dwell-drain series is called a *cycle* or an *exchange*.

Initial exchanges for markedly azotaemic or overhydrated patients are performed every 1–2 hours with 30–40 minute dwell times. This high frequency of exchanges continues for the first 24–48 hours, or until the patient is clinically stabilized with a blood urea nitrogen (BUN) of approximately 20–35 mmol/l (56–98 mg/dl) and a creatinine of approximately 350–530 µmol/l (3.96–5.99 mg/dl). At that point, a less intensive schedule is adopted, with exchanges three to

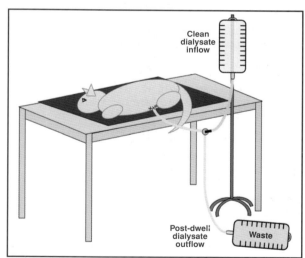

Clean dialysate inflow

Post-dwell dialysate outflow

Waste

16.7 Closed 'Y' system for drainage and infusion of dialysate in PD. The catheter is unwrapped and prepared, and the bags and lines are connected in a sterile fashion. A small amount of fresh dialysate is first flushed from the clean bag into the waste bag, and then the stopcock is turned to allow post-dwell dialysate to drain from the abdomen into the waste bag. The stopcock is then turned to allow fresh dialysate to flow into the abdomen. Following infusion, the catheter is disconnected and aseptically capped, the abdomen is wrapped, and the patient may return to its cage for the duration of the dwell time.

four times per day with 4–6 hour dwells.

The PD dialysate prescription can be quite variable, but all solutions contain sodium, chloride, a buffer (usually lactate) and varying concentrations of calcium and glucose or dextrose. Commercial PD solutions with different dextrose concentrations may be purchased, and a basic PD solution can be formulated by adding dextrose to lactated Ringer's solution (30 ml of 50% dextrose in 1 litre = 1.5% dextrose solution). Some newer commercial formulations use bicarbonate as the buffering agent, but this requires two separate dialysate bags to prevent bicarbonate and calcium components from precipitating prior to infusion. The addition of heparin (250–2000 IU/l) to the dialysate is recommended for the first days following catheter placement to minimize risk of catheter occlusion from fibrin deposition.

Maintenance of sterility in connection, disconnection, infusion and drainage is of the utmost importance, since septic peritonitis is a relatively common and often lethal complication of PD in companion animals. Scrupulous handwashing should be observed, and sterile gloves worn during connection, disconnection and bag changes, because contamination of the bag spike is the most common source of peritonitis in humans on PD. Line connections should be covered with povidone–iodine or chlorhexidine-soaked dressings. Injection ports should be cleaned with chlorhexidine and alcohol prior to use, and multidose vials for dialysate additives should be avoided.

Careful monitoring of the patient and PD procedures is critical to delivery of effective and safe treatments, and allows complications to be addressed as early as possible. Critical monitoring data for PD patients are listed in Figure 16.8, and should be collected and maintained in an organized fashion for analysis.

Physical examination parameters
Body weight every 12 hours (same scale)
Body temperature at least every 12 hours
Exit site inspection every 24 hours
Inspection for dialysate leakage or tunnel swelling/tenderness every exchange

Laboratory parameters
Haematocrit and total protein every 12 hours
Biochemistry panel every 24 hours
Cytology of drained dialysate every 24 hours

Exchange parameters

Drainage:
    Start time
    End time
    Total drain time
    Total drain volume
Inflow:
    Start time
    End time
    Total inflow time
    Total volume infused
Net balance per exchange (difference between outflow and prior inflow)

16.8 Monitoring parameters for the PD patient.

Haemodialysis

Performance of HD requires repeated large gauge vascular access, which, in animals, is achieved via jugular catheterization. A dual-lumen jugular catheter is placed, ideally with the catheter tip located in the right atrium (Figure 16.9). For acute dialysis, a temporary, non-cuffed catheter is placed percutaneously over a guidewire and provides acceptable access for 2–3 weeks (Figure 16.10a). If the need for HD exceeds the functional lifespan of the temporary catheter, a permanent HD catheter is placed (Figure 16.10b). These catheters are tunnelled subcutaneously so the cuff lies in the subcutis between the venotomy site and the skin exit site. This cuff allows tissue ingrowth, stabilizing the catheter and creating a physical barrier to bacteraemia.

Prior to each treatment, the patient is carefully assessed and the catheter exit site and ports are meticulously cleaned. The HD prescription (including dialysate formulation, dialyser and circuit selected, treatment time, ultrafiltration volume, target blood volume to process and heparinization) is designed specifically for each treatment, based on the patient's physical and biochemical status, as well as response to previous treatments. In severely azotaemic patients (BUN >70 mmol/l (>196 mg/dl)) a staged initial approach to azotaemia reduction is taken. The urea reduction ratio (URR) (Figure 16.11) is a useful concept to help plan treatments, and is calculated as:

$$1 - \left(\frac{\text{Post-treatment BUN}}{\text{Pre-treatment BUN}} \right)$$

Typically, the first HD treatment targets a URR of 0.3–0.6 (usually not to exceed a URR of >0.1 per hour), the second treatment a URR of 0.5–0.8, and the third treatment a URR 0.9–0.95 (Figures 16.12 and 16.13). Initial treatments are usually performed on consecutive days.

This type of staged reduction permits cerebral acclimatization to the decrease in plasma osmolality that accompanies resolution of severe azotaemia, diminishing the risk of dialysis disequilibrium syndrome

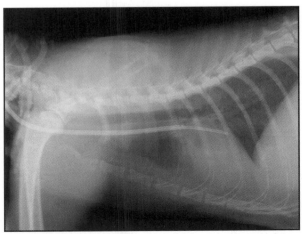

16.9 Lateral radiograph confirming placement of a temporary dual-lumen haemodialysis catheter in a cat, with the catheter tip positioned in the right atrium.

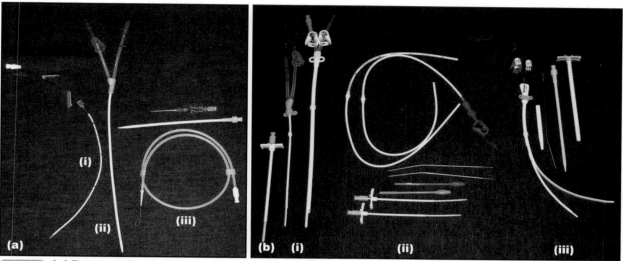

16.10 **(a)** Temporary haemodialysis catheters. **(i)** A 7 French, 20 cm, dual-lumen catheter, commonly used for parenteral nutrition and blood-sampling. **(ii)** An 11.5 French, 24 cm, dual-lumen catheter designed for temporary haemodialysis access in humans. **(iii)** A peripheral catheter (used for gaining initial venous access), a vein dilator and a guidewire coiled in its holder (top to bottom). **(b)** Three types of permanent haemodialysis catheter. **(i)** Paediatric (middle) and adult (right) dual-lumen, fixed-tip permanent catheters. On the far left is a peel-away sheath introducer for percutaneous placement. **(ii)** Tesio Cath twin catheters. An access port has been connected to only one of the catheters in this picture. Below the catheters are tunnelling devices and peel-away sheaths. **(iii)** Ash Split catheter. This catheter combines the ease of fixed-tip placement with the enhanced flows of twin catheters. Tunnelling device, vein dilator and peel-away sheath are pictured to the right of the catheter. Note the Dacron cuff at the proximal end of all permanent catheters. (Reproduced from Fischer *et al.* (2004) with permission from *Veterinary Clinics of North America: Small Animal Practice*.)

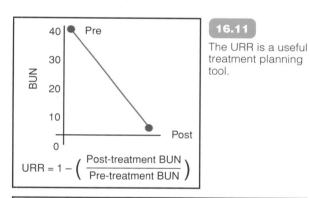

16.11 The URR is a useful treatment planning tool.

$$URR = 1 - \left(\frac{\text{Post-treatment BUN}}{\text{Pre-treatment BUN}} \right)$$

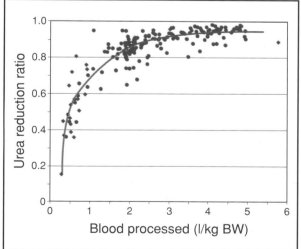

16.12 URR *versus* blood processed (l/kg). The regression line on this graph allows estimation of the amount of blood to process per kilogram body weight to achieve a desired URR in a given patient.

(DDS). DDS is the clinical manifestation of cerebral oedema, and can vary from ataxia, altered mentation and pupillary abnormalities, to seizure, coma and death from brainstem herniation. Mannitol is given during initial treatments, particularly in cats, as prophylaxis against DDS. Once renal values are lowered into the normal range, most patients can be managed with HD treatments three times per week. Mannitol is usually not needed after initial stabilization treatments. As long as renal function is minimal, azotaemia will recur between treatments, but thrice-weekly HD can usually maintain a non-uraemic state and good quality of life (Figure 16.13).

The dialysis delivery system monitors and regulates every facet of the HD treatment, including dialysate composition and temperature, rate of blood flow, heparin delivery, pressure within the extracorporeal blood circuit and ultrafiltration rate. Dialysate and bicarbonate concentrates are connected to intake hoses during machine setup. The extracorporeal circuit and dialyser are connected and primed with saline or 3% dextrans. Following systemic heparinization, the patient's catheter ports are connected to the extracorporeal circuit, and the delivery system's peristaltic pump draws the patient's blood into the circuit, then pumps it through the hollow fibres of the dialyser (Figure 16.14). The precise parameters of a given treatment are programmed into the delivery system prior to initiation of treatment. If any treatment parameters are breached, the delivery system alarms and suspends dialysis until the condition is corrected. Filters and a reverse osmosis system provide highly purified water to the dialysis delivery systems to minimize exposure of the patient's blood to harmful substances. Critical to the safe and

	Day 1	Day 2	Day 3
Pre BUN	87.5 mmol/l (245 mg/dl)	67.8 mmol/l (190 mg/dl)	35.0 mmol/l (98 mg/dl)
Reduction	30% = 26.3 mmol/l (74 mg/dl)	60% = 40.7 mmol/l (114 mg/dl)	90% = 31.5 mmol/l (88 mg/dl)
Blood to process	0.4 l/kg = 12 l	0.7 l/kg = 21 l	3 l/kg = 90 l
Treatment time	4 hours	5 hours	5 hours
Pump speed	3 l/hr = 50 ml/min	4.2 l/hr = 70 ml/min	18 l/hr = 300 ml/min
Post BUN	63.2 mmol/l (177 mg/dl)	27.1 mmol/l (76 mg/dl)	3.5 mmol/l (9 mg/dl)

(a)

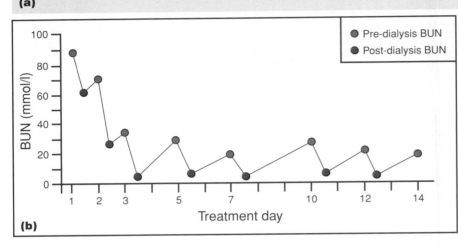

(b)

16.13 Example of a staged initial azotaemia reduction plan for a 30 kg dog. **(a)** The table shows the calculations used to plan the urea reduction (based on desired URR and body weight) and blood pump speed in the first three HD treatments for a markedly azotaemic dog. **(b)** The graph plots the BUN before (red) and after (blue) each HD treatment. Note the azotaemia rebound between treatments. The graph then shows how additional treatments performed every 48–72 hours maintain azotaemia within a tolerable range.

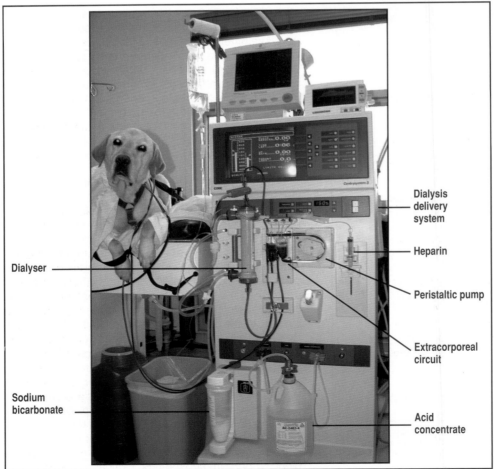

16.14 HD delivery system in use. The patient's dialysis catheter is connected to the circuit blood lines and the peristaltic pump circulates blood from the patient, through the dialyser and back to the patient. The sodium bicarbonate and acid concentrate containers are connected to uptake lines at the base of the machine. The patient wears a nylon walking harness with sewn-on clips that clip to webbing tethers anchored to the treatment table. The tethers permit movement and shifting of position, but prevent the patient jumping off the table. An ECG and oxygen saturation/haemoglobin concentration monitor sit on top of the delivery system.

effective delivery of HD treatments are personnel specifically trained in the operation of the equipment and monitoring of patients on HD.

During the treatment, the patient's physical status and treatment parameters (e.g. extracorporeal chamber pressures, ultrafiltration rate) are closely monitored. Blood pressure, heart rate and activated clotting time are monitored every 15–30 minutes as needed, and ideally venous oxygen saturation and haematocrit are continuously monitored with an in-line probe. General appearance and mentation are continuously monitored.

At the end of the treatment, the blood line connections are scrubbed and a *rinseback* procedure returns the blood in the circuit to the patient. The catheter is capped in a sterile fashion and the catheter lumens are filled with a lock solution (usually 100–5,000 IU/ml of heparin). The catheter is protected with a secure neckwrap until the next dialysis treatment. The dialysis catheter is not used or maintained by anyone other than dialysis personnel. Some dialysis catheters have been maintained successfully in dogs for a year or longer.

Discontinuation of dialysis

Dialysis, whether PD or HD, may be discontinued when the patient's kidneys can maintain normal fluid balance and have excretory function that permits clinical well-being. Azotaemia does not need to be completely resolved, but must be at a non-uraemic level. Many patients will continue to recover renal function for weeks to months after dialysis is discontinued, but may require nutritional support via feeding tube during that period.

Veterinary applications of dialysis

Dialysis can potentially provide benefit to three broad categories of veterinary patients (Figure 16.15):

- Animals with severe, intractable uraemia
- Animals with unresponsive volume overload
- Animals with some toxicoses.

Uraemia

The majority of animals considered for dialysis have acute uraemia that is unresponsive to diuresis with intravenous fluids and pharmacological manipulation (see Chapter 17). Uraemia may be due to acute renal insult, postrenal causes or acute exacerbation of an underlying chronic renal disease, and may include life-threatening hyperkalaemia and/or acidosis in addition to azotaemia. Animals may be polyuric, oliguric or anuric or have normal urine output. In dogs, common causes of acute uraemia include:

- Nephrotoxicosis
- Infectious agents
- Severe systemic illness
- Decompensation of chronic interstitial nephritis or glomerulonephritis
- Renal ischaemia.

Severe uraemia

Acute renal failure
    Refractory azotaemia (BUN ≥35.7 mmol/l (100 mg/dl) and/or creatinine ≥884 μmol/l (10 mg/dl))
    Severe electrolyte disturbance (hyperkalaemia, hypo/hypernatraemia)
    Severe metabolic acidosis
    Management of delayed graft function following transplantation
Chronic (end-stage) renal failure
    Refractory azotaemia (BUN ≥35.7 mmol/l (100 mg/dl) and/or creatinine ≥884 μmol/l (10 mg/dl)) (mainly HD)
    Preoperative conditioning for renal transplantation
    Finite extension of improved quality of life to allow client adjustment to diagnosis and prognosis

Volume overload

Unresponsive oliguria or anuric
Fulminant congestive heart failure
    Pulmonary oedema
    Circulatory overload
    Lack of response to diuretics
Iatrogenic fluid overload
Parenteral nutrition in oligoanuric animals

Acute toxicosis or drug overdose

Ethylene glycol toxicosis (acute toxicant removal and chronic management of resultant acute renal failure)
Environmental/agricultural toxins/toxicants (mainly HD)
Accidental ingestion/overdose of many chemicals and medications (mainly HD)

Miscellaneous

Pancreatitis (mainly PD)
Severe hyperthermia (mainly PD)
Severe hypothermia (mainly PD)
Hypercalcaemia

16.15 Indications for dialytic therapy.

In cats, common causes of acute uraemia include:

- Acute ureteral obstruction
- Nephrotoxicosis
- Pyelonephritis
- Lymphoma
- Acute exacerbation of chronic interstitial nephritis.

Inherent in acute uraemia is variable potential for renal recovery. For acutely uraemic patients, dialysis can provide the surrogate excretory function needed to sustain life while the kidneys undergo cellular repair or the cause of uraemia is corrected (e.g. acute ureteral obstruction). Dialysis can also mitigate the clinical manifestations of chronic, end-stage renal disease when conventional management fails, but few owners are financially able to continue such therapy indefinitely. For veterinary patients requiring chronic dialysis, HD rather than PD is currently the treatment modality of choice if it is available.

Volume overload

Life-threatening volume overload, whether due to oliguria/anuria, congestive heart failure or excessive

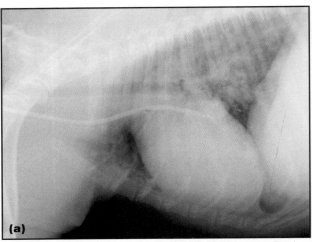 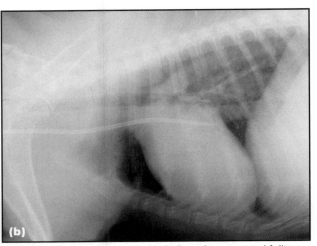

16.16 Lateral thoracic radiographs of a Labrador Retriever with oliguria from leptospirosis-induced acute renal failure. The dog was presented in an extremely overhydrated state. **(a)** This radiograph taken prior to the first HD treatment shows significant pulmonary oedema and mild cardiomegaly, as well as a dialysis catheter in place with the tip in the right atrium. **(b)** This radiograph taken immediately following the first dialysis treatment shows significant resolution of the pulmonary oedema and a more normal cardiac silhouette, due to fluid removal via ultrafiltration.

fluid administration, can be managed with ultrafiltration in a patient that is unresponsive to diuretics (Figure 16.16). Removal of excess fluid can mitigate or resolve pulmonary oedema and peripheral oedema, and help prevent re-accumulation of pleural and peritoneal effusions by decreasing capillary hydrostatic pressure. Resolution of volume overload also contributes to control of blood pressure in these often hypertensive patients.

Specific acute toxicoses

Dialysis is also uniquely suited to the management of specific acute toxicoses. Drugs and chemicals whose physical characteristics permit passage through dialyser membrane pores or across the peritoneal membrane can be removed from the bloodstream with PD or HD (Figure 16.17) (Johnson and Simmons, 2005). Of particular note, ethylene glycol and its nephrotoxic metabolites are easily removed by dialysis, and, if such

	Dialysable by HD only	Dialysable by PD and HD	Dialysable by high-flux HD only
Alcohols	Ethanol; Methanol		
Analgesics/anti-inflammatories	Paracetamol; Mesalamine (5-ASA) Pentazocine	Aspirin	Morphine
Antibacterials	Amoxicillin (most penicillins); Cefalexin (most first generation cephalosporins); Cefotetan (many second generation cephalosporins); Cefoxitin; Ceftriaxone (many third generationcephalosporins); Chloramphenicol; Cilastatin; Linezolid; Metronidazole; Nitrofurantoin; Ofloxacin; Sulbactam; Sulfamethoxazole; Trimethoprim	Amikacin; Some first generation, second generation and third generation cephalosporins; Clavulanic acid; Gentamicin; Imipenem; Kanamycin; Neomycin; Sulfisoxazole; Tobramycin	Vancomycin
Anticonvulsants	Gabapentin; Primidone	Phenobarbital	Phenytoin
Antifungals	Dapsone	Fluconazole; Flucytosine	
Antineoplastics	Busulfan; Carboplatin; Cyclophosphamide; Fluorouracil (5-FU); Ifosfamide; Methotrexate; Mercaptopurine		Cisplatin; Cytarabine
Antivirals	Aciclovir; Famciclovir; Valacyclovir	Zidovudine	
Cardiac/vasoactive medications	Atenolol; Bretylium; Captopril; Lisinopril Metoprolol; Mexilitine; Procainamide; Sotalol; Tocainide	Enalapril; Esmolol; Nitroprusside	

16.17 Readily dialysable medications and chemicals. (continues)

▶

	Dialysable by HD only	Dialysable by PD and HD	Dialysable by high-flux HD only
Chelating agents	Deferoxamine; Penicillamine	Ethylenediamine tetra-acetic acid (EDTA)	
Immunosuppressive agents	Azathioprine; Methylprednisolone		
Miscellaneous medications	Allopurinol; Chloral hydrate; Chlorphenamine; Foscarnet; Iohexol Metformin; Octreotide; Theophylline	Aminocaproic acid; Ascorbic acid; Carisoprodol; Diazoxide; Iopamidol; Lithium; Mannitol; Meprobamate; Methyldopa; Minoxidil	Ranitidine

16.17 (continued) Readily dialysable medications and chemicals.

removal is accomplished promptly and thoroughly (within 8–12 hours of ingestion in dogs), renal damage may be lessened or averted entirely.

Risks and complications

Though both PD and HD carry significant risk of morbidity and mortality, patients presented for these therapies usually have a grave prognosis if not dia-lysed. Part of determining a given patient's suitability for dialysis involves weighing potential risk *versus* potential benefit. Figures 16.18 and 16.19 present common complications and possible prevention strat-egies/management techniques for PD and HD, re-spectively.

Whether to use PD or HD in a given patient is usually a matter of availability since there are still few veterinary haemodialysis centres, but if both modalities

Complication	Prevention or management technique(s)
Catheter occlusion	Omentectomy; use of heparin in dialysate; high pressure saline flush; instillation of 15,000 units of urokinase in the catheter lumen for 3 hours; repositioning or replacement of catheter
Subcutaneous dialysate leakage	Close apposition of abdominal incision with simple interrupted sutures. Limit initial exchange volumes to quarter to half calculated volume. Stabilize catheter for good ingrowth into cuffs
Septic peritonitis	Meticulous hand hygiene; sterile gloves and excellent aseptic technique for connections, disconnections and bag changes. Monitor for pericatheter leaks. Check outflow dialysate cytology daily. If peritonitis, treat with systemic and intraperitoneal antibiotics
Exit site infection	No pursestring or other exit site sutures for longer-term catheters; dry, sterile bandages over the exit site
Tunnel infection	Stabilize catheter to allow good tissue ingrowth into cuffs
Protein loss/ hypoalbuminaemia	Ensure adequate protein/calorie nutrition. Use oesophageal feeding tubes or parenteral nutrition if necessary. Consider 1.1% amino acid dialysate
Dyspnoea	Monitor for/treat pleural effusion. Reduce infusion volumes if due to increased abdominal pressure
Overhydration	Increase concentration of dextrose in dialysate to 2.5% or 4.25% to increase ultrafiltration

16.18 Common complications and possible prevention strategies/management techniques for PD.

Complication	Prevention or management technique(s)
Catheter dysfunction	Check catheter for kinks. Resolve luminal clot with flush or by passing wire. Make sure patient is not volume depleted. Reposition or replace catheter
Bacterial catheter infection	Lock catheter with antimicrobial solution. Replace catheter over wire. Replace catheter in other jugular. In all cases, treat with systemic antimicrobials
Haemorrhage complicated by heparinization	Decrease degree of heparinization. If minor, treat with pressure; if major, consider discontinuing treatment and administering protamine. Control hypertension
Hypotension	Make sure patient is volume replete. Stop ultrafiltration. If severe and unresponsive to volume, treat with pressors or discontinue treatment
Caval thrombosis/ stenosis	If early thrombosis, may try streptokinase or tissue plasminogen activator. If organized thrombus or stenosis, remove catheter if possible
Severe circuit clotting	Manually remove clot if possible. End treatment and rinse back blood if necessary. Transfuse if necessary
Dialysis disequilibrium syndrome	Perform staged initial urea reduction. Keep initial URR below 0.1/hour. Treat markedly azotaemic patients with mannitol, especially if <10 kg. Monitor closely for pupillary abnormalities, altered mentation or bizarre behaviour

16.19 Common complications and possible prevention strategies/management techniques for HD.

Variable	Peritoneal dialysis	Haemodialysis
Equipment	Inexpensive and readily available	Expensive and very specific
Expertise	Little required	Extensive training required
Efficiency	Moderate	Extremely efficient
Toxicant/toxin removal	Moderate for some	Excellent for many
Client cost	High due to intensive care costs and labour	High if intensive care, moderate if outpatient
Labour intensiveness	Very high, especially acutely	Moderate during treatment time
Peritonitis risk	Moderate	None from procedure
Hypotension risk	None from procedure	Low to moderate (small patients)

16.20 Relative advantages and disadvantages of PD and HD.

are available Figure 16.20 presents relative advantages and disadvantages of the two techniques.

Summary

Both PD and HD have the capacity to mitigate the metabolic crises that accompany acute renal failure, and to help remove dialysable toxins from the body. PD is labour-intensive and time-consuming, and requires meticulous technique but little training or specialized equipment. Generally, veterinary PD patients remain hospitalized during therapy. HD, on the other hand, requires specialized equipment and specifically trained personnel, but is a more effective and efficient therapy which can be performed on an outpatient basis. Dialytic therapy is intensive and expensive, but for patients in need of its unique capacities, it is life-saving.

References and further reading

Burkart J (2004) Metabolic consequences of peritoneal dialysis. *Seminars in Dialysis* **17(6)**, 498–504

Chew DJ, DiBartola SP and Crisp MS (2000) Peritoneal dialysis. In: *Fluid Therapy in Small Animal Practice 2nd edn*, ed. SP DiBartola, pp. 507–527. WB Saunders, Philadelphia

Cowgill LD and Francey T (2006) Hemodialysis. In: *Fluid Electrolyte and Acid-Base Disorders in Small Animal Practice, 3rd edn*, ed. SP DiBartola, pp. 650–677. WB Saunders, Philadelphia

Crisp MS, Chew DJ, DiBartola SP and Birchard SJ (1989) Peritoneal dialysis in dogs and cats: 27 cases (1976–1987). *Journal of the American Veterinary Medical Association* **195(9)**, 1262–1266

Dzyban LA, Labato MA and Ross LA (2000) CVT update: peritoneal dialysis. In: *Kirk's Current Veterinary Therapy XIII*, ed. JD Bonagura, pp. 859–861. WB Saunders, Philadelphia

Fischer JR, Pantaleo V, Francey T and Cowgill LD (2004) Veterinary hemodialysis: advances in management and technology. *Veterinary Clinics of North America: Small Animal Practice* **34(4)**, 935–967

Fischer JR, Pantaleo V, Francey T and Cowgill LD (2004) Clinical and clinicopathological features of cats with acute ureteral obstruction managed with hemodialysis between 1993 and 2004: a review of 50 cases. *Journal of Veterinary Internal Medicine* **18**, 777 [abstract]

Johnson CD and Simmons WD (2005) *2005 Dialysis of Drugs*. Nephrology Pharmacy Associates. www.nephrologypharmacy.com

Labato MA and Ross LA (2006) Peritoneal dialysis. In: *Fluid Electrolyte and Acid-Base Disorders in Small Animal Practice, 3rd edn*, ed. SP DiBartola, 635–649. WB Saunders, Philadelphia

Langston CE, Cowgill LD and Spano JA (1997) Applications and outcome of hemodialysis in cats: a review of 29 cases. *Journal of Veterinary Internal Medicine* **11(6)**, 348–355

Pantaleo V, Francey T, Fischer JR and Cowgill LD (2004) Application of hemodialysis for the management of acute uremia in cats: 119 cases (1993–2003). *Journal of Veterinary Internal Medicine* **18**, 418 [abstract]

Tjiong HL, van den Berg JW, Wattimena JL *et al.* (2005) Dialysate as food: combined amino acid and glucose dialysate improves protein anabolism in renal failure patients on automated peritoneal dialysis. *Journal of the American Society of Nephrology* **16(5)**, 1486–1493

17

Management of acute renal failure

Gregory F. Grauer

Introduction

Acute renal failure (ARF) results from an abrupt decline in renal function and is often caused by an ischaemic or toxic insult. The kidneys are susceptible to ischaemia and toxicants because of their unique anatomical and physiological features. The large renal blood flow (approximately 20% of the cardiac output) results in increased delivery of blood-borne toxicants to the kidney compared with other organs.

The renal cortex is especially susceptible to ischaemia and toxicant exposure because it receives 90% of the renal blood flow. Within the renal cortex, the proximal tubule and thick ascending loop of Henlé epithelial cells are most frequently affected by ischaemia and toxicant-induced injury because of their transport functions and high metabolic rates. Hypoxia and substrate insufficiency associated with vasoconstriction and/or ischaemia can decrease tubular cell adenosine triphosphatase (ATP) stores causing inactivity of the Na^+/K^+ pump, cell swelling and death. In addition, in the process of reabsorbing water and electrolytes from the glomerular filtrate, tubular epithelial cells may also be exposed to increasingly high concentrations of toxicants. Toxicants that are either secreted or reabsorbed by tubular epithelial cells (e.g. gentamicin) may accumulate in high concentrations within these cells. Similarly, in the medulla, the countercurrent multiplier system may concentrate toxicants. Finally, the kidneys also play a role in the biotransformation of many drugs and toxicants. Biotransformation usually results in the formation of metabolites that are less toxic than the parent compound, however, in some cases (e.g. oxidation of ethylene glycol to glycolate and oxalate) metabolites are more toxic.

Strategies for the management of ARF in dogs and cats include preventive and supportive treatments. Treatment designed to stimulate the recovery of tubular cells damaged by ischaemic or toxic insults remains investigational. ARF has three distinct physiological phases, which are categorized as:

- Initiation
- Maintenance
- Recovery.

During the initiation phase, therapeutic measures that reduce the renal insult have the potential to prevent development of established ARF. Identification of patients at risk of developing ARF allows the clinician to increase the monitoring of these patients during procedures and therapies that may damage the kidney. This increased monitoring aids in the detection of acute tubular damage in the initiation phase of ARF. Established tubular lesions resulting in nephron dysfunction are characteristic of the maintenance phase. Fluid therapy is the cornerstone of supportive treatment for the maintenance phase of ARF. Therapeutic intervention during the maintenance phase, although potentially life-saving, usually does little to diminish existing renal lesions or attenuate dysfunction. The recovery phase is the period when reversible renal lesions are repaired and viable nephrons undergo hypertrophy resulting in improved renal function. Tubular damage associated with ARF may be reversible if the tubular basement membrane is intact and viable epithelial cells are present.

It should be noted, however, that not all lesions associated with ARF are reversible. Several retrospective studies have documented the poor prognosis associated with ARF in dogs and cats. In a study of hospital-acquired ARF, the survival rate was only 40% (Behrend et al., 1996). In another retrospective study of 99 dogs with all types of ARF, 22% died, 34% were euthanased, 24% survived but progressed to chronic kidney disease (CKD) and only 19% regained normal or adequate renal function (Vaden et al., 1997). Similarly, in a retrospective study of 25 cats with all types of ARF, 20% died, 36% were euthanased, 20% survived but progressed to CKD and only 24% regained normal or adequate renal function (Worwag and Langston, 2004). These studies underscore the importance of early detection of acute tubular damage and prevention of ARF.

Risk factors for acute renal damage and acute renal failure

In many cases, tubular damage leading to ARF inadvertently develops in the hospital setting in conjunction with diagnostic or therapeutic procedures. For example, tubular damage and ARF may result from decreased renal perfusion associated with anaesthesia and surgery or with the use of vasodilators and nonsteroidal anti-inflammatory drugs (NSAIDs). Similarly, acute tubular damage may occur in patients treated with potential nephrotoxicants, such as gentamicin,

Risk factors that may not be correctable
Pre-existing renal disease
Sepsis
Diabetes mellitus
Fever
Liver disease
Multiple organ involvement
Trauma
Advanced age
Hypoalbuminaemia
Risk factors that are potentially correctable
Dehydration
Decreased cardiac output
Electrolyte imbalances
Hypotension
Concurrent use of potentially nephrotoxic drugs
Dietary protein level
Acidosis
Hyperviscosity syndromes

17.1 Potential risk factors for ARF in dogs and cats.

amphotericin and cisplatin. Several risk factors have been identified that predispose dogs to gentamicin-induced ARF (Brown *et al.*, 1985) (Figure 17.1), however, it is likely that many of these risk factors also predispose dogs and cats to other types of toxicant-induced as well as ischaemia-induced tubular damage.

Dehydration

Dehydration is one of the most common and most important risk factors for development of ARF. Studies in people indicate volume depletion increases a patient's risk of developing ARF by a factor of ten (Brezis *et al.*, 1991). Hypovolaemia not only decreases renal perfusion, which can enhance ischaemic damage, but also decreases the volume of distribution of nephrotoxic drugs and results in decreased tubular fluid flow rates and enhanced tubular absorption of toxicants. In addition to hypovolaemia, renal hypoperfusion may be caused by decreased cardiac output, decreased plasma oncotic pressure, increased blood viscosity, systemic hypotension and decreased renal prostaglandin synthesis (e.g. use of NSAIDs). Any of these conditions can increase the risk of ARF in the hospital setting.

Pre-existing renal disease and advanced age

Pre-existing renal disease and advanced age, which is often associated with some degree of decreased renal function, can increase the potential for nephrotoxicity and ischaemic damage by several mechanisms:

- The pharmacokinetics of potentially nephrotoxic drugs can be altered in the face of decreased renal function. Gentamicin clearance is decreased in dogs with subclinical renal dysfunction (Frazier *et al.*, 1988) and the same is probably true for other nephrotoxicants that are excreted via the kidneys
- Animals with renal insufficiency have reduced urine-concentrating ability and, therefore,

decreased ability to compensate for prerenal influences
- Renal disease may also compromise the local production of prostaglandins that help maintain renal vasodilation and blood flow.

Electrolyte imbalance

Decreased serum concentrations of several electrolytes can increase the risk of renal damage and ARF. For example, hyponatraemia can potentiate intravenous contrast media-induced ARF in dogs. Additional studies in dogs have demonstrated that dietary potassium restriction exacerbates gentamicin nephrotoxicity (Brinker *et al.*, 1981), possibly because potassium-depleted cells are more susceptible to injury and necrosis. It is important to note that gentamicin administration in dogs is associated with increased urinary excretion of potassium (Brinker *et al.*, 1981). This increased urinary excretion of potassium could result in potassium depletion and increased nephrotoxicity in clinical patients. Serum electrolyte concentrations should therefore be closely monitored in patients receiving potentially nephrotoxic drugs, especially if these patients are anorexic, vomiting or have diarrhoea.

Potentially nephrotoxic drugs

Administration of potentially nephrotoxic drugs or a drug that may enhance nephrotoxicity increases the risk of ARF. Concurrent use of furosemide and gentamicin in dogs is associated with increased risk and severity of ARF (Adelman *et al.*, 1979). Furosemide probably potentiates gentamicin-induced nephrotoxicity by causing dehydration, reducing the volume of distribution of gentamicin and increasing the renal tubular absorption of gentamicin. Fluid repletion minimizes, but does not avoid, the potentiating effect of furosemide on gentamicin nephrotoxicity in the dog, because furosemide also facilitates cellular uptake of gentamicin independent of haemodynamic changes.

Similarly, the use of NSAIDs can increase the risk of ARF. Renal prostaglandin production may be compromised in patients receiving NSAIDs, which can result in decreased renal blood flow, especially if superimposed on dehydration or decreased cardiac output. Anaesthesia, hypotension, hyponatraemia, sepsis, nephrotic syndrome and hepatic disease are additional conditions in which prostaglandin-induced renal vasodilation helps maintain renal blood flow and the susceptibility to NSAIDs is increased.

Dietary protein level

Research in dogs suggests that the quantity of protein fed prior to a nephrotoxic insult can affect the subsequent renal damage and dysfunction. Feeding high dietary protein prior to and during gentamicin administration in dogs with initially normal renal function, reduces nephrotoxicity, enhances gentamicin clearance and results in a larger volume of distribution compared with feeding medium or low protein (Grauer *et al.*, 1994). The beneficial effects of high dietary protein are likely associated with increased glomerular filtration and, therefore, improved toxicant excretion. High dietary protein also results in increased urinary excretion of protein, which may compete for nephrotoxicant reabsorption by tubular epithelial cells. Similar to potential causes of decreased electrolyte stores, anorexia, vomiting and diarrhoea have the potential to decrease dietary protein assimilation and therefore increase the risk of nephrotoxicant-induced tubular damage. Dietary protein conditioning may not be a viable clinical option, but dogs with reduced protein intake should be recognized as having increased risk for developing ARF. It should be noted that these studies were conducted in dogs with normal kidney function and once renal damage has occurred, high dietary protein would probably result in increased serum urea nitrogen and phosphorus concentrations and, therefore, would not be recommended.

High-risk patients

Risk factors are probably additive and any complication occurring in high-risk patients increases the potential for tubular damage and ARF. Patients with shock, acidosis, sepsis and major organ system failure are at increased risk. These are also the patients that are likely to require aggressive treatment, including prolonged anaesthesia, surgery or chemotherapeutics, which are potentially damaging to the kidneys. For example, ARF is relatively common in dogs with pyometra and *Escherichia coli* endotoxin-induced urine-concentrating defects, especially if fluid therapy is inadequate during anaesthesia for ovariohysterectomy or during the recovery period. Trauma, extensive burns, vasculitis, pancreatitis, fever, diabetes mellitus and multiple myeloma are additional conditions associated with a high incidence of ARF. A combination of decreased renal perfusion and/or use of nephrotoxic therapeutic agents superimposed on more chronic, pre-existing renal disease is often responsible for tubular damage and ARF in the clinical setting.

Early recognition of acute renal damage

General evaluation

Since therapeutic intervention is most successful when initiated during the induction phase of ARF, early recognition of renal damage/dysfunction is important. Physical examination of the patient at risk of ARF should include thoracic auscultation and evaluation of pulse quality and hydration status. Monitoring body weight, packed cell volume (PCV) and plasma total protein in comparison with baseline values may indicate subtle changes in hydration status. Blood pressure measurement will identify hypotensive and hypertensive patients, both of whom may be at increased risk for renal injury.

Urinalysis/urine production

Numerous urine parameters can herald the development of ARF. Urine output should be monitored in all high-risk patients that undergo anaesthesia; once a patient is anaesthetized, placement of an indwelling urinary catheter (with a closed, sterile collection system) and measurement of urine production is relatively easy. Normal urine output is approximately 1–2 ml/hr/kg body weight. Decreased renal perfusion during anaesthesia can result in oliguria (<0.25 ml/hr/kg) or anuria, which signals the need for prompt treatment. Non-oliguric ARF is being recognized with increasing frequency and increases in urine production, therefore, may also signal the onset of renal damage; polyuria may occur in cases of mild renal ischaemia or very early in the course of more severe ischaemic damage. However, if oliguria or anuria occurs during anaesthesia, it requires prompt treatment. As long as cardiac function is thought to be normal, increasing the rate and volume of intravenous fluid administration is the first line of defence for hypotension and decreased urine output during anaesthesia. In addition to changes in urine volume, increased urine turbidity or changes in urine sediment (increasing numbers of renal epithelial cells, cellular or granular casts or cellular debris) are often indications of acute, ongoing tubular damage. Finally, the acute onset of tubular glucosuria (normoglycaemic glucosuria) or proteinuria may also be indicative of tubular cell damage. The interpretation of all of the above parameters is enhanced by comparison with the baseline values.

Detection of enzymes in the urine, such as gamma-glutamyl transferase (GGT) and *N*-acetyl-beta-D-glucosaminidase (NAG), has proven to be a sensitive indicator of early renal tubular damage (Greco *et al.*, 1985; Grauer *et al.*, 1994). These enzymes are too large to be normally filtered by the glomerulus, and therefore, enzymuria indicates cell leakage, usually associated with tubular epithelial damage or necrosis. Urinary GGT originates from the proximal tubule brush border and NAG is present in proximal tubule lysosomes. In studies of gentamicin-treated dogs, increased urinary GGT and NAG activity was one of the earliest markers of renal damage/dysfunction (Greco *et al.*, 1985; Grauer *et al.*, 1994). Interpretation of enzymuria is aided by baseline values obtained prior to a potential renal insult; two- to threefold increases over baseline suggest significant tubular damage. Urine enzyme:creatinine ratios have been shown to be accurate in dogs prior to the onset of azotaemia, obviating the need for timed urine collections (Grauer *et al.*, 1995). False-positive enzymuria can potentially occur with severe glomerular damage, resulting in increased glomerular filtration of serum enzymes. False-negative results can occur after severe tubular damage depletes tubular enzyme stores.

Serum antibiotic concentrations

In the specific case of aminoglycoside administration, measurement of serum trough concentrations of the antibiotic can help prevent nephrotoxicity. Renal tubular damage increases with elevated serum trough concentrations (>20 µg/l for gentamicin and >50 µg/l for amikacin) (Brown and Engelhardt, 1987). Administering the same total daily dose once or twice daily *versus* three times daily appears to maintain antimicrobial efficacy while reducing serum trough concentrations and the potential for nephrotoxicity (Frazier and Riviere, 1987). Serum aminoglycoside concentrations can be measured by many reference laboratories.

Assessment of risk factors

Knowledge of the predisposing risk factors allows the clinician to assess the risk:benefit ratio in individual cases in which an elective anaesthetic procedure is considered or the use of potentially nephrotoxic drugs is indicated. In some cases, predisposing risk factors can be corrected prior to any potential renal insults. In other cases, such as geriatric patients with suspected pre-existing renal disease, more intensive monitoring of the patient may allow detection of acute tubular damage or ARF in its initiation phase prior to the onset of established failure.

Potential protective measures

Fluid therapy sufficient to cause volume expansion and diuresis is frequently used prior to administration of amphotericin B and cisplatin to decrease the nephrotoxicity of these compounds. In a similar fashion, the prophylactic administration of diuretics and vasodilators may be protective against potential renal insults. Mannitol (1 g/kg of a 5–25% solution, i.v.) has been used to increase intravascular volume and tubular flow rates and to prevent tubular obstruction prior to potential ischaemic or toxic insults. Mannitol also has weak vasodilatory effects mediated via prostaglandins or by the release of atrial natriuretic peptide and may improve renal blood flow and glomerular filtration if given early in ARF. Administration of a constant rate intravenous infusion of dopamine (1–3 µg/kg/min) can also be effective in increasing glomerular filtration and inducing diuresis, especially when administered before the induction of ARF. Diuretics and vasodilators, however, should only be used in well hydrated patients.

Specific alterations in the dosage of medications that have nephrotoxic potential may aid in minimizing side effects. Increasing the dosage interval of drugs excreted via the kidneys by a factor related to serum creatinine or creatinine clearance is an effective means of reducing nephrotoxicity. For example, if the serum creatinine concentration is 442 µmol/l (5 mg/dl), the dosing interval for a drug normally administered every 8 hours should be 40 hours (8 hours multiplied by 5). Intravenous radiographic contrast medium administration can cause renal vasoconstriction and has been associated with ARF in the dog. Low-osmolar contrast agents (e.g. iopamidol and ioxaglate) produce less vasoconstriction in dogs than do high-osmolar contrast agents (e.g. diatrizoate); low-osmolar contrast agents should, therefore, be used in high-risk patients.

Management of prerenal azotaemia

Clinical signs associated with prerenal azotaemia are often non-specific and may be similar to those caused by ARF. Although the initial fluid therapy may be the same for all azotaemic patients, the subsequent treatment and prognosis vary greatly between prerenal azotaemia and established ARF. Any condition that decreases renal blood flow may result in prerenal azotaemia, including hypovolaemia (e.g. dehydration,

hypoadrenocorticism), hypotension (e.g. anaesthesia, shock) and aortic or renal arterial thrombus formation. In most patients with prerenal azotaemia the kidneys are structurally and functionally normal, and they respond to the decreased renal blood flow by producing hypersthenuric urine.

The differentiation between prerenal and renal azotaemia may be more difficult if urine-concentrating ability is impaired in patients with prerenal azotaemia. Examples of this situation include hypoadrenocorticism, pyometra and paraneoplastic hypercalcaemia, all of which can compromise urine-concentrating ability and result in dehydration secondary to vomiting. A potentially easy and valuable way to differentiate prerenal azotaemia from ARF is to assess response to fluid therapy. Azotaemia caused by dehydration should resolve quickly with replacement of volume deficits and restoration of renal perfusion, whereas renal azotaemia will not resolve with fluid therapy alone.

Fluid therapy for patients with suspected prerenal azotaemia should be administered intravenously with the fluid volume calculated on the basis of percentage dehydration, maintenance fluid requirements and continuing fluid losses (Figure 17.2). Many patients with suspected prerenal azotaemia have gastrointestinal fluid losses associated with vomiting and diarrhoea and therefore polyionic fluid solutions, such as lactated Ringer's solution, are good initial fluid choices. The magnitude of azotaemia as well as any electrolyte abnormalities (e.g. hypokalaemia, hyperkalaemia or hypercalcaemia) should be confirmed from serum obtained prior to initiation of fluid therapy. Rechecking a biochemistry profile to assess the patient's response to fluids can be accomplished after 12–24 hours of therapy.

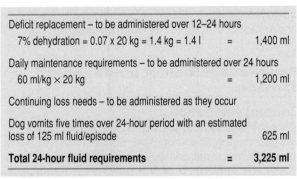

Deficit replacement – to be administered over 12–24 hours		
7% dehydration = 0.07 x 20 kg = 1.4 kg = 1.4 l	=	1,400 ml
Daily maintenance requirements – to be administered over 24 hours		
60 ml/kg × 20 kg	=	1,200 ml
Continuing loss needs – to be administered as they occur		
Dog vomits five times over 24-hour period with an estimated loss of 125 ml fluid/episode	=	625 ml
Total 24-hour fluid requirements	**=**	**3,225 ml**

17.2 Example of daily fluid requirements for a vomiting dog (20 kg) with suspected prerenal azotaemia.

Supportive treatment for established acute renal failure

Fluid therapy

Most dogs and cats with renal failure are dehydrated because of gastrointestinal fluid loss superimposed on their urine-concentrating deficits. Replacement of these volume deficits will correct the 'prerenal component' of the renal failure and help protect against any additional ischaemic renal tubular damage (Figure 17.3). Once the patient is rehydrated, establishing or augmenting diuresis can facilitate excretion of solutes that are

1. Discontinue all potentially nephrotoxic drugs, consider measures to decrease absorption (e.g. induction of emesis and administration of activated charcoal and sodium sulphate).
2. Start specific antidotal therapy if applicable (e.g. alcohol dehydrogenase inhibitors for ethylene glycol).
3. Identify and treat any prerenal or postrenal abnormalities.
4. Start intravenous fluid therapy with normal saline solution or 0.45% saline in 2.5% dextrose:
    Rehydrate patient within 4–6 hours
    Provide maintenance and continuing fluid loss needs.
5. Assess volume of urine production.
6. Correct acid–base and electrolyte abnormalities: rule out hypercalcaemic nephropathy. If necessary, to increase urine production, provide mild volume expansion while monitoring urine volume, body weight, plasma total solids, haematocrit and central venous pressure.
7. Administer diuretics, if necessary, to increase urine production (questionable efficacy):
    Mannitol
    Furosemide.
8. Consider peritoneal dialysis if no response to above treatment, perform kidney biopsy at time of dialysis catheter placement.
9. Control hyperphosphataemia:
    Phosphate-restricted diet
    Enteric phosphate binders (if necessary).
10. Treat vomiting:
    Metoclopramide
    Trimethobenzamide.
11. Treat gastric hyperacidity
    H_2 blockers
    Proton pump blockers.
12. Provide caloric requirements (70–100 kcal/kg/day).

17.3 Treatment guidelines for dogs and cats with established ARF.

Parameter	Normal	Non-oliguric ARF
Glomerular filtrate rate (l)	100	20
Tubular reabsorption (l)	99 (99%)	16 (80%)
Urine production (l)	1	4

17.4 Hypothetical comparison of daily glomerular filtration, tubular reabsorption and urine production in the normal and non-oliguric ARF state.

reabsorbed and secreted by renal tubular cells (e.g. urea nitrogen and potassium). Increasing tubular flow rates and volumes will hinder reabsorption and favour secretion of solutes.

The goal of fluid therapy for established ARF is correction of renal haemodynamic disorders and alleviation of water and solute imbalances in order to 'buy time' for nephron repair and compensation. A positive response to therapy is indicated by an increase in glomerular filtration (reduction in serum creatinine concentration) and increases in urine production (if the patient was oliguric). Induction of diuresis facilitates management of ARF by decreasing serum urea nitrogen and potassium concentrations and by lessening the tendency for overhydration to occur, however, glomerular filtration and renal blood flow are frequently unchanged. The increased urine production observed with diuresis is usually a result of a relative decrease in the tubular reabsorption of filtrate (Figure 17.4). Therefore, increased urine production alone does not indicate an improvement in glomerular filtration. It should also be noted that there are no prospective, controlled clinical trials in dogs or cats that demonstrate improved survival or enhanced or hastened recovery from ARF associated with the induction and/or maintenance of diuresis.

The large volume of fluid and rapid administration rate necessary in ARF require that fluids be given intravenously. Jugular catheters are ideal as they facilitate frequent blood sampling, infusion of hypertonic solutions (e.g. mannitol) and allow access for central venous pressure (CVP) measurement. Deficit fluid requirements should be replaced over the first 4–6 hours of treatment, unless the patient has a cardiac disorder that requires a slower administration rate. A fluid bolus challenge of 20 ml/kg body weight given intravenously over 10 minutes can help assess the possibility of a subsequent volume overload. The CVP should not increase by more than 2 cm of water if the patient's cardiovascular function is normal. The purpose of replacing volume deficits over the first 4–6 hours rather than over the normal 12–24 hours is to rapidly improve renal perfusion and decrease the likelihood of continued ischaemic damage. Normal saline (0.9% solution) is the fluid of choice for rehydration unless the patient is hypernatraemic; in this case a 0.45% saline and 2.5% dextrose solution should be used. The amount of fluid required to restore extracellular fluid deficits can be calculated by multiplying the estimated percentage dehydration by the patient's body weight in kilograms (see Figure 17.2).

During this rapid rehydration phase, the patient should be closely observed for signs of overhydration. Frequent assessment of body weight, CVP, PCV and plasma total protein will help detect early overhydration. An increase in the CVP of ≥5–7 cm of water over baseline values suggests the likelihood of overhydration. Physical manifestations of overhydration include:

- Increased bronchovesicular sounds
- Tachycardia
- Restlessness
- Chemosis
- Serous nasal discharge.

Auscultation of overt crackles and wheezes is usually a late sign indicating established pulmonary oedema. Overhydration in dogs and cats with oliguric or anuric ARF is a common complication that frequently results in pulmonary oedema. Overhydration in oliguric and anuric ARF patients is extremely difficult to correct.

Urine production should be measured and electrolyte and acid–base status assessed during the period of rehydration. Urine production (ml/kg/hr) should be measured so that maintenance fluid needs can be accurately administered. Approximately two thirds of normal maintenance fluid needs are due to fluid loss in urine, therefore oliguric and non-oliguric patients can have large variations in their maintenance fluid needs (Figure 17.5). Metabolism cages, urinary catheters and manual collection of voided urine are methods used to collect and measure urine volume. In the case of indwelling urinary catheters, strict aseptic technique and closed collection systems must be used. Because of the possibility of urinary tract infection, intermittent urinary bladder catheterization is usually recommended over indwelling catheterization for timed urine volume collections. In cats, weighing the litter pan before and after voiding is a useful, although less accurate, method for assessing urine production. Observation of urine voiding and urinary bladder palpation are the least reliable methods for determining the volume of urine produced.

Parameter	Normal	Oliguric ARF	Non-oliguric ARF
Insensible fluid loss (ml/kg/day)	20	20	20
Urine production (ml/kg/day)	40	10	160
Total maintenance fluid needs (ml/kg/day)	60	30	180

17.5 Hypothetical daily fluid requirements in oliguric and non-oliguric ARF patients compared with those of a normal animal.

Correction of electrolyte imbalances

Sodium and chloride
Initially, most patients with ARF have normal serum sodium and chloride concentrations due to isonatraemic fluid loss. Hypernatraemia can develop, however, after several days of therapy with fluids containing large amounts of sodium (0.9% NaCl, lactated Ringer's solution) and/or in association with sodium bicarbonate treatment of metabolic acidosis. If hypernatraemia occurs, the use of fluids containing 0.45% NaCl with 2.5% dextrose will usually correct the problem.

Calcium
Disorders of calcium balance can also occasionally be manifest in ARF patients. If moderate to severe hypercalcaemia is observed, a primary hypercalcaemic disorder (e.g. neoplasia or vitamin D_3 intoxication) should be considered as the cause of the renal failure. Immediate treatment for hypercalcaemia includes rehydration with 0.9% NaCl followed by diuresis induced with furosemide. Glucocorticoids will also help lower calcium concentrations by decreasing intestinal absorption and facilitating excretion, but their use may interfere with the diagnosis of the underlying disorder (e.g. lymphosarcoma). Conversely, significant hypocalcaemia can be observed in dogs and cats with ARF associated with ethylene glycol intoxication.

Potassium
Oliguric ARF patients are at risk of hyperkalaemia. Serum potassium concentrations greater than 6.5–7.0 mmol/l (6.5–7.0 mEq/l) can cause cardiac conduction disturbances (bradycardia, atrial standstill, idioventricular rhythms, ventricular tachycardia, fibrillation and asystole) and electrocardiographic changes (peaked T waves, prolonged PR intervals, widened QRS complexes or the loss of P waves). Mild to moderate hyperkalaemia is largely resolved with administration of potassium-free fluids (dilution) and improved urine flow (increased excretion). More severe hyperkalaemia (>7–8 mmol/l) or hyperkalaemia resulting in ECG abnormalities should be treated by agents that will decrease serum potassium concentrations or counteract the effects of hyperkalaemia on cardiac conduction.

Sodium bicarbonate (see dosage below) will help correct any metabolic acidosis and lower serum potassium concentration by exchanging intracellular hydrogen ions for potassium. Glucose and insulin can also be used to increase intracellular shifting of potassium. Regular (soluble) insulin is administered at a dosage of 0.1–0.25 IU/kg, i.v., followed by a glucose bolus of 1–2 g per unit of insulin given. Blood glucose monitoring should be maintained for several hours following administration of insulin since hypoglycaemia may occur. 10% calcium gluconate (0.5–1.0 ml/kg i.v. over 10–15 minutes) will counteract the cardiotoxic effects of hyperkalaemia without lowering the serum potassium and can be used in an emergency situation. The effects of the above regimes are short-lived, and fluid and acid–base therapy to initiate and maintain diuresis and maintain blood pH and bicarbonate within the normal range (see below) are important to maintain potassium excretion and normokalaemia.

Correction of acidosis
Mild to moderate metabolic acidosis also commonly resolves with fluid therapy, and specific treatment is usually not necessary unless the blood pH is less than 7.2 or total CO_2 is less than 12 mmol/l (12 mEq/l). Bicarbonate requirements can be calculated utilizing the base deficit as determined from arterial blood gas, or an estimated base deficit:

Body weight (kg) x 0.3 x base deficit or (20 − T CO_2) = mEq bicarbonate required.

Optimally, half the calculated bicarbonate dosage should be administered intravenously slowly over 15–30 minutes and then acid–base parameters reassessed. Overzealous bicarbonate administration may result in ionized calcium deficits, paradoxical cerebrospinal fluid acidosis and/or cerebral oedema.

Volume expansion
If signs of overhydration are not present and oliguria persists after apparent rehydration, mild volume expansion (3–5% of the patient's body weight in fluid) may be initiated, as dehydration of this magnitude is difficult to detect clinically. If volume expansion is attempted, the possibility of inducing overhydration increases and close patient observation is necessary. Unfortunately, most patients that present with oliguria will remain oliguric after rehydration and volume expansion.

Diuretic therapy

In the past, diuretic therapy has been frequently recommended in patients that are persistently oliguric or anuric despite appropriate fluid therapy. In comparison with those patients with diminished urine production, polyuric ARF patients are thought to have less severe tubular injury, improved excretion of solutes that are reabsorbed or secreted (e.g. urea nitrogen and potassium) and have less risk of developing overhydration and pulmonary oedema. There is, however, no evidence that diuretic therapy will hasten the recovery from ARF or decrease the mortality associated with ARF. In humans with established ARF, there is increasing evidence that diuretic therapy may actually be associated with increased risk of death and non-recovery of renal function (Kellum and Decker, 2001; Gambaro et al., 2002; Mehta et al., 2002). If the choice is to use diuretics in dogs or cats with ARF, they should only be used after dehydration has been corrected and the patient has been volume expanded. Furosemide and mannitol are probably the diuretics of choice. Dopamine is not recommended because of its unpredictable effects on renal blood flow and glomerular filtration rate.

Furosemide blocks the reabsorption of chloride and sodium in the thick ascending limb of Henlé resulting in natriuresis and an osmotic diuresis. Furosemide also has weak renovasodilatory properties that may help increase renal blood flow. The dose recommended for oliguric or anuric dogs and cats is 2–6 mg/kg i.v. q8h, however in healthy dogs, constant rate infusion of furosemide with a 0.66 mg/kg i.v. loading dose followed by 0.66 mg/kg/hr resulted in more diuresis, natriuresis, calciuresis and less kaliuresis than did intermittent bolus infusion (Adin et al., 2003). Furosemide has been shown to exacerbate gentamicin toxicity and probably should be avoided in patients with ARF caused by aminoglycoside usage.

Mannitol, in a 10% or 20% solution, has been recommended as an osmotic diuretic at a dose of 0.5–1.0 g/kg i.v., given as a slow bolus over 15–20 minutes. Urine output should increase within 1 hour if the treatment is effective. A second bolus may be attempted but the potential for volume overexpansion and complications, such as pulmonary oedema, increases considerably if urine production does not increase. As an osmotic agent, mannitol may decrease tubular cell swelling, increase tubular flow and help prevent tubular obstruction or collapse. Mannitol also has weak renal vasodilator properties that are probably mediated by prostaglandins or atrial natriuretic peptides in addition to weak free-radical-scavenging capabilities. In healthy cats, the renal effects of mannitol, when used as an adjunct to fluid therapy, are superior to those of the furosemide and dopamine combination (McCabe et al., 2004). Mannitol, compared with hypertonic glucose, is probably the better osmotic agent, since it is not metabolized or reabsorbed by the renal tubules. The use of any osmotic agent is contraindicated in an overhydrated patient because the resultant increase in intravascular volume may precipitate pulmonary oedema.

Whether or not diuresis can be established, fluid therapy should be tailored to match urine volume and other losses, including insensible losses (e.g. water loss due to respiration) and continuing losses (e.g. fluid loss due to vomiting or diarrhoea). Insensible losses are estimated at 20 ml/kg/day. Urine output is quantitated for 6–8-hour intervals and that amount is replaced over an equivalent subsequent time period. The volume of fluid loss due to vomiting and/or diarrhoea is estimated and that amount is added to the 24-hour fluid needs of the patient. If hypernatraemia and hyperkalaemia are not present and diuresis has been established, polyionic maintenance fluids should be utilized. In the recovery phase of ARF, urine volume and electrolyte losses can be great. Potassium supplementation may be necessary, especially if the patient is vomiting or anorexic.

Nausea and vomiting

Control of nausea and vomiting in dogs and cats with ARF is important in order to facilitate caloric intake. In addition, the inability to control vomiting is discouraging to owners and may result in a hastened decision for euthanasia. See Chapter 18 for specific recommendations for the treatment of nausea and vomiting.

Longer-term care

When fluid therapy is successful in inducing or maintaining diuresis, the daily volume of fluid administered to the patient will eventually need to be decreased. Indications for tapering intravenous fluid volume include:

- Significant reductions in blood urea nitrogen (BUN) and phosphorus concentrations
- Control of vomiting and diarrhoea
- The patient feeling better and showing interest in eating and drinking.

These indications rarely occur prior to 5–6 days of intense fluid therapy/diuresis and may require 10 or more days of treatment. Gradually reducing maintenance fluid requirements by 25% each day is usually recommended for fluid tapering. If the patient loses weight or increases in PCV, total protein, BUN and/or creatinine concentrations are observed, fluid therapy tapering should be discontinued, and the previous maintenance volume reinstated for at least 48 hours.

Peritoneal dialysis should be considered in patients with severe, persistent uraemia, acidosis or hyperkalaemia. Dialysis may also be used to treat overhydration and hasten elimination of dialysable toxicants (see Chapter 16). Renal biopsy should be performed if the diagnosis is in doubt, if the patient does not respond to therapy within 3–5 days or if peritoneal dialysis is considered (see Chapter 12).

The long-term prognosis for dogs or cats with ARF is usually fair to good if the patient survives the period of renal tubular regeneration and compensation; however, several weeks may be required for renal function to improve. Animals with moderate to severe renal damage may require many weeks for renal repair and this prolonged time required for recovery results in poor prognosis. The severity of the initial azotaemia/uraemia, the response to fluid therapy and assessment of renal histopathological lesions are the most important prognostic indicators early in the course of ARF.

References and further reading

Adelman RD, Spangler WL, Beasom F, Ishizaki G and Conzelman GM (1979) Furosemide enhancement of experimental gentamicin nephrotoxicity: comparison of functional and morphological changes with activities of urinary enzymes. *Journal of Infectious Diseases* **140**, 342–352

Adin DB, Taylor AW, Hill RC, Scott KC and Martin FG (2003) Intermittent bolus injection versus continuous infusion of furosemide in normal adult greyhound dogs. *Journal of Veterinary Internal Medicine* **17**, 632–636

Behrend EN, Grauer GF, Mani I, Groman RP and Greco DS (1996) Hospital-acquired acute renal failure in dogs: 29 cases (1983–1992). *Journal of the American Veterinary Medical Association* **208**, 537–541

Brezis M, Rosen S and Epstein FH (1991) Acute renal failure. In: *The Kidney*, ed. BM Brenner and FC Rector, pp. 993–1061. WB Saunders, Philadelphia

Brinker KR, Bulger RE, Dobyan DC *et al.* (1981) Effect of potassium depletion on gentamicin nephrotoxicity. *Journal of Laboratory and Clinical Medicine* **98**, 292–301

Brown SA, Barsanti JA and Crowell WA (1985) Gentamicin-associated acute renal failure in the dog. *Journal of the American Veterinary Medical Association* **186**, 686–690

Brown SA and Engelhardt JA (1987) Drug-related nephropathies. Part I: mechanisms, diagnosis and management. *Compendium on Continuing Education for the Practicing Veterinarian* **9**, 148–160

Frazier DL, Aucoin DP and Riviere JE (1988) Gentamicin pharmaco-kinetics and nephrotoxicity in naturally acquired and experimentally induced disease in dogs. *Journal of the American Veterinary Medical Association* **192**, 57–63

Frazier DL and Riviere JC (1987) Gentamicin dosing strategies for dogs with subclinical renal dysfunction. *Antimicrobial Agents and Chemotherapeutics* **31**, 1929–1934

Gambaro G, Bertaglia G, Puma G and D'Angelo A (2002) Diuretics and dopamine for the prevention and treatment of acute renal failure: a critical reappraisal. *Journal of Nephrology* **15**, 213–219

Grauer GF, Greco DS, Behrend EN *et al.* (1994) Effects of dietary protein conditioning on gentamicin-induced nephrotoxicosis in healthy male dogs. *American Journal of Veterinary Research* **55**, 90–97

Grauer GF, Greco DS, Behrend EN *et al.* (1995) Estimation of quantitative enzymuria in dogs with gentamicin-induced nephrotoxicosis using urine enzyme/creatinine ratios from spot urine samples. *Journal of Veterinary Internal Medicine* **9**, 324–327

Greco DS, Turnwald GH, Adams R *et al.* (1985) Urinary gamma-glutamyl transpeptidase activity in dogs with gentamicin-induced nephrotoxicity. *American Journal of Veterinary Research* **46**, 2332–2335

Kellum JA and Decker JM (2001) Use of dopamine in acute renal failure: a meta-analysis. *Critical Care Medicine* **29**, 1526–1531

McCabe JR, Goldstein RE, Cowgill LD and Erb HN (2004) The effects of fluids and diuretic therapies on glomerular filtration rate, renal blood flow, and urine output in healthy cats. *Journal of Veterinary Internal Medicine* **18**, 415 [abstract]

Mehta RL, Pascual MT, Soroko S and Chertow GM (2002) Diuretics, mortality, and nonrecovery of renal function in acute renal failure. *Journal of the American Medical Association* **228**, 2547–2553

Vaden SL, Levine J and Breitschwerdt EB (1997) A retrospective case-control of acute renal failure in 99 dogs. *Journal of Veterinary Internal Medicine* **11**, 58–64

Worwag S and Langston C (2004) Retrospective, acute renal failure in cats: 25 cases (1997–2002). *Journal of Veterinary Internal Medicine* **18**, 416 [abstract]

18

Management of chronic kidney disease

Scott A. Brown

Introduction

Any disease that affects the kidney is likely to alter both renal structure and function. It is the adequacy of renal function, however, that dictates the impact of this disease on the patient. While the kidney has many biological functions of importance to an animal, the most basic and central renal function is filtration; measurement of this gives the glomerular filtration rate (GFR), which serves as the 'gold standard' for assessment of the kidney in dogs and cats (see Chapter 9). In the research laboratory, renal filtration is assessed as urinary clearance of marker substances, such as inulin or creatinine. In clinical patients, urinary clearance tests are generally not practical; an approximation of GFR can be obtained by the measurement of the disappearance from plasma of renally cleared marker substances, such as creatinine, inulin, iohexol or diethylenetriaminepentaacetic acid (DTPA), following intravenous administration (Labato and Ross, 1991; Moe and Heiene, 1995; Brown et al., 1996; Gleadhill and Michell, 1996; Finco et al., 2001). Nonetheless, GFR is still usually assessed in clinical patients by the measurement of plasma concentrations of creatinine and/or urea. It is generally fair to assume that the level of most renal functions parallels changes in GFR in a clinical patient.

The accumulation of non-protein nitrogenous materials, such as creatinine and urea, is referred to as azotaemia. It may be classified as prerenal, renal, postrenal or of mixed origin:

- Prerenal azotaemia occurs whenever mean systemic arterial blood pressure declines dramatically to values below 60 mmHg and/or when dehydration causes an elevation in plasma protein concentration. Conditions that commonly lead to the development of prerenal azotaemia include dehydration, congestive heart failure and shock. Prerenal azotaemia generally resolves with appropriate treatment, as dogs and cats are resistant to adverse renal effects of hypoperfusion of the kidney
- Renal azotaemia refers to a dramatic fall in GFR produced by an intrarenal process (i.e. primary kidney disease), occurring secondary to acute or chronic kidney disease (CKD)
- Postrenal azotaemia occurs when there is a disruption of the integrity of the urinary tract

(e.g. bladder rupture) or an obstruction to urine outflow (e.g. urethral or bilateral ureteral obstruction).

Uraemia, or the uraemic syndrome, refers to that constellation of clinical signs that accompanies severe azotaemia.

Chronic kidney disease

CKD refers to a disease process in which there is a loss of functional renal tissue due to a prolonged (generally more than 2 months in duration), usually progressive, process. A CKD will generally produce dramatic changes in renal structure as well, although there is only a loose and imprecise correlation between structural and functional changes in this organ. This is partly because of the tremendous renal functional reserve, as animals can survive for long periods with only a small fraction of initial renal tissue, perhaps 5–8% in dogs and cats. Thus, a CKD often smoulders for many months or years before it becomes clinically apparent.

Most CKDs are not reversible and, once acquired, a CKD rarely resolves. Although congenital disease causes an increase in incidence of CKD in animals less than 3 years old, the prevalence of CKD increases with advancing age from 5–6 years upward. In geriatric populations at referral institutions, CKD affects up to 10% of dogs and 35% of cats (Polzin and Osborne, 1986; Krawiec and Gelberg, 1989). A reasonable estimate of the prevalence of CKD in the general small animal population is 1–3% of cats and 0.5–1.5% of dogs.

Diagnosis of chronic kidney disease

Once the GFR falls enough to cause the blood urea nitrogen (BUN) and plasma creatinine concentrations to increase, the diagnosis is generally straightforward. Usually at this time, the urine specific gravity (SG) will be <1.035 and plasma inorganic phosphorus levels are increased. Classically, CKD was diagnosed as the presence of renal azotaemia accompanied by low urine SG (<1.035). Unfortunately, these diagnostic criteria are incredibly insensitive, identifying the presence of CKD only after three quarters of the functional renal mass has been destroyed.

In early CKD, when azotaemia and clinical signs are absent, the diagnosis is sometimes made inadvertently, occurring as a result of imaging studies, laparotomy or urinalysis conducted for other purposes. Osteoporosis may be seen radiographically, but this is a late finding in CKD and is generally not useful for identifying the presence of an otherwise masked case of CKD. Where measured by one of the specific tests mentioned above, the presence of a reduced GFR is generally a highly reliable test, although it must be remembered that reductions of GFR can be caused by renal, prerenal and postrenal factors.

A potentially useful early indicator of the presence of CKD is a urine SG <1.035, despite dehydration. However, animals with early CKD, dogs with primary glomerular disease and some cats with CKD of any severity may retain the ability to concentrate urine to a SG ≥1.035. While measuring urine SG is a simple and readily available test, interpretation of a finding of a low urine SG can be complicated, as the polyuria caused by a CKD must be differentiated from diseases which cause primary polydipsia (e.g. psychogenic polydipsia and hyperthyroidism) or those interfering directly with the urine-concentrating mechanism. These interfering conditions include diseases that lead to retention of solute in tubular fluid (e.g. diuretic administration and diabetes mellitus), central diabetes insipidus and nephrogenic diabetes insipidus (e.g. hyperadrenocorticism, hypercalcaemia, pyometra and diseases causing septicaemia). Adrenal insufficiency leads to a renal concentrating defect and may thus be confused with CKD because prerenal azotaemia may be caused by the vomiting, diarrhoea and polydipsia associated with the former. Hyperkalaemia, hyponatraemia and/or a reduced plasma sodium:potassium ratio are most helpful in establishing a tentative diagnosis of adrenal insufficiency, which must be confirmed by hormonal assay(s).

Recently, tests for identification of proteinuria in veterinary patients that are both sensitive and specific have been developed (Lees *et al.*, 2005). These include the protein:creatinine ratio and species-specific albuminuria tests. The ability to identify persistent renal proteinuria with these tests offers promise as being clinically useful for identifying early CKD (see below and Chapter 6). The availability of reliable tests for proteinuria in dogs and cats makes this a very attractive approach.

Initial evaluation of animals with chronic kidney disease

For all animals with CKD, a thorough history and physical examination should be accompanied by complete clinical pathology testing, which includes a biochemical panel, haematology and urinalysis, with specific proteinuria tests and aerobic bacterial culture. Survey radiography, abdominal ultrasonography and blood pressure measurements should be performed. This initial battery of tests allows the veterinary surgeon to evaluate the severity of the disease, establish a prognosis, follow the response to subsequent therapy and identify complicating factors. As part of this evaluation, renal azotaemia should be distinguished from other causes of azotaemia and CKD should be distinguished from the more readily reversible acute kidney disease. Frequently, this latter differentiation may be accomplished with a careful history, physical examination and evaluation of laboratory findings, although occasionally a renal biopsy may be required (see below and Chapter 12).

Staging of chronic kidney disease

CKD in dogs and cats often progresses along a continuum from an initial non-azotaemic stage to end-stage uraemia. In some animals this progression occurs rapidly over days or weeks but in others it is a very slow process, taking years. Many dogs and cats with CKD will die of other causes, often before developing azotaemia or any clinically apparent consequences of CKD.

Veterinary surgeons are obliged to address the problems and patient needs that characterize that specific animal's CKD and these needs vary substantially as the disease progresses in a given animal. The International Renal Interest Society (IRIS) has proposed a classification scheme for CKD which utilizes a staged approach (Polzin *et al.*, 2005). The IRIS recognized that the degree of azotaemia in cats is not synonymous with that in dogs and proposed a separate classification scheme for dogs and cats (Figure 18.1). These classification schemes are based on the use of plasma creatinine concentration in a euvolaemic (normally hydrated) animal to estimate degree of decline of GFR caused by the CKD. The IRIS scheme is not used to identify the presence

Stage	Description	Creatinine	
		Dogs	**Cats**
I	Non-azotaemic CKD	<125 µmol/l (<1.4 mg/dl)	<140 µmol/l (<1.6 mg/dl)
II	Mild renal azotaemia	125–180 µmol/l (1.4–2.0 mg/dl)	140–250 µmol/l (1.6–2.8 mg/dl)
III	Moderate renal azotaemia	181–440 µmol/l (2.1–5.0 mg/dl)	251–440 µmol/l (2.9–5.0 mg/dl)
IV	Severe renal azotaemia	>440 µmol/l (>5.0 mg/dl)	>440 µmol/l (>5.0 mg/dl)

18.1 IRIS classification of canine and feline CKD. Due to specific prognostic and therapeutic implications regardless of stage, each case of CKD should be further categorized as to the presence, or absence, of systemic hypertension and/or proteinuria.

of CKD, but rather to categorize the disease once a diagnosis and initial evaluation of CKD are accomplished (see also Chapter 11). This classification system employs four stages:

- Stage I: non-azotaemic CKD
- Stage II: mild renal azotaemia
- Stage III: moderate renal azotaemia
- Stage IV: severe renal azotaemia.

Following staging of CKD, the diagnostic and therapeutic considerations can be put into general categories that focus on the kidney, progression of the disease and the patient, respectively. These categories are:

- Renal evaluation and specific therapy
- Evaluation of progression and renoprotective therapy
- Patient evaluation and symptomatic therapy.

Renal evaluation and specific therapy

It is a high priority, especially in stage I or early stage II CKD (Figure 18.2), to attempt to identify the primary process causing the CKD. Examples of renal evaluation that may be appropriate at these early stages include:

- Renal imaging – survey radiographs with or without contrast radiographic studies and ultrasonography
- Urinalysis with specific tests for proteinuria and urine culture
- Renal biopsy.

Known causes of CKD that may be diagnosed through this approach include diseases of the following:

- Macrovascular compartment (e.g. systemic hypertension, coagulopathies, chronic hypoperfusion)

- Microvascular compartment (e.g. systemic and glomerular hypertension, glomerulonephritis, developmental disorders, congenital collagen defects, amyloidosis)
- Interstitial compartment (e.g. pyelonephritis, neoplasia, obstructive uropathy, allergic and immune-mediated nephritis)
- Tubular compartment (e.g. tubular reabsorptive defects, chronic low-grade nephrotoxicity, obstructive uropathy).

These conditions may be acquired or heritable. A variety of breeds are afflicted with heritable CKD, which may have pathognomonic clinical and histopathological findings (see Chapter 7 for more detail). Examples of these include:

- Abyssinian cat (medullary amyloidosis)
- Persian cat (polycystic kidney disease)
- Basenji (proximal tubular reabsorptive disorder)
- Chow Chow (renal dysplasia)
- Cocker Spaniel (collagen type IV defect similar to human Alport's syndrome)
- Dobermann (familial glomerulopathy)
- Lhasa Apso (renal dysplasia)
- Norwegian Elkhound (proximal tubular reabsorptive disorder)
- Samoyed (collagen type IV defect similar to human Alport's syndrome)
- Shar Pei (amyloidosis)
- Shih Tzu (renal dysplasia)
- Soft-Coated Wheaten Terrier (renal dysplasia with proteinuria)
- Standard Poodle (glomerular atrophy).

Specific therapy is defined as a treatment that is directed at the primary cause of the kidney disease. While it is often not possible to identify the primary cause of the CKD, in the early IRIS stages use of specific therapy is a high priority (see Figure 18.2). The goal is to control the primary kidney disease, thereby reducing the magnitude of subsequent renal damage. Examples of specific therapy include (Figure 18.3):

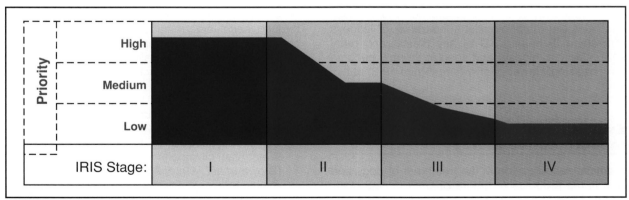

18.2 Renal evaluation and specific disease therapy. Early in CKD a diagnostic priority is to determine the primary cause (e.g. glomerulonephritis or pyelonephritis). If the primary cause of CKD is identified, employing specific therapy to ameliorate or eliminate this primary cause (e.g. immunosuppressive therapy for glomerulonephritis or antibiotics for pyelonephritis) should be a high therapeutic priority. As CKD progresses to subsequent IRIS stages, these become a lower priority (see text for further details).

Stage	Problem	Therapeutic considerations
Stage I–IV	Primary disease	*Specific therapy* for primary disease (e.g. antibiotics for pyelonephritis)
	Systemic hypertension	Antihypertensive therapy (*renoprotective and symptomatic therapy*: calcium channel blockers and/or angiotensin converting enzyme (ACE) inhibitors)
	Proteinuria	Follow 'monitor → investigate → intervene' paradigm (*renoprotective therapy*: ACE inhibitors, low-protein diet, dietary n-3 PUFA supplementation)
	Prerenal and postrenal factors	Maintain hydration at all times; treat postrenal factors, such as uroliths, where identified (*symptomatic therapy*)
Stage II–IV	Progressive loss of kidney function	Dietary phosphorus restriction ± intestinal phosphorus binders Calcitriol (dogs; cats?) Dietary n-3 PUFA supplementation ACE inhibitors (All are *renoprotective therapies*)
Stage IV	Uraemia	Low-protein/low-phosphorus diet Manage acid–base and electrolyte disorders Antiemetics Fluid therapy Calcitriol Appetite stimulants Offer variety of foods Feeding tube placement Renal replacement therapy (All are *symptomatic therapies*)

18.3 Treatment of CKD.

- Antibiotic therapy in cases of CKD caused by pyelonephritis
- Antihypertensives for animals with hypertensive nephropathy
- Dietary calcium restriction for animals with hypercalcaemic nephropathy
- Surgery for obstructive uropathy.

Interstitial fibrosis occurs in most animals with CKD (Perico *et al.*, 2005; Schnaper, 2005). The severity of interstitial fibrosis is positively correlated with the magnitude of decline of GFR and negatively correlated with the prognosis. When CKD is in the later stages (III–IV), the renal histology will probably demonstrate only this marked interstitial fibrosis, which is usually termed chronic interstitial nephritis. Chronic interstitial nephritis, also known as chronic tubulointerstitial fibrosis, describes the morphological appearance of kidneys with stage III or IV CKD of any cause, and renal evaluation (i.e. biopsy) and specific therapy become an increasingly lower priority (see Figure 18.2) at this time.

Evaluation of progression and renoprotective therapy

A critical consideration in the treatment of dogs and cats is the progressive nature of CKD (Finco *et al.*, 1999). There are several reasons that renal function will progressively deteriorate in an animal with CKD. As outlined above, of importance in stage I and early stage II is the renal damage that may be a manifestation of the primary disease process. However, in stages II–IV

other processes are activated that become more important in determining the rate of loss of renal function. These lead to what has been referred to as *inherent progression of CKD*, as these processes are intrinsic to CKD of any cause. Processes which are activated during stages II–IV of CKD and contribute to renal damage include:

- Systemic and glomerular hypertension
- Mineral imbalance
- Proteinuria
- Renal fibrosis.

Although the rate of progressive decline of renal function varies, studies to date suggest that inherent progression occurs in all animals with IRIS stages II–IV. Characterization of the rate of progression of CKD through serial determinations of plasma creatinine concentration are a high priority at this time (Figure 18.4). Measures that may slow inherent progression are referred to as *renoprotective therapies* (see Figure 18.3). These include:

- Dietary phosphorus restriction (dogs and cats) (Ross *et al.*, 1982; Brown *et al.*, 1987)
- Calcitriol administration (dogs) (Polzin, 2005)
- Dietary fish oil supplementation (dogs and cats) (Brown *et al.*, 1998a, 2000; Plantinga, 2005)
- Antihypertensive agents in animals with high blood pressure (dogs and cats) (Mathur *et al.*, 2002, 2004; Jacob *et al.*, 2003).
- Administration of ACE inhibitors (dogs and cats) (Grauer *et al.*, 2000; Gunn-Moore *et al.*, 2003).

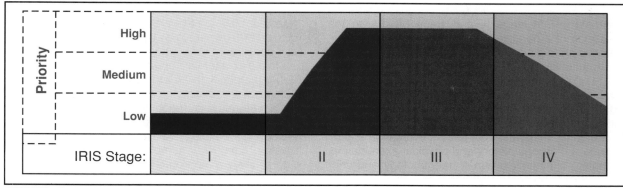

18.4 Evaluation of progression and renoprotective therapy. Generally, CKD progresses slowly in IRIS stage I. In IRIS stages II and III, a high priority of the diagnostic approach is to determine the rate of progression of CKD through serial assessments of serum creatinine and proteinuria. Therapy to delay progression, such as dietary fish oil supplementation or ACE inhibition, is a high therapeutic priority in these stages (see text for further details).

While renoprotective therapy is a high priority in IRIS stages II and III (Figure 18.4), it becomes increasingly less important in late stage IV as the focus of therapy becomes management of the complications of uraemia (see below).

Dietary restriction of phosphate and supplementation with fish oil (dogs) are important renoprotective therapies and specialized 'kidney' diets generally meet these requirements and should be utilized from stage II onward. Calcitriol administration (i.e. 0.5–1 ng/kg orally, given separately from meals to an animal that is normocalcaemic and normophosphataemic) is a renoprotective therapy in dogs (and possibly cats). If dietary restriction of phosphorus is unsuccessful in maintaining a normal level of serum phosphorus within 2–3 months, phosphate-binding gels containing calcium acetate, calcium carbonate or aluminium hydroxide should be administered with meals (initial dosage of 30 mg/kg with dosage increased as needed to achieve desired effect). Calcium-containing phosphate-binding agents should be avoided in animals receiving calcitriol.

In dogs and cats, there is a rationale for the inclusion of dietary n-3 polyunsaturated fatty acids (n-3 PUFA) and this may be accomplished with the use of special 'renal diets' that are already supplemented with n-3 PUFA and/or the addition of 1–3 g of n-3 PUFA/250 kcal of diet for dogs and 0.5–1.0 g/cat/day.

Patient evaluation and symptomatic therapy

Patient evaluations, which include efforts to identify developing complications (e.g. systemic hypertension, potassium homeostasis disorders, metabolic acidosis, proteinuria, anaemia and bacterial urinary tract infections) should be aggressively and prospectively pursued during all routine visits, regardless of IRIS stage. As CKD progresses into IRIS stage IV, clinical consequences of the reduction of GFR become apparent and thorough patient evaluations followed by appropriate symptomatic therapy (see Figure 18.3) become increasingly important (Figure 18.5).

Initially, uraemia causes occasional vomiting and lethargy. As CKD progresses within stage IV, generally over months (dogs) to years (cats), anorexia, weight loss, dehydration, oral ulceration, vomiting and diarrhoea are likely to become fully manifest. Loose teeth, deformable maxilla and mandible or pathological fractures may be seen with renal secondary osteodystrophy, but these are uncommon and are most often observed in young dogs with end-stage congenital renal disease.

Physical examination and imaging studies of animals in IRIS stages III–IV usually reveal small, irregular kidneys, although normal to large kidneys can be observed in animals with tumours, hydronephrosis,

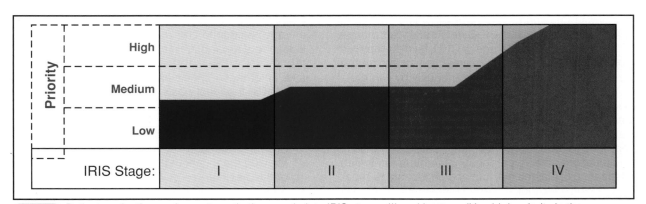

18.5 Patient evaluation and symptomatic therapy. In late IRIS stages III and in stage IV, a high priority in the diagnostic approach to CKD is identification of complications or the uraemic syndrome, such as vomiting or anaemia. Management of identified complications is a high therapeutic priority in these stages (see text for further details).

amyloidosis or glomerulonephritis. Mucous membranes are pale in late stage III and stage IV, due to the presence of a non-regenerative, normocytic, normochromic anaemia.

In animals in the severely azotaemic stage (IRIS stage IV) complications are more frequent, and patient evaluation and appropriate symptomatic therapy become an increasingly higher priority (see Figure 18.5). Affected animals at this stage should be evaluated at 1–2 monthly intervals. This patient evaluation should include a thorough history and physical examination, complete biochemical panel, haematology and urinalysis, including aerobic bacterial culture.

Symptomatic therapy is a high priority at this time (see Figure 18.5). As dietary restriction of protein may relieve some of the signs of uraemia, a high-quality protein (e.g. egg protein) should be fed at a level of 2.0–2.8 g/kg/day for dogs and 2.8–3.8 g/kg/day for cats. Commercial diets formulated for cats and dogs with CKD generally meet this recommendation.

Administration of an H_2-receptor antagonist, such as famotidine (2.5–5 mg/cat, orally once daily; 5 mg/kg, orally q6–12h in dogs), may decrease gastric acidity and vomiting. Anabolic steroids, such as oxymethalone or nandrolone, have been administered to stimulate red blood cell production in animals that are anaemic but this approach is not very effective. Recombinant erythropoietin may be given to stimulate red blood cell production (50–100 IU/kg s.c. given three times weekly initially, dosed to effect after haematocrit reaches the target range of 30–35%, with supplemental iron administration and weekly haematocrit determinations) (Cowgill, 1991; Cowgill *et al.*, 1998). Anti-erythropoietin antibodies develop in a significant percentage of animals treated with the human protein, however, and these may result in refractory anaemia; until a species-specific product becomes generally available, erythropoietin administration is now recommended only for animals showing apparent clinical signs of anaemia which generally occurs at a haematocrit ≤15%. The clinical signs of anaemia include:

- Weakness
- Marked lethargy not attributable to other factors.

Potassium citrate or sodium bicarbonate, given orally to effect, may be indicated if the animal is acidaemic (plasma bicarbonate <15 mmol/l) or if the animal remains acidaemic 2–3 weeks after diet change.

In later stage III and stage IV CKD, fluid therapy with polyionic solutions, given intravenously or subcutaneously in the hospital, or subcutaneously by owners at home (10–50 ml/kg s.c. every 1–3 days), is often beneficial in animals with intermittent signs of uraemia, particularly cats. Oral vitamin D administration (i.e. calcitriol at 0.5–1.0 ng/kg orally) is another option that may help to reduce uraemic signs. Calcitriol should be instituted only after hyperphosphataemia is eliminated. Monitoring of plasma calcium and phosphate is important during calcitriol therapy. Placement of feeding tubes (e.g. nasogastric or percutaneous endoscopic gastrostomy (PEG) tubes) can have an effective role in the management of the chronically inappetant animal

in late stage IV. Renal replacement therapy (renal transplantation and/or dialytic therapy) should be discussed with owners in early stage IV with implementation considered in late stage IV.

In the azotaemic, non-uraemic stages (IRIS stages II–III), the principles are the same for management of complications, except that the animal can be evaluated by a veterinary surgeon less frequently, generally every 3–6 months. These patient evaluations should include haematology, biochemistry panel and urinalysis. If identified, complications should be treated aggressively as appropriate. Since dogs and cats with CKD are prone to the development of bacterial urinary tract infections, urine culture should be performed twice annually.

Patient evaluation and symptomatic therapy are a lower priority in the earlier stages (I and II; see Figure 18.5). However, the systemic hypertension seen in approximately 20% of animals with CKD may be observed at any IRIS stage and this complication is not effectively controlled by feeding a low-salt diet (see Chapter 13). There is a minimal risk of target organ damage in the kidneys, eyes, brain and cardiovascular system when systolic blood pressure (BP) is 150 mmHg or less. The risk of organ injury from high BP is generally considered to be mild for systolic BP in the range of 150–159 mmHg, moderate for systolic BP in the 160–179 mmHg range and severe for systolic BP ≥180 mmHg. Because of the importance of maintaining renal perfusion in animals with CKD, the usual antihypertensive medications are vasodilatory agents. The most commonly employed agents are calcium channel blockers, such as amlodipine besylate (0.1– 0.25 mg/kg orally once daily) or ACE inhibitors, such as enalapril (0.5 mg/kg q12h in dogs and q24h in cats). While these may be co-administered at the recommended dosages, a calcium channel blocker is usually recommended as initial therapy in cats (particularly when the systolic BP exceeds 180 mmHg) (Elliott *et al.*, 2001) and an ACE inhibitor is often used as first-agent therapy in dogs.

Nutritional therapy

Nutrition plays a central role in the management of CKD (Brown *et al.*, 1998b). The response of each animal with CKD to the disease and to nutritional intervention will vary dramatically and individualized therapy is required; the only constant nutritional characteristic of renal insufficiency is inappetance and loss of body weight. Successful interventional nutrition must take all of these principles into account. For animals with CKD, the ideal goals of nutritional management are:

- Maximizing the quality and longevity of life by ensuring adequate intake of energy
- Limiting the extent of the clinical manifestations of the disease
- Slowing the rate of progression of renal disease.

Throughout all IRIS stages, non-specific supportive treatment is best managed medically at home. In addition to providing a continual supply of fresh drinking water and encouraging (and documenting) adequate dietary intake, routine use of body condition scoring should be employed to assess adequacy of intake.

Animals in late stage I should generally be fed standard, commercially available maintenance diets, unless they are proteinuric (see below). In stages II–III, nutritional modifications serve as renoprotective therapy, assuming central importance here. As noted above, the kidney is susceptible to self-perpetuating injury, and the extent of this injury may be modified by adjustments in dietary intake of phosphorus (reduced) and n-3 PUFA (supplemented).

Nutritional modifications are symptomatic therapy in late stage III and stage IV, where clinical signs of uraemia may be apparent. Most of the clinically observable abnormalities produced by the disruption of renal function are influenced by dietary intake of calories, phosphorus, sodium, potassium, protein or acid load.

Proteinuria

Recent findings have suggested that renal protein leak is not only a marker of severity of renal disease but also potentially a cause of renal injury (Lees et al., 2005) (see Chapter 6). We now recognize that proteinuria is associated with increased risk of developing end-stage CKD in dogs (Jacob et al., 2005) and cats (Syme et al., 2006); there may be an increased risk of mortality even in non-azotaemic animals. Further, studies have shown that therapies which reduce the magnitude of proteinuria are often renoprotective.

Proper management of proteinuria involves the following steps:

1. A finding of proteinuria should lead the clinician to *monitor* the patient with confirmation by a specific test for proteinuria, such as a urine protein:creatinine ratio or assessment of albuminuria. When monitoring a proteinuric patient, it is important to determine if the proteinuria is transient or persistent (at least two tests at 2-weekly intervals).
2. If persistent proteinuria is present in a patient with CKD, it is appropriate to *investigate* in order to determine the site of origin of the protein (prerenal, renal or postrenal) and determine if renal proteinuria is a sign of a complication (e.g. systemic hypertension) or evidence of a specific renal disease (e.g. glomerulonephritis) through careful patient evaluation. Proteinuria probably confers a poorer prognosis when the urine protein:creatinine ratio exceeds 0.5 in dogs or 0.4 in cats.
3. If proteinuria of this magnitude is persistent and renal in origin in an animal with CKD, the clinician should consider *intervening* by employing antiproteinuric therapy (e.g. ACE inhibitor, low-protein diet and/or n-3 PUFA supplementation). In this case, the antiproteinuric therapy is renoprotective, and is thus of higher priority in stages II, III and early stage IV (see Figure 18.4).

Serial determinations of the level of proteinuria with a specific test for albuminuria or a urine protein:creatinine ratio should be used to evaluate the success of this approach.

Summary

The proper management of a dog or cat with CKD requires a clear understanding of the diagnostic and therapeutic priorities in the stage of disease at the time the patient is being managed:

- Early in the disease process (IRIS stage I), a careful evaluation of the kidney is critical, to identify the primary disease process and specific therapy to eliminate this disease
- In the middle stages (II and III), inherent progression and renoprotective therapy are paramount
- In the final stage of CKD (IRIS stage IV), more frequent and thorough evaluations of the patient, with institution of appropriate symptomatic therapy, become the primary consideration of the veterinary surgeon.

References and further reading

Brown SA, Brown CA, Crowell WA et al. (1998a) Beneficial effects of chronic administration of dietary omega-3 polyunsaturated fatty acids in dogs with renal insufficiency. Journal of Laboratory and Clinical Medicine **131**, 447–455

Brown SA, Brown CA, Crowell WA et al. (2000) Effects of dietary polyunsaturated fatty acid supplementation in early renal insufficiency in dogs. Journal of Laboratory and Clinical Medicine **135**, 275–286

Brown SA, Finco DR, Bartges JW, Brown CA and Barsanti JA (1998b) Interventional nutrition for renal disease. Clinical Techniques in Small Animal Practice **13**, 217–223

Brown SA, Finco DR, Boudinot D et al. (1996) Evaluation of a single injection method, using iohexol, for estimating glomerular filtration rate in cats and dogs. American Journal of Veterinary Research **57**, 105–110

Brown SA, Finco DR, Crowell WA et al. (1987) Beneficial effect of moderate phosphate restriction in partially nephrectomized dogs on a low protein diet. Kidney International **31**, 380

Cowgill LD (1991) Clinical experience and the use of recombinant human erythropoietin in uremic dogs and cats. Proceedings of the 9th American College of Veterinary Internal Medicine (ACVIM) Forum, 147–149

Cowgill LD, James KM, Levy JK et al. (1998) Use of recombinant human erythropoietin for management of anemia in dogs and cats with renal failure. Journal of the American Veterinary Medical Association **212**, 521–528

Elliott J, Barber PJ, Syme HM, Rawlings JM and Markwell PJ (2001) Feline hypertension: clinical findings and response to antihypertensive treatment in 30 cases. Journal of Small Animal Practice **42**, 122–129

Finco D, Braselton W and Cooper T (2001) Relationship between plasma iohexol clearance and urinary exogenous creatinine clearance in dogs. Journal of Veterinary Internal Medicine **15**, 368–373

Finco DR, Brown SA, Brown CA et al. (1999) Progression of chronic renal disease in the dog. Journal of Veterinary Internal Medicine **13**, 516–528

Gleadhill A and Michell AR (1996) Evaluation of iohexol as a marker for the clinical measurement of glomerular filtration rate in dogs. Research in Veterinary Science **60**, 117–121

Grauer G, Greco D, Gretzy D et al. (2000) Effects of enalapril treatment versus placebo as a treatment for canine idiopathic glomerulonephritis. Journal of Veterinary Internal Medicine **14**, 526–533

Gunn-Moore D and The BENRIC Study Group (2003) Influence of proteinuria on survival time in cats with chronic renal insufficiency. Journal of Veterinary Internal Medicine **17**, 405A

Jacob F, Polzin DJ, Osborne CA *et al.* (2003) Association between initial systolic blood pressure and risk of developing a uremic crisis or of dying in dogs with chronic renal failure. *Journal of the American Veterinary Medical Association* **222**, 322–329

Jacob F, Polzin DJ, Osborne CA *et al.* (2005) Evaluation of the association between initial proteinuria and morbidity rate or death in dogs with naturally occurring chronic renal failure. *Journal of the American Veterinary Medical Association* **226**, 393–400

Krawiec D and Gelberg H (1989) Chronic renal disease in cats. In: *Current Veterinary Therapy X*, ed. RW Kirk, pp. 1170–1173. WB Saunders, Philadelphia

Labato MA and Ross LA (1991) Plasma disappearance of creatinine as a renal function test in the dog. *Research in Veterinary Science* **50**, 253–258

Lees GE, Brown SA, Elliott J, Grauer GF and Vaden SL (2005) Assessment and management of proteinuria in dogs and cats: 2004 ACVIM Forum Consensus Statement (small animal). *Journal of Veterinary Internal Medicine* **19**, 377–385

Mathur S, Brown CA, Dietrich UM *et al.* (2004) Evaluation of a technique of inducing hypertensive renal insufficiency in cats. *American Journal of Veterinary Research* **65**, 1006–1013

Mathur S, Syme H, Brown CA *et al.* (2002) Effects of the calcium channel antagonist amlodipine in cats with surgically induced hypertensive renal insufficiency. *American Journal of Veterinary Research* **63**, 833–839

Moe L and Heiene R (1995) Estimation of glomerular filtration rate in dogs with 99M-Tc-DTPA and iohexol. *Research in Veterinary Science* **58**, 138–143

Perico N, Codreanu I, Schieppati A and Remuzzi G (2005) The future of renoprotection. *Kidney International Supplement,* S95–101

Plantinga EA, Everts H, Kastelein AMC and Beynen AC (2005) Retrospective study of the survival of cats with acquired chronic renal insufficiency offered different commercial diets. *Veterinary Record* **157**, 185–187

Polzin DJ (2005) Clinical benefit of calcitriol in canine chronic kidney disease. *Journal of Veterinary Internal Medicine* **19**, 122A

Polzin DJ and Osborne CA (1986) Update: conservative medical management of chronic renal failure In: *Current Veterinary Therapy IX*, ed. RW Kirk, pp. 1167–1173. WB Saunders, Philadelphia

Polzin DJ, Osborne CA and Ross S (2005) Chronic kidney disease. In: In: *Textbook of Veterinary Internal Medicine, 6th edn,* ed. SJ Ettinger and EC Feldman, pp. 1756–1785. WB Saunders, St. Louis

Ross LA, Finco DR and Crowell WA (1982) Effect of dietary phosphorus restriction on the kidneys of cats with reduced renal mass. *American Journal of Veterinary Research* **43**, 1023–1026

Schnaper HW (2005) Renal fibrosis. *Methods in Molecular Medicine* **117**, 45–68

Syme HM, Markwell PJ, Pfeiffer D and Elliott J (2006) Survival of cats with naturally occurring chronic renal failure is related to severity of Proteinuria. *Journal of Veterinary Internal Medicine,* **20,** 528–535

19

Management of glomerulonephritis

Gregory F. Grauer

Introduction

Most canine glomerular disease is thought to be associated with the presence of immune complexes in glomerular capillary walls (DiBartola *et al.*, 1980; Jaenke and Allen, 1986; Center *et al.*, 1987; Cook and Cowgill, 1996); other examples of glomerular disease in dogs include structural abnormalities (e.g. type IV collagen defects in hereditary nephritis in Samoyed dogs), haemodynamic abnormalities (e.g. intraglomerular hypertension) and glomerular amyloid deposition. This chapter focuses on immune complex glomerular disease.

Immune complex diseases involving the glomerulus are often collectively referred to as glomerulonephritis (GN). Despite the widespread acceptance of this term, in most cases glomerular lesions associated with the presence of immune complexes do not demonstrate classic evidence of neutrophilic inflammation. In very simplistic terms, the histological changes observed in the glomerulus usually include one or more of the following:

* Cellular proliferation
* Mesangial matrix expansion
* Capillary wall thickening.

Additional histological subclassification of glomerular lesions associated with immune complexes that utilize immunohistochemical and ultrastructural studies will be necessary if we are to improve our ability to treat and provide accurate prognoses for this disease process.

Persistent proteinuria (principally albuminuria) in the face of an inactive urine sediment is the hallmark clinicopathological abnormality associated with immune complex GN. Normally plasma contains approximately 40 g/l of albumin and, due to the semipermeable nature of the healthy glomerular filter, the glomerular filtrate usually contains only 20–30 mg/l of albumin (i.e. 2000 times lower than plasma). The proximal convoluted tubular epithelial cells reabsorb much of this filtered albumin so that normal canine urine contains <10 mg/l of albumin. Pathological renal proteinuria may arise from:

* Tubulointerstitial disease (e.g. decreased tubular reabsorption)
* Glomerular disease (e.g. increased filtration) (see Chapter 6).

Use of the urine protein:creatinine ratio (UPC) to quantitatively evaluate proteinuria has greatly facilitated diagnosis of GN in veterinary medicine. Dogs with a UPC persistently >0.5 but <2.0, with normal urine sediments, usually have renal disease, either glomerular or tubular. A UPC that is persistently >2.0 and associated with a normal urine sediment is almost always indicative of glomerular disease. Beyond the diagnostic utility of proteinuria, pathophysiological consequences of persistent proteinuria in dogs may include:

* Decreased plasma oncotic pressure
* Oedema and/or ascites
* Hypercholesterolaemia
* Systemic hypertension
* Hypercoagulability
* Muscle wasting
* Weight loss.

The potential for proteinuria to be associated with renal disease progression has also been recognized, stimulating a discussion in veterinary medicine about what level of proteinuria is normal. Development of canine-specific albumin enzyme-linked immunosorbent assay (ELISA) technology that enables detection of low concentrations of albuminuria (microalbuminuria) has helped drive this re-evaluation (see Chapter 6).

Canine glomerular disease was initially thought to be uncommon and unimportant. It is now recognized, however, that glomerular disease is not only common but can also lead to chronic kidney disease in the dog. For example, in a study of 76 dogs with chronic renal disease, 40 (52%) had glomerular disease rather than non-glomerular disease as the underlying disease pathology (MacDougall *et al.*, 1986). In another study of dogs with naturally occurring end-stage renal disease that received renal allografts, glomerular disease was judged to be the underlying pathology in 7 of 15 cases (Mathews *et al.*, 2000). It is interesting to note that a UPC <5.0 was required to be eligible for the renal transplantation to help exclude underlying glomerular disease that might adversely affect the allograft. Even though the inclusion criteria were biased against proteinuria disease, 47% of the small number of dogs in this study had glomerular disease. Studies have shown the prevalence of glomerular disease in randomly selected dogs to be as high as 47–70% (Rouse and Lewis, 1975; Muller-Peddinghaus and Trautwein, 1977);

this emphasizes the need to identify and effectively treat dogs with glomerular proteinuria.

General treatment objectives for dogs with GN include reducing proteinuria and slowing disease progression. Specific treatment objectives include:

- Identification and elimination of any underlying disease process that may be producing antigen–antibody complexes
- Decreasing the angiotensin and aldosterone response
- Decreasing the platelet/thromboxane response
- Supportive care.

Pathophysiology

Soluble circulating antigen–antibody complexes may be deposited or trapped in the glomerulus, due to:

- The large proportion of cardiac output supplied to the kidneys
- The hydraulic pressure gradient across the glomerular capillary wall
- The fenestrated endothelium of the glomerular capillaries.

Glomerular deposition of preformed immune complexes often results in a 'lumpy–bumpy' or granular immunofluorescent or immunocytochemical pattern along the glomerular basement membrane. In contrast to the glomerular deposition of preformed complexes, immune complexes may also form *in situ* in the glomerular basement membrane. *In situ* immune complex formation occurs when circulating antibodies react with endogenous glomerular antigens or 'planted' non-glomerular antigens in the glomerular capillary wall. Autoimmune GN, the condition in which antibodies are directed against endogenous glomerular basement membrane material, has not been documented in dogs with naturally occurring GN. However, non-glomerular antigens may localize in the glomerular filter due to electrical charge attraction or biochemical affinity. When antibodies present in plasma react with an antigen *in situ*, a smooth, linear pattern of immune complexes is often produced. For example, studies of dogs with dirofilariasis have shown that heartworm antigens have an affinity for glomerular capillaries and that heart-worm-associated immune complexes can form *in situ* within the glomerulus (Grauer *et al.*, 1989).

The immune-mediated pathophysiology associated with either deposition or *in situ* formation of immune complexes stresses the importance of identification and correction of any underlying or concurrent disease process. Several infectious and inflammatory diseases have been associated with the presence of glomerular immune complexes (Figure 19.1). However, in many cases the antigen source or underlying disease process is not identified and the glomerular disease is referred to as idiopathic (Cook and Cowgill, 1996). Identification of endogenous immunoglobulin or complement within the glomerulus using immunofluorescence histological techniques is not difficult, but

Infectious causes
Canine adenovirus 1
Bacterial endocarditis
Brucellosis
Borelliosis
Dirofilariasis
Ehrlichiosis
Leishmaniasis
Hepatozoonosis
Rocky Mountain spotted fever
Bartonellosis
Babesiosis
Blastomycosis
Coccidiomycosis
Trypanosomiasis
Helicobacter?
Chronic bacterial infections (periodontal disease, pyoderma, pyometra, septicaemia, prostatitis)

Neoplasia

Inflammatory causes
Pancreatitis
Systemic lupus erythematosus
Other immune-mediated diseases
Prostatitis
Hepatitis
Polyarthritis
Inflammatory bowel disease

Other causes
Hyperadrenocorticism and long-term high-dose corticosteriods?
Idiopathic
Familial
Cyclic haematopoiesis (cyclic neutropenia) (grey collies)
Non-immunological hyperfiltration?
Diabetes mellitus?

19.1 Diseases associated with glomerulonephritis in dogs.

identification of the type or source of exogenous antigens within glomerular tissue is rarely accomplished.

The glomerulus provides a unique environment for injurious immune complexes to stimulate production of bioactive mediators, such as proinflammatory cytokines, vasoactive substances, growth factors and extracellular matrix proteins and proteases, that can contribute to the injury (Johnson, 1997) (Figure 19.2). These substances may be produced by endogenous glomerular cells or by platelets, macrophages and neutrophils that are attracted to the immune-mediated damage. For example, activation of the renin–angiotensin–aldosterone system (RAAS) can have haemodynamic and inflammatory/fibrotic effects on the kidney (Hilgers and Mann, 1996). The main haemodynamic effect is vasoconstriction of the efferent glomerular arteriole resulting in intraglomerular hypertension. This increased hydrostatic pressure within the glomerular capillaries helps drive plasma albumin through the injured glomerular filter. Angiotensin and aldosterone are also proinflammatory and can stimulate glomerular cell proliferation and fibrogenesis.

In addition to the RAAS, several factors, including activation of the complement system, platelet aggre-

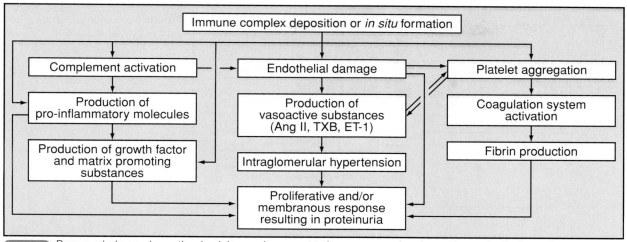

19.2 Proposed glomerular pathophysiology subsequent to immune complex deposition or *in situ* formation. Ang II = Angiotensin II; ET-1 = Endothelin-1; TXB = Thromboxane.

gation, activation of the coagulation system and fibrin deposition, also contribute to glomerular damage (Clark *et al.*, 1976). Platelet activation and aggregation occur secondarily to endothelial damage or antigen–antibody interaction (Hayslett, 1984). Platelets, in turn, exacerbate glomerular damage by release of vasoactive and inflammatory substances and by facilitation of the coagulation cascade. Platelets are also capable of releasing growth-stimulating factors that promote proliferation of vascular endothelial cells. The glomerulus responds to this injury by cellular proliferation, thickening of the glomerular basement membrane and, if the injury persists, hyalinization and sclerosis (Figure 19.3). In those cases where identification and correction of an underlying disease process is not possible, treatment is focused on decreasing this glomerular response to the immune complexes (e.g. angiotensin and platelet antagonists).

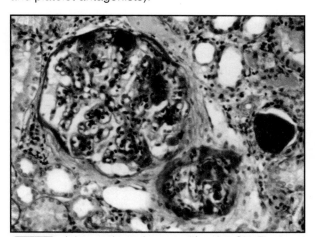

19.3 Advanced membranoproliferative GN. The large glomerulus shows hypercellularity with prominent focal accumulations of mesangial matrix material and thickened glomerular capillary walls. Adhesions to Bowman's capsule and periglomerular fibrosis are also present. The small glomerulus is irreversibly damaged and obsolescent. A hyaline cast is present in a tubule (right). (PAS stain, original magnification X200.) (Reproduced from Grauer (1991) with permission from the publisher.)

Once a glomerulus has been irreversibly damaged by GN, the entire nephron becomes non-functional. Fibrosis and scarring of irreversibly damaged nephrons may have the appearance of primary interstitial inflammation. In fact for many years renal interstitial inflammation or 'chronic interstitial nephritis' was thought to be the primary lesion that caused chronic kidney disease in dogs. As more and more nephrons become involved, glomerular filtration *in toto* decreases. Remaining viable nephrons compensate for the decrease in nephron numbers with increased individual glomerular filtration rates (GFRs) (Figure 19.4) (see also Chapter 18). This 'hyperfiltration', coupled with systemic hypertension if present, may contribute to glomerular hyalinization and sclerosis (Brenner *et al.*, 1982). Although it has not been documented in dogs with naturally occurring GN, hyperfiltration and proteinuria in remnant nephrons may result in progressive nephron loss, independent of the previously discussed immune-mediated GN.

There is increasing evidence in laboratory animals and human patients that proteinuria can cause glomerular and tubulointerstitial damage that can lead to progressive nephron loss (see also Chapter 6). Plasma proteins that have crossed the glomerular filter can accumulate within the glomerular tuft and stimulate mesangial cell proliferation and increased production of mesangial matrix (Jerums *et al.*, 1997). In addition, excessive amounts of protein in the glomerular filtrate can be toxic to human tubular epithelial cells and can lead to interstitial inflammation, fibrosis and cell death (Tang *et al.*, 1999).

Proximal tubular cells normally reabsorb protein from the glomerular filtrate by endocytosis. Albumin and other proteins accumulate in lysosomes and are then degraded into amino acids; excessive lysosomal processing, however, can result in swelling and rupture of lysosomes causing enzymatic damage to the cytoplasm (Olbricht *et al.*, 1986). Tubular injury may also occur as a consequence of tubular obstruction with proteinaceous casts (Bertani *et al.*, 1986). Increased permeability of the glomerulus to plasma results in potential contact of the tubular cell with transferrin,

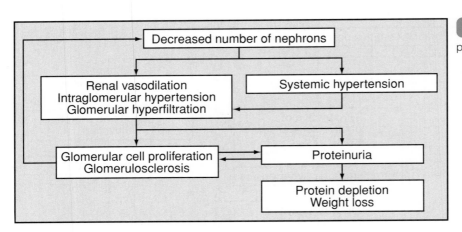

19.4 Proposed pathogenesis of nephron loss in progressive renal disease.

complement and lipoproteins, and possibly in peroxidative and/or immune-mediated damage to the tubule (Alfrey *et al.*, 1989; Camussi, 1994; Ong and Moorhead, 1994). Exposure to plasma proteins at the luminal surface of the tubular cell results in a basolateral release of growth factors, fibronectin and monocyte chemoattractant protein-1 (MCP-1) (Harris *et al.*, 1996). This process may also induce excessive tubular expression of transforming growth factor-$\beta1$ (TGF-$\beta1$) that can result in the interstitial inflammation and scarring typical of end-stage kidney disease (Remuzzi, 1995). Another mediator of tubulointerstitial damage related to excessive tubular cell protein reabsorption is the up-regulation of tubular-derived endothelin-1 (ET-1) (Benigni *et al.*, 1995). Tubular ET-1 formed in response to increasing concentrations of albumin presented to the proximal tubular epithelium is secreted towards the basolateral cellular compartment and accumulates in the interstitium, causing ischaemia. ET-1 also binds to receptors on interstitial fibroblasts and causes interstitial cellular proliferation and extracellular matrix production (Benigni *et al.*, 1995).

In dogs with naturally occurring chronic kidney disease, proteinuria resulting in a UPC ≥1.0 was associated with a threefold greater risk of development of uraemic crises and death compared with dogs with UPC <1.0. The relative risk of adverse outcome was approximately 1.5 times higher for every 1 unit increase in UPC. In addition, dogs with a UPC ≥1.0 had a decrease in renal function that was greater than that observed in dogs with a UPC <1.0 (Jacob *et al.*, 2005). Based on this evidence, it is possible that proteinuria is not only a marker of glomerular disease in the dog, but also a mediator of progressive renal injury. Based on these observational studies, and the basic understanding of cellular responses to excess protein in the glomerular filtrate, attenuation of proteinuria should be a major treatment objective in dogs with GN.

Clinical signs

There may be no clinical signs associated with low-level proteinuria; or if signs are present they are usually mild and non-specific, e.g. weight loss and lethargy. If protein loss is severe, resulting in a serum albumin concentration <10–15 g/l, oedema and/or ascites may occur (Figure 19.5). If the glomerular disease process causes loss of more than three quarters of the nephrons, clinical signs consistent with uraemia (see Chapter 5) may be present, e.g. polydipsia/polyuria, anorexia, nausea, vomiting and weight loss. Occasionally, clinical signs associated with an underlying infectious, inflammatory or neoplastic disease may be the reason why owners seek veterinary care. Rarely, dogs may be presented with acute dyspnoea or severe panting caused by a pulmonary thromboembolism.

Persistent proteinuria may lead to clinical signs of the nephrotic syndrome. This is usually defined

Manifestation	Clinical signs	Clinicopathological findings
Mild to moderate proteinuria	Lethargy, mild weight loss, decreased muscle mass	Serum albumin 15–30 g/l
Marked proteinuria (>3.5 g/day)	Severe muscle wasting, weight gain may occur, however, as result of oedema or ascites	Serum albumin <15 g/l; hypercholesterolaemia
Uraemia	Depression, anorexia, nausea, vomiting, weight loss, polyuria/polydipsia	Azotaemia, isosthenuria or minimally concentrated urine, hyperphosphataemia, non-regenerative anaemia
Pulmonary thromboembolism	Acute dyspnoea or severe panting	Hypoxaemia; normal or low PCO_2; fibrinogen >3 g/l; antithrombin III <70% of normal
Retinal haemorrhage and/or detachment	Acute blindness	Systolic blood pressure usually >180 mmHg

19.5 Signs associated with different manifestations of glomerular disease.

as a combination of proteinuria, hypoalbuminaemia, ascites or oedema, and hypercholesterolaemia. Decreased plasma oncotic pressure and hyperaldosteronism, causing sodium retention, are thought to be the primary causes of ascites and oedema. It has also been hypothesized that intrarenal mechanisms, independent of aldosterone, may also contribute to sodium retention (Brown *et al.*, 1982). The hypercholesterolaemia associated with the nephrotic syndrome probably occurs because of a combination of decreased catabolism of proteins and lipoproteins and increased hepatic synthesis of proteins and lipoproteins (Wheeler *et al.*, 1989). This results in the accumulation of large molecular weight cholesterol-rich lipoproteins, which are not as easily lost through the damaged capillary wall as are the smaller molecular weight proteins like albumin.

In addition to the previously mentioned clinical signs, systemic hypertension and hypercoagulability are frequent complications in dogs with nephrotic syndrome. A combination of activation of the RAAS and decreased renal production of vasodilators, coupled with increased responsiveness to normal vasopressor mechanisms, is likely to be involved in the pathogenesis of the systemic hypertension. Systemic hypertension has been commonly associated with immune-mediated GN, glomerulosclerosis and amyloidosis; in one study, 84% of dogs with glomerular disease were found to be hypertensive (Cowgill, 1991). Retinal changes, including haemorrhage, detachment and papilloedema, can be consequences of systemic hypertension and, rarely, blindness may be the presenting sign in hypertensive dogs. Blood pressure measurement (see Chapter 13) should be included in the evaluation and management of dogs with glomerular disease, as it is probable that control of systemic hypertension may slow the progression of the glomerular disease.

Hypercoagulability and thromboembolism associated with the nephrotic syndrome occur secondarily to several abnormalities in the clotting system. In addition to a mild thrombocytosis, a hypoalbuminaemia-related platelet hypersensitivity increases platelet adhesion and aggregation proportionally to the magnitude of hypoalbuminaemia (Green *et al.*, 1985). Loss of antithrombin III in urine also contributes to hypercoagulability (Green and Kabel, 1982).

Antithrombin III works in concert with heparin to inhibit serine proteases (clotting factors II, IX, X, XI and XII) and normally plays a vital role in modulating thrombin and fibrin production. Finally, altered fibrinolysis and increases in the concentration of large molecular weight clotting factors may lead to a relative increase in clotting factors compared with regulatory proteins. The pulmonary arterial system is the most common location for a thromboembolus to lodge. Dogs with pulmonary thromboembolisms are usually dyspnoeic and hypoxic, with minimal pulmonary abnormalities evident on radiography. Treatment of pulmonary thromboembolism is difficult, often expensive and frequently unrewarding; therefore, early prophylactic treatment to prevent thrombus formation is important.

Diagnosis

Persistent proteinuria, resulting in a UPC ≥2.0, associated with a normal urine sediment or one containing hyaline casts, is very likely to be glomerular in origin. It should be noted that a UPC <2.0 can be observed in dogs with nascent or mild GN. Persistent proteinuria was recently defined in a consensus statement commissioned by the American College of Veterinary Internal Medicine as three positive urinalyses separated by at least 2 weeks (Lees *et al.*, 2005).

If persistent proteinuria of suspected renal origin is identified, a renal biopsy is indicated. Histopathological evaluation of renal tissue will help to establish a diagnosis (e.g. GN *versus* amyloidosis or glomerulosclerosis) and aid in the formation of a prognosis. However, renal biopsy should be considered only after less invasive tests (complete blood count, serum biochemistry profile, urinalysis, quantitation of proteinuria and abdominal radiographs or renal ultrasonography) have been accomplished and an assessment of blood clotting ability has been performed. In most cases, a search for an underlying or concurrent disease process is also performed prior to obtaining a renal biopsy sample.

Renal biopsies can be performed percutaneously using the keyhole technique or by laparoscopic or ultrasonographic guidance (see Chapter 12). Frequently, the best way to perform a renal biopsy is with laparotomy where both kidneys can be visualized, haemorrhage following biopsy can be accurately assessed and treated, and adequacy of the biopsy specimen is assured. The cortical region of either kidney should be sampled in order to obtain an adequate number of glomeruli and to avoid the major vessels and renal nerves in the medullary region. Most patients will exhibit microscopic haematuria for 1–3 days following the biopsy and overt haematuria is not uncommon. Severe haemorrhage occurs less than 3% of the time (Jeraj *et al.*, 1982) and poor biopsy technique is the most frequent cause.

Consultation with the histopathology laboratory prior to the biopsy is important to ensure the appropriate fixatives are used. When possible, special stains, thin sections, immunofluorescent and/or immunocytochemical staining and electron microscopy should be used to maximize the information gained from the biopsy specimen.

Treatment

Even though GN is a major cause of chronic renal disease in the dog, its treatment has received substantially less attention in veterinary medicine than has the treatment of chronic kidney disease. Immune complexes usually initiate GN, so primary treatment objectives include:

• Identification and elimination of causative/associated antigens
• Reduction of the glomerular response to the immune complexes.

235

1. Identify and correct any underlying disease processes [a]

2. Immunosuppressive treatment?

3. Haemodynamic/antiproteinuric treatment (ACE inhibitors) [a]

4. Antiplatelet hypercoagulability treatment: aspirin 0.5 mg/kg q12–24h [a]

5. Supportive care:

Dietary –
   Sodium reduced, high-quality low-quantity protein, with n-3 fatty acid supplementation [a]

Hypertension –
   Dietary sodium reduction
   ACE inhibition (e.g. enalapril 0.5 mg/kg q12–24h) [a]

Oedema/ascites –
   Moderate dietary sodium reduction (approximately 50 mg/100 kcal)
   Cage rest
   Furosemide 1–2 mg/kg as needed. Caution: volume contraction and reduced GFR may result
   Paracentesis for patients with tense ascites and/or respiratory distress
   Plasma transfusions?

19.6 Treatment guidelines for GN ([a] denotes those treatments thought to be most important by the author).

A summary of treatment guidelines is given in Figure 19.6.

Elimination of antigens

Elimination of the source of antigenic stimulation is the treatment of choice for GN. For example, proteinuria associated with dirofilariasis in dogs often improves or resolves after successful treatment of parasitic infection. Unfortunately, elimination of the antigen source is often not possible because the antigen source or underlying disease may not be identified or may be impossible to eliminate (e.g. neoplasia). In a retrospective study of 106 dogs with GN, 43% had no identifiable concurrent disease or disorder and 19% had neoplasia (Cook and Cowgill, 1996). Infection, polyarthritis, hepatitis, hyperadrenocorticism and immune-mediated anaemia are additional commonly identified concurrent medical problems (Cook and Cowgill, 1996) (see Figure 19.1).

Immunosuppressive drugs

Based on results in humans, immunosuppressive drugs have been recommended in dogs with GN. Despite widespread use of immunosuppressive agents, there has only been one controlled clinical trial in veterinary medicine assessing the effects of immunosuppressive treatment. In this study, ciclosporin treatment was found to be of no benefit in reducing proteinuria associated with idiopathic GN in dogs (Vaden et al., 1995).

The association between hyperadrenocorticism or long-term exogenous corticosteroid administration and GN and thromboembolism in the dog, as well as the lack of consistent therapeutic response to corticosteroids, raise questions about use of corticosteroids in dogs with GN. In a retrospective study of dogs with naturally occurring GN, treatment with corticosteroids appeared to be detrimental, leading to azotaemia and worsening of proteinuria (Center et al., 1987). Similarly, prednisolone increased the UPC from 1.5 to 5.6 in carrier bitches with X-linked hereditary nephropathy (Lees et al., 2002). Consequently, routine use of corticosteroids to treat GN in dogs is not recommended. Treatment with corticosteroids would be indicated, however, if the underlying disease process were known to be steroid-responsive (e.g. systemic lupus erythematosus). As in human patients, it is also possible that there are specific subtypes of canine immune complex GN (e.g. minimal change GN) that will be shown to be steroid responsive as they are appropriately identified and treated.

Decreasing glomerular response

If an underlying or concurrent disease process cannot be identified and treated, or if immunosuppressive treatment is deemed inappropriate, treatment may be aimed at decreasing the glomerular response to the presence of immune complexes. Increased urinary excretion of thromboxane has been detected in dogs with experimentally induced GN (Longhofer et al., 1991; Grauer et al., 1992a). Thromboxane is thought to arise primarily from platelets that are attracted to the glomerulus in immune complex disease.

Furthermore, platelet survival is decreased in several types of GN in human patients, and platelet depletion attenuates GN. These findings suggest that platelets and thromboxane have an important role in the pathogenesis of GN. Thromboxane synthetase inhibitors decreased proteinuria, glomerular cell proliferation, neutrophil infiltration and fibrin deposition in dogs with experimental GN (Longhofer et al., 1991; Grauer et al., 1992a). In the absence of specific thromboxane synthetase inhibitors, aspirin may be a valuable substitute (Grauer et al., 1992b). Appropriate dosage is probably important if non-selective cyclooxygenase inhibitors, such as aspirin, are used to decrease glomerular inflammation and platelet aggregation. An extremely low dosage of aspirin (0.5 mg/kg orally q24h) may selectively inhibit platelet cyclooxygenase without preventing the beneficial effects of prostacyclin formation (e.g. vasodilation, inhibition of platelet aggregation). Low-dose aspirin is easily administered on an out-patient basis and does not require extensive monitoring, as does coumarin treatment. Because fibrin accumulation within the glomerulus is a frequent and irreversible consequence of GN, antiplatelet/anticoagulant treatment may serve a dual purpose.

Evidence indicates that angiotensin-converting enzyme (ACE) inhibitors not only reduce proteinuria but also slow disease progression in dogs with glomerular disease. In dogs with unilateral nephrectomy and experimentally induced diabetes mellitus, ACE inhibitor administration reduced glomerular transcapillary hydraulic pressure and glomerular cell hypertrophy as well as proteinuria (Brown et al., 1993). In another study, ACE inhibitor treatment of Samoyed dogs with X-linked hereditary nephritis decreased proteinuria, improved renal excretory function, decreased glomerular basement membrane splitting and prolonged survival compared with control dogs (Grodecki et al.,

1997). Recently, a double-blind, multicentre, prospective clinical trial assessed the effects of enalapril (EN) *versus* standard care in dogs with naturally occurring, idiopathic GN (Grauer *et al.*, 2000). Twenty nine adult dogs with membranous (16) and membranoproliferative (13) GN were identified for study. Dogs were randomly assigned to receive either EN (0.5 mg/kg orally q12–24h) (n=16) or placebo (n=14) for 6 months (one dog was treated first with the placebo and then with EN). All dogs were treated with low-dose aspirin (0.5–5 mg/kg orally q12–24h) and fed Hills k/d diet. After 6 months of treatment the change in UPC from baseline was different between groups, with the EN treatment group having a significantly reduced UPC. When the data were adjusted for changes in GFR (UPC × serum creatinine) a similar significant reduction was noted. The change in systolic blood pressure after 6 months of treatment was also significantly different between groups. Response to treatment was categorized as follows:

- Improvement (>50% reduction in UPC with stable serum creatinine)
- No progression (<50% reduction in UPC with stable serum creatinine)
- Progression (>50% increase in UPC and/or serum creatinine, or euthanasia due to renal failure).

Response to treatment was significantly better in the EN-treated dogs compared with the placebo-treated dogs (Grauer *et al.*, 2000).

Treatment with ACE inhibitors probably decreases proteinuria associated with glomerular disease and preserves renal function by several mechanisms:

- In dogs, administration of lisinopril decreases efferent glomerular arteriolar resistance, which results in decreased (normalized) glomerular transcapillary hydraulic pressure and decreased proteinuria (Brown *et al.*, 1993)
- In rats, administration of EN prevents the loss of glomerular heparan sulphate that can occur with glomerular disease (Reddi *et al.*, 1991)
- Administration of ACE inhibitors is thought to attenuate proteinuria by decreasing the size of glomerular capillary endothelial cell pores in people (Wiegmann *et al.*, 1992)
- The antiproteinuric and renal protective effects of ACE inhibitors in people may be, in part, associated with improved lipoprotein metabolism (Keilani *et al.*, 1993)
- Decreased production of angiotensin and aldosterone may result in decreased renal fibrosis (Epstein, 2001)
- Administration of ACE inhibitors in dogs slows glomerular mesangial cell growth and proliferation that can alter the permeability of the glomerular capillary wall and lead to glomerulosclerosis (Brown *et al.*, 1993).

Supportive therapy

Supportive therapy is important in the management of dogs with GN and should be aimed at alleviating

systemic hypertension, decreasing oedema/ascites and reducing the tendency for thromboembolism to occur. ACE inhibitors are recommended as the first line of defence for proteinuric, hypertensive dogs. In those cases where systemic hypertension is refractory to ACE inhibitor treatment, a calcium channel blocker should be added to the antihypertensive regimen.

Cage rest and dietary sodium reduction should be the primary treatment considerations for animal patients with oedema and/or ascites. Paracentesis and diuretics should be reserved for those dogs with respiratory distress and abdominal discomfort. Overzealous use of diuretics may cause dehydration and acute renal decompensation. Plasma transfusions will provide only temporary benefit. In the past, dietary protein supplementation has been recommended to offset the effects of proteinuria and reduce oedema and ascites; however, recent studies in proteinuric heterozygous bitches with X-linked nephropathy suggest that reduced dietary protein is associated with reduced proteinuria (Burkholder *et al.*, 2004). n-3 fatty acid supplementation may also be beneficial: in dogs with surgically reduced remnant kidneys, dietary supplementation with fish oil reduced proteinuria, intraglomerular pressure and glomerular lesions, and maintained glomerular filtration rate (Brown *et al.*, 1998).

Prognosis

The prognosis for dogs with GN is variable and best based on a combination of the severity of dysfunction (i.e. the magnitude of proteinuria and presence or absence of azotaemia), the response to therapy and the assessment of renal histology. Clinical experience suggests the disease is progressive in many cases. Well controlled, prospective clinical trials evaluating the efficacy of additional treatment regimens (e.g. aldosterone receptor antagonists and angiotensin receptor blockers, as well as immunosuppressive treatment of specific histological subtypes of GN) will undoubtedly provide valuable information and increase our ability to treat this disease. A major factor confounding interpretation of studies designed to assess the efficacy of treatment of GN is the variable biological behaviour of different types of GN. In human patients, for example, proliferative and membranoproliferative GN have a poor prognosis compared with that of membranous GN (Bohle *et al.*, 1992). Until results of such trials become available, if an underlying disease process cannot be identified and corrected, ACE inhibitors, moderately protein reduced diets and low-dose aspirin are recommended.

References and further reading

Alfrey AC, Froment DH and Hammond WS (1989) Role of iron in tubulointerstitial injury in nephrotoxic serum nephritis. *Kidney International* **36**, 753–759
Benigni A, Zoja C and Remuzzi G (1995) Biology of disease: the renal toxicity of sustained glomerular protein traffic. *Laboratory Investigation* **73**, 461–468
Bertani T, Cutillo F, Zoja C, Broggini M and Remuzzi G (1986) Tubulointerstitial lesions mediate renal damage in adriamycin glomerulopathy. *Kidney International* **30**, 488–496

Bohle A, Wehrmann M, Bogenschutz O et al. (1992) The long-term prognosis of the primary glomerulonephritides. *Pathology, Research and Practice* **188**, 908–924

Brenner BM, Meyer TW and Hostetter TH (1982) Dietary protein intake and the progressive nature of kidney disease: The role of hemodynamically mediated glomerular injury in the pathogenesis of progressive glomerular sclerosis in aging, renal ablation, and intrinsic renal disease. *New England Journal of Medicine* **307**, 652–659

Brown EA, Markandu ND, Roulston IE et al. (1982) Is the renin-angiotensin-aldosterone system involved in the sodium retention in the nephrotic syndrome? *Nephron* **32**, 102–107

Brown SA, Brown CA, Crowell WA et al. (1998) Beneficial effects of chronic administration of dietary n-3 polyunsaturated fatty acids in dogs with renal insufficiency. *Journal of Laboratory and Clinical Medicine* **131**, 447–455

Brown SA, Walton CL, Crawford P and Bakris GL (1993) Long-term effects of antihypertensive regimens on renal hemodynamics and proteinuria. *Kidney International* **43**, 1210–1218

Burkholder WJ, Lees GE, LeBlanc AK et al. (2004) Diet modulates proteinuria in heterozygous female dogs with x-linked hereditary nephropathy. *Journal of Veterinary Internal Medicine* **18**, 165–175

Camussi G (1994) Alternative pathway activation of complement by cultured human proximal tubular epithelial cells. *Kidney International* **45**, 451–460

Center SA, Smith CA, Wilkinson E, Erb HN and Lewis RM (1987) Clinicopathologic, renal immunofluorescent, and light microscopic features of GN in the dog: 41 cases (1975–1985). *Journal of the American Veterinary Medical Association* **190**, 81–90

Clark WF, Friesen M, Linton AL and Lindsay RM (1976) The platelet as a mediator of tissue damage in immune complex GN. *Clinical Nephrology* **6**, 287–289

Cook AK and Cowgill LD (1996) Clinical and pathologic features of protein-losing glomerular disease in the dog: A review of 137 cases. *Journal of the American Animal Hospital Association* **32**, 313–322

Cowgill LD (1991) Clinical significance, diagnosis and management of systemic hypertension in dogs and cats. In: *Managing Renal Disease and Hypertension*, pp. 35–44. Hill's Pet Products and Harmon Smith Inc.

DiBartola SP, Spaulding GL, Chew DJ and Lewis RM (1980) Urinary protein excretion and immunopathologic findings in dogs with glomerular disease. *Journal of the American Veterinary Medical Association* **177**, 73–77

Epstein M (2001) Aldosterone as a mediator of progressive renal disease: pathogenic and clinical implications. *American Journal of Kidney Disease* **37**, 677–688

Grauer GF (1991) Glomerular disease and proteinuria. In: *Small Animal Medicine*, ed. DG Allen, pp. 615–623. Lippincott, Philadelphia

Grauer GF (2005) Canine glomerulonephritis: new thoughts on proteinuria and treatment. *Journal of Small Animal Practice* **46**, 469–478

Grauer GF, Culham CA, Dubielzig RR, Longhofer SL and Grieve RB (1989) Experimental *Dirofilaria immitis*-associated GN induced in part by in situ formation of immune complexes in the glomerular capillary wall. *Journal of Parasitology* **75**, 585–593

Grauer GF, Frisbie DD, Longhofer SL and Cooley AJ (1992a) Effects of a thromboxane synthetase inhibitor on established immune complex GN in dogs. *American Journal of Veterinary Research* **53**, 808–813

Grauer GF, Greco DS, Getzy DM et al. (2000) Effects of enalapril vs placebo as a treatment for canine idiopathic glomerulonephritis. *Journal of Veterinary Internal Medicine* **14**, 526–533

Grauer GF, Rose BJ, Toolan L, Thrall MA and Colgan SP (1992b) Comparison of the effects of low-dose aspirin and specific thromboxane synthetase inhibition on whole blood platelet aggregation ATP secretion in healthy dogs. *American Journal of Veterinary Research* **53**, 1631–1635

Green RA and Kabel AL (1982) Hypercoagulable state in three dogs with nephrotic syndrome: role of acquired antithrombin III deficiency. *Journal of the American Veterinary Medical Association* **181**, 914–917

Green RA, Russo EA, Greene RT and Kabel AL (1985) Hypoalbuminemia-related platelet hypersensitivity in two dogs with nephrotic syndrome. *Journal of the American Veterinary Medical Association* **186**, 485–488

Grodecki KM, Gains MJ, Baumal R et al. (1997) Treatment of X-linked hereditary nephritis in Samoyed dogs with angiotensin converting enzyme (ACE) inhibitor. *Journal of Comparative Pathology* **117**, 209–225

Harris KP, Burton C and Walls J (1996) Proteinuria: a mediator of interstitial fibrosis? *Contributions to Nephrology* **118**, 173–179

Hayslett IP (1984) Role of platelets in GN. *New England Journal of Medicine* **310**, 1457–1458

Hilgers KF and Mann JFE (1996) Role of angiotensin II in glomerular injury: lessons from experimental and clinical studies. *Kidney and Blood Pressure Research* **19**, 254–262

Jacob F, Polzin DJ, Osborne CA et al. (2005) Evaluation of the association between initial proteinuria and morbidity rate or death in dogs with naturally occurring chronic renal failure. *Journal of the American Veterinary Medical Association* **226**, 393–400

Jaenke RS and Allen TA (1986) Membranous nephropathy in the dog. *Veterinary Pathology* **23**, 718–733

Jeraj K, Osborne CA and Stevens JB (1982) Evaluation of renal biopsy in 197 dogs and cats. *Journal of the American Veterinary Medical Association* **181**, 367–369

Jerums G, Panagiotopoulos S, Tsalamandris C et al. (1997) Why is proteinuria such an important risk factor for progression in clinical trials? *Kidney International* **52**, S87–S92

Johnson RJ (1997) Cytokines, growth factors and renal injury: Where do we go now? *Kidney International* **52**, S2–S6

Keilani T, Schlueter WA, Levin ML and Batlle DC (1993) Improvement of lipid abnormalities associated with proteinuria using fosinopril, an angiotensin-converting enzyme inhibitor. *Annals of Internal Medicine* **118**, 246–254

Lees GE, Brown SA, Elliott J et al. (2005) Assessment and management of proteinuria in dogs and cats; 2004 ACVIM Forum Consensus Statement (Small Animal). *Journal of Veterinary Internal Medicine* **19**, 377–385

Lees GE, Willard MD and Dziezuc J (2002) Glomerular proteinuria is rapidly but reversibly increased by short-term prednisone administration in heterozygous (carrier) female dogs with X-linked hereditary nephropathy (abstract). *Journal of Veterinary Internal Medicine* **16**, 352

Longhofer SL, Frisbie DD, Johnson HC et al. (1991) Effects of a thromboxane synthetase inhibitor on immune complex GN. *American Journal of Veterinary Research* **52**, 480–487

MacDougall DF, Cook T, Steward AP and Cattell V (1986) Canine chronic renal disease: prevalence and types of GN in the dog. *Kidney International* **29**, 1144–1151

Mathews KA, Holmberg DL and Miller CW (2000) Kidney transplantation in dogs with naturally occurring end-stage renal disease. *Journal of the American Animal Hospital Association* **36**, 294–301

Muller-Peddinghaus R and Trautwein G (1977) Spontaneous GN in dogs 1. Classification and Immunopathology. *Veterinary Pathology* **14**, 1–13

Olbricht CJ, Cannon JK, Garg LC and Tisher CC (1986) Activities of cathepsin B and L in isolated nephron segments from proteinuric and nonproteinuric rats. *American Journal of Physiology* **250**, F1055–F1062

Ong A and Moorhead J (1994) Tubular lipidosis: epiphenomenon or pathogenetic lesion in human renal disease. *Kidney International* **45**, 753–762

Reddi AS, Ramamurthi R, Miller M, Dhuper S and Lasker N (1991) Enalapril improves albuminuria by preventing glomerular loss of heparan sulfate in diabetic rats. *Biochemical Medicine and Metabolic Biology* **45**, 119–131

Remuzzi G (1995) Abnormal protein traffic through the glomerular barrier induces proximal tubular cell dysfunction and causes renal injury. *Current Opinion in Nephrology and Hypertension* **4**, 339–342

Rouse BT and Lewis RJ (1975) Canine glomerulonephritis: prevalence in dogs submitted at random for euthanasia. *Canadian Journal of Comparative Medicine* **39**, 365–370

Tang S, Sheerin NS, Zhou W, Brown Z and Sacks SH (1999) Apical proteins stimulate complement synthesis by cultured human proximal tubular epithelial cells. *Journal of the American Society of Nephrology* **10**, 69–76

Vaden SL, Breitschwerdt EB, Armstrong PJ et al. (1995) The effects of cyclosporin versus standard care in dogs with naturally occurring glomerulonephritis. *Journal of Veterinary Internal Medicine* **9**, 259–266

Wheeler DC, Varghese Z and Moorhead IF (1989) Hyperlipidemia in nephrotic syndrome. *American Journal of Nephrology* **9**, S78–S84

Wiegmann TB, Herron KG, Chonko AM, MacDougall ML and Moore WV (1992) Effects of angiotensin-converting enzyme inhibition on renal function and albuminuria in normotensive type I diabetic patients. *Diabetes* **41**, 62–67

20

Management of prostatic diseases

Jeanne A. Barsanti

Introduction

Both dogs and cats develop prostatic disease, but prevalence is much higher in dogs. This relates to the development of prostatic hyperplasia in dogs but not in cats. It may also relate to a greater susceptibility to bacterial infections of the genitourinary tract in dogs. This chapter focuses on prostatic diseases in dogs, but will mention cats when information is available.

Anatomy and physiology

The canine prostate gland

The prostate gland is the only accessory sex gland in the male dog. It is bilobed with a median septum on the dorsal surface (Figure 20.1a). The prostate encircles the proximal urethra at the neck of the bladder and its ducts enter the urethra throughout its circumference. The position of the prostate depends upon age, bladder distension and disease state. The prostate gland is sterile.

The purpose of the prostate gland is to produce prostatic fluid as a transport and support medium for sperm during ejaculation. Basal secretion of small amounts of prostatic fluid (<1 ml/hr) constantly enters the prostatic excretory ducts and prostatic urethra.

When neither micturition nor ejaculation is occurring, urethral pressure moves this basally secreted fluid cranially into the bladder.

The prostate gland requires the presence of testosterone to grow and maintain its size. If a dog is castrated prior to sexual maturity, normal prostatic growth is inhibited. If the dog is castrated as an adult, the prostate will involute to approximately 20% of its normal adult size.

The feline prostate gland

The feline prostate gland is also bilobed, but covers the urethra only dorsally and laterally (Figure 20.1b). Some prostatic tissue is disseminated within the urethral wall caudal to the prostate gland.

Diagnostic techniques

Diagnostic techniques for prostatic disease (Figure 20.2) include:

- History
- Physical examination with rectal palpation
- Urinalysis
- Cytological examination of any urethral discharge

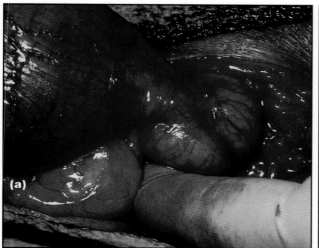

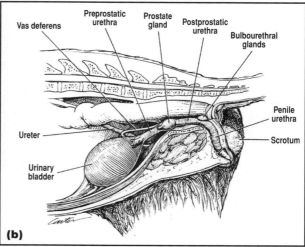

20.1 **(a)** A normal canine prostate gland viewed at surgery. The bladder has been brought out of the incision and flipped caudally, revealing the dorsal surface of the prostate gland with its medial groove and bilobed nature.
(b) The relationship of the prostate gland to other structures in the caudal abdomen of the male cat. Note that the prostate gland is more caudal to the neck of the bladder than in the dog. (Reproduced from Barsanti JA and Finco DR (1995) with permission from Elsevier.)

Disease	History	Physical examination	Urinalysis	CBC	Biochemical profile	Radiology	Ultrasonography	Prostatic fluid
Benign hyperplasia	Asymptomatic, haematuria, haemorrhagic urethral discharge, tenesmus	Symmetrical, non-painful, mild to moderate prostatomegaly	Normal or haematuria	Normal	Normal	Mild to moderate prostatomegaly	Uniformly hyperechoic, often with cysts	Normal or haemorrhagic
Squamous metaplasia	Tenesmus, dysuria	Moderate prostatomegaly, feminization, abnormal testicles	Secondary infection possible	Oestrogen toxicity possible	Normal unless abscessation also present	Prostatomegaly	Cysts or abscesses possible	Inflammation, squamous cells
Paraprostatic cysts	Tenesmus, dysuria	Large mass, abdominal or perineal	Normal	Normal	Normal	Large mass	Large, hypoechoic mass	Yellow to haemorrhagic
Acute prostatitis	Lethargy, anorexia	Fever, depression, prostatic pain	Infection	Inflammatory leucogram	Normal	Indistinct cranial prostatic border in some cases	Focal, multifocal or diffuse hyperechogenicity	Not usually collected
Chronic prostatitis	Normal to mild lethargy, infertility possible, recurrent urinary tract infection	Normal	Infection	Normal	Normal	Normal or mild granular prostatic mineralization	Focal, multifocal or diffuse hyperechogenicity	Inflammatory, infection
Abscessation	Lethargy, anorexia, tenesmus, dysuria	Moderate to marked asymmetrical prostatomegaly, fever, septic shock possible	Infection	Inflammatory leucogram	Hypoglycaemia, hypoalbuminaemia, hyperbilirubinaemia and increased alkaline phosphatase possible	Irregular, moderate to marked prostatomegaly	Assymetrical, hyperechoic with hypoechoic cavities	Inflammatory, infection
Neoplasia	Tenesmus, dysuria, occasionally hindlimb stiffness, partial anorexia, lethargy	Asymmetrical prostatomegaly, firm, not movable, fever possible	Haematuria, pyuria occasionally	Normal to mild, non-regenerative anaemia, mild leucocytosis occasionally	Increased serum alkaline phosphatase in some cases, azotaemia if obstruction	Asymmetrical prostatomegaly, granular mineralization possible, bone lesions	Asymmetrical, heterogenous hyperechogenicity	Abnormal epithelial cells, haemorrhage, inflammation possible

20.2 Expected clinical findings in dogs with prostatic diseases.

- Complete blood count (CBC) and serum biochemical profile
- Cytological and microbiological examination of prostatic fluid
- Radiography
- Ultrasonography
- Aspiration or biopsy.

The minimum database for any dog suspected of having prostatic disease includes history, physical examination, including rectal palpation of the prostate gland, and urinalysis. Other tests are added as the severity of the clinical problems dictates.

History

A complete history should be obtained including the chief complaint and a review of the dog's overall health status. It should be established whether urination and defecation are normal.

Physical examination

The prostate is best examined with a two-handed approach, using digital rectal palpation and caudal abdominal palpation (Figure 20.3). The prostate should be evaluated for size, symmetry, surface contour, consistency, pain and whether it is fixed or movable. The normal prostate gland is smooth, symmetrical, non-painful on palpation and movable. The normal gland does not compromise the rectal canal or push the bladder cranially. If an increase in size is suspected, estimated measurements should be recorded so that progression can be followed.

The physical examination may uncover related abnormalities in other systems, such as icterus in some cases of abscessation, heart murmurs associated with bacteraemia, or an abnormal gait associated with prostatic pain or spinal metastasis from neoplasia.

Urinalysis/urine culture

Finding haematuria, pyuria and/or bacteriuria in urinalysis from an intact male dog should always prompt consideration of prostatic disease. Urine culture from a sample collected by cystocentesis is indicated in cases of suspected prostatic infection.

Complete blood count/serum biochemical profile

A CBC and biochemical profile are indicated in cases with systemic signs of illness. Because many dogs with prostatic disease are old, the biochemical profile is important in screening for occult diseases of aged animals. There are currently no serum tests specifically for prostatic disease in dogs.

Evaluation of prostatic fluid

If a clinically significant prostatic disease is suspected to be present in a dog, evaluation of prostatic fluid is indicated to determine whether and what type of prostatic disease exists.

Urethral discharge

A urethral discharge must be distinguished from a preputial discharge by physical examination. In addition to prostatic diseases, urinary incontinence and urethral diseases must be considered as potential causes of a urethral discharge.

Any urethral discharge should be collected for microscopic examination (Figure 20.4). A urethral discharge is generally not cultured for bacteria because of potential contamination by the normal resident bacterial flora of the distal urethra and prepuce. Occasionally a urethral discharge of prostatic origin will increase with prostatic palpation.

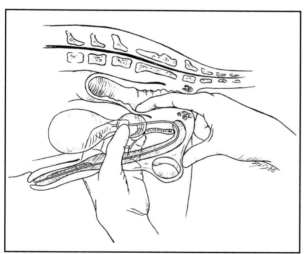

20.3 Rectal palpation of the prostate gland in male dogs. One hand should apply pressure on the caudal abdomen while the other palpates rectally. The prostate gland, when abdominal, can be palpated in the caudal abdomen as well as per rectum. The hand palpating the caudal abdomen can both evaluate the cranial aspects of the gland and push the prostate into or near the pelvic canal for better palpation per rectum. (Reproduced from Barsanti JA (1992) with permission.)

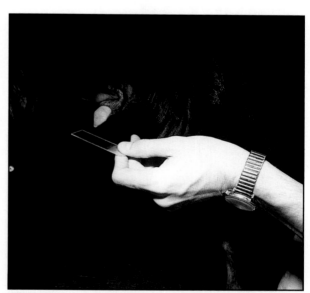

20.4 Collection of a discharge from the urethral orifice for examination. Note that the prepuce has been retracted and any preputial discharge gently removed before collection. The sample is allowed to drip on to the slide. If a larger volume is present, it can be collected into a larger, clean container. (Reproduced from Barsanti JA and Finco DR (1995) with permission from Elsevier.)

Semen evaluation

In intact male dogs, an ejaculate is valuable in assessing prostatic disease since prostatic fluid comprises more than 95% of semen volume. In dogs, semen is composed of three fractions, of which the first and third fractions originate in the prostate gland (Figure 20.5). For diagnostic purposes, 2–3 ml of the third fraction should be collected (Figure 20.6). Both cytology and culture must be assessed for accurate interpretation. Quantitative culture is essential, since the distal urethra has a normal bacterial flora.

In some dogs with prostatic disease, the entire ejaculate appears to be abnormal (Figure 20.7). In these cases, testicular or epididymal diseases are possible causes of the abnormal semen.

Prostatic fluid from an ejaculate from a normal dog has occasional white blood cells. A few squamous cells

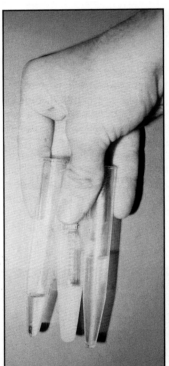

20.5 The three fractions of the normal canine ejaculate. The first fraction is clear and small in volume (0.1–2 ml). The second fraction is white and cloudy due to the large number of sperm. The volume of the second fraction is 0.1–4 ml. Both the first and second fractions are ejaculated over the first 1–3 minutes. The third fraction of the ejaculate, following the sperm-rich fraction, is normally clear, 1–16 ml in volume, and released over 3–35 minutes. The third fraction is the easiest to collect cleanly, as it drips from the urethral orifice after the dog completes any thrusting motion. (Reproduced from Barsanti JA and Finco DR (1995) with permission from Elsevier.)

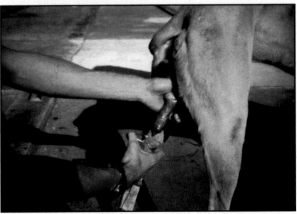

20.6 Collection of a semen sample to evaluate a dog for prostatic disease. Note that the dog has stepped over the collector's arm and is in the 'tie' position, during which the majority of prostatic fluid is expelled.

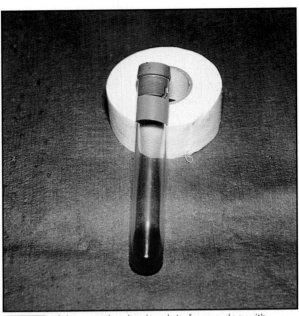

20.7 A haemorrhagic ejaculate from a dog with benign prostatic hyperplasia.

may also be found. Contaminating bacteria may be free or within squamous cells. The pH of normal canine semen is 6.0–6.7. Significant findings include:

- Large numbers of white blood cells indicate inflammation
- Large numbers of red blood cells indicate haemorrhage
- Macrophages containing haemosiderin indicate chronic haemorrhage
- Bacteria, especially if within white blood cells or macrophages, suggest infection.

Bacteria can be cultured from normal ejaculates due to contamination with urethral organisms. Contaminant bacteria usually number fewer than 100,000/ml and are usually Gram-positive. Culturing more than one species of bacteria also suggests contamination. High numbers (>100,000/ml) of Gram-negative organisms with large numbers of white blood cells indicate infection. High numbers of Gram-positive organisms with large numbers of white blood cells also indicate infection if preputial contamination did not occur. Lower numbers of Gram-negative or Gram-positive organisms must be correlated with clinical signs, results of urinalysis and urine culture and ejaculate cytology to determine significance.

Prostatic massage

In cases of suspected prostatic neoplasia with involvement of the prostatic urethra, prostatic massage specimens are more likely to contain abnormal cells than ejaculates. With the increased use of ultrasonography, direct aspiration of prostatic cysts and abnormal prostatic tissue has largely replaced prostatic massage. However, the prostatic massage/catheter biopsy technique is useful in dogs with suspected prostatic neoplasia involving the urethra.

Radiography

Survey radiography (see Chapter 10) is of limited benefit in the diagnosis of specific prostatic diseases. In many cases the prostate can be palpated more accurately than it can be visualized on survey radiographs. However, helpful findings include the following:

- Poor contrast of caudal abdominal structures may exist with abscessation, carcinoma and paraprostatic cysts
- Asymmetrical shape is noted with abscess, neoplasia and cysts
- Granular mineralization can be seen with inflammation or neoplasia
- Marked prostatic enlargement is most often associated with abscess, cysts and neoplasia.

If prostatic neoplasia is a likely possibility, thoracic and abdominal radiographs should be examined for evidence of metastasis.

Distension retrograde urethrocystography is the contrast study of choice for prostatic disease when the dog is dysuric. A narrowed prostatic urethra can be noted with neoplasia, abscessation, large parenchymal cysts and, rarely, with hyperplasia. If the prostatic urethra is markedly irregular, neoplasia is most likely. If the prostate is markedly asymmetrical in relation to the urethra, abscessation, parenchymal cysts or neoplasia are most likely.

Ultrasonography

Ultrasonography (see Chapter 10) provides more information about prostatic structure than radiography does, but is less sensitive in imaging the prostatic urethra. The normal prostate is uniformly hyperechoic compared to surrounding structures, with a small hypoechoic area in the centre, which is the urethra. There is considerable overlap in ultrasonographic appearance with different prostatic diseases (see Figure 20.2 and Chapter 10). Doppler ultrasonography could not differentiate a normal prostate from one with inflammation in asymptomatic dogs (Newell *et al.*, 1998). Nevertheless, some ultrasonographic patterns are more typical of some diseases than others:

- A focal, multifocal or diffuse hyperechogenicity is associated with prostatic inflammation
- Neoplasia tends to produce a complex combination of hyperechoic and hypoechoic areas with some unaffected parenchyma
- With abscess formation, the prostate gland is usually hyperechoic with parenchymal hypoechoic cavities with irregular outlines and asymmetrical shapes. The cavitary areas exhibit distal enhancement, but abscesses cannot be distinguished from uninfected prostatic cysts, cavitary neoplasias or haematomas.

The sublumbar lymph nodes should be evaluated as enlargement and/or change in echogenicity may be seen with prostatic infection or neoplasia.

Urethroscopy

The prostatic urethra can be visualized via urethroscopy in male dogs over 12 kg in weight, using flexible endoscopic equipment (Threlfall and Chew, 1999). It may be possible to verify that an exudate or haemorrhage is entering the prostatic urethra and to exclude non-prostatic urethral lesions as a cause for a urethral discharge.

Prostatic aspiration

Aspiration can be used to collect fluid from intraprostatic cavitary lesions or to collect cells for cytology. Needle aspiration is usually performed by the transabdominal route under ultrasound guidance. Needle aspiration is generally avoided in dogs with suspected abscessation, since bacteraemia or localized peritonitis may develop. If an abscess is aspirated, intravenous antibiotics should be started immediately and continued for at least 24 hours, followed by oral antimicrobial therapy. Other than the inadvertent penetration of abscesses, complications of aspiration are rare. Occasionally, mild transient haematuria, lasting less than 4 days, has been noted.

If prostatic fluid is obtained by aspiration, it should be examined microscopically and cultured for aerobic bacteria. Culture for anaerobic bacteria should also be considered in cases of abscessation. Cytological examination should include evaluation for haemorrhage, purulence or neoplasia. One must be cautious in diagnosing neoplasia from cytology alone, as normal epithelial cells vary in appearance. It must be remembered that fine needle aspirates provide a very small sample, so a negative aspirate does not rule out neoplasia.

Prostatic biopsy

Percutaneous prostatic biopsy

Percutaneous prostatic biopsy is usually performed transabdominally under ultrasound guidance with sedation. An automatic spring-loaded biopsy device with a 14–18 gauge needle makes the procedure easier. Abscessation is a contraindication to a percutaneous biopsy. Parenchymal cystic lesions, identifiable by ultrasonography, should be aspirated rather than have biopsy samples taken. Dogs should be observed closely for several hours after biopsy to detect any complications. The most common complication is mild haematuria, although significant haemorrhage is possible. Orchitis and scrotal oedema were reported in one dog.

Ultrasound-guided aspiration and/or biopsy of the prostate resulted in an accurate diagnosis in 14 of 17 cases (82%) in one survey (Barr, 1995). One difficulty with diagnosis by aspiration or biopsy is that the prostate may be affected by more than one disease process. This possibility necessitates that all the data about a clinical case be evaluated. A diagnosis must be reconsidered if response to therapy is not as predicted.

Surgical prostatic biopsy

Prostatic biopsies can be performed surgically, with a biopsy needle or by resection of a wedge of prostatic parenchyma. Cystic or potentially abscessed areas should be aspirated before performing a biopsy. Multiple sites can be sampled, depending on visual and palpable abnormalities detected. The sublumbar lymph nodes should also be sampled. Potential complications of a surgical biopsy include haemorrhage, dissemination of infection or neoplasia and trauma to the urethra. If the urethra is in the area of the wedge biopsy, a urethral catheter should be passed into the prostatic urethra prior to biopsy, so that the location of the urethra can be precisely determined and avoided.

Prostatic diseases

Diseases discussed include benign hyperplasia, squamous metaplasia, paraprostatic cysts, infection and neoplasia. Prostatic pain with a stilted gait has been noted in dogs exposed to, but unable to breed, a bitch in oestrus. This has been attributed to vascular engorgement. This condition is rarely described in the literature, either because it is uncommon or because it resolves within 24 hours without intervention.

Benign hyperplasia/cystic hyperplasia

Pathophysiology
Prostatic hyperplasia is the most common canine prostatic disease, with almost 100% of intact dogs developing histological evidence of prostatic hyperplasia with aging. Benign prostatic hyperplasia is an increase in epithelial cell number (hyperplasia) as well as epithelial cell size (hypertrophy), but the increase in number is more marked. Hyperplasia and hypertrophy usually lead to a symmetrical increase in prostatic size. The vascularity of the prostate is increased with hyperplasia and the gland has a tendency to bleed (Figure 20.8).

Hyperplasia is associated with an altered androgen:oestrogen ratio, and requires the presence of the testes. Dihydrotestosterone within the gland serves as the main hormonal mediator. The condition begins as glandular hyperplasia as early as 2.5 years of age. Intraparenchymal fluid cysts may develop in association with hyperplasia. The tendency to cystic hyperplasia begins after 4 years of age. Intra-

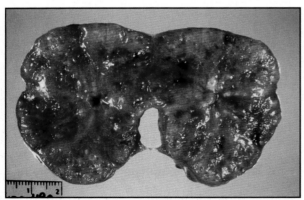

20.8 A prostate gland with cystic hyperplasia; note the multifocal cystic areas and the mildly irregular 'cobblestone' contour. (Courtesy of Drs WA Crowell and LA Cowan; reproduced from Barsanti JA (1992) with permission.)

parenchymal cysts may communicate with the urethra via the prostatic ducts. The cysts vary in size and contain a thin, clear, colourless to amber fluid. Asymptomatic intraprostatic cysts were found by ultrasonography in 14% of a population of intact male dogs over 3 years of age (Black *et al.*, 1998).

Clinical findings
Most affected dogs are asymptomatic. Common signs in symptomatic animals are a haemorrhagic/sanguineous urethral discharge, haematuria, haematospermia and/or difficult defecation in an otherwise normal dog (see Figures 20.2 and 20.7). Dysuria and lethargy are reported (Root-Kustritz and Merkel, 1998), but rarely. On rectal palpation, the prostate gland is non-painful, symmetrically enlarged and movable, with a variable consistency (normal to mildly irregular). Rarely, the prostate is asymmetrical (Gilson *et al.*, 1992; Root-Kustritz and Merkel, 1998). On ultrasonography, the prostate may be diffusely hyperechoic with parenchymal cavities (Figure 20.9). The cavitary areas are typically well defined and smoothly marginated. In one study, 4 of 12 dogs with asymptomatic intraprostatic cysts detected by ultrasonography had an asymptomatic urinary tract infection; culture of prostatic cyst fluid from these dogs revealed the same organism as that causing the urinary tract infection. Thus, a culture of urine is indicated in all dogs with intraprostatic cysts.

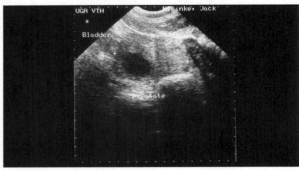

20.9 A transabdominal ultrasound image from an intact male dog with benign prostatic hyperplasia. Note the general, mild hyperechogenicity and the hypoechoic cavitary area.

Diagnosis
Definitive diagnosis is by biopsy, but a definitive diagnosis is not needed if the clinical findings are typical. A positive response to castration confirms the diagnosis. Prostatic hyperplasia accompanies most other prostatic diseases in older, intact male dogs. It may be difficult to distinguish prostatic hyperplasia from early neoplasia and from chronic infection on the basis of history and physical examination alone. Prostatic neoplasia, however, does not respond to castration. Chronic prostatic infection results in urinary tract infection and inflammatory prostatic fluid.

Treatment
Treatment is only required if abnormal signs are present.

Castration: The most effective treatment is castration, which will result in a 75% decrease in prostate size over

8–9 weeks. Involution begins within days, with a 50% reduction in size in 3 weeks. Prostatic secretion becomes minimal at 7–16 days after castration. There is no medical therapy as effective as castration.

Oestrogen: Oestrogens cause prostatic atrophy by reducing androgen concentrations by depressing gonadotropin secretion from the pituitary gland. Short courses of therapy decrease prostatic secretory capability for months. Effective doses of oestrogen have not been determined and various protocols have been used.

Oestrogen toxicity can be fatal and occurs due to overdosage, repeated administration or, more rarely, idiosyncratically. Toxicity is characterized by an initial leucocytosis with a left shift, followed by severe bone marrow depression with resultant anaemia, thrombocytopenia and leucopenia. Repeated administration can cause growth of the fibromuscular stroma of the prostate, metaplasia of prostatic glandular epithelium and secretory stasis.

Anti-androgens: Flutamide is an orally administered non-steroidal anti-androgen that competitively binds to dihydrotestosterone receptors in the prostate gland. Flutamide causes a significant decrease in prostatic size in dogs within 10 days. When administered to research dogs at 5 mg/kg/day orally for 1 year, there was no change in libido or sperm production. Hyperplasia recurred within 2 months of discontinuing the drug.

Finasteride is a 5-alpha-reductase inhibitor (the final enzyme in the synthetic pathway for dihydrotestosterone). Doses of 0.1–0.5 mg/kg/day caused as much suppression of serum dihydrotestosterone concentrations as higher doses and decreased prostatic volume approximately 40% after 8 weeks (Sirinarumitr et al., 2001). There was a decrease in semen volume but no adverse effect on semen quality, libido or fertility. Clinical signs of prostatic hyperplasia resolved within 4 weeks in most dogs. This drug can cause anomalies in male fetuses when it reaches the uterus at 3 months of gestation, presenting a risk to pregnant women. Finasteride is present in semen, urine and faeces of treated dogs. The tablets are coated to prevent contact with finasteride when handling the tablets, but this protection is lost if the tablets are crushed or broken.

Megestrol reduces serum testosterone concentrations, competitively inhibits dihydrotestosterone binding to its receptors, decreases dihydrotestosterone concentrations and decreases the number of prostatic androgen receptors. Megestrol acetate at a dose of 0.55 mg/kg/day orally for 4 weeks resulted in resolution of clinical signs of hyperplasia with no decrease in sperm production. Medroxyprogesterone acetate has been used subcutaneously at 3 mg/kg. Sixteen of 19 dogs responded and most remained symptom free for 10 months, after which time relapse was common. Diabetes mellitus developed in one of the 19 treated dogs. In the UK an injectable product containing delmadinone acetate is authorized for treatment of this condition; recommended dose is 1–2 mg/kg by intra-

muscular or subcutaneous injection. In animals that respond, the recommendation is to repeat the dose every 3–4 weeks.

Herbs: Products containing extracts of the saw palmetto plant, *Serenoa repens*, are available over the counter for prostatic hyperplasia in men. The author was unable to document any beneficial or harmful effects (Barsanti et al., 2000).

Patient monitoring

- If the dog is asymptomatic, the owner is advised to watch for typical clinical signs.
- If the dog is neutered, the dog's prostate gland should be palpated 2–3 weeks postoperatively to be sure it is involuting as expected. If it is not, a more serious prostatic disease may be present.
- If medical therapy is chosen, the dog is monitored for changes in prostatic size and for development of adverse effects, according to the drug chosen.

Squamous metaplasia

Pathophysiology

Squamous metaplasia refers to a change in the appearance of prostatic epithelium secondary to exogenous or endogenous hyperoestrogenism. The major endogenous cause is a functional Sertoli cell tumour. Oestrogens also cause secretory stasis. The epithelial change and secretory stasis predispose to cyst formation, infection and abscessation.

Clinical findings

With endogenous hyperoestrogenism, the testicles may be palpably abnormal with one testicle enlarged and the other atrophied. With exogenous hyperoestrogenism, both testicles atrophy. Other physical signs of hyperoestrogenism, including alopecia, hyperpigmentation, gynaecomastia and pendulous prepuce, may be present (see Figure 20.2). The prostate is enlarged to a variable degree. Haematology may reflect oestrogen toxicity. Squamous cells may be numerous in an ejaculate (Figure 20.10). Ultrasonography may identify filling defects within the prostate gland (cysts or abscesses). If retrograde urethrography is performed,

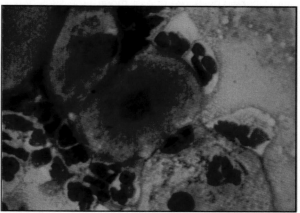

20.10 Squamous cells in the prostatic fluid of a dog with squamous metaplasia of the prostate gland.

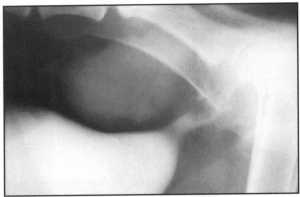

20.11 Retrograde urethrogram in a dog with prostatomegaly, cryptorchidism and gynaecomastia. The colliculus seminalis is evident as a filling defect in the urethra. A Sertoli cell tumour of the testicle and squamous metaplasia of the prostate were identified in tissue specimens removed surgically.

reflux of contrast material into cavities within the prostate gland and a persistent radiolucent filling defect in the prostatic urethra (enlarged colliculus seminalis) may be observed (Figure 20.11).

Diagnosis
Definitive diagnosis is by biopsy. Presumptive diagnosis is based on the history of oestrogen therapy or the finding of a Sertoli cell tumour in association with prostatomegaly.

Treatment
Treatment requires castration in endogenous hyperoestrogenism or discontinuation of oestrogen therapy.

Patient monitoring
If the prostate is cystic, but uninfected, patient monitoring should include repeat ultrasonographic imaging approximately 1 month after treatment to ensure that the cysts are resolving. If the prostate is abscessed, the patient should be monitored as described under abscessation.

Paraprostatic cysts

Pathophysiology
Paraprostatic cysts are one or more large sacs of fluid found adjacent to the prostate and attached to it via a stalk (patent or non-patent) or adhesions. Most do not communicate with the urethra. These large cysts may be prostatic in origin or may be remnants of the uterus masculinus. Paraprostatic cysts can have a thin or thick wall with a smooth or calcified lining. Cases of cystic uterus masculinus have been reported in cats. A cyst of apparently prostatic origin has also been reported in a cat.

Clinical findings
Clinical signs are related to cyst size, with encroachment on the urethra or colon resulting in dysuria or tenesmus (see Figure 20.2). Urinary incontinence has also been noted, associated with bladder overdistension due to partial urethral obstruction. If the cyst is sufficiently large, abdominal distension may be seen (Figure 20.12a).

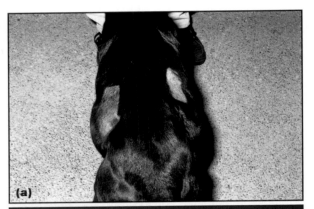

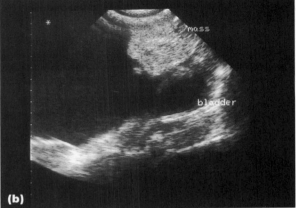

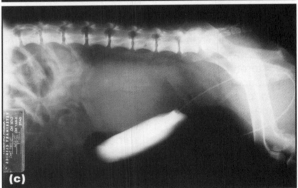

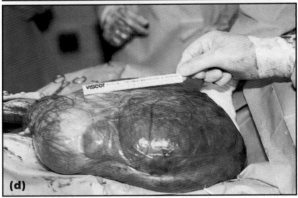

20.12 **(a)** Dog with abdominal distension due to a large paraprostatic cyst. Abdominal distension was the presenting complaint. **(b)** Ultrasound image of the large paraprostatic cyst. The ultrasound image was made with the dog standing. **(c)** Positive contrast cystogram showing a paraprostatic cyst as the large structure dorsal to the bladder. **(d)** The large paraprostatic cyst at surgery.

Alternatively, the cyst may extend into the perineal region. The cysts may be palpable in the caudal abdomen or perineal area; if calcified, they feel firm.

Urinalysis is usually normal, although haematuria is possible if haemorrhage occurs into the cyst and the cyst communicates with the urethra. Urinary tract infections are sometimes present, especially with infected cysts. Haematological findings are usually normal, but a neutrophilic leucocytosis was noted in about 30% of cases in one series.

Fluid can be aspirated under ultrasound guidance (Figure 20.12b). Prostatic cyst fluid is usually yellow to serosanguineous to brown. It has low numbers of white blood cells, variable numbers of red blood cells, variable numbers of epithelial cells and is usually sterile. If cyst fluid becomes infected, the cyst may become an abscess.

On survey radiographs, two bladder-like structures may be evident. A cystogram is often necessary to determine which structure is the bladder (Figure 20.12c).

Diagnosis

Exploratory laparotomy with cyst drainage and excisional biopsy is usually indicated for definitive diagnosis and therapy (Figure 20.12d).

Treatment

Treatment is surgical. Castration is recommended. Antibiotic therapy as for a prostatic abscess is indicated if the cyst is infected.

Patient monitoring

The caudal abdomen should be monitored for cyst recurrence with ultrasonography for several months. If the cyst was infected, urinalysis and urine culture should be performed 1 week after discontinuing antibiotic therapy and monthly for 2–3 months to check for recurrence of infection.

Prostatitis: acute, chronic, abscessation

Pathophysiology

Prostatitis is an inflammatory disease of the prostate gland, most commonly associated with bacterial infection. *Escherichia coli* is the most common infectious agent. Prostatitis is the second most common canine prostatic disease to cause clinical signs. Prostatitis may be acute or chronic. Chronic infections are more common. Approximately 42% of parenchymal prostatic cysts developing in dogs with prostatic hyperplasia are infected and the same organism is usually found in the urine (Black *et al.*, 1998). Abscesses develop when the infection is severe and encapsulation of purulent material occurs (Figure 20.13). Prostatic infections are mainly a problem in intact male dogs or dogs neutered after infection develops.

The pathogenesis of prostatic infections is incompletely understood. Most infections are assumed to be secondary to migration of bacteria up the urethra, although spread via blood, urine, semen and rectal flora (via direct extension or lymphatics) is also postulated. The close anatomical relationship between the bladder, proximal urethra and prostate gland is re-

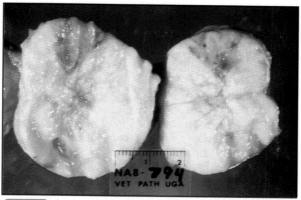

20.13 A prostate gland with multifocal abscessed areas. (Courtesy of Drs WA Crowell and LA Cowan; reproduced from Barsanti JA (1992) with permission.)

flected in the high frequency with which all three are simultaneously infected. Any condition that increases bacterial numbers in the prostatic urethra predisposes to infection. Examples include urethral urolithiasis, neoplasia, trauma or stricture.

Acute bacterial prostatitis and abscess formation may result in septicaemia, which is responsible for the severity of clinical signs in some cases. Chronic prostatitis may be a sequel to acute infection or may develop insidiously. Abscess formation is thought to result from chronic infection and from infection of prostatic cysts.

Clinical findings

Signs associated with acute bacterial prostatitis include fever, depression, anorexia, urethral discharge and pain on prostatic palpation (see Figure 20.2). Vomiting is possible because of localized peritonitis. Less common signs are constipation from avoidance of defecation and a stiff, stilted hindlimb gait (Figure 20.14). The size, symmetry and contour of the prostate gland are normal, unless it is enlarged as a result of hyperplasia.

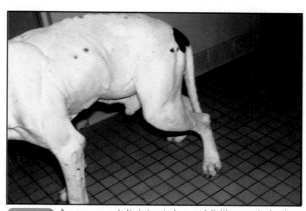

20.14 A young, adult, intact dog exhibiting pain in the hindlimbs by standing up on its toes and squatting slightly. The pain was localized to the prostate gland by rectal palpation. The concurrent presence of fever, leucocytosis and urinary tract infection, with only mild prostatomegaly supported a presumptive diagnosis of acute bacterial prostatitis. (Reproduced from Barsanti JA (1992) with permission.)

Chronic bacterial prostatitis is usually not associated with signs of illness, although some dogs may be more lethargic than normal. A purulent or haemorrhagic urethral discharge may be present. In some dogs, the only indication of chronic bacterial prostatitis is recurrent urinary tract infection or mild haematuria. Chronic prostatitis should be considered in dogs with infertility. The prostate gland is not painful on palpation and infection alone does not affect prostatic size, although there may be some variation in consistency associated with increased fibrous tissue.

The most common signs of prostatic abscessation in dogs are fever and lethargy, associated with caudal abdominal pain. The prostate is often enlarged and asymmetrical, causing tenesmus and constipation. A constant or an intermittent urethral discharge, which is haemorrhagic and/or purulent, may be present. Dysuria can occur as a result of interference with normal urethral function. Chronic partial urethral obstruction can result. About 10% of dogs have signs of septic shock (tachycardia, pale mucous membranes, delayed capillary refill, weak pulse, icterus). Rupture of a prostatic abscess can cause localized or diffuse peritonitis with signs of abdominal pain and vomiting.

In the one reported case of chronic prostatitis with abscessation in a cat, the presenting sign was dys-chezia due to constipation from encroachment on the colon by the enlarged prostate (Roura *et al.*, 2002). There were no signs of systemic disease.

Diagnosis

Associated clinical signs and physical examination findings, in conjunction with CBC, urinalysis and urine culture results, are often sufficient to establish a tentative diagnosis of acute prostatitis. Evaluation of prostatic fluid is usually necessary in cases of chronic prostatitis to localize the site of infection to the prostate gland (Figure 20.15a). Findings on prostatic ultrasonography (Figure 20.15b) in conjunction with signs of systemic illness indicate the presence of an abscess.

Therapy

Acute bacterial prostatitis: An antibiotic based on urine culture results should be administered for 28 days. Because the blood–prostatic fluid barrier is damaged in acute inflammation, a wide choice of antibiotics, similar to that used for urinary tract infection, is acceptable for initial treatment. If the presenting signs are severe, the antimicrobial is initially given intravenously. Supportive therapy should be given as needed. Once the dog's condition is stable, an oral antimicrobial with prostatic penetrance is preferred for the remainder of therapy.

Chronic bacterial prostatitis: Cases of chronic bacterial prostatitis are difficult to treat successfully since the blood–prostatic fluid barrier is intact. This barrier is related to the pH difference between the blood and the prostatic fluid and the characteristics of the prostatic acinar epithelium. A drug's ability to enter prostatic fluid depends upon its lipid solubility, its degree of ionization in plasma (pKa), its molecular size if it is water soluble and its plasma protein-binding characteristics.

The pH of the blood and the prostatic interstitium is 7.4, whereas the pH of normal and infected prostatic fluid in dogs is less than 7.4. Most antimicrobial agents are weak acids or weak bases and ionized to varying degrees in biological fluids. The degree of ionization is determined by the dissociation constant (pKa) of the drug and the pH of the fluid. Since canine prostatic fluid is usually more acidic than plasma and extracellular fluid, basic antibiotics, such as erythromycin, clindamycin and trimethoprim, will enter prostatic fluid becoming ion trapped and so attaining higher concentrations within prostatic fluid than other antibiotics.

Lipid solubility is also an important factor in determining drug movement across the prostatic epithelium. Chloramphenicol, macrolide antibiotics, trimethoprim and fluoroquinolones are examples of lipid-soluble drugs that can cross the barrier effectively. In general, diffusion of tetracyclines into canine prostatic fluid is minimal. Although clinical studies in men with prostatitis demonstrated efficacy of minocycline and doxycycline, these lipid-soluble drugs do not penetrate well into canine prostatic fluid (Baumueller and Madsen, 1977). Drugs with low lipid solubility, such as penicillin, ampicillin, cephalosporin and aminoglycosides, cannot cross into the prostatic acini.

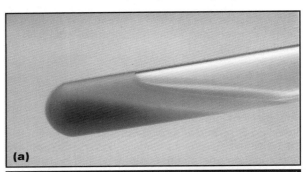

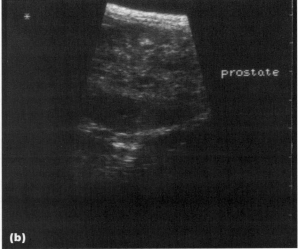

20.15 **(a)** Purulent prostatic fluid collected by ejaculation from a dog with recurrent urinary tract infections associated with chronic prostatitis. (Reproduced from Barsanti JA and Finco DR (1989) with permission from Elsevier.) **(b)** Ultrasonogram of a dog with a prostatic abscess. Note the multiple, varying sized hypoechoic cavities, the largest of which displays posterior shadowing. The overall echogenicity of the gland is quite variable.

Current recommendations for the treatment of chronic bacterial prostatitis are based on whether a Gram-positive or Gram-negative organism is the infective agent:

- If the causative organism is Gram-positive, erythromycin, clindamycin or trimethoprim can be given, depending on the organism's susceptibility
- If the causative organism is Gram-negative, trimethoprim or a quinolone are recommended. Although trimethoprim is often combined with a sulphonamide, sulphonamides do not diffuse into the prostate gland. Fluoroquinolones typically have a small molecular size, high lipid solubility and low protein binding, which makes them useful in chronic prostatic infections.

Because a higher maximum concentration is more important in efficacy than duration of time above the mean inhibitory concentration (MIC) with fluoroquinolones, a higher once daily dose is considered more effective than a lower twice daily dose. Antibiotic therapy should be continued for 6 weeks. If a urinary tract infection is present, urine should be re-evaluated by culture during therapy to be sure that the administered drug eliminates the urinary tract infection.

Castration in dogs is beneficial, and may be essential to resolve chronic prostatic infection.

Prostatic abscesses: Prostatic abscesses require surgical drainage. Relatively small (<1.5 × 2.4 cm), infected prostatic cysts in asymptomatic dogs may be cured with ultrasound-guided drainage and antimicrobial therapy (Black *et al.*, 1998). Larger abscesses in dogs whose owners have financial limitations have been managed with ultrasound-guided drainage and long-term antimicrobial therapy, but this therapy is unlikely to be curative. Note that ofloxacin, administered by intraprostatic injection, produced a prostatic tissue concentration similar to that of orally administered ofloxacin, even though a much lower dose was injected than that given orally (Bahk *et al.*, 2000).

Intracapsular prostatic omentalization is considered the surgical approach of choice. Partial prostatectomy with an ultrasonic surgical aspirator has few complications and allows an equally rapid recovery, but the equipment is expensive (Rawlings, 1997).

If prostatic enlargement has resulted in partial urethral obstruction, bladder and urethral function should be carefully assessed. Prolonged bladder distension may have resulted in bladder atony. An indwelling urinary catheter may be necessary to allow the detrusor muscle to recover. If the bladder wall has been chronically distended and infected, it may be irreversibly damaged.

Castration is recommended as adjunctive therapy. Castration without abscess drainage leads to reduction of prostatic tissue but continuation of the abscess pockets.

An affected dog should be treated with antibiotics as described previously for chronic prostatitis. The antibiotic choice should be modified based on the results of culture and susceptibility and the presence or absence of bacteraemia. Intravenous antimicrobials should be provided when the dog is systemically ill and during surgery. If possible, surgery should be delayed until culture results are obtained.

Polyuria and polydipsia, similar to those expected with nephrogenic diabetes insipidus, have been noted in a few dogs with prostatic abscesses. These problems resolved within 1 month after surgery. Evidence of hepatopathy also resolved postoperatively. It is assumed that these signs are due to secondary septicaemia/endotoxaemia.

Patient monitoring

Because acute infections may become chronic, re-examination should be performed 7 days after antibiotic therapy is finished. This examination should include physical examination, urinalysis, urine culture and prostatic fluid cytology and culture.

With chronic prostatitis, urine should be recultured 1 week, 1 month and 3 months after antimicrobial therapy is completed.

With abscessation, the prostate gland should be re-examined by palpation and ultrasonography at monthly intervals until abscess resolution is confirmed. In one survey 31% of dogs with successful surgical outcome had urinary tract infection recurrence within 1 year (Rawlings *et al.*, 1997). These dogs are usually asymptomatic so detection requires urinalysis and urine culture.

Neoplasia

Pathophysiology

The aging prostate gland is subject to neoplastic transformation, most commonly carcinoma, either adenocarcinoma or transitional cell carcinoma. These are often difficult to distinguish (LeRoy *et al.*, 2004). The prostate may serve as a metastatic or primary site for tumours that are more common elsewhere, such as lymphosarcoma, squamous cell carcinoma and haemangiosarcoma. Benign tumours of the prostate, such as leiomyoma, are rarely reported (Hayden *et al.*, 1999). One case of nodular, benign hyperplasia that appeared very similar to a benign tumour has also been reported (Gilson *et al.*, 1992).

Prostatic carcinoma occurs in both intact and neutered male dogs (Teske *et al.*, 2002). Prostatic carcinoma is the most common prostatic disease diagnosed in dogs neutered before the onset of a prostatic disease. With any type of neoplastic invasion, the prostate becomes enlarged and often asymmetrical. Prostatic carcinoma tends to metastasize through the external and internal iliac lymph nodes to vertebral bodies as well as to the lungs. The urethra may become obstructed. The tumour may grow into the neck of the bladder and obstruct the ureters. The colonic and pelvic musculature may be invaded via direct extension. Cysts, abscesses and areas of haemorrhage can be found in association with neoplasia. Prostatic neoplasia has been reported in cats (LeRoy and Lech, 2004).

Clinical findings

Dogs with carcinoma have a mean age of 9–10 years and tend to be medium to large breeds. Historical problems include tenesmus, dysuria, haemorrhagic urethral discharge, hindlimb weakness, stiffness or pain and chronic weight loss and anorexia (see Figure 20.2). Haematuria, signs of urethral obstruction and obstipation are the findings reported in cats.

One or more firm, irregular nodules may be palpated on a routine rectal examination prior to development of clinical signs. Most affected dogs are identified after onset of clinical signs. In these cases, the gland will be enlarged and asymmetrical with increased firmness. It may be painful on palpation and is often fixed. In determining whether the prostate is enlarged or not, the examiner must consider the dog's reproductive status. The prostate in a neutered dog involutes to a very small size. Palpation of a prostate gland that would be normal for an intact dog is abnormal in a neutered dog (Figure 20.16). Systemic signs may include depression, cachexia and pyrexia.

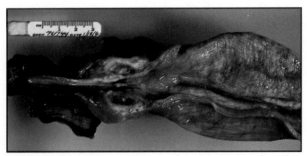

20.16 Necropsy specimens of the bladder and urethra opened on the midline from a castrated dog presented for overflow incontinence. Note the flaccid appearance of the bladder. The cause of the incontinence was urethral obstruction due to prostatic carcinoma. Note that the prostate is not grossly enlarged but is larger than expected for a dog neutered as a puppy. (Reproduced from Barsanti JA and Finco DR (1989), with permission from Elsevier.)

Haematuria is the predominant abnormality on urinalysis. Atypical cells are occasionally found in urine sediment. Urinary tract and prostatic infections may occur concomitantly. The white blood cell count is usually normal, but a neutrophilic leucocytosis with or without a left shift may be present due to necrosis and inflammation associated with tumour growth. A mild non-regenerative anaemia is found in about one fifth of cases. Azotaemia may be present due to obstruction of both ureters or to urethral obstruction. Approximately 50% of affected dogs have an increase in serum alkaline phosphatase. Abnormal epithelial cells may be detected following prostatic massage.

Asymmetrical, irregular prostatic enlargement may be evident on survey abdominal radiography. Occasionally prostatic carcinomas are associated with multifocal, granular, poorly defined mineral densities. The lumbar vertebral bodies and the pelvic bones should be examined for areas of lysis or proliferative changes suggestive of metastasis or reactive osteoarthropathy (Figure 20.17). Metastasis may also occur to other vertebral bodies, long bones, scapula, ribs and

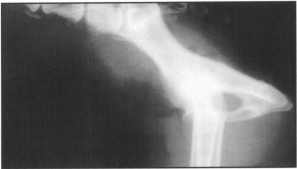

20.17 Osteoproliferative lesions to the sixth and seventh lumbar vertebrae, sacrum and medial aspect of the left ilium in a dog with prostatic carcinoma. Also note the ventral deviation and compression of the colon by a soft tissue mass in the area of the sublumbar lymph nodes. (Reproduced from Barsanti and Finco (1995) and Barsanti JA (1995) with permission from Elsevier.)

digits. Thoracic radiographs are indicated to check for metastasis to the lungs. Even if thoracic radiographs show no evidence of metastasis, there is a 40% chance that lung metastases are present in dogs with prostatic carcinoma.

Ultrasonography usually shows focal or multifocal hyperechoic parenchyma with asymmetry and irregular prostatic outline (Figure 20.18). Echogenicity tends to be very heterogenous with poorly defined hyperechoic foci that seem to coalesce. There may be multifocal irregularly distributed areas of mineralization. Occasionally cavitary lesions may also be noted which can represent infarction, necrosis, haemorrhage or oedema.

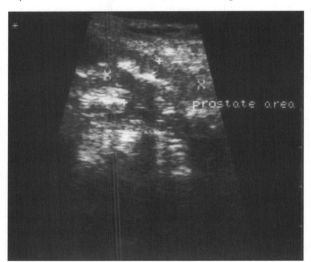

20.18 Transabdominal ultrasonographic image of the prostate of a dog with prostatic carcinoma. Note the heterogenous echogenicity.

Diagnosis

If the dog was neutered as a young dog and prostatomegaly is evident, neoplasia is the most likely prostatic disease. The presence of metastatic disease makes the diagnosis of neoplasia as the cause of prostatomegaly highly likely. If metastasis is not evident, a presumptive diagnosis of neoplasia should always be confirmed by aspiration or biopsy (Figure 20.19).

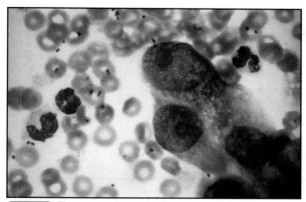

20.19 Two prostatic epithelial cells which appear abnormally large in size with prominent nucleoli and chromatin. Numerous similar cells were found, suggestive of neoplasia, but such a diagnosis should be based on all clinical findings since epithelial cells can be variable in appearance. Red blood cells and a few white blood cells are also seen. A biopsy confirmed prostatic carcinoma in this dog. (With appreciation to Dr Keith Prasse; reproduced from Barsanti JA and Finco DR (1995) with permission from Elsevier.)

In intact dogs with marked prostatomegaly, neoplasia must be distinguished from prostatic abscessation and paraprostatic cysts by laboratory tests and imaging techniques. In earlier stages in intact dogs, neoplasia must be differentiated from hyperplasia. This is usually done by palpation and imaging, as the prostate tends to be irregular and asymmetrical in neoplasia, and symmetrical and regular in hyperplasia. Response to castration can also be used to differentiate these two diseases.

Treatment
Most dogs with prostatic carcinoma are euthanased within 2 months of diagnosis because of progressive disease. However, one reported case survived 19 months without therapy. Therefore the decision with regard to euthanasia should be based on the animal's quality of life. Radiation therapy has been used. With intraoperative orthovoltage radiation, median and mean survival times for 10 dogs were 114 and 196 days, respectively (Turrel, 1987). The usual goal is temporary control of the tumour and amelioration of clinical signs; cure is unlikely. Prostatectomy is another therapy, but the owner must be willing to accept the probable postsurgical development of urinary incontinence. The longest reported postoperative survival in dogs with adenocarcinoma is 9 months. This dog had only a few small nodules in the prostate at the time of diagnosis.

Castration has little beneficial effect in affected dogs. Castration also did not reduce the size of the prostate in a cat with prostatic carcinoma (LeRoy and Lech, 2004). Some response to cisplatin combined with piroxicam has been reported (Kutzler and Yeager, 2005). Treatment with piroxicam alone (0.3 mg/kg/day) may lead to improved quality of life, especially with transitional cell carcinomas, although cure is unlikely.

References and further reading

Bahk JY, Hyun JS, Lee JY *et al.* (2000) Concentration of ofloxacin in canine prostate tissue and prostate fluid after intraprostatic injection of biodegradable sustained-releasing microspheres containing ofloxacin. *Journal of Urology* **163**, 1560–1564

Barr F (1995) Percutaneous biopsy of abdominal organs under ultrasound guidance. *Journal of Small Animal Practice* **36**, 105–113

Barsanti JA (1992) Diagnosis and medical therapy of prostatic disorders. In: *Urologic Surgery of the Dog and Cat*, ed. EA Stone and JA Barsanti, pp. 215–226. Lea & Febiger, Philadelphia

Barsanti JA (1995) Diseases of the prostate gland. In: *Canine and Feline Nephrology and Urology*, ed. CA Osborne and DR Finco, pp. 726–755. Lea & Febiger, Baltimore

Barsanti JA (2003) Diseases of the prostate gland. In: *Handbook of Small Animal Practice, 4th edn*, ed. R Morgan, R Bright and M Swartout, pp. 570–580. WB Saunders, Philadelphia

Barsanti JA (2006) Genitourinary infections. In: *Infectious Diseases of the Dog and Cat, 3rd edn*, ed. C Greene, pp. 935–961. Elsevier Saunders, St. Louis

Barsanti JA and Finco DR (1989) Canine prostatic diseases. In: *Textbook of Veterinary Internal Medicine*, ed. S Ettinger, pp. 1859–1880. WB Saunders, Philadelphia

Barsanti JA and Finco DR (1995) Canine Prostatic Diseases. In: *Textbook of Veterinary Internal Medicine, 4th edn*, ed. S Ettinger and E Feldman, pp. 1662–1685. WB Saunders, Philadelphia

Barsanti JA, Finco DR, Mahaffey MM *et al.* (2000) Effects of an extract of *Serenoa repens* on dogs with hyperplasia of the prostate gland. *American Journal of Veterinary Research* **61**, 880–885

Baumueller A and Madsen PO (1977) Secretion of various antimicrobial substances in dogs with experimental prostatitis. *Urological Research* **5**, 215–218

Black GM, Ling GV, Nyland TG and Baker T (1998) Prevalence of prostatic cysts in adult, large-breed dogs. *Journal of the American Animal Hospital Association* **34**, 177–180

Gilson SD, Miller RT, Hardie EM and Spaulding KA (1992) Unusual prostatic mass in a dog. *Journal of the American Veterinary Medical Association* **200**, 702–704

Hayden DW, Klausner JS and Waters DJ (1999) Prostatic leiomyosarcoma in a dog. *Journal of Veterinary Diagnostic Investigation* **11**, 283–286

Kutzler MA and Yeager A (2005) Prostatic diseases. In: *Textbook of Veterinary Internal Medicine, 6th edn*, ed. S Ettinger and E Feldman, pp.1809–1819. Elsevier Saunders, St. Louis

LeRoy BE and Lech ME (2004) Prostatic carcinoma causing urethral obstruction and obstipation in a cat. *Journal of Feline Medicine & Surgery* **6**, 397–400

LeRoy BE, Nadella MVP, Toribio RE, Leav I and Rosol TJ (2004) Canine prostate carcinomas express markers of urothelial and prostate differentiation. *Veterinary Pathology* **41**, 131–140

Newell SM, Neuwirth L, Ginn PE *et al.* (1998) Doppler ultrasound of the prostate in normal dogs and in dogs with chronic lymphocytic-lymphoplasmocytic prostatitis. *Veterinary Radiology & Ultrasound* **39**, 332–336

Rawlings CA, Mahaffey MB, Barsanti JA *et al.* (1997) Use of partial prostatectomy for treatment of prostatic abscesses and cysts in dogs. *Journal of the American Veterinary Medical Association* **211**, 868–871

Root-Kustritz MV and Merkel L (1998) Theriogenology question of the month. *Journal of the American Veterinary Medical Association* **213**, 807–809

Roura X, Camps-Palau MA, Lloret A, Garcia F and Espada I (2002) Bacterial prostatitis in a cat. *Journal of Veterinary Internal Medicine* **16**, 593– 597

Sirinarumitr K, Sirinarumitr T, Johnston SD, Sarkar DK and Kustritz MV (2001) Effects of finasteride on size of the prostate gland and semen quality in dogs with benign prostaic hypertrophy. *Journal of the American Veterinary Medical Association* **218**, 1275–1280

Stone EA and Barsanti JA (1992) *Urologic surgery of the dog and cat*. Lea & Febiger, Philadelphia

Teske E, Naan EC, van Dijk EM *et al.* (2002) Canine prostatic carcinoma: epidemiological evidence of an increased risk in castrated dogs. *Molecular and Cellular Endocrinology* **197**, 251–255

Threlfall WR and Chew DJ (1999) Diagnosis and treatment of canine bacterial prostatitis. *Compendium on Continuing Education for the Practicing Veterinarian* **21**, 73–87

Turrel JM (1987) Intraoperative radiography of carcinoma of the prostate gland in 10 dogs. *Journal of the American Veterinary Medical Association* **190**, 48–52

21

Management of urolithiasis

Jody P. Lulich and Carl A. Osborne

Introduction

Urolithiasis is a general term referring to the causes and effects of stones anywhere in the urinary tract. Urolithiasis should not be viewed conceptually as a single disease with a single cause but rather as a sequela of multiple interacting underlying abnormalities. Thus, the syndrome of urolithiasis may be defined as the occurrence of familial, congenital or acquired pathophysiological factors that, in combination, progressively increase the risk of precipitation of excretory metabolites in urine to form stones (i.e. uroliths).

Naturally occurring urolithiasis is affected by many risk factors, some of which are known and some of which are unknown. Some risk factors that are known to influence urolith formation include breed, gender, age, anatomical and functional abnormalities of the urinary tract, abnormalities of metabolism, urinary tract infections (UTIs), diet, urine pH and body water homeostasis. Each factor may play a limited or significant role in the development or prevention of different types of uroliths. Therefore, recognition and control of lithogenic risk factors should minimize urolith formation and recurrence.

Anatomy of a stone

The term *urolith* is derived from the Greek *uro*, meaning urine, and *lith*, meaning stone. Unlike the gastrointestinal tract, solids that form in the urinary tract are abnormal, because the urinary system is designed to dispose of body wastes in liquid form. Under less than optimal conditions, some wastes, especially minerals, precipitate out of solution to form crystals. If these crystallized minerals are retained in the urinary system, they may grow and aggregate to form stones.

A crystal that forms within the urinary system may be viewed as a microlith; however, crystalluria (microlithuria) is not synonymous with the formation of macroliths (uroliths) and the clinical signs associated with them. Nor is crystalluria irrefutable evidence of a stone-forming tendency. In fact, the crystalluria that occurs in individuals with anatomically and functionally normal urinary tracts is often harmless. Identification of crystals in such individuals does not itself justify therapy. On the other hand, detection of some types of abnormal crystals or aggregates of crystals commonly observed in healthy individuals may be of diagnostic,

prognostic and therapeutic significance. For example, ammonium urate crystalluria may be indicative of portovascular disorders or primary hepatic disorders.

A macroscopic urolith is primarily composed of one or more crystallized biogenic minerals in combination with relatively small quantities of organic matrix. Although one mineral usually predominates, the composition of many uroliths is mixed. Combinations of minerals may be unevenly mixed throughout the urolith or they may be deposited in layers (laminations). Each urolith may contain a nidus, a stone, a shell and surface crystals (Figure 21.1). The Minnesota Urolith Center uses the following terminology when reporting the results of urolith analysis (Osborne *et al.*, 1999c):

- The nidus or nucleus of a urolith is an area of obvious initiation of urolith growth
- Stone refers to the major body of the urolith
- Shell designates a layer of precipitated material that completely surrounds the body of the stone
- Surface crystals are an incomplete covering of the outermost surface of the urolith.

In the authors' studies, a urolith that contained 70% or more of one type of mineral, without a nidus or a shell, was identified by that mineral. A urolith with less than 70% of one mineral was identified as a 'mixed' urolith. A urolith with a nidus or stone with one or more surrounding layers of different mineral composition was called a 'compound' urolith (Figure 21.1).

Knowledge of urolith composition is important because contemporary methods of treatment are primarily based on this information. Several types of uroliths are commonly recognized in dogs and cats (Figure 21.2). The authors use a protocol to predict urolith

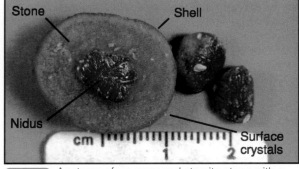

21.1 Anatomy of a compound struvite stone with a nidus composed of calcium oxalate dihydrate.

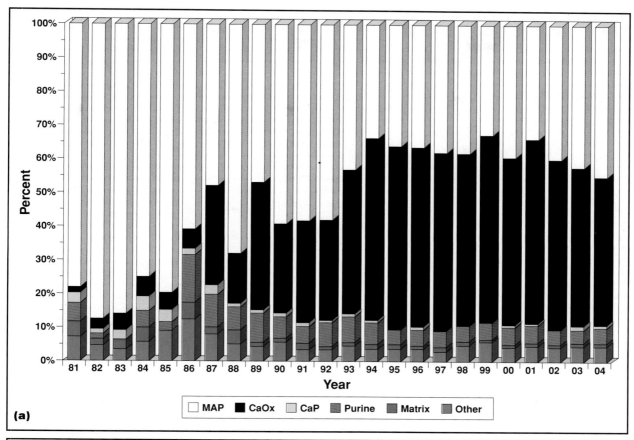

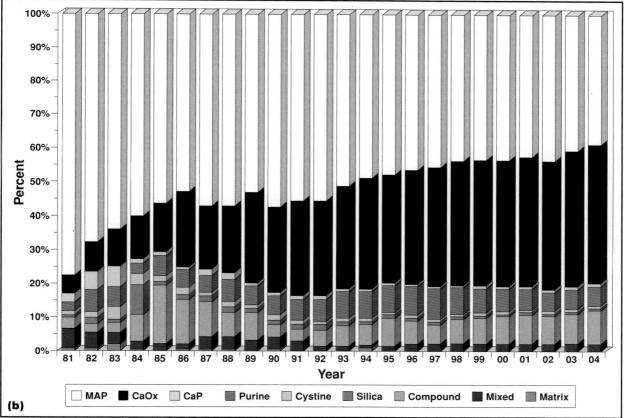

21.2 **(a)** Changes in the prevalence of uroliths in cats between 1981 and 2004 (64,288 submissions). **(b)** Changes in the prevalence of uroliths in dogs between 1981 and 2004 (241,274 submissions). CaOx = Calcium oxalate; CaP = Calcium phosphate; MAP = Magnesium ammonium phosphate.

composition (Figure 21.3) prior to determination by quantitative analysis. Small uroliths may also be retrieved from the urinary bladder for quantative mineral analysis without surgical intervention (Figure 21.4)

(Lulich and Osborne, 1992). Urolith dissolution and prevention protocols devised on the basis of their quantitative mineral analysis typically provide the most consistent therapeutic results.

Mineral type	Predictors					
	Urine pH	**Crystal appearance**	**Urine culture** (ᵃunless complicated by a secondary urinary tract infection)	**Radiographic density**	**Radiographic contour**	**Serum abnormalities**
Magnesium ammonium phosphate (struvite)	Neutral to alkaline	Four- to six-sided colourless prisms	Urease-producing bacteria (*Staphylococcus, Proteus, Enterococcus, Mycoplasma*)	+ to + + + +	Smooth, round or faceted; may assume shape of bladder or urethra	None
Calcium oxalate	Acid to neutral	Dihydrate salt: colourless, envelope or octahedral shape. Monohydrate salt: spindles or dumbbell shape	Negative ᵃ	+ + to + + +	Dihydrate salt: rough or spiculated. Monohydrate salt: small, smooth, round; sometimes jackstone	Occasional hypercalcaemia
Urate	Acid to neutral	Yellow–brown amorphous shapes or spheres (ammonium urate)	Negative ᵃ	– to + +	Smooth round or oval	Low urea nitrogen and serum albumin in dogs with hepatic shunts
Calcium phosphate	Alkaline to neutral (brushite forms in acidic urine)	Amorphous or long thin prisms	Negative ᵃ	+ + to + + +	Smooth, round or faceted	Occasional hypercalcaemia
Cystine	Acid to neutral	Flat colourless, hexagonal plates	Negative ᵃ	+ to + +	Smooth to slightly irregular, round to oval	None
Silica	Acid to neutral	None observed	Negative ᵃ	+ + to + + +	Round centre with radial spoke-like projections (jackstone)	None

21.3 Predicting mineral composition of uroliths.

Method	Suitable application	Considerations
Spontaneous voiding	Small (<3–5 mm), asymptomatic urocystoliths with a relatively slow growth rate (i.e. calcium oxalate, calcium phosphate, uric acid) in female patients	Patients with uroliths larger than the urethral lumen may develop urethral obstruction. Concomitant urinary tract infection should be eradicated
Medical dissolution	Sterile struvite (see Figure 21.6), infection-induced struvite (see Figure 21.7), allopurinol-induced xanthine (seeFigure 21.8), uric acid (see Figure 21.9) and cystine (see Figure 21.10) stones are amenable to medical dissolution	Sterile struvite and allopurinol-induced xanthine uroliths dissolve within weeks. Large infection-induced struvite stones may take 2–3 months to dissolve. Stones in kidney require longer dissolution time than stones in the bladder. Urethral obstruction is uncommon during dissolution of struvite stones for the following reasons: • Sruvite uroliths commonly occur in females • The wide urethra of females is less likely to result in obstruction • Bacterial infection promoting dysuria which may promote urolith movement into the urethra is easily controlled with appropriate antibiotic administration

21.4 Methods of urolith removal. Methods are listed from least invasive to most invasive. (continues) ▶

Method	Suitable application	Considerations
Catheter retrieval (see Figure 21.11)	To retrieve small urocystoliths (<3 mm) for quantitative mineral analysis	Can be performed without anaesthesia
Voiding urohydropropulsion (VUH) (see Figure 21.12)	To evacuate small to moderate size (<5–7 mm) urocystoliths of any composition	Not suitable for male cats unless they have a perineal urethrostomy Not suitable for patients with a urethral obstruction Not ideal for patients that have recently undergone bladder surgery Eradicate urinary infection prior to performing VUH
Stone basket retrieval	Urocystoliths smaller than the distended diameter of the urethra (<5–7 mm)	Performed during cystoscopy
Urolith evacuators	Small urocystoliths or urolith fragments following lithotripsy in large female dogs	Most evacuators are designed to fit only the sheath of human cystoscopes Can remove urolith fragments in large dogs too heavy to lift for VUH
Intracorporeal lithotripsy	Urocystoliths in female dogs and cats and urethroliths in male dogs	Performed during cystoscopy The flexibility of probes for laser lithotripsy permits fragmentation of urocystoliths in male dogs The urethra of the male cat will rarely accommodate cystoscopy equipment to perform lithotripsy Large hard uroliths (calcium oxalate monohydrate) in male dogs require considerably longer times to fragment
Extracorporeal shock wave lithotripsy (ESWL)	Ureteroliths and nephroliths in dogs	Uroliths in the renal pelvis are easier to fragment than ureteroliths The ability to perform ESWL without damaging the feline kidney is controversial – newer generation lithotriptors may prove safer
Laparoscopic assisted cystotomy	Urocystoliths in dogs	Requires training in cystoscopy and laparoscopic surgery
Cystotomy/ urethrotomy/ urethrostomy	Urocystoliths or uroliths lodged in the urethra	Consider retrograde urohydropropulsion of urethroliths prior to urethrotomy or urethrostomy With cystotomy there is failure to remove all uroliths in 15–20% of cases
Ureterotomy/ ureteroneocystotomy/ ureteroneoureterotomy	Clinically active ureteroliths	High degree of surgical skill required when performed on cats Surgery performed on dilated ureters has been associated with greater success than that performed on normal sized ureters
Pyelotomy/nephrotomy	Nephroliths or ureteroliths flushed back into the kidney	Some reduction in kidney function should be anticipated following surgery Difficult to locate some stones in renal pelvis

21.4 (continued) Methods of urolith removal. Methods are listed from least invasive to most invasive.

Clinical consequences of uroliths

Uroliths may spontaneously pass through various parts of the urinary tract, spontaneously dissolve, continue to grow or become inactive (no growth occurs). Not all persistent uroliths are associated with clinical signs. In the authors' experience, most inactive uroliths are not associated with UTIs. Nonetheless, if uroliths remain in the urinary tract, dysuria, UTI, partial or total urinary obstruction and polyp formation are potential sequelae.

UTI is both a cause and consequence of uroliths. Infections with urease-producing bacteria commonly cause struvite urolith formation in dogs. In turn, the presence of other urolith types can facilitate initiation of UTI. Factors contributing to the increased risk of UTI include:

- Traumatic disruption of the mucosal lining of the urinary bladder
- Incomplete urine voiding
- Sequestration of microorganisms.

Infections with urease-producing bacteria can result in the deposition of magnesium ammonium phosphate on the surface of other urolith types, confounding diagnostic and management efforts to resolve the initial lithogenic events that are ultimately responsible for disease (Lulich and Osborne, 2000).

Polyp formation has been documented in several cases of dogs with urocystoliths. The events promoting polyp formation are unknown; however, it is logical to assume that chronic irritation to the urinary bladder mucosa and bacterial infection contribute to mucosal hyperplasia. Although polyps have been routinely managed surgically, inflammatory polyps have also spontaneously regressed following eradication of uroliths and urinary infection.

Small uroliths located in the urinary bladder commonly pass into the urethra during the voiding phase of micturition. Uroliths whose diameter is slightly larger than the dilated proximal urethral lumen can become lodged in the urethra. Uroliths associated with complete and persistent obstruction affecting both kidneys result in uraemia. Complete obstruction to urine outflow associated with UTI may result in rapid destruction of renal parenchyma and septicaemia. If treatment is not provided, death can be expected to occur within 2–4 days.

Urolith management

Managing urethral obstruction

Once uroliths become lodged in the urethra, it is unlikely that they can be removed non-surgically by antegrade voiding hydropropulsion (Lulich *et al.*, 1993). However, lithotripsy can be used to break the urethrolith into fragments small enough to pass through the urethra (Wynn *et al.*, 2003; Davidson *et al.*, 2004). To avoid urethral surgery when lithotripsy is not available, flushing urethroliths back into the bladder lumen by retrograde urohydropropulsion can, with a few exceptions, restore urethral patency (Osborne *et al.*, 1999b). The efficacy of this technique depends on dilating the portion of the urethral lumen containing the urethroliths with fluid under pressure. To be consistently successful, one must be familiar with all aspects of the technique (Figure 21.5).

Managing ureteral obstruction

Upper tract uroliths pose unique management problems, partly because most are composed of calcium oxalate (Lekcharoensuk *et al.*, 2005; Kyles *et al.*, 2005). Medical protocols that promote dissolution of calcium oxalate uroliths have not yet been developed. Difficulty in managing ureteroliths is magnified in cats because ureteral surgery is associated with significant risks, especially irreparable damage to the ureters and kidneys (Kyles *et al.*, 2005). For these reasons, the authors recommend managing cats with renal failure and ureteroliths by initially using non-invasive medical protocols designed to restore fluid volume, correct electrolyte and acid–base imbalances associated with uraemia and promote migration of ureteroliths into the urinary bladder.

Surgical removal of uroliths that obstruct a ureter should decrease the magnitude of renal dysfunction. However, determining when the benefits of ureteral surgery outweigh the risks is often difficult. The timing of surgical intervention depends on the following:

- The severity and rate of progression of renal dysfunction
- The potential for reversing renal dysfunction
- The potential for urolith migration through the ureter
- The presence of infection or uncontrollable pain
- Risks associated with surgery of the ureters.

A urolith may obstruct a ureter in a patient with previously compensated renal failure and cause an abrupt decline in renal function. This may be associated with life-threatening hyperkalaemia and/or acidaemia that can only be controlled by peritoneal dialysis or haemodialysis. In such a case, surgical intervention should be considered. Placement of nephrostomy tubes to bypass obstructed ureters may be considered as a method of temporarily improving renal function, but maintaining nephrostomy tube position, seal and patency for longer than 24 hours is often technically difficult (Nwadike *et al.*, 2000; Hardie and Kyles, 2004). In addition to severe unresponsive azotaemia, if infection and pain cannot be appropriately managed, surgi-

1. Decompress urinary bladder. Urethroliths cannot be safely flushed back into a bladder over-distended with urine. To empty the bladder, use a 22-gauge, 37 mm (1.5 inch) needle attached to intravenous extension tubing, a three-way stopcock and a large-volume syringe. By using the intravenous extension tubing and the three-way stopcock, the urinary bladder will not have to be repunctured after emptying a full syringe of urine. Excessive digital pressure should not be applied to the bladder wall while the needle is in its lumen in case urine is forced around the needle into the peritoneal cavity. Attempting complete evacuation of the bladder lumen is undesirable because the sharp point of the needle may then damage the bladder wall. 10–15 ml of urine should remain in the bladder.

2. Lubricate around the urethroliths. Fill one 12 ml syringe with 5 ml of saline and another 12 ml syringe with 5 ml of sterile water-soluble lubricant. Attach these two syringes with a three-way stopcock. Mix the contents of both syringes by emptying one syringe into the other several times. After inserting a urethral catheter, inject 3–8 ml of mixture to lubricate around uroliths. This step is not always necessary.

3. Insert a lubricated large-bore flexible catheter. The tip of the catheter should remain distal to the urethroliths.

4. Occlude pelvic urethra. Insert a gloved index finger into the rectum and occlude the urethral lumen by compressing the urethra against the floor or side of the bony pelvis.

5. Occlude distal urethra. With a moistened gauze sponge, occlude the distal urethra by compressing the distal tip of the penis around the catheter.

6. Forcefully flush fluid through catheter. Fill a large syringe (20–35 ml) with sterile isotonic solution (e.g. saline, lactated Ringer's solution). The normal bladder holds approximately 7–11 ml/kg body weight. With the syringe attached to the catheter, turn it upside down, and place the top of the plunger against the tabletop. Hold the syringe by the barrel and forcefully push it down over the plunger with the goal of dilating the urethral lumen with saline.

7. Relieve occlusion of pelvic urethra. Once the urethra becomes dilated, digital pressure applied to the pelvic urethra (but not the penile urethra) should be rapidly released.

8. Continue flushing fluid through the catheter and urethral lumen to propel the urethroliths into the urinary bladder. Use caution not to over-distend the bladder lumen with saline. If the technique is repeated, accumulation of saline in the bladder lumen necessitates repeating decompressive cystocentesis.

9. Medical imaging. Radiography is used to assess whether or not all of the uroliths have been flushed into the bladder lumen. Transurethral catheterization is not a reliable method of verifying that all uroliths have been flushed out of the urethra.

21.5 Technique for retrograde urohydropropulsion.

cal ureterolith removal should be considered. Due to the high risk of irreparable ureteral damage associated with ureterotomy, surgical removal of ureteroliths is not recommended if:

- Ureteroliths are migrating through the ureter
- Azotaemia is resolving
- The associated kidney is non-functional
- Surgeons are unfamiliar with appropriate surgical techniques.

Methods of urolith removal

For decades, treatment of patients with uroliths has been the province of the surgeon. However, within the past 10 years, a variety of non-surgical protocols has been developed to manage uroliths (see Figure 21.4). The type of management selected will vary with the characteristics of the urolith (composition, size, con-

tour and location), the effects of the urolith on the patient and the veterinary surgeon's familiarity with available procedures. The techniques are described in Figures 21.5–21.12.

Diagnostic plan

1. Perform appropriate diagnostic studies including urinalysis (e.g. pH >6.5, magnesium ammonium phosphate (MAP) crystalluria), diagnostic radiography (radiodense urolith) and urine culture (infection-induced struvite uroliths are usually caused by staphylococcal species of bacteria) supporting the diagnosis of sterile MAP uroliths.
2. Determine mineral composition of voided or retrieved uroliths. If unavailable, predict mineral composition by evaluating clinical data (see Figure 21.3).

Therapeutic plan

1. Consider mechanical removal (see Figure 21.4) if uroliths obstructing urine flow cannot be dislodged, or if patients with a high risk of urine outflow obstruction cannot be monitored.
2. Initiate therapy with a diet designed to dissolve MAP uroliths (e.g. Hills Prescription diet s/d, Innovative Veterinary Diets (IVD) dissolution formula). No other food, supplements or treats should be fed. Continue dietary therapy 3–4 weeks after radiographically detected dissolution.

Monitor efficacy of therapy

1. Evaluate serial urinalyses. Urine pH should be acidic, urine specific gravity should be low (<1.015 in dog and <1.035 in cat (lower if using the canned food)) and struvite crystalluria should be absent.
2. Continue calculolytic diet therapy for at least 1 month after radiographic disappearance of uroliths. The rationale is to provide therapy of adequate duration to dissolve small uroliths that cannot be detected by survey radiography.
3. If uroliths increase in size during dietary management or do not begin to decrease in size after approximately 2–4 weeks of appropriate medical management, alternative methods should be considered. Difficulty in inducing complete dissolution of uroliths by creating urine that is undersaturated with the suspected calculogenic crystalloid should prompt consideration that either:
   • The wrong mineral component was identified
   • The nucleus of the urolith is of different mineral composition than other portions of the urolith
   • The owner of the patient is not complying with medical recommendations.

21.6 Dissolution of sterile struvite uroliths.

Diagnostic plan

1. Perform appropriate diagnostic studies including urinalysis (e.g. pH >6.5, magnesium ammonium phosphate (MAP) crystalluria, bacteriuria), quantitative urine culture (e.g. usually staphylococcal bacteria when infection-induced), diagnostic radiography (radiodense urolith) supporting the diagnosis of infection-induced MAP uroliths.
2. Determine mineral composition of voided or retrieved uroliths. If unavailable, predict mineral composition by evaluating clinical data (see Figure 21.3).

Therapeutic plan

1. Consider mechanical removal (see Figure 21.4) if uroliths obstructing urine flow cannot be dislodged, or if patients with a high risk of urine outflow obstruction cannot be monitored.
2. Eradicate urinary tract infection with appropriate antibiotics. Maintain antimicrobial therapy at the full dose during dissolution of uroliths and for 3–4 weeks after dissolution.
3. Initiate therapy with a diet designed to dissolve MAP uroliths (e.g. Hills Prescription diet s/d, IVD dissolution formula). Other food, supplements or treats should not be fed. Continue dietary therapy 3–4 weeks after radiographic confirmation of dissolution.

Monitor efficacy of therapy

1. Evaluate serial urinalyses. Urine pH should be acidic, urine specific gravity should be low (<1.015 in dog and <1.035 in cat (lower if using the canned food)) and MAP crystalluria should be absent.
2. Perform urine cultures to determine whether bacteria have been eradicated. Cultures are especially important in patients that are infected before therapy and those that are catheterized during therapy.
3. Perform radiography monthly to assess urolith number, size, and position. If uroliths increase in size during therapy or do not begin to decrease in size after approximately 4–8 weeks of appropriate medical management, alternative management strategies (i.e. surgery, lithotripsy) can be considered. Difficulty in inducing complete dissolution of uroliths by creating urine that is undersaturated with the suspected calculogenic crystalloid should prompt consideration that either:
   • The wrong mineral component was identified
   • The nucleus of the urolith is of different mineral composition than other portions of the urolith
   • The owner of the patient is not complying with medical recommendations
   • There is a persistent urinary tract infection.

21.7 Recommendations for medical dissolution of infection-induced struvite uroliths.

Diagnostic plan

1. Perform appropriate diagnostic studies including urinalysis (e.g. pH <6.5, amorphous crystalluria), diagnostic radiography (marginally radiodense urolith requiring contrast cystourethrography or ultrasonography) and a history of allopurinol administration supporting the diagnosis of xanthine uroliths.
2. If possible, verify mineral composition of voided or retrieved uroliths.

Therapeutic plan

1. Consider mechanical removal (see Figure 21.4) if uroliths obstructing urine flow cannot be dislodged, or if patients with a high risk of urine outflow obstruction cannot be monitored.
2. Discontinue allopurinol administration.
3. Initiate therapy with a calculolytic diet (e.g. Hills Prescription Diet Canine canned u/d). Other food or mineral supplements should not be fed.

Monitor efficacy of therapy

1. Evaluate serial urinalyses. Urine pH should be alkaline, urine specific gravity should be low (<1.015 in dog and <1.035 in cat (lower if using the canned food)) and crystalluria should be absent.
2. Perform radiography monthly to assess urolith number, size and position. If uroliths grow during medical management or do not begin to dissolve in 4 weeks, alternative methods should be considered (see Figure 21.4).

21.8 Recommendations for medical dissolution of allopurinol-induced xanthine uroliths.

Diagnostic plan

1. Perform appropriate diagnostic studies including urinalysis (e.g. pH <7, urate or amorphous crystalluria), diagnostic radiography (marginally radiodense urolith requiring contrast cystourethrography or ultrasonography) supporting the diagnosis of urate uroliths. In breeds other than Dalmatians or English Bulldogs, consider liver function tests (provocative serum concentrations of bile acids and liver size). Decreased liver function is rarely associated with urate uroliths in cats.
2. Determine mineral composition of voided or retrieved uroliths. If unavailable, predict mineral composition by evaluating clinical data (see Figure 21.3).

Therapeutic plan

1. Consider mechanical removal (see Figure 21.4) if uroliths obstructing urine flow cannot be dislodged, or if patients with a high risk of urine outflow obstruction cannot be monitored.
2. Initiate therapy with a low purine calculolytic diet (Hills Prescription Diet Canine u/d, l/d or d/d). Other food supplements should not be fed to the patient.
3. Initiate therapy with allopurinol at a dosage of 15 mg/kg q12h orally (a lesser dose will be required in azotaemic patients).
4. If necessary, administer potassium citrate or sodium bicarbonate orally in order to eliminate aciduria. Strive for a urine pH of approximately 7.

Monitor efficacy of therapy

1. Try to minimize follow-up studies that require urinary catheterization; if it is necessary, give appropriate antimicrobial agents to prevent iatrogenic catheter-induced UTI.
2. Evalute serial urinalyses. Urine pH should be >7, urine specific gravity should be <1.020 and crystals should be absent.
3. Perform serial radiography at monthly intervals to evaluate reductions in urolith number and size.
4. Continue calculolytic diet and allopurinol for approximately 1 month after disappearance of uroliths as detected by medical imaging.

21.9 Recommendations for medical dissolution of urate uroliths in dogs.

Diagnostic plan

1. Perform appropriate diagnostic studies including urinalysis (e.g. pH <6.5, cystine crystalluria) and diagnostic radiography (marginally radiodense urolith requiring contrast cystourethrography or ultrasonography) supporting a diagnosis of cystine uroliths.
2. Determine mineral composition of voided or retrieved uroliths. If unavailable, predict mineral composition by evaluating clinical data (see Figure 21.3).

Therapeutic plan

1. Consider mechanical removal (see Figure 21.4) if uroliths obstructing urine flow cannot be dislodged, or if patients with a high risk of urine outflow obstruction cannot be monitored.
2. Initiate therapy with calculolytic diet (e.g. Hill's Prescription Diet Canine canned u/d). Other food or mineral supplements should not be fed.
3. Initiate therapy with N-(2-mercaptopropionyl)-glycine (2-MPG), approximately 15 mg/kg q12h orally. Other thiol containing drugs (D-penicillamine, captopril and bucillamine) are available to augment cystine dissolution; however, because of their unproven efficacy or increased toxicity they require more careful monitoring.
4. If necessary, administer potassium citrate orally (75 mg/kg q12h) to induce alkaluria. Titrate dose to achieve a pH of approximately 7–7.5.

21.10 Recommendations for medical dissolution of cystine uroliths. (continues) ▶

Monitor efficacy of therapy (4–6 week intervals)

1. Try to minimize follow-up studies that require urinary catheterization, but if they are required give appropriate antimicrobial agents to prevent iatrogenic catheter-induced UTI.
2. Evaluate serial urinalyses. Urine pH should be >7, urine specific gravity should be <1.020 and crystals should be absent.
3. Perform serial radiography at monthly intervals to evaluate reductions in urolith number and size.
4. Continue calculolytic diet, 2-MPG and alkalinizing therapy for approximately 1 month after disappearance of uroliths as detected by radiography.

21.10 (continued) Recommendations for medical dissolution of cystine uroliths.

---

1. Sedation. For most dogs sedation is unnecessary; however, sterile lubricant with topical anaesthetics (e.g. lidocaine) can improve patient comfort. Transurethral catheterization of most cats requires sedation.
2. Catheter selection. Select the largest catheter that can be easily inserted into the urethra. The authors commonly use sterile, 8 French diameter or larger catheters in dogs. The distal tip is cut smoothly so that the catheter is open at the end.
3. Determine the length of catheter that must be inserted so that the open end reaches the trigone. This distance is easily determined by measuring urethral length from a radiograph.
4. Place catheter transurethrally. The well lubricated, sterile catheter from step 2 is advanced through the urethra into the bladder lumen and the patient is placed in lateral recumbency.
5. Fill the urinary bladder. If the urinary bladder is not distended with urine, it should be moderately distended with sterile physiological solutions (e.g. lactated Ringer's solution, normal saline).
6. Agitate the bladder while removing fluid. While aspirating fluid from the bladder through the catheter into a syringe, vigorously and repeatedly agitate the bladder. The bladder is agitated by placing your hand (palm up) between the patient (in the area of the bladder) and the table. Repeatedly flex and extend your fingers to move the animal's abdomen (i.e. urinary bladder) up and down. This manoeuvre will disperse uroliths throughout the fluid in the bladder lumen. Small uroliths in the vicinity of the catheter tip are usually aspirated into the catheter along with the fluid.
7. Repeat steps 5 and 6. It may be necessary to repeat this sequence of steps several times before a sufficient quantity of uroliths is retrieved. Difficulty in aspirating fluid may be caused by poor catheter position (position catheter tip in trigone of bladder) or occlusion of the catheter lumen with uroliths (injecting fluid back through the catheter should clear the catheter lumen).

21.11 Catheter retrieval of uroliths.

---

1. Anaesthetize the patient. The type of anaesthesia selected may vary based on the likelihood of success and gender of the patient. Consider reversible short-acting anaesthetics for patients with very small uroliths that are easily removed. Patients likely to go to surgery/lithotripsy should be placed under inhalation anaesthesia. Consider epidural anaesthesia to facilitate relaxation of the urethra in male dogs.
2. Attach a three-way stopcock to the end of the urinary catheter. This facilitates control of the volume of fluid entering the bladder and containment of fluid once the bladder is filled.
3. Fill the urinary bladder and remove the catheter. Sterile physiological solutions (e.g. lactated Ringer's solution, normal saline) are injected through a transurethral catheter to distend the bladder. If fluid is expelled prematurely around the catheter prior to adequate bladder filling, the vulva and/or urethra can be gently occluded using your thumb and first finger. Placement of additional fluid may not be needed.
4. Position the patient so that the spine is approximately vertical. Repositioning the patient allows uroliths to accumulate at the neck of the bladder facilitating their expulsion. Anatomically, the urethra does not become vertical until the caudal spine is 20–25 degrees anterior of vertical, but this may not be clinically important.
5. Agitate the bladder left and right to dislodge uroliths loosely adhered to the bladder mucosa.
6. Express the urinary bladder. Apply steady digital pressure to the urinary bladder to induce micturition. Once voiding begins, the bladder is more vigorously compressed. Compress the urinary bladder dorsally and cranially (toward the back and head of the patient). Movement of the urinary bladder caudally toward the pelvic canal may cause the urethra to kink preventing maximal urethral dilation.
7. Repeat steps 2–6. The bladder is flushed repeatedly until no uroliths are expelled.
8. Medical imaging. Radiography provides an appropriate method of assessing successful expulsion of uroliths. Consider double-contrast cystography to enhance detection of remaining small uroliths (only the lateral view is needed).

21.12 Performing voiding urohydropropulsion.

Preventing urolith recurrence

Uroliths tend to recur. Prevention of recurrent uroliths, which reduces the need for medical therapy and surgery, is therefore cost effective. In general, preventative strategies are designed to eliminate or control the underlying causes of various types of uroliths. When causes cannot be identified, preventative strategies should aim to minimize risk factors associated with calculogenesis. These strategies commonly include dietary modification (Figures 21.13–21.16).

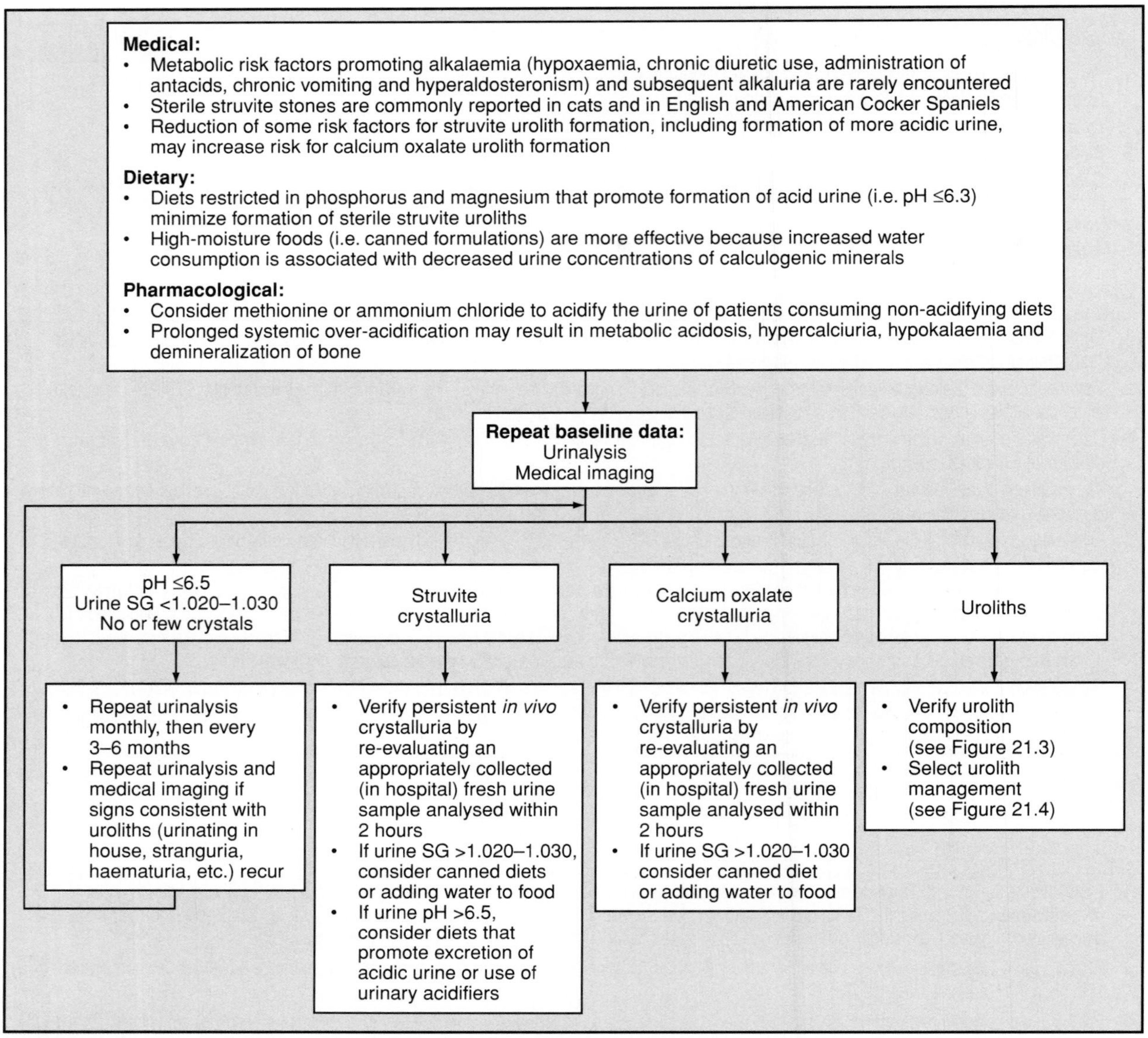

Medical:
- Metabolic risk factors promoting alkalaemia (hypoxaemia, chronic diuretic use, administration of antacids, chronic vomiting and hyperaldosteronism) and subsequent alkaluria are rarely encountered
- Sterile struvite stones are commonly reported in cats and in English and American Cocker Spaniels
- Reduction of some risk factors for struvite urolith formation, including formation of more acidic urine, may increase risk for calcium oxalate urolith formation

Dietary:
- Diets restricted in phosphorus and magnesium that promote formation of acid urine (i.e. pH ≤6.3) minimize formation of sterile struvite uroliths
- High-moisture foods (i.e. canned formulations) are more effective because increased water consumption is associated with decreased urine concentrations of calculogenic minerals

Pharmacological:
- Consider methionine or ammonium chloride to acidify the urine of patients consuming non-acidifying diets
- Prolonged systemic over-acidification may result in metabolic acidosis, hypercalciuria, hypokalaemia and demineralization of bone

Repeat baseline data:
Urinalysis
Medical imaging

pH ≤6.5 Urine SG <1.020–1.030 No or few crystals	Struvite crystalluria	Calcium oxalate crystalluria	Uroliths

- Repeat urinalysis monthly, then every 3–6 months
- Repeat urinalysis and medical imaging if signs consistent with uroliths (urinating in house, stranguria, haematuria, etc.) recur

- Verify persistent *in vivo* crystalluria by re-evaluating an appropriately collected (in hospital) fresh urine sample analysed within 2 hours
- If urine SG >1.020–1.030, consider canned diets or adding water to food
- If urine pH >6.5, consider diets that promote excretion of acidic urine or use of urinary acidifiers

- Verify persistent *in vivo* crystalluria by re-evaluating an appropriately collected (in hospital) fresh urine sample analysed within 2 hours
- If urine SG >1.020–1.030 consider canned diet or adding water to food

- Verify urolith composition (see Figure 21.3)
- Select urolith management (see Figure 21.4)

21.13 Strategies to prevent sterile struvite uroliths. SG = Specific gravity.

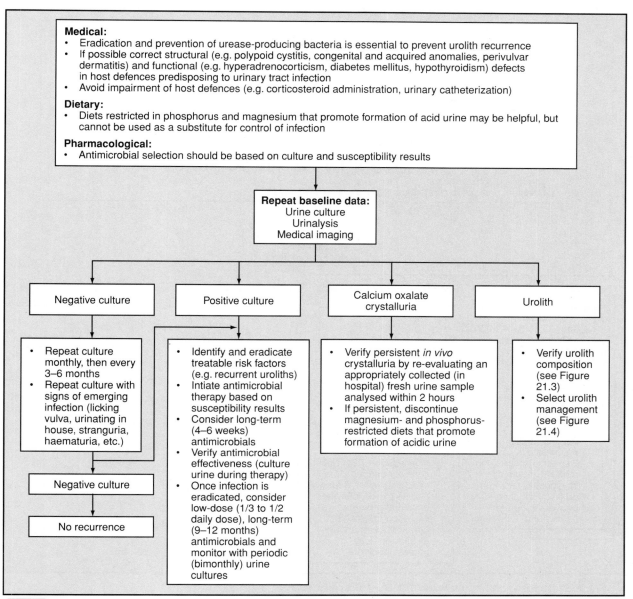

Medical:
- Eradication and prevention of urease-producing bacteria is essential to prevent urolith recurrence
- If possible correct structural (e.g. polypoid cystitis, congenital and acquired anomalies, perivulvar dermatitis) and functional (e.g. hyperadrenocorticism, diabetes mellitus, hypothyroidism) defects in host defences predisposing to urinary tract infection
- Avoid impairment of host defences (e.g. corticosteroid administration, urinary catheterization)

Dietary:
- Diets restricted in phosphorus and magnesium that promote formation of acid urine may be helpful, but cannot be used as a substitute for control of infection

Pharmacological:
- Antimicrobial selection should be based on culture and susceptibility results

Repeat baseline data:
Urine culture
Urinalysis
Medical imaging

Negative culture
- Repeat culture monthly, then every 3–6 months
- Repeat culture with signs of emerging infection (licking vulva, urinating in house, stranguria, haematuria, etc.)

Negative culture

No recurrence

Positive culture
- Identify and eradicate treatable risk factors (e.g. recurrent uroliths)
- Intiate antimicrobial therapy based on susceptibility results
- Consider long-term (4–6 weeks) antimicrobials
- Verify antimicrobial effectiveness (culture urine during therapy)
- Once infection is eradicated, consider low-dose (1/3 to 1/2 daily dose), long-term (9–12 months) antimicrobials and monitor with periodic (bimonthly) urine cultures

Calcium oxalate crystalluria
- Verify persistent *in vivo* crystalluria by re-evaluating an appropriately collected (in hospital) fresh urine sample analysed within 2 hours
- If persistent, discontinue magnesium- and phosphorus-restricted diets that promote formation of acidic urine

Urolith
- Verify urolith composition (see Figure 21.3)
- Select urolith management (see Figure 21.4)

21.14 Strategies to prevent infection-induced struvite uroliths.

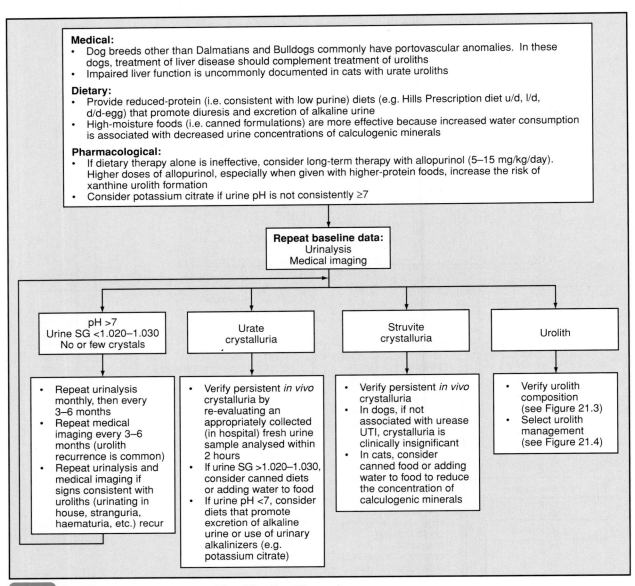

Medical:
- Dog breeds other than Dalmatians and Bulldogs commonly have portovascular anomalies. In these dogs, treatment of liver disease should complement treatment of uroliths
- Impaired liver function is uncommonly documented in cats with urate uroliths

Dietary:
- Provide reduced-protein (i.e. consistent with low purine) diets (e.g. Hills Prescription diet u/d, l/d, d/d-egg) that promote diuresis and excretion of alkaline urine
- High-moisture foods (i.e. canned formulations) are more effective because increased water consumption is associated with decreased urine concentrations of calculogenic minerals

Pharmacological:
- If dietary therapy alone is ineffective, consider long-term therapy with allopurinol (5–15 mg/kg/day). Higher doses of allopurinol, especially when given with higher-protein foods, increase the risk of xanthine urolith formation
- Consider potassium citrate if urine pH is not consistently ≥7

Repeat baseline data:
Urinalysis
Medical imaging

| pH >7 Urine SG <1.020–1.030 No or few crystals | Urate crystalluria | Struvite crystalluria | Urolith |

pH >7 / Urine SG <1.020–1.030 / No or few crystals
- Repeat urinalysis monthly, then every 3–6 months
- Repeat medical imaging every 3–6 months (urolith recurrence is common)
- Repeat urinalysis and medical imaging if signs consistent with uroliths (urinating in house, stranguria, haematuria, etc.) recur

Urate crystalluria
- Verify persistent *in vivo* crystalluria by re-evaluating an appropriately collected (in hospital) fresh urine sample analysed within 2 hours
- If urine SG >1.020–1.030, consider canned diets or adding water to food
- If urine pH <7, consider diets that promote excretion of alkaline urine or use of urinary alkalinizers (e.g. potassium citrate)

Struvite crystalluria
- Verify persistent *in vivo* crystalluria
- In dogs, if not associated with urease UTI, crystalluria is clinically insignificant
- In cats, consider canned food or adding water to food to reduce the concentration of calculogenic minerals

Urolith
- Verify urolith composition (see Figure 21.3)
- Select urolith management (see Figure 21.4)

21.15 Strategies to prevent urate uroliths. SG = Specific gravity.

Medical:
- Hypercalcaemia is uncommon; if detected, its cause should be investigated and controlled
- Hypercalciuria, a risk factor for calcium oxalate urolithiasis, has been associated with hyperadrenocorticism, exogenous glucocorticoid administration and metabolic acidosis

Dietary:
- Avoid calcium supplements and foods containing high quantities of oxalate (e.g. chocolate, peanuts)
- Provide reduced-protein diets (e.g. Hills Prescription diet u/d, g/d) that promote diuresis and formation of alkaline urine
- High-moisture foods (i.e. canned formulations) are more effective because increased water consumption is associated with decreased urine concentrations of calculogenic minerals

Pharmacological:
- Consider potassium citrate if urine pH is not consistently 6.5–7
- Consider vitamin B6 (2–4 mg q24–48h) in patients consuming primarily human diets or diets with unknown or insufficient B6 content
- Consider thiazide diuretics (hydrochlorothizide 2mg/kg q12h) in dogs with highly recurrent disease

Repeat baseline data:
Urinalysis
Medical imaging

pH >7
Urine SG <1.020–1.030
No or few crystals

Calcium oxalate crystalluria

Struvite crystalluria

Urolith

- Repeat urinalysis monthly, then every 3–6 months
- Repeat medical imaging every 3–6 months (urolith recurrence is common)
- Repeat urinalysis and medical imaging if signs consistent with uroliths (urinating in house, stranguria, haematuria, etc.) recur

- Verify persistent *in vivo* crystalluria by re-evaluating an appropriately collected (in hospital) fresh urine sample analysed within 2 hours
- If urine SG >1.020–1.030, consider canned diets or adding water to food
- If urine pH <6.5–7, consider diets that promote formation of less acidic urine or use of urinary alkalinizers (e.g. potassium citrate)

- Verify persistent *in vivo* crystalluria
- In dogs, if not associated with urease UTI, crystalluria is clinically insignificant
- In cats, consider canned food or adding water to food to reduce the concentration of calculogenic minerals

- Verify urolith composition (see Figure 21.3)
- Select urolith management (see Figure 21.4)

21.16 Strategies to prevent calcium oxalate uroliths. SG = Specific gravity.

References and further reading

Davidson EB, Richey JW, Higbee RD, Lucroy MD and Bartels KE (2004) Laser lithotripsy for treatment of canine uroliths. *Veterinary Surgery* 33, 56–61

Hardie EM and Kyles AE (2004) Management of ureteral obstruction. *Veterinary Clinics of North America* 34, 989–1010

Kyles AE, Hardie EM, Wooden BG *et al.* (2005) Management and outcome of cats with ureteral calculi: 153 cases (1984–2002). *Journal of the American Veterinary Medical Association* 226, 937–944

Lekcharoensuk C, Osborne CA, Lulich JP *et al.* (2005) Evaluation of trends in the frequency of calcium oxalate uroliths in the upper urinary tract of cats. *Journal of the American Animal Hospital Association* 41, 39–46

Lulich JP and Osborne CA (1992) Catheter-assisted retrieval of urocystoliths from dogs and cats. *Journal of the American Veterinary Medical Association* 201, 111–113

Lulich JP and Osborne CA (2000) Compound uroliths: treatment and prevention. In: *Current Veterinary Therapy, Vol XIII*, ed. JD Bonagura, pp. 874–877. WB Saunders, Philadelphia

Lulich JP, Osborne CA, Unger LK *et al.* (1993) Nonsurgical removal of urocystoliths by voiding urohydropropulsion. *Journal of the American Veterinary Medical Association* 203, 660–663

Nwadike BS, Wilson LP and Stone EA (2000) Use of temporary nephrosotomy catheters for emergency treatment of bilateral ureter transection in a cat. *Journal of the American Veterinary Medical Association* 217, 1862–1865

Osborne CA, Lulich JP and Bartges JW (ed) (1999a) The Rocket Science of Canine Urolithiasis. *Veterinary Clinics of North America: Small Animal Practice*

Osborne CA, Lulich JP and Polzin DP (1999b) Canine retrograde urohydropropulsion: 25 years of experience. *Veterinary Clinics of North America: Small Animal Practice* 29(1), 267–281

Osborne CA, Lulich JP, Polzin DJ *et al.* (1999c) Analysis of 77,000 canine uroliths: perspectives from the Minnesota Urolith Center. *Veterinary Clinics of North America: Small Animal Practice* 29, 17–39

Wynn VM, Davidson EB, Higbee RD *et al.* (2003) In vitro effects of pulsed holmium laser energy on canine uroliths and porcine cadaveric urethra. *Lasers in Surgery and Medicine* 33, 243–246

22

Management of non-obstructive idiopathic/interstitial cystitis in cats

C.A. Tony Buffington and Dennis J. Chew

Introduction

The vague terms feline urological syndrome (FUS) and feline lower urinary tract disease (FLUTD) were coined to describe cats with signs of lower urinary tract distress and irritative voidings. There was some advantage to these terms in that they did not specify how much of the process was from the urinary bladder, urethra or both. It can be exceedingly difficult to rule lower urinary tract (LUT) inflammation in or out in male cats, as diagnostic evaluation of these organs is limited with presently available technology. Unfortunately, for many veterinary surgeons, the use of these terms came to mean a specific disorder rather than the possibility of several distinct diagnoses.

The term idiopathic cystitis focuses attention on abnormal voiding behaviour after exclusion of other disorders, such as urolithiasis, bacterial urinary infection, anatomical abnormalities and neoplasia. Idiopathic cystitis can be acute or chronic. Interstitial cystitis is a chronic disorder associated with either persistence or frequent recurrence of clinical signs without an obvious cause after a minimal level of diagnostic evaluation.

Interstitial cystitis of cats shares many similarities to interstitial cystitis of humans. A diagnosis of interstitial cystitis in people requires cystoscopic evaluation, revealing the presence of characteristic lesions (submucosal petechial haemorrhages, referred to as glomerulations), although the need for this criterion is under debate. Many cats with idiopathic cystitis also have glomerulations. Urethroscopic lesions are not usually present in affected female cats; urethroscopic lesions are more commonly seen in affected males than in females, although the occurrence is still low. It is likely that the term idiopathic or interstitial cystitis in cats will be supplanted by more specific diagnoses as we improve our understanding of this frustrating syndrome. Results of studies over the past decade indicate that idiopathic cystitis in cats is the result of complex interactions between the bladder, nervous system, adrenal glands, husbandry practices and the environment in which the cat lives (further detailed under Pathophysiology). Idiopathic cystitis is not just a bladder disorder. Moreover, indoor housing and stress have been associated with a number of other common disorders of cats, including behavioural problems, diabetes, dental disease, hyperthyroidism, obesity, separation anxiety disorder and urolithiasis.

Differential diagnosis

In cats less than 10 years of age:

- Idiopathic cystitis is the diagnosis that accounts for clinical signs of irritative urinary voiding in about 60–70% of cats
- Urolithiasis is encountered in about 10–20% of cases, with most being associated with either calcium oxalate or struvite
- About 10% may have an associated structural abnormality, such as urachal diverticulum or urethral stricture
- About 10% have what appears to be a behavioural disorder
- Less than 2% of cases will be associated with urinary infection
- Less than 1% can be expected to have bladder or urethral neoplasia
- Very rarely, LUT signs can be associated with cytoxan treatment that induces cystitis from a metabolite (acrolein), or with parasitic cystitis associated with *Capillaria felis*.

In cats over 10 years of age at time of presentation:

- About 5% of cases can be expected to be idiopathic
- Over 50% of cases will have bacterial urinary infection either alone or in association with urolithiasis. Many of these cats with positive quantitative bacterial cultures will have renal disease and submaximally concentrated urine.

Diagnosis

Signalment

Idiopathic cystitis affects males and females equally, although neutered males and females have increased risk compared with their intact counterparts. Typically, an affected cat is 1–10 years of age (peak risk 2–6 years), spends nearly all of its time living indoors with humans, is expected to use a litter tray for urination and defection and eats 75–100% dry food. Obesity and inappropriate urination are comorbid associations. Owners sometimes note that an affected cat is quite nervous and over-reactive to the environment compared with other cats. Cats with access to the outdoors can still be affected, especially if the cat population in the outdoor area is dense.

History and clinical signs

Signs of idiopathic cystitis are related to voiding urgency due to inflammation (Figure 22.1) and include:

- Increased frequency of urination
- Inappropriate urination
- Stranguria
- Haematuria (Figure 22.2)
- Possibly howling during urination.

Inappropriate urination (urinating in the house outside the litter tray – periuria) is the clinical sign most commonly reported by owners and may sometimes be the only reported sign (22% in one series). It is important to determine if the presenting episode is the cat's first episode of idiopathic cystitis or if it is a recurrent bout. In chronic idiopathic cystitis, documentation of the frequency and severity of the LUT signs is important, as this will be used later to check for the degree of improvement following treatment.

Answers to detailed history questions regarding location of urination, number and type of litter trays, litter substrate, tray cleaning schedule and mechanics are important in identifying risk factors for periuria.

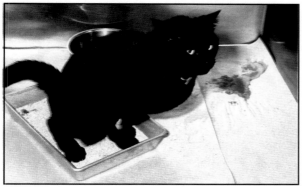

22.1 Stranguria, dysuria and haematuria (stained area on cage papers) in a cat with idiopathic cystitis.

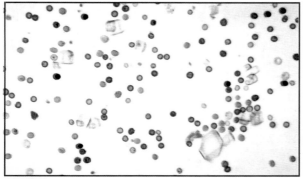

22.2 Urinary sediment with findings typical of cats with idiopathic cystitis. Notice that nearly all the cells are red blood cells. Very few white blood cells are observed in urinary sediment from cats with idiopathic cystitis. A few struvite crystals are also observed in this urinary sediment, but they have no pathological significance in cats with idiopathic cystitis. (Original magnification X100)

Stress in the cat's or owner's lives is often identified during detailed history, and may contribute to creating or perpetuating clinical signs.

Toileting is the deposition of apparently normal urine or faeces in the litter tray without signs of irritative voidings. When toileting occurs outside the litter tray, the volume of deposited urine may be moderate and in one spot, rather than small volumes in several spots that are often produced by cats with idiopathic cystitis. Cats may decide to toilet in particular locations because they have a preference for the substrate there (carpet texture) or have an aversion to the available litter tray and litter type. Aversion to a specific litter type can develop in cats that associate this litter with painful attempts to urinate during acute episodes of idiopathic cystitis. Alternatively, the cat may not use the litter tray because it is not being cleaned adequately or frequently enough.

If the history includes deposition of both faeces and urine outside the litter box, problems related to behaviour or litter tray management are more likely. The locations of urine soiling can provide helpful clues as to the cause. Vertical locations of urine soiling usually indicate spraying and marking behaviour – although spraying with blood-tinged urine has been reported. Urination just outside or near the litter tray suggests suboptimal litter tray management. Are the urine spots single and large, or multiple and small? Single large spots could be a normal urination in an unusual location, again suggesting suboptimal litter tray management. Paw markings on the carpet around the soiled area suggest an attempt to cover the area, a behaviour associated with normal urination in an unusual location. Avoidance of the litter tray or substrate preference (e.g. shag rug) may be the cause. Urination outside the tray in only one location suggests litter tray avoidance or preference of substrate.

Answers to the following questions should be determined for all cats with periuria or signs of irritative voiding:

- How many litter trays are being offered for use and where are they located? The adequate number of litter trays depends on the number of cats in the household. Too few litter trays is often overlooked as a possible cause for not using the litter tray. Easy and private access to litter trays in different locations may be important for providing adequate toileting opportunities for some cats
- What size and depth of trays are being provided? Some trays may not be big enough for specific cats. Some trays may be too high for arthritic or small cats
- Are the trays hooded or uncovered? Some cats prefer the privacy offered by hooded trays, but these trays are often not adequately cleaned by owners since there are few obvious clues from sight or odour
- Is an electrical automated cleaning litter tray used? This type of tray can dramatically increase the cleanliness of the litter, but some cats may become frightened by the noises created by the mechanics of the device
- What type of litter is being used (clumping, non-clumping, scented, silica, paper, corncob, plastic

beads, etc.)? Is the litter type consistent or is the type changed frequently?

- Does the cat fully cover faeces and urine in the tray? Failure to do so suggests less than optimal experience of the cat with the litter substrate (again a toileting issue) that makes the cat less likely to use the litter tray. Failure to cover faeces and urine adequately suggests litter aversion or inadequate depth of litter in the tray

- How frequently is the litter tray cleared of faeces and urine? How often is the litter tray thoroughly emptied of litter and washed? It is important to get a clear picture of the cleaning pattern, as inadequate cleaning and litter maintenance contribute to failure to use the litter tray.

Figure 22.3 provides a detailed survey for indoor-housed cats regarding food and water, litter tray man-

	Yes	No
Food and water		
Each cat has its own food and water bowl in a convenient location that provides some privacy while eating or drinking, and there is an 'escape' route		
Bowls are located such that another animal cannot sneak up on the cat while it eats		
Bowls are located away from appliances or air ducts that could come on unexpectedly while the cat eats or drinks		
Food and water are kept fresh (daily)		
Bowls are washed regularly (at least weekly) with a mild detergent		
The brand or type of food purchased is changed infrequently (less than monthly)		
If a new food is offered, it is put in a separate dish next to the familiar food so the cat can choose to eat it if it wants to		
Litter tray management		
Trays are located on more than one level in multi-level houses		
Trays are located so another animal cannot sneak up on the cat while it uses the tray		
Trays are located away from appliances or air ducts that could come on unexpectedly while the cat uses the tray and there is an 'escape' route		
The litter is kept clean, scooped as soon after use as possible (just like we flush after each use); at least daily		
Trays are washed regularly (at least weekly) with a mild detergent (like dishwashing liquid), rather than strongly scented cleaners		
Unscented clumping litter is used		
The brand or type of litter purchased is changed infrequently (less than monthly)		
If a new type of litter is offered, it is put in a separate tray so the cat can choose to use it if it wants to		
Each cat has its own litter tray in a convenient, well ventilated location that still gives the cat some privacy while using it		
Environmental considerations		
Scratching posts are provided		
Toys are provided, rotated or replaced regularly		
Each cat has the opportunity to move to a warmer or cooler area if it chooses to		
Each cat has a hiding area where it can get away from threats if it chooses to		
Each cat has its own space that it can use if it chooses to		
Rest		
Each cat has its own resting area in a convenient location that still provides some privacy, and an 'escape' route		
Resting areas are located such that another animal cannot sneak up on the cat while it rests		
Resting areas are located away from appliances or air ducts that could come on unexpectedly while the cat rests		
If a new bed is provided, it is placed next to the familiar bed so the cat can choose to use it if it wants to		
Movement		
Each cat has the opportunity to move about freely, explore, climb, stretch and play if it chooses to		
Social contact		
Each cat has the opportunity to engage in play with other animals or the owner if it chooses to		

22.3   Environmental survey for indoor-housed cats. Analysis of answers to these questions is helpful in tailoring individual needs for environmental enrichment.

agement, environmental considerations, resting opportunities, movement and social contact. Responses to these questions will be helpful in prescribing environmental enrichment (see below).

Physical examination

Abdominal palpation may reveal urinary bladder pain and/or thickening of the bladder wall in some affected cats. The bladder is usually small during active bouts of cystitis. The rest of the examination is usually normal. On rare occasions, chewing of hair on the caudal ventral abdomen may be observed, possibly as a reflection of referred pain. Although not reported, it is the authors' opinion that cats with idiopathic cystitis have an increased frequency of heart murmurs and gallop rhythms on auscultation; hypertrophic cardio-myopathy (HCM) is one condition reported to occur in cats with idiopathic cystitis.

Philosophy of how many diagnostics to pursue and when

If this is a young cat's first episode of LUT signs, it can be argued that diagnostics are not needed unless the clinical signs have failed to abate after at least a week. Many cats with idiopathic cystitis will show spontaneous remission of clinical signs during this time. It is, however, customary to evaluate at least a survey abdominal radiograph and urinalysis. The diagnosis of idiopathic cystitis results following exclusion of urolithiasis, urinary tract infection (UTI) and neoplasia, as well as inclusionary findings of clinical history and results from laboratory testing and imaging as noted below.

Urinary tract imaging

Urinary tract imaging is recommended for all cats with recurrent LUT signs. Survey radiographs are helpful to identify radiodense calculi, such as calcium oxalate or struvite, which are usually visible if ≥2–3 mm in size (Figures 22.4 and 22.5). In those cats with multiple

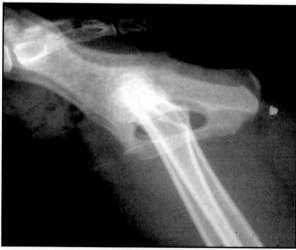

22.5 Caudal abdominal radiograph of a male cat with stranguria and haematuria. It is important to ensure that the perineal region is included in the field of view. Note one radiopaque calculus in the region of the post-prostatic urethra.

recurrences or persistence of clinical signs, advanced urinary tract imaging should be pursued if the survey radiographs were normal, in order to exclude radiolucent calculi and anatomical defects.

Contrast cystourethrography is normal in about 85% of cats with recurrent idiopathic cystitis. Abnormalities that can be identified during double-contrast cystography include focal or diffuse thickening of the bladder wall, permeation of contrast agent into the bladder wall, permeation of contrast medium through the bladder and into the abdomen and filling defects in the contrast medium pool (blood clots and cellular debris) (Figure 22.6). Positive-contrast urethrography in male cats will occasionally document the presence of a focal urethral stricture, although this may be difficult to determine depending on the degree of bladder filling and rate of injection of contrast medium into the urethra (Figure 22.7). Symmetrical annular urethral stricture is very difficult to diagnose. It is important to perform contrast urethrography in male cats that have undergone previous urethral catheterization and now have recurrence of LUT signs.

Ultrasonography can be useful as a less invasive method of imaging than contrast urethrocystography. Bladder wall thickness can be readily measured if the bladder is adequately distended with urine (overestimation of bladder wall thickness occurs when there is minimal distension with urine) (Figure 22.8). Ultrasonography can document the presence of bladder calculi regardless of their radiodensity if they are of sufficient size (>2 mm) (Figure 22.9). Discrimination between urinary debris that settles to dependent bladder locations, urinary 'sand' and small stones is difficult and frustrating even for experienced ultrasonographers. Small stones may not 'shadow' and sometimes debris that piles up appears to shadow. Ultrasonography of affected and normal cats sometimes reveals highly echogenic acoustic interfaces of both suspended and gravitating particles – the origin of these echogenic particles remains to be determined, but they do not

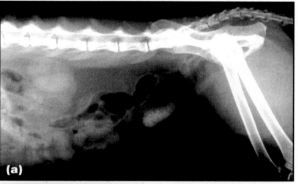

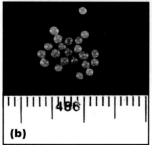

22.4 **(a)** Lateral radiograph of male cat with sudden onset of stranguria. Note the many radiopaque cystic calculi. **(b)** Many small stones were collected following voiding urohydropulsion from the cat in (a). Quantitative stone analysis revealed 100% calcium oxalate. Scale is in millimetres.

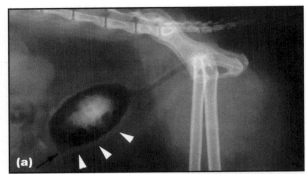

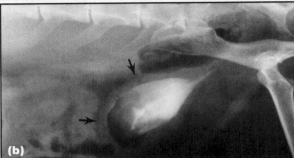

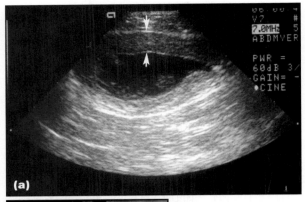

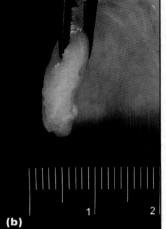

22.6 **(a)** Double-contrast cystogram of male cat with chronic LUT signs. Notice the thickening of the bladder wall (arrowheads). Also notice the outpouching of the cranioventral bladder typical of urachal diverticulum (arrowed). There are numerous irregular filling defects of the central contrast medium pool, probably due to blood clots. A urachal diverticulum can be acquired following obstruction in male cats – it can resolve following relief of obstruction. It is controversial whether a urachal diverticulum is a significant disorder in cats that are not obstructed. This cat does not qualify for a diagnosis of idiopathic cystitis since a structural abnormality was found. **(b)** Double-contrast cystogram of a female cat with chronic LUT signs from idiopathic cystitis. In addition to some filling defects in the central contrast medium pool, there is considerable thickening of the bladder wall throughout all regions of the bladder. Arrows outline the serosal surface of the bladder. Focal or diffuse thickening of the bladder wall occurs in about 15% of cats with chronic idiopathic cystitis that undergo contrast urography. (Courtesy of Dr Paul Barthez.)

22.8 **(a)** Ultrasonogram of the urinary bladder from a cat with chronic LUT signs. Thickening of the bladder is severe in this case (arrowed). The assessment of thickening of the bladder wall on ultrasonography is exaggerated when the bladder contains little urine. Bladder thickening in this case was from idiopathic cystitis. Partial obstruction of the urethra can cause bladder wall thickening that is identical, so it is important to ensure that there are no urethral calculi or strictures. (Courtesy of Dr. Paul Barthez.) **(b)** Thickened bladder wall from a cat that was euthanased for chronic LUT signs from idiopathic cystitis that did not respond to treatment. Much of the thickening was caused by oedema within the bladder wall. Scale is in millimetres. (Courtesy of Dr Jodi Westropp.)

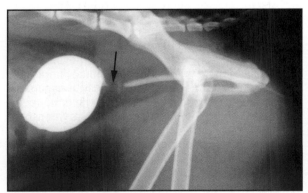

22.7 Positive-contrast urethrogram and cystogram in a male cat with recurrent signs of pollakiuria. This cat was treated 2 months before with an indwelling urinary catheter for urethral obstruction. Notice the filling defect in the proximal urethra – this finding is compatible with a urethral stricture. It is important to perform contrast radiography in cats with recurrent LUT signs, especially males that have previously been treated with indwelling urinary catheters. (Courtesy of Dr Paul Barthez.)

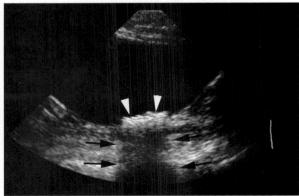

22.9 Ultrasonogram of a female cat after several weeks of haematuria and stranguria. Note multiple small urinary calculi (arrowheads) that create shadowing (arrowed). Although the calculi are obvious in this case, detection of small calculi can be very difficult if the stones do not pile up on each other.

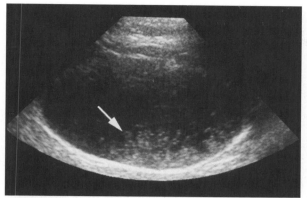

22.10 Ultrasonogram of the bladder of a cat with acute LUT signs from idiopathic cystitis. Notice the highly echogenic acoustic interfaces (arrowed). Urinalysis did not reveal crystals in this case. The nature of these interfaces has yet to be determined, but in the vast majority of cats it is not crystalline (personal observations). (Courtesy of Dr Paul Barthez.)

represent crystals in the vast majority of cases (Figure 22.10). The proximal urethra can be examined with ultrasonography, but most of the urethra cannot be examined.

Uroendoscopy (cystoscopy) is available at some referral centres. Urethroscopy of male cats is possible with the use of very small fibrescopes. Excellent evaluation of the urethra is usually possible. Verification of suspected urethral stricture and evaluation of the urethral mucosa for erosions and haemorrhages can be readily achieved. Detailed evaluation of the bladder mucosa is sometimes possible if there is no bleeding. Excellent evaluation of the urethra and bladder is usually possible in female cats >3 kg using a rigid paediatric cystoscope. The vestibule and urethra are normal in most instances. The bladder of cats with idiopathic cystitis will often display a varying degree of increased vessel numbers, increased vascular tortuosity, oedema and submucosal petechial haemorrhages (glomerulations) (Figure 22.11). Increased number or size of glomerulations and increasing oedema can be observed when higher bladder filling pressure is used during the scoping. These findings are not seen in cats with normal bladders.

Laboratory evaluation

Complete blood count (CBC) and routine serum biochemistry are normal in cats affected with idiopathic cystitis. T4 concentrations and serology for feline leukaemia virus (FeLV) and feline immunodeficiency virus (FIV) should be analysed, as hyperthyroidism or infections with FeLV or FIV can result in abnormal urination behaviour.

Urinalysis

Findings from urinalysis are useful, but are neither sensitive nor specific. The classical findings of haematuria and proteinuria in cats affected with idiopathic cystitis often wax and wane between days and even within the same day. Additionally it is impossible to know with certainty that red cells and protein in the urine did not enter during collection when cystocentesis

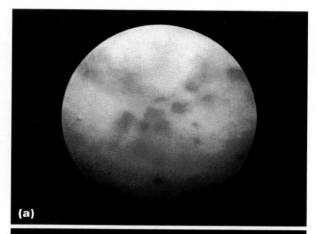

(a)

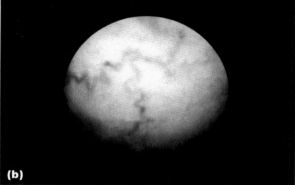

(b)

22.11 **(a)** Cystoscopic view of a female cat with chronic LUT signs from idiopathic cystitis. The round blotches are called 'glomerulations' – submucosal petechial haemorrhages. Not all cats with chronic idiopathic cystitis have glomerulations. Notice also that blood vessel detail has been completely lost due to severe oedema. **(b)** Cystoscopic view of a female cat with chronic idiopathic cystitis. In this case, there are no glomerulations but the bladder is still highly abnormal. Notice the tortuosity of the blood vessels and the bladder wall oedema that causes the vessels to come into and out of view.

is used. The classical positive finding is 'haemorrhagic inflammation', which means that there is a preponderance of red blood cells with few neutrophils in the urine sediment.

Crystals often are not present when fresh urine is evaluated. If crystals are observed, they are usually present in low numbers. Refrigeration can cause the generation of *ex vivo* crystalluria that was not present *in vivo*. Regardless, the presence of crystals has no known diagnostic or pathophysiological impact on non-obstructive forms of idiopathic cystitis. Struvite or calcium oxalate crystals do not damage a healthy urothelium. Conventional wisdom previously held that crystals formed and subsequently caused damage, but it is more likely that sterile inflammation occurs first, plasma proteins exude into urine, urinary pH increases and then struvite crystals precipitate as a secondary event. It is physiologically normal to observe a few crystals in urinary sediment, especially when the urine is highly concentrated.

Urine specific gravity (SG) in healthy cats should be >1.025 in those eating mostly canned foods and >1.035 in those eating exclusively dry foods. In cats with LUT signs and urine SG <1.025, some systemic disease (renal disease, renal failure, hyperthyroidism, diabetes mellitus) may be present that is interfering with the formation of more concentrated urine. Though not specifically studied, it has been the authors' impression that cats with an extremely high urine SG (1.060–1.080) are at higher risk for perpetuation of idiopathic cystitis once initiated if urine concentration is not reduced.

There is no evidence that urine pH has any impact on the pathophysiology or management of cats with idiopathic cystitis. Urine pH depends on a complex interaction of factors, including diet, postprandial alkaline tide, stress-induced acute respiratory alkalosis, the presence of urease-producing bacterial UTI and the degree of entry of plasma proteins (pH 7.3–7.4) into urine from the inflammatory process. Most cats in North America consume foods that tend to acidify the urine. The finding of neutral urine in cats affected with idiopathic cystitis does not necessarily reflect a failure of the diet to acidify the urine.

Microbiology

In urine collected by cystocentesis from young cats with LUT signs, quantitative bacterial culture reveals growth in 1–2 % of the samples. Special cultures for *Ureaplasma* and *Mycoplasma* are routinely negative. It may not be necessary to perform urine culture in cats less than 10 years of age with LUT signs that have a urine SG >1.040, and fewer than five white blood cells (WBC)/high power field (hpf) on urinary sediment examination. Urine culture is recommended for all cats with the following:

- Recurrent LUT signs
- Urine SG <1.040
- Azotaemia
- Previous perineal urethrostomy or history of urethral catheterization within the past 6 months.

Histopathology

Histopathology of the bladder is not usually needed in cats suspected to have idiopathic cystitis. In cats with a very thickened bladder in which bladder cancer cannot be excluded, full thickness bladder biopsy is recommended. The diagnosis is still very likely to be idiopathic cystitis in younger cats even with marked bladder thickening that is asymmetrical. Toluidine blue staining of the tissues should be requested in addition to routine haematoxylin and eosin (H&E) staining in order to reveal the presence, if any, of mast cells which can contribute a component of inflammatory cell infiltration in some cats. Non-specific findings consistent with, but not pathognomonic for, idiopathic cystitis are described under Pathophysiology (below).

Pathophysiology

Risk factors for development of idiopathic cystitis include:

- Neutering (but not age at neutering)
- Indoor living
- Consumption of mostly dry food
- Living in multicat households
- Obesity
- Sedentary life style.

Cats that are obese and sedentary have been shown to have a higher incidence of LUT signs, as do cats that are fed solely dry food or fed intermittently throughout the day. One study found an association between the development of LUT signs and the use of a litter tray coupled with restriction outdoors, recent moves and decreased water intake. Environmental factors, such as interactions with owners, multicat households and changes in routine, have been associated with LUT signs. Breed predispositions found in some epidemiological studies suggest that a genetic component may be important in some cats.

Idiopathic cystitis can be acute or chronic. Clinical signs associated with an initial episode of idiopathic cystitis or a recurrent episode of idiopathic cystitis often resolve with or without treatment within about 7 days. Nearly 50% of cats with idiopathic cystitis will have recurrent signs within 1 year based on recent studies (Kruger *et al.*, 1991; Gunn-Moore and Shenoy, 2004). It appears that most cats with recurrence have episodic signs of idiopathic cystitis, but some have persistent clinical signs that do not abate.

Not much is known about the pathophysiology of the first episode of acute idiopathic cystitis. Clinical signs of the first episode usually resolve quickly so that detailed diagnostics, including bladder histopathology, are not performed. Most of the authors' studies have been in cats with either frequently recurrent idiopathic cystitis or those with persistent idiopathic cystitis (clinical signs may wax and wane but never completely go away). It appears that cats with recurrent idiopathic cystitis may never really be normal even in the absence of clinical signs. Studies of cats with documented idiopathic cystitis that have recovered from detectable clinical signs of their disease still have abnormalities of urothelial integrity, bladder permeability, glycosaminoglycan (GAG) excretion, adrenal hypofunction during stress and a variety of central nervous system changes. Part of the overarching concept in recurrent idiopathic cystitis is the persistence of these abnormalities with or without clinical signs. The development of clinical signs requires predisposing intrinsic abnormalities within a specific cat (bladder, nervous system, adrenal gland) plus extrinsic factors (stressors) that bring the cat to a threshold so that clinical signs will be exhibited.

The pathophysiology of chronic idiopathic cystitis is not fully understood and appears to involve complex interactions between a number of body systems. Abnormalities have been found in the bladder, nervous system, hypothalamic–pituitary–adrenal axis and other body systems in cats with idiopathic cystitis.

Bladder

Histological changes, urothelial abnormalities and decreased excretion of both total urinary GAG and a specific GAG, GP-51, have been identified in the bladders of cats with idiopathic cystitis. Histological changes associated with interstitial cystitis are generally non-specific, and may include:

- An intact or damaged urothelium with submucosal oedema
- Dilation of submucosal blood vessels with marginated neutrophils
- Submucosal haemorrhage
- Sometimes increased mast cell infiltration
- A paucity of neutrophilic infiltration, but there may be a minor increase in lymphoplasmacytic cells in the submucosa.

Scanning electron microscopy reveals patches devoid of superficial epithelial cells and disruption of tight junctions that worsens after hydrodistension. Urothelial abnormalities include hypersensitivity to mechanical stimuli and altered neurotransmitter release. GAG and GP-51 contribute to the surface mucus covering the urothelium that is believed to inhibit bacterial adherence and urothelial injury from the constituents of the urine. Decreased urinary GAG excretion may reflect decreased synthesis of GAG or increased adherence of GAG to damaged urothelial cells. De-

creased urothelial coating with GAG could contribute to increased bladder permeability to constituents of urine.

No correlation between histology and cystoscopic lesions and clinical signs has been identified. In fact, owners' have reported complete remission of LUT signs at times when cystoscopic visualization of their cat's bladder mucosa revealed glomerulations and other abnormalities.

Nervous system

Abnormalities of sensory neurons are present. Sensory neurons reach the bladder via the pelvic and hypogastric nerves, and the central processes of these nerves synapse in the dorsal horn of the sacral and lumbar spinal cord, respectively. These neurons include unmyelinated nociceptive fibres, commonly referred to as C-fibres (Figure 22.12). Recent studies in cats with idiopathic cystitis have identified that these fibres are more sensitive to distension, and have a variety of altered neural properties. These abnormalities were not specific to bladder neurons, however, suggesting that the changes in afferent neuron excitability may be associated with a more general abnor-

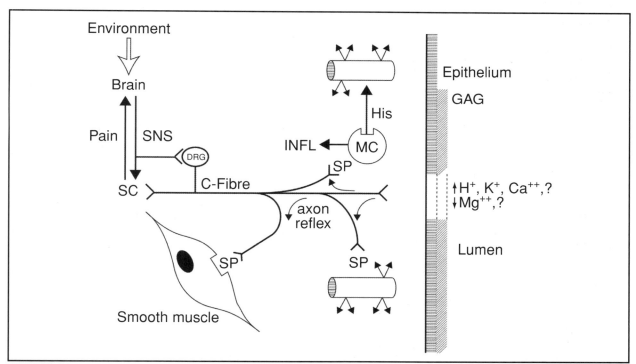

22.12 Neurogenic inflammation as it affects the urinary bladder in interstitial cystitis. Sensory neurons (C-fibres) seem to play a central role in transmission of action potentials via the dorsal root ganglia (DRG). These signals are transmitted by the spiral cord (SC) and may be perceived as painful by the brain. Sensory fibres also can propagate a local axon reflex without transmission of an axon potential. The axon reflex results in release of peptide neurotransmitters such as substance P (SP) by the nerve endings. Interaction of SP with receptors on vessel walls results in vascular leakage that can be augmented by SP-induced release of histamine by mast cells (MC). These actions may give rise to the submucosal petechial haemorrhages observed at cystoscopy. Receptors for SP also occur on smooth muscle, and they stimulate muscle contraction when activated. Also shown are the urothelium (epithelium) and the overlying glycosaminoglycan (GAG) layer adjacent to the bladder lumen. Damage or malfunction of either or both of these layers may permit constituents of the urine, such as protons, potassium ions or hyperosmolar (>2,000 mOsm/l) fluid, to activate the sensory fibres. The effects of stress on sensory fibres may be related to descending efferent sympathetic (SNS) signals stimulating the DRG and inducing peripheral release of neuropeptides. Local release of neurotransmitters by bladder sympathetic fibres could also stimulate sensory fibres. Another factor probably involved in chronic bladder inflammation, but not shown, is local and systemic release of nerve growth factors, which may promote sensory fibre terminal sprouting to increase the size of sensory fibre receptive fields.

mality in the nervous system. This may explain the observation that symptoms of idiopathic cystitis extend beyond the bladder, affecting other organs in the body. Normal cats have far fewer C-fibres that respond to bladder distension compared with cats with idiopathic cystitis.

In the brain, a significant increase in tyrosine hydroxylase (TH) immunoreactivity has been identified in the locus coeruleus (LC) (Barrington's nucleus) as well as the paraventricular nucleus of the hypothalamus in cats with idiopathic cystitis. TH is the rate-limiting enzyme of catecholamine synthesis. Bladder distension stimulates neuronal activity in the LC, and the LC is the origin of the descending excitatory pathway to the bladder. Chronic activation of the stress response system can increase TH activity in the LC, with accompanying increases in autonomic outflow. The LC contains the largest number of noradrenergic neurons, and is the most important source of noradrenaline (norepinephrine) in the feline central nervous system. It is involved in global brain functions, such as vigilance, arousal and analgesia, and appears to mediate visceral responses to stress. The increased TH immunoreactivity observed in the LC of cats with interstitial cystitis may provide a clue to the observation that clinical symptoms of interstitial cystitis follow a waxing and waning course, and can be aggravated by environmental stressors.

In addition to increased LC activity, increased plasma noradrenaline and cerebrospinal fluid (CSF) catecholamine concentrations and their metabolites have been documented in cats with idiopathic cystitis compared with healthy cats, when measured during stressful situations. Alpha 2-adrenoceptors also seem to play a role in the development of interstitial cystitis. Centrally, alpha 2-adrenoceptors are found in the LC and spinal cord, where they inhibit catecholamine release and nociceptive input to the brain. Peripherally, alpha 2-adrenoceptors are found in the bladder mucosa, where they are believed to regulate blood flow. Desensitization of the central alpha 2-receptors as a result of chronic stimulation and enhanced catecholamine release from the bladder of cats with idiopathic cystitis may potentiate the inflammatory response.

Increased noradrenergic outflow may alter urothelial permeability, increasing C-fibre activity, and activate local neurogenic inflammatory mechanisms. Increased epithelial permeability could permit constituents of urine to gain greater access to sensory afferent neurons in the bladder wall, which could result in increased sensory afferent firing and local inflammation. Sympathoneural-epithelial interactions appear to play an important role in bladder permeability, but this does not require direct interaction with epithelial cells.

Hypothalamic–pituitary–adrenal axis

In addition to the sympathetic nervous system, abnormalities in the hypothalamic–pituitary–adrenal axis (HPA) have been observed in cats with idiopathic cystitis. Increased concentrations of corticotropin releasing factor (CRF) from the hypothalamus and adrenocorticotrophic hormone (ACTH) from the anterior pituitary gland have been documented at times of

decreased serum cortisol response to ACTH stimulation during periods of stress in cats with idiopathic cystitis; this indicates reduced adrenocortical reserve in this population. CRF stimulates both the release of ACTH from the anterior pituitary and activation of the sympathetic nervous system in the brainstem.

Reduced adrenal volume (both absolute and relative to body weight) determined by computed tomography (CT) and gross histopathological evaluation have been reported, but no correlation could be found between adrenal size and cortisol production. The areas consisting of the zonae fasciculata and reticularis were significantly smaller in sections of glands from cats with idiopathic cystitis than from healthy cats, whereas the relative area of the adrenal medulla was slightly larger. Although the adrenal glands were small, no obvious histological abnormalities were identified.

During chronic stress in cats with idiopathic cystitis, it appears that there is a disproportionate activation of noradrenergic outflow in the absence of a parallel increase in outpouring of adrenocortical steroids (ACS). This phenomenon may be important, since cortisol and other ACS normally restrain sympathetic nervous system outflow from the LC, and also inhibit their own release by feedback inhibition at the level of the anterior pituitary and hypothalamus to terminate the stress response (Figure 22.13). Decreased ACS activity may adversely affect epithelial permeability, as cortisol is known to enhance tight junction integrity to reduce permeability in other tissues. Since cats with idiopathic

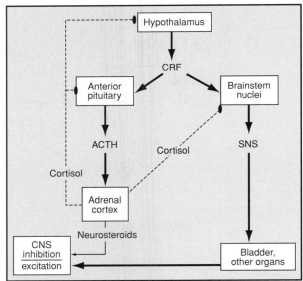

22.13 Imbalanced neuroendocrine system of cats with idiopathic cystitis. Excitatory sympathetic nervous system (SNS) outflow is inadequately restrained by cortisol. This enhanced activity can increase tissue permeability, resulting in increased sensory afferent activity. Feedback inhibition at the level of the anterior pituitary and hypothalamus is also reduced, which tends to perpetuate corticotropin releasing factor (CRF) output. Neurosteroid production by the adrenal cortex, which generally enhances central nervous system (CNS) inhibitory tone during chronic stress, may also be reduced. The solid lines indicate stimulation, the dotted lines indicate inhibition. Line thickness is intended to indicate intensity of the signal.

cystitis do not experience long-term benefits of gluco-corticoid therapy, inadequate production of other ACS (sex steroids, neurosteroids) might play a role in the pathophysiology of this disease, but only cortisol has been studied so far.

Treatment

The waxing and waning natural history of cats with idiopathic cystitis has made it difficult to determine which treatments, if any, are effective. The goals of treatment are:

- To decrease the severity and duration of signs during an acute episode (intra-episode)
- To increase the interval between episodes in those with recurrent idiopathic cystitis (inter-episode)
- To decrease severity of signs in those with persistent idiopathic cystitis.

Based on the pathophysiology described above, it is crucial to reduce the output of the sympathetic nervous system since enhanced noradrenergic outflow appears to potentiate clinical signs by a variety of mechanisms. Based on the premise that cats with idiopathic cystitis are 'sensitive cats in a provocative environment', the goal is to identify and modify provocateurs (diet, water, indoor living with humans, suboptimal animal husbandry, stress, inactivity).

Since chronic pain perception activates noradrenergic outflow, it is important to consider treatments that provide analgesia. Breaking the pain–inflammation cycle can be an important step in the management of some cats with chronic idiopathic cystitis. Providing analgesia centrally appears to be more important than analgesia within the bladder locally.

Evidence-based outcomes of treatment for idiopathic cystitis in cats have recently begun to emerge. Unfortunately, the effect of specific drugs compared with an active placebo has not yet been demonstrated. A high positive response rate to the placebo often occurs when cats enter any study, possibly because the standard of care is increased for all cats that participate, together with regression to the mean, positive owner expectations and classical conditioning. Similar findings have been shown in treatment studies of humans with idiopathic cystitis, in which 50% of the positive outcomes occur in those receiving placebo.

What is a realistic expectation for successful treatment or management of a particular cat with chronic idiopathic cystitis? That will depend to some degree on the specific cat, the ability of the owner and veterinary surgeon to identify risk factors and the owner implementing treatments and changes in husbandry practices. Cats with severe signs of long-standing idiopathic cystitis are often more difficult to manage successfully than those with earlier intervention. The owner's ability and willingness to implement recommendations for the cat's husbandry and changes in the environment will be a big factor determining success or failure. In cats with very high internal risk factors, it may not be possible to bring them below the threshold for develop-

ment of clinical signs despite maximal efforts to decrease or eliminate the external risk factors.

From the veterinary surgeon's point of view, success may be rated based on the history of resolution of clinical signs plus resolution of abnormalities discovered during previous diagnostic work-up, such as haematuria, proteinuria, bladder wall thickening and bladder pain during palpation (although these changes may or may not match resolution of clinical signs). Microscopic haematuria and proteinuria may persist despite resolution of clinical signs.

Most cats can undergo substantial improvement, as perceived by their owners. Success ultimately is defined by the owner's perception of the cat using the litter tray more often (fewer episodes of urinating in the house), less macroscopic haematuria, fewer painful behaviours (stranguria, dysuria, howling, pain when picked up) and improved interactions with the owners. Although it is possible to have resolution of all the LUT signs following treatment for long periods, the owner may still perceive success when only partial improvement is achieved. It is important to remember that events perceived as stressful by the cat can lead to an acute flare of clinical signs.

Different tiers of treatment are prescribed based on the response to initial management recommendations. Additional treatments are given to those cats that fail the first tier of treatment recommendations as noted below. All cats affected with idiopathic cystitis should receive the first tier of recommendations. Their owners should be instructed on how to:

- Clean up urinary house soiling
- Enhance the management of the litter tray
- Provide pain relief
- Enhance water intake
- Reduce the cat's perception of stress
- Provide environmental enrichment when the cat lives mostly indoors with people.

The authors often prescribe a mild dose of tranquillizers (e.g. acepromazine maleate) for severely affected cats with an acute episode or flare. Subsequent tiers of treatment may require more advanced measures of environmental enrichment and drugs.

Prognosis

The prognosis for diseases affected by environmental factors may depend on parameters of the patient, the housing situation and the client.

Patient factors include:

- The animal's genetic predisposition and prior individual experience
- The duration of the problem
- The frequency of occurrences
- The number of areas and different types of surfaces soiled (for inappropriate urination).

Housing factors include:

- The number of cats in the household
- The number of affected cats

- The advisability of allowing limited outdoor access
- The feasibility of rearranging the environment.

Client factors include:

- The owner's ability to identify modifiable causes
- The strength of bond to affected cats
- Their willingness to pay for treatment
- The amount of time available to devote to solving the problem
- The willingness to accept and use adjunctive medications as indicated.

Prognosis for successful treatment of recurrent or chronic idiopathic cystitis will vary with the degree of empowerment attained by the owners. Empowerment of the owner with knowledge, resources and encouragement allows reduction of external risk factors for some cats.

Treatment of a first episode or an infrequent acute flare

Resolution of clinical signs in this population occurs in an estimated 85% of cats within 1 week, often without treatment. However, the recurrence rate for clinical signs is high within the next 6–12 months with conventional treatment. If clinical signs last longer than 7 days spontaneous resolution is unlikely for most cats, so specific recommendations are justified.

Cleaning soiled areas

It is important to clean areas of carpet and furniture that have urine soiling, otherwise other cats in the household may start urinating at these places or the cat with idiopathic cystitis may continue to use these areas for toileting. Counteracting urine that has seeped into carpet padding can be difficult or impossible. Injector kits are available to inject enzymes into padding beneath carpets to breakdown the urine. Although it is tempting to use chemical deodorizers, these products render enzyme treatments useless. Products with strong odours also lessen the effects of feline facial pheromones should they be chosen for use at the same time. In situations with extensive urine soiling, it may not be possible to neutralize urine in the carpet; tearing up the carpet and underlying pad may be the only solution.

Treatment of the cleaned area with aluminium foil, sticky tape or citrus-fragranced deodorants will deter cats from using these areas for toileting.

Analgesia

Relief of bladder pain during acute episodes or flares of chronic idiopathic cystitis is recommended. Although not specifically studied, oral buprenorphine at 5–20 µg/kg q6–12h for 3–5 days has been helpful in providing relief to affected cats in the authors' practice. It is not known whether provision of analgesia for acute episodes affects development of future episodes.

The best regimen of analgesia for bladder pain (visceral) has yet to be determined. Butorphanol has been used but its effect is not as long-lived nor as potent as that of buprenorphine. Fentanyl patches have been used in rare cases in which bladder pain was assessed as severe. There are many anecdotal reports of the usefulness of non-steroidal anti-inflammatory drugs (NSAIDs), especially meloxicam and ketoprofen, but no studies of safety or effectiveness are available for review. Some specialists have prescribed piroxicam for use on alternate days but there are no reports of its effectiveness or safety. NSAIDs are not effective for treatment of idiopathic cystitis in humans. NSAIDs that are licensed for use in cats usually list pre-emptive pain management as a single treatment before anaesthesia and surgery. Chronic use of NSAIDs in cats can be dangerous due to the possibility of development of acute intrinsic renal failure, especially should the cat become dehydrated for any reason at the time of NSAID administration.

Environmental enrichment – level 1

The overarching premise of environmental enrichment is that some cats suffer adverse consequences of indoor housing, especially when cats are forced to spend nearly all of their time indoors in association with people and other animals. Ethological and behavioural studies demonstrate that captivity may elicit a stress response in some cats. The indoor environment of some house cats may be monotonous and predictable, which could be stressful. If we are to continue to recommend indoor housing to reduce the risks of exposure to accidents and infectious agents, recommendations to enrich the indoor environment from the cat's point of view should be developed. Many indoor-housed cats appear to survive adequately by accommodating to less than perfect surroundings. The neuroendocrine abnormalities in cats with recurrent idiopathic cystitis suggest a suboptimal response to stress, indicating that these cats may have greater needs.

Environmental enrichment and modification can reduce stress responses and decrease the severity and intervals of interstitial cystitis episodes. Environmental enrichment strategies consist of:

- Owner education about their cat's disease
- Optimal or enhanced litter tray management routines
- Dietary alterations
- Methods to increase water intake
- Modification of the indoor environment to reduce anxiety
- Working with owners in multicat households to reduce conflict.

Environmental modification may also extend to the manner in which food and water are provided to the cat. The individual cat's preferences are determined for food and feeding, water and watering, litter trays and litter substrates, space and interactions with people and other animals. Increased access to resources can decrease competition for food and water and opportunities for elimination that otherwise contribute to LUT signs. Environmental enrichment is designed to simulate activities that are natural and enjoyable to the cat.

Especially sensitive cats may perceive any change in routine, feeding schedule, owner work schedule, addition or removal of people or pets from the household and the owner's emotions as threatening. Therefore, changes in the environment of a sensitive cat should be kept to a minimum, made gradually and tailored for each individual cat according to the needs and limitations of each cat, owner and household.

Owners of cats and their veterinary surgeons have an obligation to maximize the quality of the indoor living experience for cats that spend most of their time indoors. Indoor housing in unenriched environments does not create idiopathic cystitis, but it can contribute to its development and maintenance by unmasking the tendency of a particular cat to develop idiopathic cystitis in response to external risk factors. The goal of environmental enrichment is to provide excellent environmental modifications that will allow the cat to fall below the threshold for clinical signs of idiopathic cystitis. When environmental enrichment is successfully implemented, activation of the stress response system will decrease, which helps decrease clinical signs of idiopathic cystitis.

Successful environmental enrichment may obviate the need for drug therapy in many instances. Based on uncontrolled prospective studies at the authors' hospital, we estimate that 80% of cats with recurrent idiopathic cystitis will have dramatic reductions in clinical signs over the following year when the first level of environmental enrichment can be successfully implemented. A website devoted to environmental enrichment called 'The Indoor Cat Initiative' can be accessed online at www.indoorcat.org and may be useful both for clients and veterinary surgeons to gain further knowledge in general about idiopathic cystitis and for further resources on enrichment.

Most of the authors' experience has been with implementation of environmental enrichment in cats with recurrent idiopathic cystitis. The concepts espoused here seem likely to benefit cats with a first episode of idiopathic cystitis (actually all cats living mostly indoors). Optimal litter tray management and increased water intake can be considered part of environmental enrichment though they were discussed separately above as part of general husbandry improvements.

How is environmental enrichment provided for cats that live extensively indoors? Understanding some basic concepts regarding cat behaviour and husbandry is important in the development of indoor housing strategies that minimize perception of stress for a particular cat. Although not antisocial, cats evolved as solitary hunters in relatively large spaces. Unlike dogs and people, cats are not pack animals. In the wild, cats eat up to 20 small meals (birds, rodents, insects) per day and display no apparent rhythm to their activities. Dogs and primates are their natural predators. Indoor housing seriously reduces the area available for hunting and roaming activities, no prey are provided and cats are expected to adapt to the rhythmic activities of humans with which they share space. Cats also often live with dogs. In households with cats in the USA, the average have more than two cats per household.

Living with other cats in confinement is inherently stressful for some cats. Owners of cats living with other cats inside rarely note that these animals are stressed, but it is likely that owners or veterinary surgeons poorly recognize conflict and stress in these situations. Some sensitive cats, more than dogs, seem to be affected by living indoors with humans.

Stress in an individual cat can emanate from cat to cat, people to cat, environment to cat or combinations of these. Identification and quantification of stress in cats is quite difficult but strategies for stress reduction are important if successful outcomes in reduction of severity or length of clinical signs of idiopathic cystitis are to be achieved. Cats that perceive chronic threat activate the stress response system, which adversely affects both the physiology and behaviour of some sensitive cats.

Litter tray management: Enhanced management of the litter tray is essential for cats with idiopathic cystitis and for those with toileting problems. The goal is to make the litter tray a pristine place for the cat to eliminate. Nothing should discourage the cat from frequent trips to the litter tray – anything that discourages use of the litter tray may also encourage longer periods of urine retention. This may have adverse effects on cats with idiopathic cystitis, as longer periods of urine retention may facilitate constituents of urine gaining access to the bladder wall (see Pathophysiology), which will amplify the inflammatory response.

A complete discussion of litter trays, types of litter and management is beyond the scope of this chapter. For cats that stay indoors extensively, the number of litter trays that are provided and their locations are extremely important management issues. The general rule for number of litter trays is to have one tray more than the number of cats (n) in the household (i.e. n + 1). The litter trays need to be easily and safely accessible to the cats. Placing litter trays in different locations (and on different levels in multilevel houses) is recommended so that ample toileting opportunities are provided. Placing litter trays in quiet, convenient locations that provide an escape route if necessary for the cat could help improve conditions for normal elimination behaviour. This also reduces the effect of dominant cats that otherwise can prevent access to the elimination area. Whatever schedule of litter tray scooping and cleaning has been previously used, it should be increased. The authors recommend scooping the litter tray twice daily and a full litter exchange weekly for sensitive cats that might be deterred from litter tray use by less vigorous cleaning. The value of providing enough litter trays that are frequently cleaned cannot be overemphasized. Cleaning of litter trays with detergents that leave a strong or citrus odour can discourage some cats from willingly entering the litter tray.

The nature of the tray and the substrate preferred (or avoided) are also important considerations, and optimal use by the cat varies with the individual. Consequently, it may take a while to find the litter tray and litter substrate that are the best for a specific cat. In general, the litter tray needs to be large enough to accommodate the cat completely. Hooded litter trays are problematic in that some cats prefer the privacy, but owners often do not clean them as often, as the odours are contained within. Unscented clumping litter is recommended. It appears that scenting of some litter deters use of the litter tray by some cats. The use of clumping litter has been associated with improved use of the litter tray by cats in some settings; whether all cats prefer clumping litter is debatable. It is also likely that owners clean litter trays more frequently or adequately when clumping litter is used.

Trials with different litter substrates may reveal preferences for one type over another. Having two litter trays next to each other with different substrates is one way to determine which litter may be preferred – multiple tests may be required before a substrate is identified that the affected cat really seems to enjoy. If urine and faeces are not well covered in the litter tray, it is likely that the litter is not something the cat is willing to paw in order to cover the excrement. Well covered faeces and urine spots usually mean that the cat is willing to use that particular litter.

Increasing water intake: Some cats with idiopathic cystitis have extremely concentrated urine based on specific gravity (1.060–1.080), especially if they eat nearly exclusively dry formulations of commercial cat food. Highly concentrated urine is likely to be more irritating to the bladder wall as it gains access from increased bladder permeability that is characteristic of chronic idiopathic cystitis. Changing to the highest percentage of canned food that the cat will eat, or adding water to dry food or to semi-moist food pouches, may be the most powerful single treatment in the prevention of recurrence of the signs of idiopathic cystitis. When water is added to pouches of semi-moist foods, gravy forms that many cats will consume before they eat the wet portion of the more solid food. Cats with recurrent idiopathic cystitis that consumed canned formulations of a veterinary diet compared with a similar formulation of the dry product had far fewer recurrences over the next year. The benefit from canned food has been thought to be due to a substantially lower urine SG compared with that while fed dry foods. With the same renal solute load for excretion, cats with a lower SG must form a larger urine volume and presumably will urinate more frequently than cats with higher SG. Other reasons associated with the feeding of canned foods could include the hedonics (feeling or sensation in the mouth) of this food (altered mood or noradrenergic outflow) and enhanced interactions surrounding feeding between the cat and owners.

To ensure adequate water intake, the cat's water bowl preferences should be determined for freshness, taste and movement (Figure 22.14). Depth of water, type of bowl, flavouring, freshness and the use of fountains all may need to be adjusted until the individual cat's preferences are determined. The use of water fountains, dripping faucets, flavoured water (tuna or clam juice) and bottled water (especially if in heavily mineralized water or chlorinated tap water areas) may increase water intake in some cats. Some cats will drink more water when the water bowl is filled to the top several times a day; other cats prefer to find water in

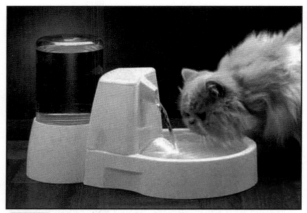

22.14   Water fountain for cats. Running water may increase water intake in some cats. Increased water intake is an important treatment for cats with idiopathic cystitis.

obscure places. Salting the food can increase water intake in cats. Concerns exist about long-term treatment with salt supplementation in cats with regard to chronic renal disease, hypertension and hypercalciuria, which are known to occur in other species on such treatment.

The target urine SG is 1.030 or less to decrease recurrence of clinical signs. It is difficult to impossible to achieve such a low SG in cats that continue to consume mostly dry food. Even when the desired target zone cannot be achieved, any reduction from the previously higher levels has the potential to be helpful.

Food and feeding: Dietary modification should be recommended to increase water intake and decrease the concentration of noxious substances in urine, as described above. However, some cats and owners prefer dry foods and become very stressed by forced transition to canned foods. Attempts to acidify urine further and minimize struvite crystalluria often are not indicated as there is no evidence that struvite crystalluria damages normal urothelium or worsens existing cystitis in non-obstructive forms of idiopathic cystitis. Perhaps more important is maintaining the constancy, consistency and composition of the diet that is being fed.

Constancy refers to minimizing changes in the diet that is being fed. If a change in diet is deemed advisable, it should be the cat's choice to switch to the new diet. For example, if a change is made from dry to moist food, both diets should be made available during feeding. If the cat chooses the moist diet, the dry food can be slowly removed. Consistency refers to the water content of the food. Composition refers to the nutrient content of the diet being fed. Feeding of certain diets may result in excretion of noxious substances in the urine. Highly acidic urine may activate sensory nerve fibres in the urothelium. The optimal diet for cats with interstitial cystitis has yet to be determined, and no commercially available cat foods are specifically designed for the treatment of interstitial cystitis.

Cats prefer to eat individually in a quiet location where they will not be startled by other animals, sudden movement or activity of an air duct or appliance that may begin operation unexpectedly. Natural cat feeding behaviour also includes predatory activities such as stalking and pouncing. These may be simulated by hiding small amounts of food around the house, or by putting dry food in a container, which the cat has to extract individual pieces from or move to release the food pieces, if such interventions appeal to the cat.

Conflict: Inter-cat conflict commonly occurs when several cats are housed indoors together and health problems are present. Conflict among cats can develop because of threats to the cats' perception of their overall status or rank in the home, from other animals in the home or from outside cats. The goal is to reduce conflict to a more manageable level for the cats involved.

Signs of open conflict are easy to recognize. The signs of silent conflict can be so subtle they are easily missed. Threatened cats may attempt to circumvent agonistic encounters by avoiding other cats, by decreasing their activity or both. Threatened cats often spend increasingly large amounts of time away from the family, staying in areas of the house that others do not use, or they attempt to interact with family members only when the assertive cat is elsewhere. Although cats engaged in conflict may spray or eliminate outside the litter tray, threatened cats are more likely to develop elimination problems.

The most common cause of conflict between indoor-housed cats appears to be competition for resources. Cats may engage in open or silent conflict over space, food, water, litter trays, perches, sunny areas, safe places where the cat can watch its environment or attention from people. There may be no obvious limitation to access of resources and conflict can still develop. Open conflict is most likely to occur when a new cat is introduced into the house. Conflict-related urine marking can be exhibited by either the assertive or threatened cat, but idiopathic cystitis usually occurs in the threatened cat.

Treatment for conflict between indoor cats involves providing a separate set of resources for each cat, preferably in locations where the cats can use them without being seen by other cats. Neutering all of the cats can also reduce conflict. Trimming all nails may also be helpful. Whenever the cats involved in the conflict cannot be directly supervised, the threatened cat should be provided a refuge in a separate protected space. Conflict between indoor-housed cats and outside cats can occur when a new cat enters the area around the house where the affected cat lives. To cats, windows are no protection from a threatening cat outside. If outside cats are the source of the problem, a variety of strategies are available to make one's garden less desirable to them.

Toys/prey/play: Environmental enrichment involves providing resources and interactions for cats that simulate some of the activities that they would encounter in the wild. Simulations of prey, including laser lights, lures and feathered fishing pole toys, can be useful interactions for some cats (Figure 22.15). Cats often enjoy playing with toys, particularly those that are

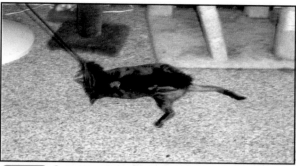

22.15 Cat vigorously playing with a toy that resembles an animal with a furry tail. A variety of toys are available for play activities; some resemble rodents, birds, or insects that simulate some prey of cats. Enhanced play activities for some indoor cats appear to reduce the stress response and LUT signs in those with idiopathic cystitis. (Courtesy of Dr Patricia Schenck.)

small, that move and that mimic prey characteristics. Use of containers or toys that intermittently release food during play may simulate hunting behaviour.

Identifying a cat's 'prey preference' allows one to buy or make toys that the cat will be more likely to play with. Prey preference can be identified by paying close attention to the cat's reaction to toys with specific qualities, such as those that resemble birds (feather toys), small mammals ('furry mice') or insects (laser pointers, pieces of dry food) presented one at a time or together. Expandable tunnels provide opportunities for cats to play by themselves and for hiding. Many cats also prefer novelty, so a variety of toys should be provided and rotated or replaced regularly to sustain their interest.

Play activities with the owners may decrease stress in a cat's life if the owners are not the source of the stress in the first place. Some cats seem to prefer to be petted and groomed, whereas others may prefer play interactions with owners. Cats also can be trained to perform behaviours ('tricks'); cats respond much better to praise than to force, and seem to be more amenable to learning if the behaviour is shaped before feeding.

Although not specifically studied, herbal treatments of toys, scratching posts and bedding may alter behaviour and mood of some cats. Catnip, honeysuckle and valerian root exert dramatic behavioural changes that appear to be very relaxing for some cats.

Space: Cats generally prefer more space than the average house or apartment provides. Cats interact with both the physical structures and other animals, including humans, in their environment. The physical environment should include opportunities for scratching (both horizontal and vertical may be necessary), climbing, hiding and resting undisturbed (Figure 22.16). Cats seem to prefer to monitor their surroundings from elevated vantage points, so climbing frames, hammocks, platforms, raised walkways, shelves or window seats may appeal to them. The addition of elevated spaces, such as shelves, 'kitty condos', cardboard boxes, beds or crates, may provide enough space to reduce conflict in multicat households to a tolerable level and to provide increased stimulation to housed

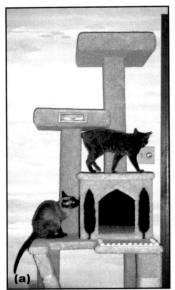

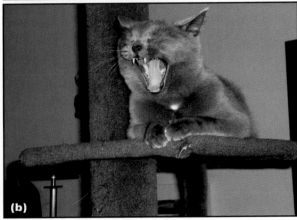

22.16 **(a)** Cat climbing tree designed to enhance activities for cats that live extensively indoors. Many cats enjoy these kinds of devices that provide elevated spaces for them to climb. (Courtesy of Dr. Patricia Schenck.) **(b)** This cat spends a considerable amount of time surveying the area from this height and relaxes here. Providing elevated spaces appears to be important in reduction of stress in some cats that live indoors. (Courtesy of David Beauvais.)

cats in general. Playing a radio to habituate cats to sudden changes in sound and human voices has also been recommended. Videotapes to provide visual stimulation from possible prey are available and seem to be captivating for some cats.

Pheromonotherapy

Synthetic feline facial pheromones are marketed to reduce urine marking or spraying behaviours in cats. Natural pheromones from the head and cheeks are rubbed by cats on to objects in their environment as a means of communicating familiarity and noting them as non-threatening. The pheromones exert a calming effect and reduce the vigilance of the cat so that the need to mark or spray territory is reduced. Since vigilance of cats is maintained largely by activity of the sympathetic nervous system, it is possible that use of these pheromones contributes to decreased adrenergic outflow from the brainstem in some cats. If so, they could be useful for treatment of chronic idiopathic cystitis in cats. A statistically significant effect could not be demonstrated in a study of affected idiopathic cystitis cats between facial pheromones and placebo, though there appeared to be a positive trend (Gunn-Moore and Shenoy, 2004). There appears to be a powerful salutary effect of these pheromones in some

cats (personal observations) and the authors continue to prescribe their use. The authors prefer the electric room diffuser form which continually disperses the pheromone (Figure 22.17). One or more diffusers should be placed in rooms where the cat may be the most stressed: near windows and doors, soiled furniture and/or the litter tray. The authors recommend the use of pheromonotherapy in cats with recurrent idiopathic cystitis during implementation of environmental enrichment (including enhanced water and litter tray dynamics) or after environmental enrichment has failed.

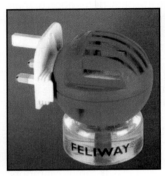

22.17 Pheromone room diffuser. Feline facial pheromones are useful in the reduction of urine marking in cats. Some cats are believed to benefit from the calming effect induced by these pheromones, although they are not definitively proven to be helpful in cats with idiopathic cystitis.

Frequent recurrence or persistence of signs

Further environmental enrichment – level 2

If initial implementation of environmental enrichment at level 1 was not helpful in adequately reducing the signs of idiopathic cystitis, it is important to go back and review what was implemented and what was not. Alternative attempts at enrichment should be suggested for those that were not initially implemented. Additional enrichments may be added at this time.

Increased exposure to the outdoors can be helpful in the management of some cats. A dramatic improvement occurs in some cats that are allowed at least a few hours of outdoor activities daily. Partial access to the outdoors can be attempted in contained yards or with the use of enclosures on patios or special fences designed to keep pet cats inside and prevent access of other outside cats. In some areas, increased exposure to the outdoors may actually be damaging if the density of cats in that area is particularly high.

Drugs

Drug therapy is not attempted until analgesics have been administered and level 1 environmental enrichment implemented without adequate resolution of clinical signs (including low-grade persistent signs or frequent recurrence of clinical signs). A summary of drugs used in treatment of idiopathic cystitis is given in Figure 22.18.

Tricyclic analgesics/antidepressants: Tricyclic analgesics/antidepressants (TCA) can exert powerful effects that decrease clinical signs in cats with recurrent idiopathic cystitis (Chew *et al.*, 1998), even in the absence of change in cystoscopic appearance. Although many different mechanisms could account for a salutary effect of TCA, none has been proven in a

Analgesic	Class	Indications	Dose	Potential side effects
Acute therapy				
Butorphanol	Synthetic partial opioid agonist	Acute episodes	0.2–0.4 mg/kg orally, s.c. q8h	Sedation
Buprenorphine	Synthetic partial opioid agonist	Acute episodes	0.01–0.02 mg/kg q8–12h; 0.015 mg/kg orally q8–12h (anecdotal)	Sedation
Fentanyl	Opioid agonist	Acute episodes	25 µg/hour	Respiratory depression; bradycardia
Bladder/urethral contractility				
Acepromazine maleate	Phenothiazine derivative	For sedation and antispasmodic for urethral obstruction	0.05 mg/kg s.c. q8h	Hypotension; sedation
Prazosin	α1-adrenoceptor antagonist	Sedation, antispasmodic for urethral obstruction	0.05 mg/kg s.c. q8h	Hypotension
Phenoxybenzamine	α1-adrenoceptor antagonist	Sedation, antispasmodic for urethral obstruction	2.5 mg orally q12h	Hypotension
Chronic therapy				
Amitriptyline	Tricyclic antidepressant	Idiopathic cystitis	5–12.5 mg orally q12–24h	Sedation; weight gain; urine retention; urolith formation
Clomipramine	Tricyclic antidepressant	Idiopathic cystitis; urine spraying	0.5 mg/kg orally q24h	Sedation; anticholinergic effects
Buspirone	A non-benzodiazepine anxiolytic agent	Idiopathic cystitis; urine spraying; anxiety	2.5–5 mg orally q12h	Rare but sedation or other neurological effects
Fluoxetine	Antidepressant	Idiopathic cystitis; urine spraying	1 mg/kg orally q24h	Decreased food intake; vomiting and lethargy are rare
Pentosan polysulphate sodium	Glycosaminoglycan (GAG) supplement	Idiopathic cystitis	50 mg orally q12h	Diarrhoea; vomiting (rare)
F3 fraction of feline facial pheromone	Synthetic pheromone	Anxiety Idiopathic cystitis	1 spray in affected area q24h or room diffuser	None reported

22.18 Drugs commonly used to treat and manage cats with idiopathic cystitis.

setting of natural disease in cats. Possible mechanisms for the effects of TCA on bladder inflammation include:

- Stabilization of mast cells which may infiltrate the bladder wall during idiopathic cystitis
- Reduced contractions of detrusor muscle from anticholinergic effects
- Decreased sensory nerve pain fibre sensations from the bladder
- Effects on sodium, potassium and glutamate channels
- Downregulation of noradrenaline outflow from the brain due to its effects as a central noradrenaline-reuptake inhibitor.

There is no benefit from the use of TCA to treat acute bouts of idiopathic cystitis, as shown in two recent studies (Kraijer *et al.*, 2003; Kruger *et al.*, 2003). Abrupt cessation of TCA administration after 7 days increased the severity of clinical signs and frequency of recurrence in one study of amitriptyline for treatment of acute idiopathic cystitis (Kruger *et al.*, 2003).

Amitriptyline caused resolution of clinical signs in 60% of cats with severe recurrent idiopathic cystitis for one year during administration of 10 mg once daily orally at the owner's bedtime. Despite the decrease in clinical signs there was no improvement in the cystoscopic appearance of the bladder mucosa (Chew *et al.*, 1998).

The use of TCA is considered only when other treatments described above have not been helpful. Cats often have markedly decreased clinical signs of idiopathic cystitis during such treatment with amitriptyline, the TCA with which the authors have had the most experience. Despite the improvement in clinical signs, the behaviour of these cats is different and is associated with weight gain and poor grooming. If the situation is desperate for the owner and the clinical signs severe, the authors recommend starting with 10 mg amitriptyline once daily. If there is less urgency for immediate improvement, one may start with 5 mg once daily and either decrease or increase the dose to an eventual 2.5–12.5 mg total daily dose of amitriptyline.

Sometimes TCA can be given while environmental enrichment is being implemented. If environmental enrichment is successful in reducing the cat's stress, it may be possible to taper the dose of TCA gradually and, in some instances, to stop this form of medication.

Some cats have a better resolution of clinical signs of idiopathic cystitis when treated with clomipramine rather than with amitriptyline. Treatment with fluoxetine has also been effective in treatment of idiopathic cystitis in some cats. Treatment with behaviour-modifying drugs has the possibility of decreasing the activity of the sympathetic nervous system that could exert benefits on chronic idiopathic cystitis.

Due to possible effects on liver enzymes or function during administration of TCA, a serum biochemical panel is recommended prior to starting the drug and again at 1, 3 and 6 months during treatment. A complete blood count (CBC) is also recommended to ensure no adverse effects of chronic treatment are occurring (thrombocytopenia and neutropenia). TCA should be used cautiously, if at all, in cats with serious heart disease.

Glycosaminoglycan supplementation: Since GAG excretion in cats affected with idiopathic cystitis is decreased compared with healthy cats, it was hypothesized that supplemental GAG treatment might heal the highly permeable bladder that is encountered in idiopathic cystitis. Studies to date have not shown a benefit of glucosamine or pentosan polysulphate (PPS) supplementation over that of placebo in cats with idiopathic cystitis. In humans with idiopathic cystitis, PPS treatments appear to work in about 10% more patients than does placebo. Whether GAG supplementation has a benefit in combination with other treatments, such as TCA or environmental enrichment, has not been investigated in cats. Diarrhoea at routine doses and coagulopathy at high doses are possible side effects of GAG supplementation, but are rare.

Antibiotics: Since bacterial urinary infections are exceedingly uncommon in cats less than 10 years of age, it is very unlikely that antibiotics have a role in treatment of most LUT conditions in cats. An exception would be in male cats that have previously undergone perineal urethrostomy or those that have been catheterized within the previous 6 months. In these populations, as well as in cats with submaximally concentrated urine (SG <1.030), much greater risk of a true bacterial urinary tract infection exists.

Conclusions

Converging evidence from a variety of studies suggests that idiopathic cystitis in some cats is more likely to be a disorder affecting the bladder than a primary bladder disorder. Thus, idiopathic cystitis in these cats may be more comparable to diabetes or spinal cord injury than to a urinary tract infection or bladder tumour. The fact that the clinical signs of all these (and other) conditions are similar may be related more to the limited number of responses the bladder is capable of mounting than to the location of the insult.

Cats with idiopathic cystitis have variably severe involvement of the stress response system (internal factors), and are exposed to a range of environmental stimuli (external factors). Given the current state of our knowledge, we have limited capacity to treat the internal factors, and so therefore have focused on modification of external factors pending development of strategies to modulate the activity or output of the stress response system.

Although many indoor-housed cats appear to accommodate to a wide range of surroundings, the neuro-endocrine abnormalities in cats with idiopathic cystitis do not seem to permit them the adaptive capacity of healthy cats. Although environments may appear adequate for healthy cats, we should focus on external factors to accommodate the limitations of cats with idiopathic cystitis. Moreover, since external factors have been shown to unmask susceptibility to many common chronic diseases in cats, environmental enrichment is recommended as preventative healthcare for all cats, just as appropriate vaccination and provision of satisfactory nutrition are recommended.

References and further reading

Barsanti JA, Brown J, Marks A *et al.* (1996) Relationship of lower urinary tract signs to seropositivity for feline immunodeficiency virus in cats. *Journal of Veterinary Internal Medicine* **10(1)**, 34–38

Buffington CA (2002) External and internal influences on disease risk in cats. *Journal of the American Veterinary Medical Association* **220(7)**, 994–1002

Buffington CA (2004) Comorbidity of interstitial cystitis with other unexplained clinical conditions. *Journal of Urology* **172(4)**, 1242–1248

Buffington CA, Chew DJ and DiBartola SP (1996) Interstitial cystitis in cats. *Veterinary Clinics of North America: Small Animal Practice* **26(2)**, 317–326

Buffington CA, Chew DJ, Kendall MS *et al.* (1997) Clinical evaluation of cats with nonobstructive urinary tract diseases. *Journal of the American Veterinary Medical Association* **210(1)**, 46–50

Buffington CA, Chew DJ and Woodworth BE (1999) Feline interstitial cystitis. *Journal of the American Veterinary Medical Association* **215(5)**, 682–687

Cameron ME, Casey RA, Bradshaw JW, Waran NK and Gunn-Moore DA (2004) A study of environmental and behavioural factors that may be associated with feline idiopathic cystitis. *Journal of Small Animal Practice* **45(3)**, 144–147

Chew DJ, Buffington CA, Kendall MS, DiBartola SP and Woodworth BE (1998) Amitriptyline treatment for severe recurrent idiopathic cystitis in cats. *Journal of the American Veterinary Medical Association* **213(9)**, 1282–1286

Gunn-Moore DA and Cameron ME (2004) A pilot study using synthetic feline facial pheromone for the management of feline idiopathic cystitis. *Journal of Feline Medicine and Surgery* **6(3)**, 133–138

Gunn-Moore DA and Shenoy CM (2004) Oral glucosamine and the management of feline idiopathic cystitis. *Journal of Feline Medicine and Surgery* **6(4)**, 219–225

Hostutler RA, Chew DJ and DiBartola SP (2005) Recent concepts in feline lower urinary tract disease. *Veterinary Clinics of North America: Small Animal Practice* **35(1)**, 147–170

Kraijer M, Fink-Gremmels J and Nickel RF (2003) The short-term clinical efficacy of amitriptyline in the management of idiopathic feline lower urinary tract disease: a controlled clinical study. *Journal of Feline Medicine and Surgery* **5(3)**, 191–196

Kruger JM, Conway TS, Kaneene JB *et al.* (2003) Randomized controlled trial of the efficacy of short-term amitriptyline administration for treatment of acute, nonobstructive, idiopathic lower urinary tract disease in cats. *Journal of the American Veterinary Medical Association* **222(6)**, 749–758

Kruger JM, Osborne CA, Goyal SM *et al.* (1991) Clinical evaluation of cats with lower urinary tract disease. *Journal of the American Veterinary Medical Association* **199(2)**, 211–216

Lavelle JP, Meyers SA, Ruiz WG *et al.* (2000) Urothelial pathophysiological changes in feline interstitial cystitis: a human model. *American Journal of Physiology. Renal Physiology* **278(4)**, F540–553

Markwell PJ, Buffington CA, Chew DJ *et al.* (1999) Clinical evaluation of commercially available urinary acidification diets in the management of idiopathic cystitis in cats. *Journal of the American Veterinary Medical Association* **214(3)**, 361–365

Osborne CA, Kruger JM, Lulich JP and Polzin DJ (1999) Feline urologic syndrome, feline lower urinary tract disease, feline interstitial cystitis: what's in a name? *Journal of the American Veterinary Medical Association* **214(10)**, 1470–1480

Westropp JL and Buffington CA (2002) In vivo models of interstitial cystitis. *Journal of Urology* **167(2)**, 694–702

Westropp JL and Buffington CA (2004) Feline idiopathic cystitis: current understanding of pathophysiology and management. *Veterinary Clinics of North America: Small Animal Practice* **34(4)**, 1043–1055

Westropp JL, Welk KA and Buffington CA (2003) Small adrenal glands in cats with feline interstitial cystitis. *Journal of Urology* **170(6)**, 2494–2497

23

Management of urinary tract infections

David F. Senior

Introduction

Urinary tract infection (UTI) is most commonly a consequence of ascending migration of bacteria through the genital tract and urethra to the bladder. Colonization can subsequently extend to the ureters and kidneys. Host defences against UTI are usually effective and the proximal urethra, bladder, ureters and kidneys are normally sterile. The distal urethra and external genitalia have a normal flora and are constantly exposed to potential colonization by enteric organisms. Cultures of the vaginal and preputial flora usually grow a wide variety of bacteria, some of which may be potential uropathogens. Occurrence of UTI is determined by the balance between two opposing forces: bacterial invasiveness and host defences.

Bacterial virulence

Uropathogens are derived from the faecal flora and gain access by colonization of the perineum and external genitalia followed by ascending infection (Low *et al.*, 1988; Wadas *et al.*, 1996; Chen *et al.*, 2003). Properties of bacteria that enable them to colonize, penetrate tissue and induce disease are called virulence factors (Figure 23.1). Important factors often expressed by uropathogenic microorganisms include (Senior *et al.*, 1992; Yuri *et al.*, 1998; Chen *et al.*, 2003):

- Expression of adhesins, which enable bacteria to attach to uroepithelial cell binding sites
- Toxin production
- Urease production
- Expression of certain O:K:H serotypes in coliform bacteria
- Production of bacteriocins, which inhibit the growth of other bacteria
- Production of haemolysins and iron-chelating agents that enable bacteria to scavenge iron, an essential requirement for bacterial growth.

Vaginal colonization by uropathogens involves interaction with the normal flora. Bacteriocins produced by one strain of bacteria interfere with metabolism of other strains and different strains compete for epithelial binding sites and essential nutrients, e.g. iron. Virulent bacteria tend to produce haemolysin and iron-binding molecules, such as aerobactin. Following genital colo-

Expression of fimbriae
Expression of specific adhesins
Serotypes
Haemolysin production
Aerobactin production
Endotoxin and exotoxin production
Urease production
Colicin production

23.1 Bacterial virulence factors.

nization, bacterial uropathogens must travel along the urethra to the bladder. The intrinsic motility of some bacteria may aid in their retrograde migration through the excretory pathway but even if they are not motile, bacteria can progressively grow along the urethral wall. Turbulent urine flow caused by anatomical defects can assist ascent of bacteria into the bladder.

Recent evidence strongly supports a major role of bacterial adherence in colonization of vaginal and urethral surfaces and uroepithelial cells. Bacterial adherence to epithelial surfaces is achieved by molecular binding between bacterial structures and specific receptor sites on the uroepithelial surface. Specific molecular structures, adhesins, bind with complementary receptor sites on epithelial cell surfaces. Once a sufficient number of adhesin–receptor interactions occur, bacteria are firmly attached. The molecular structure of a number of adhesins and receptors has been established. Lipotechoic acid appears to be the adhesin of group A streptococci. The complementary epithelial receptor site remains unknown, but evidence suggests that it may be an albumin-like membrane protein or lipoprotein. Strains of *Escherichia coli* give rise to fimbriae with adhesins that bind to carbohydrate and sialic acid components expressed on the surface of host epithelial cells (Senior *et al.*, 1992; Backhed *et al.*, 2003). Further protein-to-protein binding can occur between bacterial fimbriae and host extracellular matrix to facilitate colonization of subepithelial tissue (Westerlund *et al.*, 1993).

Bacteria can express more than one adhesin at the same time or may vary expression of adhesins based on environmental conditions. This phenomenon may be important in different phases of tissue invasion because mannose-sensitive adhesins render bacteria more susceptible to phagocytosis. Bacteria that undergo rapid phenotypic variation, so that adhesins are not expressed once tissue invasion begins, are less susceptible to phagocytosis. The on–off switch for expression of bacterial adhesins is located in DNA.

Bacterial adherence is essential to subsequent tissue invasion. Toxins produced by attached bacteria more readily interact with toxin receptor sites on the uroepithelial cell surface rather than being inactivated by urine and mucus. Among the most important toxins are:

- Bacterial endotoxin, which induces a major immune-system response via tumour necrosis factor, interleukin-1 and interleukin-6
- Urease, which induces high ammonium (NH_4^+) levels in urine. High NH_4^+ levels promote bacterial attachment by disrupting the surface protective glycosaminoglycan (GAG) layer on the uroepithelium (Parsons *et al.*, 1984) and bacterial urease production facilitates renal colonization and tissue damage (Johnson *et al.*, 1993).

The clonal theory of bacterial virulence is based on the observation that the majority of UTIs caused by *E. coli* are due to four to six main serotypes, both in humans and dogs (Senior *et al.*, 1992; Kurazono *et al.*, 2003). These data suggest that certain O:K:H serotypes are more virulent, although the virulence may not be attributable to the antigenic properties of the strains *per se* but rather to other properties genetically associated with expression of these particular serotypes.

Host defence mechanisms

A wide range of host defence mechanisms to prevent bacterial colonization have been identified or hypothesized (Figure 23.2).

Normal micturition

The hydrodynamics associated with voiding urine are thought to represent one of the most important natural defence mechanisms against infection of the urinary tract. The effectiveness of voiding as a defence is dependent on the rate of urine production and flow, the frequency of voiding and the completeness of emptying (the amount of residual volume). Disorders that impair the frequency or volume of micturition, or that permit residual urine to remain in the urinary bladder following micturition predispose to infection. Urethral stricture secondary to fibrosis, hypertrophy and tumours may interfere with normal urine outflow and ulcerated areas of tumours and polyps provide sites for microbial colonization. Furthermore, incomplete bladder emptying secondary to spinal lesions and acquired or congenital atonic bladder will predispose to UTI. Urine retention for prolonged periods in apartment-dwelling pets expected to go for long periods between voiding may also be a factor.

Anatomical structures

The presence of a high-pressure zone in the urethra of bitches has been hypothesized to inhibit the migration of bacteria from the distal urethra into the proxi-

Normal micturition
Adequate urine flow
Frequent voiding
Complete voiding

Anatomical structures
Urethral high-pressure zone
Surface characteristics of urethral urothelium
Urethral peristalsis
Prostatic antibacterial fraction
Length of urethra
Ureterovesical flap valves and ureteral peristalsis

Mucosal defence barriers
Antibody production
Surface glycosaminoglycan layer
Intrinsic mucosal antimicrobial properties
Bacterial interference
Exfoliation of cells

Antimicrobial properties of urine
Extremes (high or low) of urine pH
Hyperosmolality
High concentration of urea
Organic acids

Renal defences
Glomerular mesangial cells?
Extensive blood supply and large blood flow

23.2 Host defence mechanisms.

mal urethra and bladder. Further inhibition of movement of bacteria towards the bladder may be provided by symmetrical peristaltic contractions of the urethra which have been identified in male dogs. The oblique passage of the ureters through the bladder wall prevents vesicoureteral reflux; however, manual bladder compression to express urine may induce vesicoureteral reflux. Any disease that causes excessive intravesicular pressure, e.g. outflow obstruction, can induce reflux.

Congenital anomalies may lead to increased susceptibility to infection. Ascending infections with pyelonephritis frequently accompany ectopic ureters (Lamb and Gregory, 1998). Although infrequent in dogs, urachal diverticula may provide a site for bacterial colonization and chronic UTI. Vulval involution is thought to predispose dogs to recurrent UTI (Crawford and Adams, 2002). Devitalized skin in the involuted vulval folds leads to the establishment of an abnormal bacterial flora adjacent to the opening of the vulva. Vulvovaginal stricture has also been implicated as an anatomical abnormality predisposing to UTI but the precise mechanism for this is not clear (Crawford and Adams, 2002).

Cats with perineal urethrostomy tend to develop UTI, presumably because the altered anatomy promotes the establishment of an abnormal microbial flora in the vicinity of the newly constructed urethral opening, and also because defence factors intrinsic to the normal anatomy of the distal urethra have been lost.

Mucosal defence barriers

Local antibody production is thought to be important in the prevention of UTI because bacteria coated by antibodies are less able to attach to the uroepithelium. Urine contains a significant quantity of IgG and secretory IgA, which may be important in the prevention of UTI (Uelling *et al.*, 1999). Bacterial attachment to the uroepithelium also appears to be impaired by surface layer GAGs (Parsons *et al.*, 1988). In some species normal GAG production is controlled by oestrogen and progesterone. Normal epithelial exfoliation may further contribute to mucosal resistance to permanent bacterial colonization.

Direct trauma caused by urethral catheterization, urolithiasis, neoplastic invasion and chemical irritants, such as cyclophosphamide, are all capable of disrupting the normal mucosal defence mechanisms. Long-term catheterization (more than 4 days) causes a high percentage of dogs to develop UTI (Smarick *et al.*, 2004).

Antimicrobial properties of urine

Urine appears to inhibit bacterial growth at extremely high pH, extremely low pH and when very concentrated. A tendency toward more alkaline urine, a normal consequence of some diets, may enhance growth of some bacteria, such as *Proteus* species. Dilute urine tends to support bacterial growth better and will predispose to UTI. Paradoxically, a high urine output will tend to inhibit bacterial colonization of the kidney. Inhibitory effects in hyperosmolar urine may be related to the high concentration of urea. The extremely concentrated urine of younger cats may enhance the antimicrobial properties of urine and render them resistant to UTI. In cats, UTI is quite rare in animals under 7 years old. As cats get older, renal concentrating capacity can be reduced and the lower urine concentration seen in older cats may explain in part why UTI is more common in this life stage. A high incidence of UTI (39%) has been recorded in dogs given corticosteroids and affected animals exhibited minimal to no clinical signs with little evidence of inflammation in the urine sediment (Ihrke *et al.*, 1985). The high rate of infection could be due in part to dilute urine, but other factors related to immunosuppression and altered skin microflora could be involved.

Hepcidin, a recently identified cysteine-rich peptide that is produced in the liver and excreted in the urine appears to inhibit growth of some uropathogens (Park *et al.*, 2001; Fry *et al.*, 2004). Hepcidin is conserved in many species, including the dog, and is known to regulate iron metabolism (Park *et al.*, 2001; Fry *et al.*, 2004).

The consequences of UTI are variable. In many cases, infection will be transient, signs will be minimal and the condition responds readily to treatment. In some cases, however, infection persists or frequent recurrences occur. Severe acute or chronic renal infection can lead to renal failure.

Causative organisms

The most frequent isolates are shown in Figure 23.3. *E. coli* is the most common isolate with *Staphylococ-*

Bacterial isolate	Percentage of total isolates (n = 8,354)
Escherichia coli	44.1
Staphylococcus spp.	11.6
Proteus spp.	9.3
Streptococcus spp.	5.4
Klebsiella spp.	9.1
Enterococcus spp.	8.0

23.3 Bacterial isolates in canine urinary tract infection (Ling *et al.*, 2001).

cus spp., *Streptococcus/Enterococcus* spp. and *Proteus* spp. less common (Ling *et al.*, 2001). *Mycoplasma canis* has been reported to cause UTI with the most complete description of this infection reported in Norway (L'Abbee-Lund *et al.*, 2003). Fungal infections, including *Candida* spp., have been described in immunocompromised patients (Pressler *et al.*, 2003). *Aspergillus terreus* has been identified in the urine sediment and on urine culture of dogs with disseminated fungal infection that also involved the kidneys (Kabay *et al.*, 1985).

Management of simple urinary tract infection

Diagnosis

When an active infection causes irritation, animals exhibit urgency to urinate, pollakiuria, unproductive straining to urinate at the end of urination and haematuria. A strong urine stream may not be developed. Owners can also report urinary incontinence between urinations and an offensive odour to the urine. However, in subacute, long-standing infections and in dogs with hyperadrenocorticism, clinical signs may be present but attenuated. A large proportion of canine patients with UTI exhibit minimal clinical signs.

On physical examination, there may be increased sensitivity to palpation of the bladder and the animal may be febrile if there is significant acute renal or prostatic involvement or the inflammation of the bladder is massive. When inflammation is confined to the lower urinary tract, fever does not generally occur. The bladder is often painful on palpation in acute cystitis and, in both acute and chronic cystitis, the bladder tends to feel thickened.

The interpretation of urinalysis and bacterial culture results depends upon the method of collection. Urine samples for urinalysis and culture are best obtained by cystocentesis because results are much easier to interpret. However, this procedure can be difficult to perform in patients with UTI because they tend to pass small volumes of urine frequently and the bladder may remain small and not readily palpable. Although catheterization can be used to collect urine for urinalysis and culture, the procedure introduces bacteria into the urinary tract and traumatizes the uroepithelium. Mid-stream voided samples may be suitable for routine screening evaluation of urine, but this method of collection is not recommended for urine culture.

On urinalysis, bacteria, white blood cells, red blood cells, proteinuria, strands of mucus and increased numbers of epithelial cells may be seen. If the inflammation involves the kidney, white blood cell casts and granular casts may be observed but this is an inconsistent finding. When significant bacteriuria is present, bacteria generally can be observed in the urine sediment. The identification of bacteria in the urine sediment is facilitated and made more accurate if the urine sediment is stained with modified Wright's stain (Swenson et al., 2004). The observation of white blood cells in the urine sediment without bacteria should alert the clinician to the possibility of an inflammatory process that does not involve bacterial infection, e.g. tumours and sterile uroliths. However, cultures should still be performed because positive cultures can be grown even when bacteria are not obvious in the urine sediment.

Clinicians may or may not wish to undertake the expense of culture and sensitivity tests depending on the economic circumstances of their practice and individual clients. However, emerging resistance is becoming more of a problem; recognition that the faecal flora of pets and owners may serve as mutual reservoirs of antimicrobial resistance for infections in either species makes antimicrobial identification and sensitivity testing, followed by specific antimicrobial treatment, more a public health imperative than a management option. Thus, definitive diagnosis by urine culture and sensitivity testing is highly recommended. Urine should be cultured as soon as possible after collection and certainly after no longer than 4 hours. With cystocentesis samples any bacterial growth is considered significant, but it has been suggested that 10^4 colonies per millilitre for catheterized samples and 10^5 cfu/ml for voided samples must be present to be considered significant. Voided specimens are not satisfactory for urine culture.

Occasionally non-traditional microorganisms may be observed in the urine sediment or isolated on urine culture. Mycoplasma spp. infection may be suspected in animals with evidence of urinary tract inflammation where no bacteria can be isolated using common microbiological culture techniques and where treatment with usually effective antibiotics is unsuccessful. However, Mycoplasma spp. that were readily isolated on standard blood agar plates have been identified from UTI in dogs (L'Abee-Lund et al., 2003).

The presence of funguria may be an indication of a localized UTI secondary to multiple predisposing factors, such as diabetes mellitus, previous antimicrobial treatment or immunosuppression. However, in some instances funguria may be an indication of generalized systemic fungal infection.

Sensitivity testing and selection of antimicrobials

Antimicrobial sensitivity tests using the Kirby–Bauer disc-diffusion method are based on antimicrobial concentrations achievable in tissue and serum. When an isolate appears sensitive to an antimicrobial, the result is most likely to be reliable. However, when an isolate appears resistant, the result may be erroneous because the antimicrobial concentration attainable in urine may be up to 100 times the serum level. For this reason the minimum inhibitory concentration (MIC) antimicrobial sensitivity technique is preferred when selecting the appropriate antimicrobial in lower urinary tract infection. Sensitivity patterns of the major uropathogens for a number of commonly used antimicrobials are shown in Figure 23.4. Recommended doses, dosing frequency, route of administration, mean urinary concentration found in normal dogs and the corresponding 'breakpoint' for sensitivity are shown in Figure 23.5. The 'breakpoint' is the maximum MIC for which the drug shown is likely to be effective. MIC levels above the 'breakpoint' usually indicate that the microorganism will be resistant to that particular drug. For the more recently released antimicrobials, the manufacturer's product insert includes mean urinary concentration (MUC) levels for the standard recommended dosages. Note that patients forming dilute urine may not achieve these levels.

	Ampicillin	Cefalexin	Potentiated sulphonamide	Chloramphenicol	Gentamicin [a]	Unpredictable
Escherichia coli						X
Staphylococcus spp.	X (≥ 90% of isolates will be sensitive to standard doses)	X	X	X	X	
Streptococcus spp.	X	X	X	X	X	
Enterococcus spp.	X	X	X			
Proteus spp.	X	X	X	X	X	
Klebsiella spp.						X
Pseudomonas spp.					X	X
Enterobacter spp.						X

23.4 Sensitivity of frequent isolates from dogs with previously untreated UTI. [a] Note that aminoglycosides should not be routinely used to treat UTI due to their nephrotoxic potential.

Antimicrobial	Dose and route of administration	Mean (± 1 SD) urine concentration (µg/ml)	Breakpoint (MUC/4) (µg/ml)
Amoxicillin	11 mg/kg q8h orally	202 ± 93	50
Ampicillin	25 mg/kg q8h orally	309 ± 55	75
Cefalexin	10 mg/kg q8h orally	805 ± 421	200
Enrofloxacin	2.5 mg/kg q12h orally	40	10
Gentamicin [a]	2 mg/kg q8h s.c.	107 ± 33	25
Marbofloxacin	2 mg/kg q24h orally	41 ± 9.3	10
Nitrofurantoin	4.4 mg/kg q8h orally	100	25
Sulfisoxazole	22 mg/kg q8h orally	1466 ± 832	350
Tetracycline	18 mg.kg q8h orally	137 ± 64	35
Trimethoprim/sulfadiazine	15 mg/kg q12h orally	55 ± 19 (based on the trimethoprim fraction)	14

23.5 Mean urinary concentration of commonly used antimicrobial drugs. [a] Note that aminoglycosides should not be routinely used to treat UTI due to their nephrotoxic potential.

When considering more specific antimicrobial treatment based on culture and sensitivity results, an understanding of MIC sensitivity results and MUC of common antimicrobials is required. In human studies, clinical cure of UTI was achieved in 90% of patients when antimicrobial concentrations were four times the MIC of the bacteria involved. However, clinical cure of UTI occurred in less than 20% of patients when urinary antibiotic concentration was less than twice the MIC of the bacteria involved. Similar results have been observed in the dog. Predictions of success of antimicrobial treatment can be more accurately defined by more exacting pharmacokinetic/pharmacodynamic criteria, including the duration that serum concentrations of antimicrobial exceed the MIC, the ratio of peak antimicrobial concentration to the MIC, and the ratio of the area under the curve for antimicrobial levels and the MIC (Jacobs, 2003). However, such precise data are not currently available in veterinary medicine. Oral tetracycline has been used in the treatment of urinary infections caused by *Pseudomonas* spp. in humans with a success rate of about 80%, and observations in dogs suggest a success rate of approximately 60%. The surprising success of oral tetracycline in this setting is attributed to the fact that the MIC of tetracycline for most urinary isolates of canine *Pseudomonas* spp. is less than 40 µg/ml, whereas the mean 8-hour canine urinary concentration of tetracycline given orally at standard doses is about 140 µg/ml. However, enrofloxacin and other fluoroquinolones are more suitable antimicrobials for *Pseudomonas* infections. The MUCs of commonly used antimicrobials are shown in Figure 23.5. These data can predict the likelihood of success with various drugs once MIC values for the isolated bacteria are known.

Antimicrobial sensitivity results for infections that involve the kidney and prostate must be based on plasma-achievable antimicrobial levels because antimicrobials diffuse into the parenchyma of these tissues from plasma, not urine. In the prostate of the dog, the pH of acinar fluid remains acidic even in the face of infection, so antimicrobials that are weak bases (high pKa), lipid soluble and/or poorly bound to plasma protein tend to be the most effective because of high prostatic penetration. Acidic and hydrophilic antimicrobials, such as penicillins and cephalosporins, tend to be less effective because of poor prostatic penetration.

Localization of infection

It can be challenging to establish whether UTI is confined to the lower urinary tract or has extended to involve the kidneys. The presence of white blood cell casts in the urine sediment is diagnostic of pyelonephritis, but their absence does not rule out pyelonephritis because they tend to be present in urine intermittently. Pyelonephritis often causes production of dilute urine because of reduced urine-concentrating capacity. A peripheral leucocytosis may be present in acute pyelonephritis, but this is not a consistent finding. In contrast, leucocytosis does not develop in cystitis unless the inflammation is massive, which is a rare occurrence. On intravenous pyelography examination of advanced chronic pyelonephritis, the kidneys appear small and irregular with pelvic dilation, and the renal diverticula are widened, divergent and have irregular borders (Figure 23.6). These findings may not

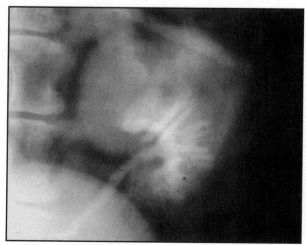

23.6 Radiographic appearance of pyelonephritis on intravenous pyelography.

be present if the renal infection is recent. Furthermore, finding dramatic morphological changes does not prove that active renal infection is present at the time of the study.

Various special techniques have been developed in an attempt to define the presence or absence of renal infection. Bacterial washout techniques, the demonstration of bacteria coated by antibodies in urine, and urinary enzyme levels have all been used in human medicine with variable success. For practical purposes, the possibility of upper UTI should always be considered, particularly if the urine is dilute and if infection recurs after initial short-term therapy. For this reason, follow-up rechecks of urine from animals treated for infection should be performed routinely. In intact male dogs with UTI the prostate is almost always colonized and treatment must be designed to address the unique antimicrobial diffusion characteristics of this organ (see Chapter 21).

Treatment

Frequently, the diagnosis of UTI has been based on clinical history and physical examination, supported by the presence of white blood cells and bacteria in the urine sediment. Antimicrobial medications have been prescribed on the basis of probable cause and past success. This approach was well established in veterinary medicine and suited the economic and time limitations of small animal practice. Furthermore, even if a urine culture is taken, treatment is almost always instituted prior to knowledge of the antimicrobial sensitivity test results. Fortunately, some bacterial species have predictable sensitivity patterns that may be applied to empirical antimicrobial treatment. In one study, more than 90% of the isolates of *Staphylococcus* spp., *Enterococcus* spp., *Streptococcus* spp. and *Proteus* spp. were susceptible to ampicillin and trimethoprim–sulphonamide (Rohrich *et al.*, 1983). While this situation is likely to vary depending on previous antimicrobial use in the patient and in the practice area, the point is made that these bacterial species tend to have predictable sensitivity patterns that can guide empirical treatment. Thus, if cocci (*Staphylococcus*, *Enterococcus*, *Streptococcus*) or rods in very alkaline urine (*Proteus*) are observed in the urine sediment, the sensitivity of the infecting organisms is likely to be more predictable based on previous antimicrobial sensitivity surveys in a practice area. However, if rods are seen in the urine sediment of neutral or acidic urine (*Escherichia coli*, *Klebsiella*, *Enterobacter*, *Pseudomonas*), the antimicrobial sensitivity of the infecting organism is likely to be less predictable.

Antimicrobial treatment should continue for 10–14 days in acute infections and 4–6 weeks in chronic infections and where prostatic or renal involvement appears likely. When an empirical approach to treatment is taken, follow-up urinalysis and urine culture should be performed both during treatment and several days after the end of treatment to ensure that the medication was successful. Clinical improvement can be misleading because many dogs with chronic UTI fail to exhibit obvious signs.

An extremely high proportion of intact male dogs

with UTI appear to have concurrent colonization of the prostate gland. Thus, treatment of these patients must always be instituted with consideration of the special antimicrobial penetration characteristics of prostatic tissue in mind. Most fluoroquinolones, but particularly marbofloxacin, enrofloxacin, trimethoprim and chloramphenicol all penetrate the prostate well. The beta-lactam classes of antimicrobials, including all penicillins and cephalosporins, do not penetrate well and should not be used.

Mycoplasma-induced UTI does not appear to be common. *Mycoplasma* UTI in dogs has been reported to respond to treatment with tylosin, tetracycline and doxycycline. For *Candida* spp. infections confined to the lower urinary tract, elimination of the underlying cause in some instances can result in clearance of the infection (Pressler *et al.*, 2003). Mild alkalinization of the urine is also thought to inhibit fungal growth. Many drugs have been used to treat funguria with limited success. Amphotericin B used as a local irrigant into the bladder has been suggested for persistent infections localized to the lower urinary tract. Fluconazole is effective in humans for the treatment of fungal infections of the urinary tract but the drug is very expensive. Intravesicular clotrimazole was reported to clear a candidal infection in a cat (Toll *et al.*, 2003).

Management of recurrent urinary tract infection

Diagnosis

Distinguishing between persistence of an initial infection after treatment (relapse) and reinfection by another strain can be difficult. If the bacterial strain isolated after treatment is different from the initial isolate (e.g. *Escherichia coli versus Staphylococcus* spp.), then the interpretation is easy. However, if both before and after treatment isolates are *E. coli*, distinguishing between the first and second isolate may require serotyping, enzymatic profiling, pulsed-field gel electrophoresis and polymerase chain reaction (PCR) (Drazenovich *et al.*, 2004).

Treatment failure in urinary infections should be analysed so that errors or omissions in medical diagnosis or management or instructions to the owner may be avoided in similar situations in the future. Failure of an antimicrobial agent to sterilize the urine (relapses) should alert the clinician to one or more of the following possibilities:

- Inappropriate drug, dose, or duration of therapy. Owner compliance is very important in this respect
- Failure of the drug to reach sufficient concentrations in urine despite drug administration, e.g. intestinal malabsorption of the drug, impaired renal concentrating capacity and therefore failure to concentrate the drug in urine to inhibitory concentrations, development of antimicrobial resistance
- The presence of a nidus of infection which is capable of colonizing the urinary tract as soon as

antimicrobial therapy is withdrawn, e.g. pyelonephritis, prostatitis, neoplasia, infected urachal remnant and urolithiasis

- The presence of some defect in the anatomical or functional characteristics of the urinary tract that lowers resistance to bacterial colonization, but is undetectable by presently available clinical methods of diagnosis.

In male dogs a routine work-up for prostatic disease should be performed, including cytology and culture of a prostatic wash or ejaculate, ultrasonographic examination and possibly prostatic aspiration or biopsy. Plain and contrast radiographic studies, including intravenous pyelography, double-contrast cystography and retrograde and voiding urethrography, should be sufficient to diagnose or rule out the presence of major anatomical defects. Urolithiasis is a frequent cause of recurrent signs of lower urinary tract inflammation in dogs and cats of any age, while neoplasia of the bladder, urethra or prostate is often the underlying problem in older dogs.

Treatment

Identification of a specific anatomical abnormality should be addressed, especially when reinfections occur. Vulval involution should be corrected by episioplasty; vulvovaginal stricture should be resected (Lightner *et al.*, 2001; Hammel and Bjorling, 2002). Infected urachal remnants should be resected. Uroliths should be eliminated either medically or surgically. Bladder polyps and tumours should be resected if possible. Hyperadrenocorticism and diabetes mellitus should be controlled (Forrester *et al.*, 1999). Intact male dogs should be treated for at least 30 days with antimicrobials that penetrate the prostate.

When an animal suffers frequent recurrences of UTI despite adequate treatment and in the absence of detectable or correctable anatomical and functional disturbances, long-term management with antimicrobials may be necessary to prevent additional recurrences. Substances that interfere with bacterial expression of fimbrial adhesins could also prevent attachment and colonization. *In vitro*, sub-minimum inhibitory concentration levels of penicillin G suppressed fimbrial expression of resting group A streptococci and caused them to lose their adherence capacity. Similarly, sub-minimum inhibitory concentration urine levels of penicillin, ampicillin and amoxicillin prevented fimbria formation and adherence of growth phase *Escherichia coli* to human epithelial cells. In humans and dogs, single daily administration of antibiotics at one half to one eighth the normal daily dose is well recognized as a preventive strategy for chronic recurrent bacterial UTI. The success of this regimen may be partially due to interference with fimbria formation by bacteria.

A potentiated sulphonamide or amoxicillin–clavulanic acid given for 6 months at 25–30% of the total daily dose at night after the last void prevents recurrence (Ling, 1984). By giving the treatment after the last void at night, the urine concentration of the antimicrobial will be high enough during the 8–10-hour period of sleeping to kill ascending susceptible pathogenic bacteria. A full course of antimicrobial treatment should be used first to eliminate the infection.

Resistant faecal and vaginal bacteria are always a risk in long-term dosing and there is mounting evidence that pets may serve as a reservoir for uropathogens, some of which may be pathogenic in humans (Johnson *et al.*, 2001). The steady development of resistance to fluoroquinolone antimicrobials in some strains of bacteria is of concern (Cohn *et al.*, 2003). Patients undergoing long-term low-dose antimicrobial treatment should always have urine culture and sensitivity tests repeated monthly throughout treatment. Follow-up specimens of urine taken from patients with a history of recurrent UTI should always be collected by cystocentesis. Urethral catheterization should be avoided in this circumstance because trauma to the urethral mucosa may facilitate reinfection.

Possible additional approaches

A substance in cranberry juice may block attachment of bacteria to mannose residues in the uroepithelial surface, a major mechanism of attachment in *Escherichia coli* cystitis in dogs. Although cranberry extract is available in a powder form that can be given in oral capsules, urine from dogs treated with cranberry extract did not inhibit *E. coli* attachment to canine bladder epithelial cells (Suksawat *et al.*, 1996).

The surface GAG layer on uroepithelial surfaces is a major natural barrier to bacterial colonization. In an experimental model of bacterial UTI, bladder infusion of heparin, a synthetic GAG, reduced bacterial attachment in rabbits after the natural GAG layer had been damaged by povidone–iodine treatment. Because heparin must be instilled into the bladder directly, its use in the clinical situation is limited. The synthetic GAG, pentosan polysulphate, prevented bacterial adherence following acid damage of the endogenous GAG layer in rabbits. Pentosan polysulphate is excreted in the urine of dogs after oral administration but in preliminary studies with experimentally induced UTI it failed to improve the rate of clearance of infection.

A vaccine composed of fimbriae could cause production of an antifimbrial antibody. Secretory antibodies could bind with the fimbriae and interfere with adhesin-mediated adherence. A fimbrial vaccine prevented experimental pyelonephritis due to *E. coli* expressing type 1 fimbriae in rats. A fimbrial vaccine prevented experimental pyelonephritis due to P-fimbriated *E. coli* in monkeys (Roberts *et al.*, 2004). Such products, however, are not currently available for therapeutic use.

References and further reading

Backhed F, Alsen B, Roche N *et al.* (2003) Identification of target tissue glycosphingolipid receptors for uropathogenic, F1C-fimbriated *Escherichia coli* and its role in mucosal inflammation. *Journal of Urology* **169(4)**, 1613–1614
Chen YM, Wright PJ, Lee CS and Browning GF (2003) Uropathogenic virulence factors in isolates of *Escherichia coli* from clinical cases

of canine pyometra and feces of healthy bitches. *Veterinary Microbiology* **94(1)**, 57–69

Cohn LA, Gary AT, Fales WH and Madsen RW (2003) Trends in fluoroquinolone resistance of bacteria isolated from canine urinary tracts. *Journal of Veterinary Diagnostic Investigation* **15(4)**, 338–343

Crawford JT and Adams WM (2002) Influence of vestibulovaginal stenosis, pelvic bladder, and recessed vulva on response to treatment for clinical signs of lower urinary tract disease in dogs: 38 cases (1990–1999). *Journal of the American Veterinary Medical Association* **221(7)**, 995–999

Drazenovich N, Ling GV and Foley J (2004) Molecular investigation of *Escherichia coli* strains associated with apparently persistent urinary tract infection in dogs. *Journal of Veterinary Internal Medicine* **18(3)**, 301–306

Forrester SD, Troy GC, Dalton MN, Huffman JW and Holtzman G (1999) Retrospective evaluation of urinary tract infection in 42 dogs with hyperadrenocorticism or diabetes mellitus or both. *Journal of Veterinary Internal Medicine* **13(6)**, 557–560

Fry MM, Liggett JL and Baek SJ (2004) Molecular cloning and expression of canine hepcidin. *Veterinary Clinical Pathology* **33(4)**, 223–227

Hammel SP and Bjorling DE (2002) Results of vulvoplasty for treatment of recessed vulva in dogs. *Journal of the American Animal Hospital Association* **38(1)**, 79–83

Ihrke PJ, Norton AL, Ling GV and Stannard AA (1985) Urinary tract infection associated with long-term corticosteroid administration in dogs with chronic skin diseases. *Journal of the American Veterinary Medical Association* **186(1)**, 43–46

Jacobs MR (2003) How can we predict bacterial eradication? *International Journal of Infectious Diseases* **7(Suppl 1)**, S13–20

Johnson DE, Russell RG, Lockatell CV *et al.* (1993) Contribution of *Proteus mirabilis* urease to persistence, urolithiasis, and acute pyelonephritis in a mouse model of ascending urinary tract infection. *Infection and Immunity* **61(7)**, 2748–2754

Johnson JR, Stell AL, Delavari P *et al.* (2001) Phylogenetic and pathotypic similarities between *Escherichia coli* isolates from urinary tract infections in dogs and extraintestinal infections in humans. *Journal of Infectious Diseases* **183**, 897–906

Kabay MJ, Robinson WF, Huxtable CR and McAleer R (1985) The pathology of disseminated *Aspergillus terreus* infection in dogs. *Veterinary Pathology* **22(6)**, 540–547

Kurazono H, Nakano M, Yamamoto S *et al.* (2003) Distribution of the *usp* gene in uropathogenic *Escherichia coli* isolated from companion animals and correlation with serotypes and size-variations of the pathogenicity island. *Microbiology and Immunology* **47(10)**, 797–802

L'Abee-Lund TM, Heiene R, Friis NF, Ahrens P and Sorum H (2003) *Mycoplasma canis* and urogenital disease in dogs in Norway. *Veterinary Record* **153(3)**, 231–235

Lamb CR and Gregory SP (1998) Ultrasonographic findings in 14 dogs with ectopic ureter. *Veterinary Radiology and Ultrasound* **39(3)**, 218–223

Lightner BA, McLoughlin MA, Chew DJ, Beardsley SM and Matthews HK (2001) Episioplasty for the treatment of perivulvar dermatitis or recurrent urinary tract infections in dogs with excessive perivulvar skin folds: 31 cases (1983–2000). *Journal of the American Veterinary Medical Association* **219(11)**, 1577–1581

Ling GV, Norris CR, Franti CE *et al.* (2001) Interrelations of organism prevalence, specimen collection method, and host age, sex, and breed among 8,354 canine urinary tract infections (1969–1995). *Journal of Veterinary Internal Medicine* **15(4)**, 341–347

Ling GV (1984) Therapeutic strategies involving antimicrobial treatment of the canine urinary tract. *Journal of the American Veterinary Medical Association* **185(10)**, 1162–1164

Low DA, Braaten BA, Ling GV, Johnson DL and Ruby AL (1988) Isolation and comparison of *Escherichia coli* strains from canine and human patients with urinary tract infections. *Infection and Immunity* **56(10)**, 2601–2609

Park CH, Valore EV, Waring AJ and Ganz T (2001) Hepcidin, a urinary antimicrobial peptide synthesized in the liver. *Journal of Biological Chemistry* **276(11)**, 7806–7810

Parsons CL, Stauffer C, Mulholland SG and Griffith DP (1984) Effect of ammonium on bacterial adherence to bladder transitional epithelium. *Journal of Urology* **132(2)**, 365–366

Parsons CL, Stauffer CW and Schmidt JD (1988) Reversible inactivation of bladder surface glycosaminoglycan antibacterial activity by protamine sulfate. *Infection and Immunity* **56(5)**, 1341–1343

Pressler BM, Vaden SL, Lane IF, Cowgill LD and Dye JA (2003) *Candida* spp. urinary tract infections in 13 dogs and seven cats: predisposing factors, treatment, and outcome. *Journal of the American Animal Hospital Association* **39(3)**, 263–270

Roberts JA, Kaack MB, Baskin G *et al.* (2004) Antibody responses and protection from pyelonephritis following vaccination with purified *Escherichia coli* PapDG protein. *Journal of Urology* **171(4)**, 1682–1685

Rohrich PJ, Ling GV, Ruby AL, Jang SS and Johnson DL (1983) In vitro susceptibilities of canine urinary bacteria to selected antimicrobial agents. *Journal of the American Veterinary Medical Association* **183(8)**, 863–867

Senior DF, deMan P and Svanborg C (1992) Serotype, hemolysin production, and adherence characteristics of strains of *Escherichia coli* causing urinary tract infection in dogs. *American Journal of Veterinary Research* **53(4)**, 494–498

Smarick SD, Haskins SC, Aldrich J *et al.* (2004) Incidence of catheter-associated urinary tract infection among dogs in a small animal intensive care unit. *Journal of the American Veterinary Medical Association* **224(12)**, 1936–1940

Suksawat J, Cox HU, O'Rielly KL, Oliver JL and Senior DF (1996) Inhibition of bacterial adherence to canine uroepithelial cells using cranberry juice extract. *Journal of Veterinary Internal Medicine* **10**, 167 (abstract)

Swenson CL, Boisvert AM, Kruger JM and Gibbons-Burgener SN (2004) Evaluation of modified Wright-staining of urine sediment as a method for accurate detection of bacteriuria in dogs. *Journal of the American Veterinary Medical Association* **224(8)**, 1282–1289

Toll J, Ashe CM and Trepanier LA (2003) Intravesicular administration of clotrimazole for treatment of candiduria in a cat with diabetes mellitus. *Journal of the American Veterinary Medical Association* **223(8)**, 1156–1158

Uehling DT, Johnson DB and Hopkins WJ (1999) The urinary tract response to entry of pathogens. *World Journal of Urology* **17(6)**, 351–358

Wadas B, Kuhn I, Lagerstedt AS and Jonsson P (1996) Biochemical phenotypes of *Escherichia coli* in dogs: comparison of isolates isolated from bitches suffering from pyometra and urinary tract infection with isolates from faeces of healthy dogs. *Veterinary Microbiology* **52(3-4)**, 293–300

Westerlund B, Van Die I, Hoekstra W, Virkola R and Korhonen TK (1993) P fimbriae of uropathogenic *Escherichia coli* as multifunctional adherence organelles. *Zentralblatt für Bakteriologie* **278(2-3)**, 229–237

Yuri K, Nakata K, Katae H, Yamamato S and Hasegawa A (1998) Distribution of uropathogenic virulence factors among *Escherichia coli* strains isolated from dogs and cats. *Journal of Veterinary Medical Science* **60(3)**, 287–290

Appendix

Conversion table for units

	SI unit	Conversion factor	Conventional unit
Haematology			
Red blood cell count	10^{12} / l	1	10^6 / μl
Haemoglobin	g / l	0.1	g / dl
MCH	pg / cell	1	pg / cell
MCHC	g / l	0.1	g / dl
MCV	fl	1	μm^3
Platelet count	10^9 / l	1	10^3 / μl
White blood cell count	10^9 / l	1	10^3 / μl
Biochemistry			
Alanine transferase	IU / l	1	IU / l
Albumin	g / l	0.1	g / dl
Aldosterone	nmol / l	0.0277	ng / dl
Alkaline phosphatase	IU / l	1	IU / l
Antiduirectic hormone	pmol / l	0.923	pg / ml
Aspartate transaminase	IU / l	1	IU / l
Bilirubin	μmol / l	0.0584	mg / dl
BUN	mmol / l	2.8	mg / dl
Calcitriol	pmol / l	0.417	pg / ml
Calcium	mmol / l	4	mg / dl
Carbon dioxide (total)	mmol / l	1	mEq / l
Cholesterol	mmol / l	38.61	mg / dl
Chloride	mmol / l	1	mEq / l
Cortisol	nmol / l	0.362	ng / ml
Creatine kinase	IU / l	1	IU / l
Creatinine	μmol / l	0.0113	mg / dl
Erythropoietin	IU / l	1	mIU / ml
Glucose	mmol / l	18.02	mg / dl
Insulin	pmol / l	0.1394	μIU / ml
Iron	μmol / l	5.587	μg / dl
Magnesium	mmol / l	2	mEq / l
Parathyroid hormone	ng / l	1	pg / ml
Phosphorus	mmol / l	3.1	mg / dl
Potassium	mmol / l	1	mEq / l
Renin	pmol / l	0.0237	pg / ml
Sodium	mmol / l	1	mEq / l
Total protein	g / l	0.1	g / dl
Thyroxine (T4) (free)	pmol / l	0.0775	ng / dl
Thyroxine (T4) (total)	nmol / l	0.0775	μg / dl
Tri-iodothyronine (T3)	nmol / l	65.1	ng / dl
Triglycerides	mmol / l	88.5	mg / dl

AP1 SI and conventional units. Measurements in SI units are multiplied by the conversion factor to give concentrations in conventional units.

Index

Index

Index

Index

Index

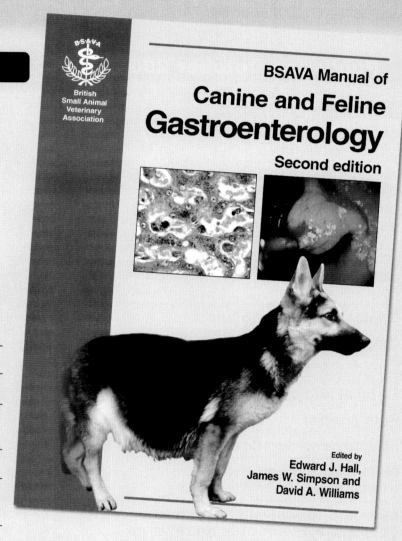
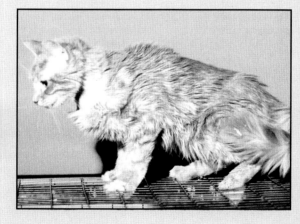

BSAVA Manual of Canine and Feline
Oncology
Second edition

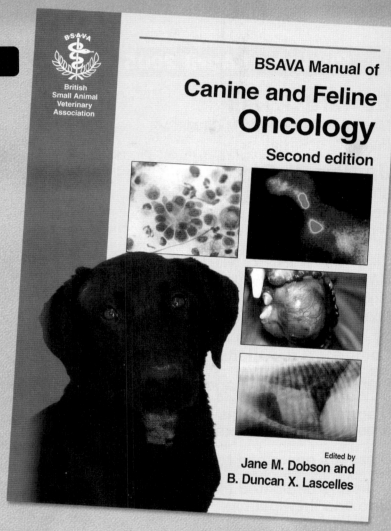
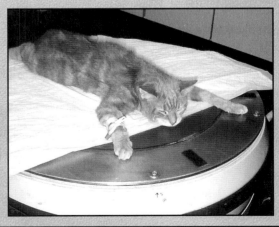